American Academy of Pediatrics

Developmental and Behavioral Pediatrics

2ND EDITION

Section on Developmental and Behavioral Pediatrics
American Academy of Pediatrics

EDITOR

Robert G. Voigt, MD, FAAP

ASSOCIATE EDITORS

Michelle M. Macias, MD, FAAP
Scott M. Myers, MD, FAAP
Carl D. Tapia, MD, MPH, FAAP

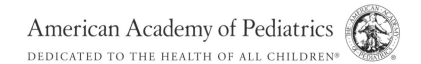

American Academy of Pediatrics
DEDICATED TO THE HEALTH OF ALL CHILDREN®

American Academy of Pediatrics Publishing Staff

Mark Grimes, *Vice President, Publishing*
Eileen Glasstetter, MS, *Senior Editor, Professional/Clinical Publishing*
Theresa Wiener, *Production Manager, Clinical and Professional Publications*
Linda Diamond, *Manager, Art Direction and Production*
Mary Lou White, *Chief Product and Services Officer/SVP, Membership, Marketing, and Publishing*
Linda Smessaert, MSIMC, *Senior Marketing Manager, Professional Resources*
Mary Louise Carr, MBA, *Marketing Manager, Clinical Publications*

345 Park Blvd
Itasca, IL 60143
Telephone: 630/626-6000
Facsimile: 847/434-8000
www.aap.org

The American Academy of Pediatrics is an organization of 66,000 primary care pediatricians, pediatric medical subspecialists, and pediatric surgical specialists dedicated to the health, safety, and well-being of infants, children, adolescents, and young adults.

The recommendations in this publication do not indicate an exclusive course of treatment or serve as a standard of care. Variations, taking into account individual circumstances, may be appropriate.

Listing of resources does not imply an endorsement by the American Academy of Pediatrics (AAP). The AAP is not responsible for the content of external resources. Information was current at the time of publication.

Brand names are furnished for identification purposes only.
No endorsement of the manufacturers or products mentioned is implied.

Every effort has been made to ensure that the drug selection and dosages set forth in this text are in accordance with the current recommendations and practice at the time of publication. It is the responsibility of the health care professional to check the package insert of each drug for any change in indications and dosages and for added warnings and precautions.

The publishers have made every effort to trace the copyright holders for borrowed materials. If they have inadvertently overlooked any, they will be pleased to make the necessary arrangements at the first opportunity.

This publication has been developed by the American Academy of Pediatrics. The authors, editors, and contributors are expert authorities in the field of pediatrics. No commercial involvement of any kind has been solicited or accepted in the development of the content of this publication. Disclosures: Dr Larson disclosed an advisory board relationship with Human Code. Dr Blum disclosed an editorial relationship with the American Board of Pediatrics.

Every effort is made to keep *American Academy of Pediatrics Developmental and Behavioral Pediatrics* consistent with the most recent advice and information available from the American Academy of Pediatrics.

Special discounts are available for bulk purchases of this publication. E-mail Special Sales at aapsales@aap.org for more information.

Printed in the United States of America

3-339/0418   2 3 4 5 6 7 8 9 10

MA0844
ISBN: 978-1-61002-134-0
eBook: 978-1-61002-135-7
EPUB: 978-1-61002-239-2
Mobi: 978-1-61002-240-8
Library of Congress Control Number: 2017935587

American Academy of Pediatrics
Section on Developmental and Behavioral Pediatrics
2017–2018

Executive Committee Members

Carol C. Weitzman, MD, FAAP, Chairperson
Nerissa S. Bauer, MD, MPH, FAAP
David O. Childers Jr, MD, FAAP
Jack M. Levine, MD, FAAP
Ada Myriam Peralta-Carcelen, MD, MPH, FAAP
Peter J. Smith, MD, MA, FAAP

Immediate Past Chairperson

Nathan J. Blum, MD, FAAP

Liaisons

Marilyn Augustyn, MD, FAAP
Rebecca A. Baum, MD, FAAP
Beth Ellen Davis, MD, MPH, FAAP
Alice Meng, MD, FAAP

Program Chairperson

Carolyn Bridgemohan, MD, FAAP

Newsletter Editor

Robert G. Voigt, MD, FAAP

Web Site Editor

Kimberlly L. Stringer, MD, FAAP

Staff

Linda B. Paul, MPH

Editors and Contributors

Editor in Chief

Robert G. Voigt, MD, FAAP

Professor of Pediatrics
Head, Section of Developmental Pediatrics
Baylor College of Medicine
Director, Meyer Center for Developmental Pediatrics and Autism Center
Texas Children's Hospital
Houston, TX

Associate Editors

Michelle M. Macias, MD, FAAP

Professor of Pediatrics
Chief, Division of Developmental-Behavioral Pediatrics
Medical University of South Carolina
Charleston, SC

Scott M. Myers, MD, FAAP

Neurodevelopmental Pediatrician
Associate Professor of Pediatrics
Geisinger Autism & Developmental Medicine Institute
Lewisburg, PA

Carl D. Tapia, MD, MPH, FAAP

Assistant Professor, Department of Pediatrics
Baylor College of Medicine
Texas Children's Hospital
Houston, TX

Contributors

Kruti R. Acharya, MD, FAAP

Assistant Professor of Disability and Human Development
University of Illinois at Chicago
Chicago, IL

Ch 26: Transition to Adult Medical Care

William J. Barbaresi, MD, FAAP

Director, Developmental Medicine Center
Wade Family Foundation Chair in Developmental Medicine
Boston Children's Hospital
Professor of Pediatrics
Harvard Medical School
Boston, MA

Ch 17: Learning Disabilities
Ch 21: Disruptive Behavior Disorders

Nathan J. Blum, MD, FAAP

Chief, Division of Developmental and Behavioral Pediatrics
The Children's Hospital of Philadelphia
William H. Bennett Professor of Pediatrics
Perelman School of Medicine at the University of Pennsylvania
Philadelphia, PA

*Ch 7: Basics of Child Behavior and Primary Care Management
of Common Behavioral Problems*

Thomas D. Challman, MD, FAAP

Medical Director
Geisinger Autism & Developmental Medicine Institute
Lewisburg, PA

Ch 19: Autism Spectrum Disorder
Ch 24: Complementary Health Approaches in Developmental and Behavioral Pediatrics

Eugenia Chan, MD, MPH, FAAP

Assistant Professor of Pediatrics
Division of Developmental Medicine
Boston Children's Hospital
Harvard Medical School
Boston, MA

Ch 23: Basics of Psychopharmacological Management

Viola Cheung, DO, FAAP
Developmental Behavioral Pediatrician
TJH Medical Services
Medisys Child Development and Education Center
Flushing Hospital Medical Center
Flushing, NY
Ch 22: Anxiety and Mood Disorders

David O. Childers Jr, MD, FAAP
Associate Professor of Pediatrics
Chief, Division of Developmental Pediatrics
Chief, Division of General Academic Pediatrics
Chief, Division of Child Neurology
Director Regional Early Intervention Program
University of Florida College of Medicine–Jacksonville
Jacksonville, FL
Ch 6: Early Intervention

Peter J. Chung, MD, FAAP
Assistant Clinical Professor of Pediatrics
Division of Developmental-Behavioral Pediatrics
Center for Autism & Neurodevelopmental Disorders
University of California, Irvine
Santa Ana, CA
Ch 23: Basics of Psychopharmacological Management

Stephen H. Contompasis, MD, FAAP
Emeritus Professor of Pediatrics
Larner College of Medicine
University of Vermont
Burlington, VT
Ch 26: Transition to Adult Medical Care

Benard P. Dreyer, MD, FAAP
Professor of Pediatrics
Director of Developmental-Behavioral Pediatrics
NYU School of Medicine and Hassenfeld Children's Hospital at NYU Langone
Director of Pediatrics
Bellevue Hospital Center
New York, NY
Ch 3: Environmental Influences on Child Development and Behavior

John C. Duby, MD, FAAP, CPE
Professor and Chair, Department of Pediatrics
Wright State University Boonshoft School of Medicine
Vice President of Academic Affairs and Community Health
Dayton Children's Hospital
Dayton, OH
Ch 12: Social and Emotional Development

Ellen R. Elias, MD, FAAP, FACMG
Professor of Pediatrics and Genetics
University of Colorado School of Medicine
Aurora, CO
*Ch 4: Biological Influences on Child Development and Behavior and Medical Evaluation
of Children With Developmental-Behavioral Disorders*

Jason M. Fogler, MA, PhD
Staff Psychologist
Codirector of ADHD Services
The Division of Developmental Medicine
Boston Children's Hospital
Instructor in Psychiatry
Harvard Medical School
Boston, MA
Ch 17: Learning Disabilities

Jill J. Fussell, MD, FAAP
Professor
Developmental Behavioral Pediatrics Fellowship Director
Medical Director of the James L. Dennis Developmental Center
Section of Developmental Pediatrics and Rehabilitative Medicine
University of Arkansas for Medical Sciences
Arkansas Children's Hospital
Little Rock, AR
Ch 15: Cognitive Development and Disorders

Dinah L. Godwin, MSW, LCSW
Assistant Professor of Pediatrics
Baylor College of Medicine
Meyer Center for Developmental Pediatrics
Texas Children's Hospital
Houston, TX
*Ch 25: Social and Community Services for Children With Developmental Disabilities
and/or Behavioral Disorders and Their Families*

Elizabeth B. Harstad, MD, MPH
Assistant Professor of Pediatrics
Division of Developmental Medicine
Boston Children's Hospital
Boston, MA

Ch 21: Disruptive Behavior Disorders

Pamela C. High, MD, FAAP
Director, Developmental-Behavioral Pediatrics
Hasbro Children's Hospital
Warren Alpert Medical School, Brown University
Providence, RI

Ch 3: Environmental Influences on Child Development and Behavior

Carrie Kelly, MD, FAAP
Division of Developmental-Behavioral Pediatrics
Hasbro Children's Hospital
Warren Alpert Medical School, Brown University
Providence, RI

Ch 3: Environmental Influences on Child Development and Behavior

Desmond P. Kelly, MD, FAAP
Professor of Pediatrics
University of South Carolina School of Medicine Greenville
Vice Chair for Academic Affairs, Department of Pediatrics
Greenville Health System Children's Hospital
Greenville, SC

Ch 13: Sensory Impairments: Hearing and Vision

Mary C. Kral, PhD
Associate Professor of Pediatrics
Division of Developmental-Behavioral Pediatrics
Medical University of South Carolina
Charleston, SC

Ch 20: Interpreting Psychoeducational Testing Reports, Individualized Family Service Plans (IFSP), and Individualized Education Program (IEP) Plans

Angela C. LaRosa, MD, MSCR, FAAP
Professor of Pediatrics
Division of Developmental-Behavioral Pediatrics
Medical University of South Carolina
Charleston, SC

Ch 16: Speech and Language Development and Disorders

Austin A. Larson, MD

Instructor, Department of Pediatrics
Section on Genetics
University of Colorado School of Medicine
Aurora, CO

Ch 4: Biological Influences on Child Development and Behavior and Medical Evaluation of Children With Developmental-Behavioral Disorders

Michele L. Ledesma, MD, FAAP

Fellow, Developmental & Behavioral Pediatrics
Department of Pediatrics
Yale School of Medicine
New Haven, CT

Ch 22: Anxiety and Mood Disorders

Mary L. O'Connor Leppert, MB, BCh, FAAP

Director, Center for Development and Learning
Kennedy Krieger Institute
Assistant Professor of Pediatrics
Johns Hopkins University School of Medicine
Baltimore, MD

Ch 10: Developmental Evaluation

Paul H. Lipkin, MD, FAAP

Kennedy Krieger Institute
Johns Hopkins University School of Medicine
Baltimore, MD

Ch 9: Developmental and Behavioral Surveillance and Screening Within the Medical Home

Michelle M. Macias, MD, FAAP

Professor of Pediatrics
Chief, Division of Developmental-Behavioral Pediatrics
Medical University of South Carolina
Charleston, SC

Ch 1: Child Development: The Basic Science of Pediatrics

Ch 9: Developmental and Behavioral Surveillance and Screening Within the Medical Home

Ch 16: Speech and Language Development and Disorders

Shruti Mittal, MD, FAAP
Division of Developmental-Behavioral Pediatrics
Medical University of South Carolina
Charleston, SC
Ch 16: Speech and Language Development and Disorders

Catherine Morgan, PhD
Senior Research Fellow
Cerebral Palsy Alliance Research Institute, School of Medicine
University of Sydney
Sydney, NSW
Australia
Ch 14: Motor Development and Disorders

Michael E. Msall, MD, FAAP
Professor of Pediatrics, University of Chicago
Co-director Kennedy Research Center on Intellectual and
Neurodevelopmental Disabilities
Chief of Developmental and Behavioral Pediatrics
Comer Children's Hospital
Chicago, Illinois
Ch 14: Motor Development and Disorders

Scott M. Myers, MD, FAAP
Neurodevelopmental Pediatrician
Associate Professor of Pediatrics
Geisinger Autism & Developmental Medicine Institute
Lewisburg, PA
Ch 1: Child Development: The Basic Science of Pediatrics
Ch 19: Autism Spectrum Disorder
Ch 24: Complementary Health Approaches in Developmental and Behavioral Pediatrics

Mary E. Pipan, MD, FAAP
Clinical Director, Trisomy 21 Program
Attending Physician, Developmental Behavioral Pediatrics
The Children's Hospital of Philadelphia
Philadelphia, PA
Ch 7: Basics of Child Behavior and Primary Care Management
of Common Behavioral Problems

Jennifer K. Poon, MD, FAAP
Associate Professor of Pediatrics
Division of Developmental-Behavioral Pediatrics
Medical University of South Carolina
Charleston, SC
Ch 6: Early Intervention

Michael I. Reiff, MD, FAAP
Professor, Department of Pediatrics
Division of Pediatric Clinical Neuroscience
University of Minnesota
Minneapolis, MN
Ch 18: Attention-Deficit/Hyperactivity Disorder

Marie Reilly, MD
Instructor in Pediatrics
Division of Developmental Medicine
Boston Children's Hospital
Harvard Medical School
Boston, MA
Ch 8: Development and Disorders of Feeding, Sleep, and Elimination

Ann M. Reynolds, MD, FAAP
Associate Professor of Pediatrics
Section of Developmental Pediatrics
University of Colorado School of Medicine
Children's Hospital Colorado
Aurora, CO
Ch 15: Cognitive Development and Disorders

Julie Ribaudo, LMSW, IMH-E(IV)
Clinical Associate Professor
University of Michigan School of Social Work
Ann Arbor, MI
Ch 5: Interviewing and Counseling Children and Families

Angelica Robles, MD, FAAP
Division of Developmental-Behavioral Pediatrics
Hasbro Children's Hospital
Warren Alpert Medical School, Brown University
Providence, RI
Ch 3: Environmental Influences on Child Development and Behavior

Alison Schonwald, MD, FAAP
Assistant Professor of Pediatrics, Harvard Medical School
Assistant in Medicine, Boston Children's Hospital
Boston, MA
Ch 8: Development and Disorders of Feeding, Sleep, and Elimination

Prachi E. Shah, MD, MS
Associate Professor, Pediatrics
Division of Developmental and Behavioral Pediatrics and
Center for Human Growth and Development
University of Michigan
Ann Arbor, MI
Ch 5: Interviewing and Counseling Children and Families

Peter J. Smith, MD, MA, FAAP
Associate Professor, Pediatrics
Section of Developmental-Behavioral Pediatrics
University of Chicago
Chicago, IL
Ch 26: Transition to Adult Medical Care

Martin T. Stein, MD, FAAP
Professor of Pediatrics Emeritus
Developmental-Behavioral Pediatrics
University of California San Diego
Rady Children's Hospital San Diego
San Diego, CA
Ch 18: Attention-Deficit/Hyperactivity Disorder

Carl D. Tapia, MD, MPH, FAAP
Assistant Professor, Department of Pediatrics
Baylor College of Medicine
Texas Children's Hospital
Houston, TX
Ch 1: Child Development: The Basic Science of Pediatrics

Stuart W. Teplin, MD, FAAP
Developmental-Behavioral Pediatrician
Associate Professor, Emeritus
Department of Pediatrics
University of North Carolina School of Medicine
Chapel Hill, NC
Ch 13: Sensory Impairments: Hearing and Vision

Bridget Thompson, DO, FAAP
Division of Developmental-Behavioral Pediatrics
Hasbro Children's Hospital
Warren Alpert Medical School, Brown University
Providence, RI
Ch 3: Environmental Influences on Child Development and Behavior

Katherine A. Trier, MD, FAAP
Fellow, Developmental and Behavioral Pediatrics
Division of Developmental Medicine
Boston Children's Hospital
Harvard Medical School
Boston, MA
Ch 23: Basics of Psychopharmacological Management

Sherry Sellers Vinson, MD, MEd, FAAP
Assistant Professor of Pediatrics
Baylor College of Medicine
Neurodevelopmental Specialist
Meyer Center for Developmental Pediatrics
Texas Children's Hospital
Houston, TX
Ch 25: Social and Community Services for Children With Developmental Disabilities and/or Behavioral Disorders and Their Families

Robert G. Voigt, MD, FAAP
Professor of Pediatrics
Head, Section of Developmental Pediatrics
Baylor College of Medicine
Director, Meyer Center for Developmental Pediatrics and Autism Center
Texas Children's Hospital
Houston, TX
Ch 1: Child Development: The Basic Science of Pediatrics
Ch 11: Making Developmental-Behavioral Diagnoses

Paul Wang, MD, FAAP
Deputy Director, Clinical Research
Simons Foundation
New York, NY
Associate Clinical Professor of Pediatrics
Yale University School of Medicine
New Haven, CT
Ch 2: Nature, Nurture, and Their Interactions in Child Development and Behavior

Lynn Mowbray Wegner, MD, FAAP
Clinical Professor, Emerita
University of North Carolina School of Medicine
Chapel Hill, NC
*Ch 27: Billing and Coding for Developmental and Behavioral Problems
in Outpatient Primary Care*

Carol C. Weitzman, MD, FAAP
Professor of Pediatrics and Child Study Center
Director, Developmental-Behavioral Pediatrics
Yale School of Medicine
New Haven, CT
Ch 22: Anxiety and Mood Disorders

American Academy of Pediatrics
Reviewers

Board of Directors Reviewer
David I. Bromberg, MD, FAAP

Committees, Councils, and Sections

Committee on Bioethics
Committee on Coding and Nomenclature
Committee on Continuing Medical Education
Committee on Drugs
Committee on Medical Liability and Risk Management
Committee on Nutrition
Committee on Psychosocial Aspects of Child and Family Health
Committee on Substance Use and Prevention
Council on Children With Disabilities
Council on Early Childhood
Council on Environmental Health
Council on Genetics
Council on School Health
Disaster Preparedness Advisory Council
Private Payer Advocacy Advisory Committee
Section on Breastfeeding
Section on Gastroenterology, Hepatology, and Nutrition
Section on Home Care
Section on Ophthalmology
Section on Oral Health
Section on Otolaryngology–Head and Neck Surgery
Section on Pediatric Pulmonology and Sleep Medicine
Section on Urology
Surgery Advisory Panel

Contents

CHAPTER 1

Child Development: The Basic Science of Pediatrics

Robert G. Voigt, MD, FAAP

Michelle M. Macias, MD, FAAP

Scott M. Myers, MD, FAAP

Carl D. Tapia, MD, MPH, FAAP

More than 50 years ago, Julius B. Richmond, MD, characterized child development as the basic science of pediatrics.[1] The processes of child development and behavior affect all primary pediatric health care professionals* and pediatric subspecialists, and these fundamentally differentiate pediatrics from all other areas of medicine. In addition to being experts in childhood wellness and illness, parents expect primary pediatric health care professionals to be experts in all aspects of childhood and adolescence, especially in the domains of development and behavior. Thus, clinical competence in child development and behavioral health is vital to the success of all pediatric health care encounters.

Despite child development's role as the basic science of pediatrics, the Accreditation Council for Graduate Medical Education unfortunately requires all pediatric residents to receive a total of only 32 half-day sessions' experience in developmental-behavioral pediatrics during their residency training.[2] Thus, even though most practicing primary care general pediatricians will rarely step inside a pediatric or neonatal critical care unit or even provide direct care for hospitalized patients after they have graduated from residency, they will rarely make it through even a half-day in their general pediatric practices without a question from a parent about a child's development or behavior, for which, unfortunately, they are required to receive a total of only 16 days of training. This clearly represents a distressing mismatch between the amount of training and future demands in daily pediatric practice.[3] Given this limited experience, it is not unexpected that surveys of pediatricians in practice continue to indicate that pediatricians feel ill-prepared in this distinguishing domain of pediatric practice.[4,5] In addition, family medicine residents, family and pediatric nurse practitioners, and physician assistants, who will provide medical homes for at least one-third of all children in the United States,[6] generally receive little, if any, training in this basic science. As illustrated in Table 1.1, and even more concerning in this setting of limited training, developmental disorders are the most prevalent chronic medical conditions encountered in primary care, and psychosocial and behavioral issues are even more ubiquitous in day-to-day pediatric practice.[7–9]

---

*Throughout this manual, the term *primary pediatric health care professionals* is intended to encompass pediatricians, family physicians, nurse practitioners, and physician assistants who provide primary care to infants, children, and adolescents.

Table 1.1. Prevalence of Developmental-Behavioral Disorders and Other Chronic Medical Conditions in Children[a]

Condition	Prevalence
Slower learning (IQ between 70 and 89)	23%
Asthma	8.4%
Learning disabilities	7.7%
Attention-deficit/hyperactivity disorder	6.7%
Other developmental delays/intellectual disabilities	4.4%
Autism spectrum disorder	1.5%
Epilepsy	1%
Congenital heart disease	1%
Cerebral palsy	0.4%
Inflammatory bowel disease	0.4%
Juvenile rheumatic diseases	0.4%
Diabetes	0.2%
Cancer	0.02%
Cystic fibrosis	0.04%
Chronic renal disease	0.008%

[a] Data derived from Boyle CA, Boulet S, Schieve LA, et al. Trends in the prevalence of developmental disabilities in US children, 1997–2008. *Pediatrics.* 2011;127(6):1034–1042; Christensen DL, Baio J, Van Naarden Braun K, et al. Prevalence and characteristics of autism spectrum disorder among children aged 8 years—Autism and Developmental Disabilities Monitoring Network, 11 sites, United States, 2012. *MMWR Surveill Summ.* 2016;65(3):1–23; and Centers for Disease Control and Prevention National Center for Health Statistics. http://www.cdc.gov/nchs. Accessed January 18, 2018.

Of the 118,292 pediatricians currently certified by the American Board of Pediatrics, only 775 are subspecialty board-certified in Developmental-Behavioral Pediatrics and only 255 are subspecialty board-certified in Neurodevelopmental Disabilities.[10] This does not represent 1,030 different subspecialists, as some individuals have both certifications. To illustrate the critical dearth of developmental-behavioral subspecialists, consider that congenital heart disease affects approximately 1% of the pediatric population. Currently, there are 3,218 board-certified pediatric cardiologists to care for these children.[10] However, if this is the number of subspecialists required to provide subspecialty care for this 1% of the population, then it would require nearly 80,000 board-certified developmental-behavioral pediatricians (not the current 775) to provide the same level of subspecialty care for the approximately 25% of the pediatric population with developmental-behavioral concerns (see Table 1.1).

This combination of a very high prevalence of developmental-behavioral disorders and an enormously critical shortage of subspecialists to whom patients may be referred creates extremely long waiting lists at tertiary care developmental-behavioral evaluation centers; this makes subspecialty referral a futile proposition for the vast majority of children with developmental or behavioral concerns.[3] Thus, most children with developmental or behavioral concerns must be managed within their primary care medical homes. Clinical judgment and confidence in evaluation and management of developmental-behavioral concerns need to be considered as basic to general pediatric practice as are evaluation and management of asthma and other common chronic medical conditions encountered daily in pediatric practice.[3]

This second edition of *American Academy of Pediatrics Developmental and Behavioral Pediatrics* continues to represent a cooperative effort of the American Academy of Pediatrics Section on Developmental and Behavioral Pediatrics and Council on Children With Disabilities. While it certainly cannot provide the experiential learning that an expansion of required subspecialty exposure to developmental-behavioral pediatrics during pediatric or family medicine residency training or in the training of future primary care nurse practitioners or physician assistants would provide, given the crucial need to enhance the education of all primary pediatric health care professionals in this basic science of pediatrics, this manual attempts to blend the overlapping perspectives of both Neurodevelopmental Disabilities and Developmental-Behavioral Pediatrics with the goal of improving care for all children.

Finally, this manual is intended to be neither an exhaustive reference geared for the subspecialist nor a cursory introductory list of developmental and behavioral pediatric topics. Instead, this expanded second edition aims to be a resource that provides the essentials of what all primary pediatric health care professionals need to know to successfully care for children with developmental and behavioral concerns in their practices and to identify those who truly require subspecialty referral. It is hoped that with the assistance of this manual, primary pediatric health care professionals will gain more confidence in evaluating and managing children with developmental and behavioral concerns and provide evidence-based developmental-behavioral pediatric care within the medical home.

References

1. Richmond JB. Child development: a basic science for pediatrics. *Pediatrics*. 1967;39(5):649–658
2. Accreditation Council for Graduate Medical Education Program Requirements for Graduate Medical Education in Pediatrics. http://www.acgme.org/Portals/0/PFAssets/ProgramRequirements/320_pediatrics_2017-07-01.pdf?ver=2017-06-30-083432-507. Accessed January 18, 2018
3. Voigt RG, Accardo PJ. Formal speech-language screening not shown to help children. *Pediatrics*. 2015;136(2):e494–e495
4. Sices L, Feudtner C, McLaughlin J, Drotar D, Williams M. How do primary care physicians identify young children with developmental delays? A national survey. *J Dev Behav Pediatr*. 2003;24(6):409–417
5. Halfon N, Regalado M, Sareen H, et al. Assessing development in the pediatric office. *Pediatrics*. 2004;113(6)(suppl 5):1926–1933
6. Phillips RL, Bazemore AW, Dodoo MS, Shipman SA, Green LA. Family physicians in the child health care workforce: opportunities for collaboration in improving the health of children. *Pediatrics*. 2006;118(3):1200–1206
7. Boyle CA, Boulet S, Schieve LA, et al. Trends in the prevalence of developmental disabilities in US children, 1997–2008. *Pediatrics*. 2011;127(6):1034–1042
8. Christensen DL, Baio J, Van Naarden Braun K, et al. Prevalence and characteristics of autism spectrum disorder among children aged 8 years—Autism and Developmental Disabilities Monitoring Network, 11 sites, United States, 2012. *MMWR Surveill Summ*. 2016;65(3):1–23
9. Centers for Disease Control and Prevention National Center for Health Statistics. http://www.cdc.gov/nchs. Accessed January 18, 2018
10. American Board of Pediatrics, Inc. *Pediatric Physicians Workforce Data Book 2015-2016*. Chapel Hill, NC: American Board of Pediatrics, Inc; 2016

CHAPTER 2

Nature, Nurture, and Their Interactions in Child Development and Behavior

Paul Wang, MD, FAAP

Nature and nurture have long been regarded as rival influences on child development and behavior. One school of thought has contended that a child's behaviors and developmental outcome are determined by nature—that is, by innate biology—while a rival school has argued that nurture—a child's environment and experiences—is dominant in determining the child's developmental outcome. While the nature-nurture debate raged among academics, intuitive parents and primary pediatric health care professionals have long known that both sets of factors—the innate and the experiential—are important in the complex processes of child development and behavior. Over the last several decades, science has amassed substantial evidence to document the importance of both nature and nurture.[1] Moreover, current research is elucidating the complex ways in which nature and nurture interact throughout the childhood years.

This chapter attempts to provide a framework in which to consider how nature, nurture, and their interactions shape children's lives. Many examples are provided of both innate and experiential factors that influence children's development and behavior, and of the mechanisms through which those factors are believed to act. Throughout the chapter, the reader is asked to hold 2 overarching concepts in mind: *individual variability* and *developmental plasticity*. Because of individual variability, children differ in how any factor may shape their development and behavior regardless of whether that factor is innate or environmental. As research is beginning to show, much of this variability may be rooted in the interaction of nature and nurture, also known as gene by environment interaction or GxE. Because of developmental plasticity, the effects of both innate and experiential factors can be either augmented or ameliorated by other factors over time. No developmental influence, whether innate or environmental, should be regarded as deterministic, strictly consigning a child to a certain fate. Rather, the processes of development continue throughout childhood, adolescence, and even adulthood, allowing biological and behavioral interventions to shape later outcomes.

Innate Factors in Child Development and Behavior

Nature can be variably construed in either a narrow or a broad manner. From the narrow perspective, a child's nature is defined as the child's innate biological endowment and heredity and, thus, consists primarily of genetics. From the broader perspective, all factors that are believed to operate through a direct biological mechanism are construed as being within the category of nature.

Genetics

Research on the influence of nature on children's behavior and development started in earnest with twin studies, which examine the resemblance of monozygotic (identical) twins to each other and the resemblance of dizygotic (fraternal) twins to each other. Data from these twin studies are commonly summarized in a numerical parameter known as *heritability*, which can range from 0 to 1.00 and is symbolized as h^2. For example, studies of attention-deficit/hyperactivity disorder (ADHD) estimate its heritability to be between 0.60 and 0.90, while IQ studies estimate the heritability of intelligence 0.50 to 0.85 with values tending higher with increasing age (ie, genetic factors have a larger influence in older ages).[2] It should be understood that heritability is an abstract mathematical parameter that does not translate easily to tangible interpretation. That is, if the heritability of reading disability is 0.75, it does not imply that 75% of all cases of dyslexia have an exclusively genetic etiology, or that the child of a person with dyslexia has a 75% chance of having dyslexia, or any such implication. Heritability merely describes the proportion of the statistical variance in a trait that was attributable to genetics in a particular research study.

Behavioral genetic studies commonly yield estimates of heritability that are greater than 0.50 for many developmental-behavioral diagnoses and traits,[3] leading some commentators to claim that biology is more important than environment. Such a claim is misleading at best. First, the word *more* is confusing in this context. Even when the estimate of heritability is high, it cannot be concluded that any particular case of a disease is "more" caused by genetic or environmental factors or that more cases of that disease are caused by genetics than environment. Since no study of any trait has shown complete genetic heritability (ie, heritability has always been found to be <1.00), and since even identical twins do not show 100% concordance for any diagnosis or trait (eg, autism, schizophrenia, reading skills; Figure 2.1), it implies that environmental factors can make a clinically significant difference even when 2 individuals are genetically identical. It seems much more likely that all or almost all cases of a disease have both genetic and environmental influences in their pathogenesis. Robert Plomin, one of the most prominent researchers in the field, has commented that behavioral genetic studies can be regarded as providing some of the best evidence of the importance of environmental factors in shaping health and disease.[4]

A further argument against the overinterpretation of heritability parameters is that they are dependent on the amounts of genetic and environmental variation in the populations under study. For example, if all the subjects in a study had identical environments,

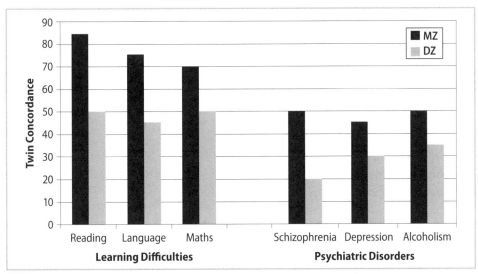

Figure 2.1. Twin concordances for learning disabilities and for psychiatric disorders.

Abbreviations: MZ, monozygotic; DZ, dizygotic.

Reproduced from Haworth C, Plomin R. Quantitative genetics in the era of molecular genetics: learning abilities and disabilities as an example. *J Am Acad Child Adolesc Psychiatry.* 2010;49(8):783–793, with permission from Elsevier.

the study would show misleadingly high estimates of genetic heritability and low estimates of environmental influence. In fact, it is well known that extreme environmental manipulation can have enormous effects on behavior and development. Common, real-life variability in the environment also affects estimates of heritability, as Turkheimer and colleagues[5] demonstrated. They found that estimates of the heritability of IQ are higher in populations with higher socioeconomic status (SES), while heritability is near zero in populations of lower SES. Explanations for this finding are only speculative, but it seems possible that families with higher SES provide a more consistently beneficial environment to their children, thus minimizing the environmental differences between them and thereby making genetics a larger source of variance. In populations with lower SES, on the other hand, some children may encounter more beneficial environments (eg, a particularly nurturing teacher) while others do not, which results in higher estimates of environmental variance in IQ and minimal genetic heritability.

With the advent of molecular genetic methods, twin studies have been supplanted by research that examines specific genes and their effects on child behavior and development. Genome-wide association studies (GWASs) provide one example of this new approach. In these studies, single nucleotide polymorphisms, which are commonly found in the general population, are studied in relation to phenotypic traits. In general, GWASs are suited to finding genetic differences that are relatively common but have relatively weak effects on the risk of having a medical condition, whether that disease is emphysema or a reading disability. More recently, next-generation genetic sequencing methods have been applied to the task of finding the genetic roots of behavior and development. These methods include whole exome sequencing and whole genome sequencing, in which every base pair in a person's genome is sequenced, whether it is found in an exon, in an intron, or in the intervening segments that comprise 98% of our DNA (formerly referred to as "junk DNA"). These "next-gen" studies are finding variations that are rare in the population as a whole but that may carry much stronger disease risk.[6] (It is reasoned that if a genetic difference carried a high risk for a serious medical condition, then it could not be common in the population, as it would decrease the fitness of individuals who have it.) Even when differences in genotype are found, science is faced with the daunting task of understanding how these differences in genetic sequence give rise to seemingly dramatic phenotypic differences. Genes and their protein products interact in enormously complex networks, regulating the expression and effect of other genes and proteins, and scientists will be busy for many decades unraveling this complexity.

Genetic factors can have either large or subtle influences on child development and behavior. Examples of the former include genetic diagnoses that are associated with intellectual disability or severe behavioral abnormalities. These disorders can result from single gene mutations (eg, in the *FMR1, HPRT1,* or *MECP2* genes associated with fragile X syndrome, Lesch-Nyhan syndrome, and Rett syndrome, respectively) or from genetic conditions that affect multiple genes (eg, contiguous gene deletion syndromes such as Williams syndrome or velocardiofacial syndrome, chromosomal aneuploidies such as Down syndrome and segmental chromosomal deletions or duplications). In some of these disorders, the exact pathogenic mechanism is not fully understood. For example, it is still not conclusively known which genes on the triploid chromosome 21 have significant roles in causing the neurobiological differences associated with Down syndrome. In other disorders, including fragile X syndrome and many metabolic conditions, such as Lesch-Nyhan syndrome, the pathogenesis is understood to a greater extent.

In contrast to the large effects of mutations in genes such as *FMR1, HPRT1,* and *MECP2,* mutations and variants in other genes are believed to have more subtle effects on the risk for conditions such as reading disability, ADHD, and other learning disabilities. For some conditions, such as autism spectrum disorder (ASD), research suggests that there are both large-effect and small-effect genes. Mutations in the *SHANK3* and *CHD8* genes, for example, are associated with a large risk for autism, but mutations in large-effect genes such as these are estimated to account for only 30% to 40% of all cases of ASD, at most, while most cases of ASD are believed to be associated with small-effect mutations or common variants in other genes.[7] These genetic differences may not give rise to autism on their own but may work with other genetic risk factors or with yet-unspecified environmental factors to cause autism. Because of the smaller effects of these genes, however, and their complex interactions with other factors, they have been difficult to identify and to confirm.

Individual variability in clinical manifestations is present both for small-effect common variant genetic differences but also for the large-effect genes. For instance, only 25% to 30% of individuals with fragile X syndrome, associated with the *FMR1* gene, meet full diagnostic criteria for autism. Even the level of intellectual disability seen in fragile X syndrome varies widely among those with the full mutation. Similarly, mutations in

CHD8 are not fully penetrant in causing autism; perhaps only 50% of those with mutations are diagnosed with autism, while other affected individuals may have other developmental-behavioral disorders (see Chapter 11, Making Developmental-Behavioral Diagnoses). The same general pattern is seen with copy number variations, in which a segment of DNA is either deleted, duplicated, or repeated more than 2 times. For example, among individuals with deletions of the 16p11.2 region, about 25% have ASD, more than half have a language-related disability, and a small percentage do not meet criteria for any developmental or psychiatric disorder at all.[8] Related research has shown that the genetic risk factors for many psychiatric disorders, from schizophrenia to mood disorders to ASD to ADHD, overlap widely, suggesting that individual variability in outcome is a universal rule rather than an exception.

What is the source of this variability? One undeniable answer is that environmental factors interact in very important ways with genetics, even for the classic, severe genetic disorders. These disorders were long thought to result in preordained, minimally changeable developmental outcomes. But for many metabolic disorders, with phenylketonuria serving as a particularly well-known example, early diagnosis and careful nutritional management can greatly enhance outcome. Even in chromosomal disorders such as Down syndrome where a very large number of genes are affected, the past decades have yielded powerful evidence for developmental variation that depends on environmental factors. When Down syndrome was first recognized in the medical literature, almost all affected individuals had moderate or severe intellectual disability, and virtually all were confined to state-run residential institutions. Today, children with Down syndrome typically grow up with their own families; they receive extensive early intervention and special educational support, and their cognitive and functional capacities are far greater than they were a generation ago.[9]

Epigenetics

Even from the narrow perspective of what "nature" means, it is now recognized that, besides genes, there are epigenetic factors that must be considered a part of every child's biological endowment. Epigenetic factors are biological differences related to genes but not involving the sequence of base pairs in a person's DNA. The best understood example of this is imprinting, by which a child's DNA is somehow marked as having come from either the mother or the father. For example, the genetic syndromes of Prader-Willi and Angelman both can result from a deletion at chromosome 15q11-q13. If this deletion occurs on the chromosome 15 that was inherited from the father, then the child is affected by Prader-Willi syndrome, but if the deletion occurs on the maternally inherited chromosome 15, then the child will have Angelman syndrome.

Fragile X syndrome provides another example of an epigenetic phenomenon. In almost all cases, the mutation that causes the syndrome, which is found in the promoter region of the *FMRP* gene, is accompanied by methylation of the *FMRP* gene. This methylation blocks the gene from being expressed, causing the affected child to fully manifest fragile X syndrome. In rare cases, however, the mutated gene is not methylated, allowing some FMRP to be produced and resulting in less severe symptoms.

A third possible example of an epigenetic modification is found in Turner syndrome.[10] In Turner syndrome, girls have only one X chromosome, which can be inherited from either their father or their mother. According to some reports, social and cognitive skills in girls with Turner syndrome may differ depending on whether their only X chromosome comes from their father or from their mother. Other medical characteristics, such as body mass index, cholesterol levels, and the presence of renal malformations, may also be a function of the parent-of-origin of the X chromosome. Researchers hypothesize that there may be a gene or genes on the X chromosome that are active in males (who have only one X chromosome) but may be methylated and turned off on one of the female X chromosomes, and that some differences may also be found after the X chromosome is passed on to the child with Turner syndrome.

Intriguing research has shown that monozygotic twins, who by definition have identical genetic sequences, can have differences in their epigenetic states.[11] As a corollary, the twins can have differences in the extent to which the epigenetically regulated genes are expressed, which would lead to differences in their phenotypes. The data show that twins' epigenetic differences increase with age, particularly if the twins live apart from each other. The tentative conclusion is that the different environments that the twins experience are the cause of their epigenetic divergence and, thus, of the phenotypic differences that arise between identical twins. This conclusion is supported by findings in animal research that an individual's epigenetic state can change during life as a consequence of specific environmental experiences.

Biological Experiences

The broad perspective on nature's influences includes not only genetic and epigenetic factors but also biological events that are experienced either prenatally or postnatally. Examples include traumatic brain injury, hypoxic-ischemic encephalopathy, meningoencephalitis, congenital brain malformations, and prenatal drug exposures. Scientists recently established that prenatal exposure to tobacco smoking leaves a biological signature on the child's epigenome—specifically, the pattern of DNA methylation remains different, even at age 3 to 5 years, in children whose mothers smoked during pregnancy.[12] Because these factors have a well-defined biological mechanism, they often have been thought to have a strongly constraining influence on developmental-behavioral outcomes. The fallacy in such reasoning can be found in conditions such as malnutrition, in utero infections, and chronic illness. These conditions are among the most common biological insults experienced by children worldwide, with protein malnutrition and deficiencies of iron and iodine as prime examples. Each of these conditions also has a clear biological mechanism, but each is associated with a range of developmental-behavioral outcomes. It is widely appreciated that the outcome in this second set of conditions depends on the success of interventions directed either to the underlying conditions or to their developmental-behavioral consequences. We are now learning that the same is true for genetic differences and for biological conditions that were previously regarded more fatalistically. It seems very likely that future research will point the way to interventions that may help to treat the biological conditions that were historically regarded as resistant to treatment. As an example, constraint therapy, a possible therapy for focal brain injury and cerebral palsy, is discussed in the Extraordinary Manipulations of the Environment section below.

Environmental Factors in Child Development and Behavior

The variety of environmental, or experiential, factors affecting development and behavior is wide. As is evident from even a short listing of these factors—from birth order, maternal educational level, and family dynamics to poverty, child abuse, and strength of religious affiliation—experiential factors can be either beneficial or dele-terious in their effects, and they can be either direct or indirect in their mechanisms. In almost all cases, the mechanisms by which these factors exert their effects are still unknown, but it is an unstated assumption that experiential factors act through brain plasticity, whether or not we know the exact mechanisms. That is, the brain has the potential to be molded (nurtured) by environmental factors in either a beneficial, func-tionally positive direction or in a deleterious, functionally negative direction. Stated in yet another way, it can be expected that experiential factors ultimately act through neurobiological mechanisms to shape the status and the function of children's brains, just as Freud himself hypothesized that the action and effects of his psychotherapy were made manifest through neurobiological processes.

Neurobiological Effects of Environmental Enrichment

A classic, early demonstration of the neurobiological effect of environmental enrich-ment is found in the work of Volkmar and Greenough[13] on rats. This research built on earlier work that showed superior problem-solving abilities in rats raised as pets com-pared with rats raised without such extensive human interaction. These experiments showed that environmental enrichment is associated with greater cerebral volumes, a larger number of synapses, and increased complexity of dendritic branching. Thus, differences in environmental variables were translated into changes in neurobiological characteristics.

Maternal Education, Socioeconomic Status, and Poverty

In this light, it is no surprise that maternal education level (or analogous variables such as maternal SES or maternal IQ) has been shown repeatedly to be one of the strongest predictors of developmental outcome, regardless of the primary risk factor being studied (eg, prematurity, meningitis, adoption after institutionalization). The specific mechanism through which maternal educational level exerts its action on the child is not known, but it may take the form of an enriched environment, whether that enrichment is provided directly by the mother or indirectly through other aspects of the environment that the mother shapes. More recently, many studies have begun to look beyond demographic variables such as SES to make a detailed assessment of observable environmental variables, such as the presence of books in the home, hours of electronic media exposure, types of conversation in which the child is engaged, and/or the sheer volume of words that a child is exposed to.[14,15] These studies suggest that the demographic variables that are associated with child development may be mediated at least partially through these concrete, more proximal factors.

Other environmental factors that influence child development, such as poverty and institutionalization, may operate at least partly through similar mechanisms, though there has been little study to date of the detailed mechanisms of these environmental factors. Poverty has been hypothesized to exert its effects through nutritional status, toxin exposure, stress, or other pathways. Recent data suggest that poverty is associated with changes in brain structure and brain activation patterns that are evident on neuro-imaging and with impairments in executive functions, such as attention and inhibition.[16] These data provide further evidence that environmental factors are associated with changes in neurobiological processes in children's brains.

The mechanisms by which environmental factors influence behavioral health outcomes are even less well understood. As suggested in the literature on the effects of poverty, stress-related physiology may underlie the effects of many environmental factors, ranging from child abuse or neglect, familial dysfunction and divorce, or exposure to violence, while resilience factors may mitigate such stress.[17] Alternatively or additionally, some such factors may shape children's behavior by providing a behavioral model that, unfortunately, is assimilated and later recapitulated.

Sensitive Periods

The extremely rare cases of "wild" or "feral" children have contributed greatly to the concept of *sensitive* or *critical* periods of child development. In these tragic cases, children are severely deprived of human interaction, and they grow up to be pervasively impaired.[18] In addition to these unusual cases, there are also commonly encountered conditions that give insight into sensitive periods and illustrate the importance of environmental influences and their interactions with biological factors. The example that is best understood on a neurobiological level is strabismus. Neural inputs from both eyes are known to converge in the primary visual cortex of the occipital lobe. In children with strabismus, the connections from one of the two eyes to specific cortical cells are lost, and the capacity for binocular vision is lost with them. The pathogenic mechanism for amblyopia secondary to refractive errors is analogous. Related animal research has studied other unusual constraints on visual input, such as exposing young animals to an environment that has only vertical stripes. Such animals lose much of their capacity to perceive visual features other than stripes. As is the case for strabismus and amblyopia in humans, this research demonstrates how normal brain development requires appropriate environmental inputs and how these inputs must occur around a certain age.

Language development provides another common example of a sensitive period for environmental stimulation in child development. The cases of feral children again provide an extreme example, in which it is argued that language cannot be acquired if there is an absence of appropriate language stimulation in the first few years of life.

More prosaically, it is widely observed that children tend to acquire a second language much more easily and proficiently than adults do. While there are exceptions to this rule, there is likely to be a combination of biological and environmental explanations for children's advantage over adults in second language learning. Besides having brains that may be more receptive to a second language, children typically learn a second language in a different social and psychological environment than adults do—they tend to be immersed with other children who provide plentiful, possibly simpler and more concrete language input, and children may be less embarrassed than adult learners to practice their emerging language skills.

More generally, primary pediatric health care professionals, , psychologists, parents, educators, and policy makers understand that the first few years of life constitute a very important period for child development. This belief is rooted in the rapid biological development of the brain in those years. Recent research on children adopted internationally illustrates this principle clearly.[19] Whether they are from Romania, Russia, China, or elsewhere, children who remain in institutions past 24 months of age show more severe and more enduring developmental impairments than those adopted before age 2 years. Ongoing research suggests that the prognosis of all institutionalized orphans improves when they are placed in foster care or its equivalent, even if they remain in their country of origin.[20]

While the term *critical period* was used frequently in the older literature, the term *sensitive period* now is used more commonly, reflecting the fact that most developmental processes are not completely limited to a specific window in time. Rather, while specific developmental processes might proceed most quickly and efficiently during their sensitive periods, they can still move forward later in life. Even in the case of strabismus and loss of stereovision, there are many case reports of adults who were able to acquire stereovision later in life.[21]

Education as Nurture

Many of the innate and experiential factors discussed previously are inadvertent (ie, the affected child and his or her parents did not seek out traumatic brain injury, malnutrition, or a deleterious gene mutation) and have negative influences, but there are, of course, many environmental factors that are positive in their influence and that are actively sought by children and their caregivers. Education is a prime example of a positive environmental experience that is deliberately sought, with early intervention and the Head Start program being 2 specific examples within the larger category of educational experiences. Very few parents would deny the importance of formal education, and the data supporting the general benefits of early intervention and Head Start are now unassailable (see Chapter 6, Early Intervention). Indeed, the effects of Head Start have been demonstrated on multiple levels of outcome, from brain electrophysiology to behavior and academic achievement.[22]

Education researchers continually engage in the refinement and development of new curricula that might be more effective than previously used curricula. Recently, these efforts have turned their focus beyond just academic skills to include the teaching of fundamental cognitive skills. In one example, preschool curricula have been created that are successful in promoting better executive functions (eg, working memory, inhibition, attention) in children.[23]

Extraordinary Manipulations of the Environment

Therapeutic environmental experiences can also take very unusual approaches in their efforts to tailor interventions to specific populations of children. To return to the example of amblyopia, monocular occlusion (patching) of the better-sighted eye seems as extreme as the manipulations imposed on research animals in the study of vision, as discussed previously, but its value is proven. A relatively unknown and still incompletely proven therapy for cerebral palsy takes a related approach. In constraint therapy, individuals with a hemiplegia have their better-functioning limb restrained or immobilized, forcing them to use their affected limb more intensely, just as eye patching forces the use of the impaired eye. It is hypothesized that the more intense use of the impaired limb results in faster and more thorough remapping of brain circuits, culminating in better recovery of function. A large, randomized trial of constraint therapy is now under way in children with cerebral palsy.[24]

The discrete trial/applied behavioral analytic (ABA) approach to autism intervention might also be considered an extraordinary manipulation of the environment. The rigid programming and massed trials approach that ABA uses bears little resemblance to the typical environment in which children develop. Nonetheless, ABA appears to be beneficial for many children with autism, and it is regarded as the most strongly evidence-based intervention for autism that is available, though its benefits may not always generalize easily to regular life contexts (see Chapter 19, Autism Spectrum Disorder). Another intervention approach for autism, known as the Early Start Denver Model (ESDM), incorporates ABA principles and other therapeutic and educational approaches as well. A controlled study of ESDM showed not only that it improved behavioral outcomes but that brain electrophysiological responses to pictures of faces also normalized after treatment.[25]

Environmental Factors and Behavioral Development

While much of the previous discussion has focused on children's cognitive development, it is well known that environmental factors can have enormous effects on children's behavioral development. Many factors discussed in relation to cognitive development also have very important influences on child behavior. A dramatic example is that of institutionalization and its effects on attachment-related behavior. Early and severe deprivation from typical bonding and attachment experiences has enduring effects on later behavior in this domain.[20] Thus, there seems to be a very important sensitive period for newborns, infants, and toddlers to experience normative formation of close interpersonal relationships.

Children more commonly encounter other environmental factors that are less dramatic but can also have important influences on behavioral development. Birth order, parental age, and the parents' marital status are among the demographic variables known to be associated with child behavioral outcomes. Examples of other variables that are associated with behavioral outcomes and that are more proximal to children's day-to-day lives are parenting style, the parents' mental health, parental substance abuse, and exposure to violence in the home, media, or community. A substantial body of research also has identified positive environmental factors that support resilience in behavioral and developmental outcomes.[17] Findings from an early but still influential study of resilience, the Kauai Longitudinal Study,[26] indicate that both internal (eg, temperament and academic competence) and external (eg, membership in a religious community and a close relationship with a supportive adult) factors can modulate outcomes in a positive direction, in the face of various risk factors.

The Interaction of Nature and Nurture

As the landmark publication *From Neurons to Neighborhoods* concluded,[1] "[T]he longstanding nature versus nurture debate is over-simplistic and scientifically obsolete." Instead, the book's authors went on to explain, "the question is… how early experiences and genetic predispositions interact." Researchers have only recently acquired the tools and underlying knowledge needed to answer this question, but their early efforts are beginning to elucidate how nature and nurture interact at a fundamental level.

Much of the research on the interaction between genetic and environmental factors is particularly relevant to pediatrics. For example, one pioneering study investigated the relationship between childhood experiences of maltreatment and violent or antisocial behavior in adulthood. By performing genotyping studies on a very large cohort of children who had been victims of abuse in childhood, Caspi et al[27] found an interaction between the *MAOA* gene and child maltreatment (Figure 2.2). Boys who had one version of the gene (the version associated with lower enzyme activity) had a much higher risk of developing antisocial behavior themselves. In a group of control subjects with no history of childhood abuse, the *MAOA* gene was not associated with a higher risk of adult antisocial behavior. Thus, a synergistic interaction between gene and environment was critical in determining outcomes; neither factor alone showed nearly the effect as did the 2 risk factors in combination.

Attempts to replicate the finding of Caspi et al have been inconsistent, and there currently is no clear consensus on whether *MAOA* interacts with childhood maltreatment. However, there is strong evidence across 22 studies that another genetic factor—the VAL66MET substitution in the gene for *BDNF*—interacts with stressful life events to increase the risk for major depression in adulthood.[28] *BDNF* codes for the protein brain-derived neurotrophic factor, which is important in neuronal growth and survival and in synaptic plasticity.

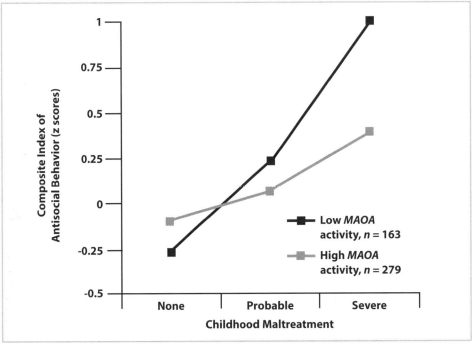

Figure 2.2. Interaction of *MAOA* genotype and exposure to maltreatment. Exposure to maltreatment increases the severity of antisocial behavior in boys, but this effect is much larger in boys with the low-activity version of the gene for MAOA than for boys with the high-activity version of this gene.

Reprinted from Caspi A, McClay J, Moffitt TE, et al. Role of genotype in the cycle of violence in maltreated children. *Science.* 2002;297(5582):851–854, with permission from the American Association for the Advancement of Science (AAAS).

Lead intoxication provides another example of gene-environment interaction. Even at levels that are below the previously accepted limit of 10 mcg/dL, population studies show that lead exposure is associated with lower IQ scores, after accounting for maternal IQ, various home environment factors, and other confounding factors. However, it may also be true that some individuals are more severely affected than others at any given level of lead exposure. This thesis has been articulated by many, perhaps most elegantly by Ruff,[29] but it is only recently that researchers have begun to explain why this may be so. A study of the effects of lead on executive functions (which are a diverse set of frontal lobe–dependent functions that include attention, inhibition, cognitive flexibility, and more) suggests that for some of these functions, the deleterious effects of lead exposure only appear in children with a specific allele of a gene for a dopamine neurotransmitter receptor.[30] These results require replication, but they again point to the intricate interplay between environmental and genetic factors in child development and behavior.

Intraventricular hemorrhage (IVH) is a neurobiological injury with which primary care pediatric health care professionals and families of neonates who are born preterm, are too familiar. Preterm birth is well known as a risk factor associated with IVH and a variety of other medical and developmental conditions, from necrotizing enterocolitis to cerebral palsy; however, these morbidities affect some neonates born preterm, but not all.

A collection of recent studies suggests that several different genes may increase susceptibility to IVH among neonates born preterm. These genes have a role in processes ranging from coagulation (the gene for factor V Leiden) to vascular structure (collagen 4A1, *COL4A1*).[31]

A final example of gene-environment interaction is widely appreciated in clinical medicine but perhaps not usually thought of in this context: pharmacogenomics. Physicians understand that individual patients often respond differently to any given drug therapy, and these differences may be rooted in genetic differences. Individual differences in hepatic metabolism are one mechanism through which genetics interact with the effects of drug therapy. For patients treated with atomoxetine, for example, those who are "poor metabolizers" through the *CYP2D6* pathway have a higher incidence of side effects than patients who are "extensive metabolizers," and they also show a trend toward greater efficacy.[32] Genetic differences in neurotransmitter receptors or neurotransmitter metabolism may be associated with differences in efficacy and tolerability for specific patient subpopulations, as pilot studies suggest about the effects of methylphenidate on hyperactivity in children with ASD.[33]

Yet another line of current research examines the effect of environment on the epigenome. Data in rats have shown that maternal grooming and nurturing can lead to changes in gene methylation. This, in turn, results in changes in gene expression that subsequently increase grooming and nurturing in the offspring when it matures.[34] Analogous research in humans is only just beginning, but one study has reported that childhood stress is associated with changes in DNA methylation that are still present in adolescence. These differences are presumably associated with changes in DNA expression patterns in the affected individuals.[35]

Fragile X Syndrome: An Example of Nature, Nurture, and Their Interactions

Fragile X syndrome is the most common inherited cause of intellectual disability (see Chapter 15, Cognitive Development and Disorders), and it is the subject of very active research on multiple levels. That research, from the molecular to the behavioral, provides examples of the effects on child development and behavior of nature, nurture, and their interactions.[36]

The single gene mutation that defines fragile X syndrome causes intellectual disabilities and behavioral problems in most affected individuals. As with essentially all genetic conditions causing intellectual disability, however, there is a significant range of cognitive and behavioral function within the population of individuals with fragile X syndrome. The biological and environmental factors that account for this variability are starting to be illuminated. First, while all affected individuals have a "full mutation" (>200 repeats of a CGG triplet) in the *FMR1* gene, the epigenetic factor of gene methylation is absent in a small percentage of individuals. In these individuals, the *FMRP* gene is still partially expressed, some protein product is made, and the cognitive impairment is moderated. Second, as is the case for many other genetic conditions, genetic mosaicism occurs in some individuals such that some cells carry the fragile X syndrome mutation, but others do not. A closely related phenomenon, random X inactivation (also known as lyonization), is also associated with variability in symptom severity. As a result of random X inactivation, females who are heterozygous for the fragile X syndrome mutation can have either an uncommonly high or low percentage of cells in which the active X chromosome has the fragile X syndrome mutation. The behavioral and developmental symptoms of individuals with fragile X syndrome varies as a function of all of these factors: methylation, mosaicism, and lyonization.

Investigators recently examined the role of other genes, besides the *FMRP* gene itself, on response to drug treatment among patients with fragile X syndrome. Their preliminary results suggest that a polymorphism in the gene for *BDNF* is predictive of positive response (in language development) to serotonin reuptake inhibitors.[37] These results need replication before they can be regarded as definitive, but they show the direction of current research and its potential to elucidate how genes interact with each other to affect child development and behavior.

Environmental factors are also of great importance in shaping the development and behavior of children with fragile X syndrome. As many had suspected might be the case, the effect of having a mother who also has fragile X syndrome is very important. More generally, it has been found that home environment, as assessed by a multidimensional, direct-observation instrument, has a significant influence on cognitive and adaptive outcomes in children with fragile X syndrome. The IQ of males with fragile X syndrome was most strongly predicted by the home environment, which included such dimensions as parental responsiveness to the child, presence of learning materials in the home, and parental efforts to provide developmental enrichment.[38] In fact, the association of home environment with IQ was numerically larger than for any other variable, including the child's levels of FMRP and mean parental IQ (which was not a statistically significant predictor). For adaptive behavior, the association between home environment and total score on the Vineland Adaptive Behavior Scale was numerically larger than for any other predictor, including the child's own IQ.[39]

Conclusion

Nature and nurture both have profound effects on child development and behavior. Genetic differences can be associated with either subtle or dramatic effects, and the field of genomics is starting to unravel the complex interactions among the many genes involved in brain development and behavior. Environmental factors also can have either subtle or profound effects, and in contrast to genetic factors, many environmental influences are typically thought of in the context of their beneficial or protective effects. Education and other behavioral interventions are rightly regarded as environmental influences on child development and behavior. Newer approaches to intervention may be expanding the range of influence of educational efforts.

While many behavioral genetic studies have attempted to quantify the relative influence of genetic versus environmental influences, this endeavor is unavoidably compromised by interpretative limitations and is of little relevance to individual patient cases. Of greater research and clinical interest is the burgeoning understanding of gene-environment interactions. This research is beginning to show that the variability of genetic and environmental influences may often arise because of their interaction. In the future, clinicians may need to integrate genetic and environmental information on their patients to best understand the effect of both sets of factors.

References

1. Committee on Integrating the Science of Early Childhood Development. *From Neurons to Neighborhoods: The Science of Early Childhood Development.* Washington, DC: National Academies Press; 2000
2. Sternberg RJ. Improving fluid intelligence is possible after all. *Proc Natl Acad Sci U S A.* 2008;105(19):6791–6792
3. Boomsma D, Busjahn A, Peltonen L. Classical twin studies and beyond. *Nat Rev Genet.* 2002;3(11):872–882
4. Plomin R, Owen MJ, McGuffin P. The genetic basis of complex human behaviors. *Science.* 1994;264(5166):1733–1739
5. Turkheimer E, Haley A, Waldron M, D'Onofrio B, Gottesman II. Socioeconomic status modifies heritability of IQ in young children. *Psychol Sci.* 2003;14(6):623–628
6. Feero WG, Guttmacher AE. Genomics, personalized medicine, and pediatrics. *Acad Pediatr.* 2014;14(1):14–22
7. Gaugler T, Klei L, Sanders SJ, et al. Most genetic risk for autism resides with common variation. *Nat Genet.* 2014;46(8):881–885
8. Hanson E, Bernier R, Porche K, et al. The cognitive and behavioral phenotype of the 16p11.2 deletion in a clinically ascertained population. *Biol Psychiatry.* 2015;77(9):785–793
9. Roizen NJ, Patterson D. Down's syndrome. *Lancet.* 2003;361(9365):1281–1289
10. Bondy CA, Hougen HY, Zhou J, Cheng CM. Genomic imprinting and Turner syndrome. *Pediatr Endocrinol Rev.* 2012;9(Suppl 2):728–732
11. Fraga MF, Ballestar E, Paz MF, et al. Epigenetic differences arise during the lifetime of monozygotic twins. *Proc Natl Acad Sci U S A.* 2005;102(30):10604–10609
12. Ladd-Acosta C, Shu C, Lee BK, et al. Presence of an epigenetic signature of prenatal cigarette smoke exposure in childhood. *Environ Res.* 2016;144(Pt A):139–148
13. Volkmar FR, Greenough WT. Rearing complexity affects branching of dendrites in the visual cortex of the rat. *Science.* 1972;176(4042):1445–1447
14. Tong S, Baghurst P, Vimpani G, McMichael A. Socioeconomic position, maternal IQ, home environment, and cognitive development. *J Pediatr.* 2007;151(3):284–288, 288.e1
15. Hart B, Risley TR. *Meaningful Differences in the Everyday Experience of Young American Children.* Baltimore, MD: Paul H. Brookes Publishing Co; 1995
16. Johnson SB, Riis JL, Noble KG. State of the art review: poverty and the developing brain. *Pediatrics.* 2016;137(4):e20153075
17. Bonanno GA, Mancini AD. The human capacity to thrive in the face of potential trauma. *Pediatrics.* 2008;121(2):369–375
18. Rymer R. *Genie: A Scientific Tragedy.* New York, NY: HarperCollins Publishers; 1994
19. Juffer F, van Ijzendoorn MH. Behavior problems and mental health referrals of international adoptees: a meta-analysis. *JAMA.* 2005;293(20):2501–2515
20. Rutter M, O'Connor TG; English and Romanian Adoptees (ERA) Study Team. Are there biological programming effects for psychological development? Findings from a study of Romanian adoptees. *Dev Psychol.* 2004;40(1):81–94
21. Levi DM, Knill DC, Bavelier D. Stereopsis and amblyopia: a mini-review. *Vision Res.* 2015;114:17–30
22. Neville HJ, Stevens C, Pakulak E, et al. Family-based training program improves brain function, cognition, and behavior in lower socioeconomic status preschoolers. *Proc Natl Acad Sci U S A.* 2013;110(29):12138–12143
23. Diamond A, Ling DS. Conclusions about interventions, programs, and approaches for improving executive functions that appear justified and those that, despite much hype, do not. *Dev Cogn Neurosci.* 2016;18:34–48
24. Chorna O, Heathcock J, Key A, et al. Early childhood constraint therapy for sensory/motor impairment in cerebral palsy: a randomised clinical trial protocol. *BMJ Open.* 2015;5(12):e010212
25. Dawson G, Jones EJ, Merkle K, et al. Early behavioral intervention is associated with normalized brain activity in young children with autism. *J Am Acad Child Adolesc Psychiatry.* 2012;51(11):1150–1159
26. Werner EE. Vulnerable but invincible: high-risk children from birth to adulthood. *Acta Paediatr Suppl.* 1997;422:103–105

27. Caspi A, McClay J, Moffitt TE, et al. Role of genotype in the cycle of violence in maltreated children. *Science.* 2002;297(5582):851–854

28. Hosang G, Shiles C, Tansey KE, McGuffin P, Uher R. Interaction between stress and the BDNF Val66Met polymorphism in depression: a systematic review and meta-analysis. *BMC Med.* 2014;12:7

29. Ruff HA. Population-based data and the development of individual children: the case of low to moderate lead levels and intelligence. *J Dev Behav Pediatr.* 1999;20(1):42–49

30. Froehlich TE, Lanphear BP, Dietrich KN, Cory-Slechta DA, Wang N, Kahn RS. Interactive effects of a DRD4 polymorphism, lead, and sex on executive functions in children. *Biol Psychiatry.* 2007;62(3):243–249

31. Ment LR, Adén U, Lin A, et al. Gene-environment interactions in severe intraventricular hemorrhage of preterm neonates. *Pediatr Res.* 2014;75(1–2):241–250

32. Michelson D, Read HA, Ruff DD, Witcher J, Zhang S, McCracken J. CYP2D6 and clinical response to atomoxetine in children and adolescents with ADHD. *J Am Acad Child Adolesc Psychiatry.* 2007;46(2):242–251

33. McCracken JT, Badashova KK, Posey DJ, et al. Positive effects of methylphenidate on hyperactivity are moderated by monoaminergic gene variants in children with autism spectrum disorders. *Pharmacogenomics J.* 2014;14(3):295–302

34. Weaver IC, Cervoni N, Champagne FA, et al. Epigenetic programming by maternal behavior. *Nat Neurosci.* 2004;7(8):847–854

35. Essex MJ, Boyce WT, Hertzman C, et al. Epigenetic vestiges of early developmental adversity: childhood stress exposure and DNA methylation in adolescence. *Child Dev.* 2013;84(1):58–75

36. Hagerman RJ, Berry-Kravis E, Kaufmann WE, et al. Advances in the treatment of fragile X syndrome. *Pediatrics.* 2009;123(1):378–390

37. Al Olaby RR, Sweha SR, Silva M, et al. Molecular biomarkers predictive of sertraline treatment response in young children with fragile X syndrome. *Brain Dev.* 2017;39(6):483–492

38. Dyer-Friedman J, Glaser B, Hessl D, et al. Genetic and environmental influences on the cognitive outcomes of children with fragile X syndrome. *J Am Acad Child Adolesc Psychiatry.* 2002;41(3):237–244

39. Glaser B, Hessl D, Dyer-Friedman J, et al. Biological and environmental contributions to adaptive behavior in fragile X syndrome. *Am J Med Genet A.* 2003;117A(1):21–29

CHAPTER 3

Environmental Influences on Child Development and Behavior

Pamela C. High, MD, FAAP

Carrie Kelly, MD, FAAP

Angelica Robles, MD, FAAP

Bridget Thompson, DO, FAAP

Benard P. Dreyer, MD, FAAP

How the Environment Stimulates Early Brain Development

The amazing newborn brain is composed of 100 million neurons and 10 times as many glial elements. These organize, migrate, connect, and specialize in response to dopaminergic, adrenergic, and serotonergic neurotransmitter systems. Newborns have 50 trillion synapses connecting these neurons at birth, and an explosion in synaptogenesis leads them to develop 20 times that number by their first birthday. This overproduction is followed by a period of synaptic pruning. Synapses that are used become stronger, and those neglected are pruned away. By the time a person reaches 20 years of age, that person has only half the number of synapses he or she had at 1 year of age. This process happens in a sequential way, with the number of synapses in sensory and motor areas peaking as early as 4 months, followed by stabilization in the number of synapses by preschool age. However, not every area of the brain follows this timeline. For example, in the prefrontal cortex, where executive functions are controlled, the number of synapses peaks at 1 year of age but does not stabilize until late adolescence or early adulthood. Myelination of neuronal sheaths also occurs early in motor and sensory areas and later in the prefrontal cortex.[1,2]

Thus synaptic pruning and myelination are 2 mechanisms by which an individual neurobiologically adapts to his or her environment. These are also mechanisms by which the environment shapes brain architecture. Often-used examples of this are the images of small and underdeveloped brains of children raised under circumstances of extreme neglect experienced in some orphanages.[2] Recently, more subtle neuroimaging confirms this impact of environment on brain structure. For example, maternal support observed in the preschool years has been found to be strongly predictive of hippocampal volume at school age.[3]

The Impact of Early Childhood Adversity and Toxic Stress on Child Development and Behavior

The field of pediatrics has continued to evolve since it emerged as a specialized entity in clinical medicine in the late 19th century. Initially, pediatricians focused on optimizing nutrition, treating infectious diseases, and preventing premature death. As advances in antibiotics, effective immunizations, and public health initiatives have diminished or, in some cases, eradicated many childhood illnesses, increased focus has been placed on child development, behavior, and family functioning. Over this time, parental substance abuse and mental illness, as well as exposure to violence, have been identified as factors that negatively impact children's health and development. More recently, societal concerns, such as the adverse effects of watching excessive amounts of television, the influence of new technologies, epidemic increases in obesity, and the persistent economic, racial, and ethnic disparities in health status, have been brought to the forefront of pediatrics.[4] In fact, a recent American Academy of Pediatrics (AAP) technical report reviewing 58 years of published studies characterized racial and ethnic disparities in children's health to be extensive, pervasive, persistent, and, in some cases, worsening.[5]

As the practice of pediatrics has evolved, so has the understanding of the process of child development. As described in Chapter 2, (Nature, Nurture and Their Interactions in Child Development and Behavior), a child's learning, behavior, and physical and mental health are influenced both by his or her genetic predisposition and by the environment. The relatively new field of epigenetics has allowed us to understand that environmental influences occurring prenatally and in early life can start to shape development before birth, throughout childhood, and beyond, potentially affecting subsequent generations. It is in this context that early childhood adversity and toxic stress in the lives of young children can be understood as a significant risk factor for poor outcomes in development, behavior, and learning across the life course.

Physiological responses to stress are well studied and defined.[6-8] During the stress response, the hypothalamic-pituitary-adrenocortical axis and the sympathetic-adrenomedullary system are activated, resulting in increased levels of stress hormones, such as corticotrophin-releasing hormone (CRH), cortisol, norepinephrine, and adrenaline. At the same time, other mediators, such as inflammatory cytokines, are released. Meanwhile, the parasympathetic nervous system responds to provide a counterbalance and attempt to achieve homeostasis within the body. Transient increases in these hormones in response to stress are protective and essential for survival. In contrast, excessively high or prolonged elevations in stress hormones are harmful and can be considered toxic, leading to chronic changes in brain architecture and bodily function, including alterations in physiological and emotional regulation and in executive function.[6-8] The AAP describes 3 distinct types of stress in young children: positive, tolerable, and toxic stress.[4]

A **positive stress** is of mild to moderate intensity, and it elicits a physiological response that is brief and of mild to moderate magnitude. This might occur with an immunization or on the first day of school, when a caring adult is present to help ease a child's distress. Positive stress with appropriate scaffolding by caregivers can be seen as growth-promoting and important for healthy development.

Tolerable stress is associated with exposure to an experience that presents a greater magnitude of adversity or threat, such as the death of a family member, a natural disaster, or a contentious divorce, and so it elicits a much stronger physiological stress response. If effectively buffered by supportive and nurturing adults, the risk that it will cause prolonged activation of the stress response system, negatively impacting health and learning, is significantly reduced. Therefore, this form of stress response is tolerable depending on the extent to which protective adult relationships can facilitate the child's adaptive coping and sense of control, thereby promoting a return of the child's physiological stress response to its baseline.

In contrast to positive or tolerable stress, **toxic stress** is the result of strong, frequent, or prolonged activation of the body's stress response systems in the absence of the buffering protection of supportive and enduring adult relationships. Examples of these kinds of stressors include child abuse and neglect, parental mental health concerns, and the cumulative burden of persistent financial hardship. The key elements differentiating the type of stressors and a child's response to them are the intensity and persistence of the stress and the lack of availability of a caring and responsive adult whose comfort can serve as a protective factor, facilitating the return of the stress response to its baseline equilibrium state.

Toxic stress can stimulate a child's reticular activating system and lead to sleep disturbances. Elevated circulating catecholamines can also produce anxiety, suppression of the satiety center (leading to overeating or failure to thrive), enuresis, and encopresis. Toxic stress can impact working memory and lead to slow acquisition of milestones or learning challenges. It can decrease inhibitory control, causing tantrums or fighting. Its impact on cognitive flexibility may result in difficulty with frustration tolerance, organization, concentration, and activity level.[9]

Toxic stresses are the kinds of risk factors studied in the Adverse Childhood Experiences (ACE) Study[10] of more than 17,000 adults for more than 20 years. This work has shown a strong and graded association between the number of these childhood stressors and a higher risk of poor outcomes in health and educational achievement in adulthood. A recent AAP technical report summarizes the growing evidence that links childhood toxic stress with the subsequent development of unhealthy lifestyles, persistent socioeconomic inequality, and poor health.[4]

In addition to short-term changes in observable behavior in young children, toxic stress can lead to outwardly visible and permanent changes in brain structure and function.[7,8] Both human and animal studies demonstrate that persistently elevated levels of stress hormones can disrupt the brain's developing architecture.[7,8] Therefore, this altered brain architecture in response to toxic stress in early childhood can explain, at least in part, the strong association between early adverse experiences and subsequent deficits in educational and health outcomes.

Toxic stress early in life plays a critical role in changing the course of development by disrupting brain circuitry and other important regulatory systems in ways that continue to influence physiology, behavior, and health decades later.[4] Some degree of childhood adversity is inevitable, and learning to manage mild to moderate levels of stress is important for healthy development. As the central element of toxic stress is the absence of buffers needed to return the physiological stress response to baseline, pediatric health care professionals play an important role in recognizing risk factors, supporting families through anticipatory guidance, strengthening families' social support systems, and encouraging a family's adoption of positive parenting techniques. These actions can facilitate a child's emerging social, emotional, and language skills. In addition to the AAP currently recommended developmental screenings at 9, 18, 24, and 30 months of age, pediatric practices should consider implementing standardized measures to identify other family- or community-level factors that place children at risk for toxic stress (eg, maternal depression, parental substance abuse, domestic or community violence, food scarcity, poor social connectedness).[11,12] See also Figure 3.1.

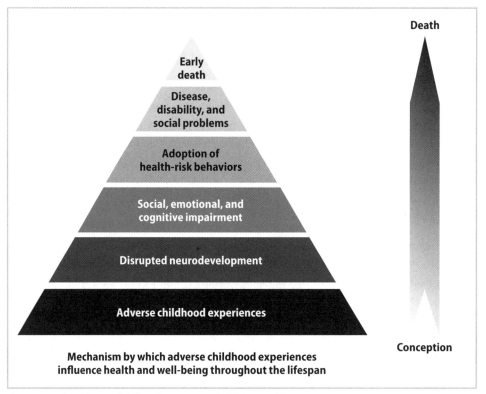

Figure 3.1. The Adverse Childhood Experiences (ACE) Pyramid.[13]

Important Examples of Environmental Factors That Affect Child Development and Behavior

The Impact of Poverty on Child Development, Behavior, and Academic Achievement

One in 5 children grows up poor in the United States, and 42% of children are poor or near poor.[14] Children are the poorest age group in our society. In comparison, only 9% of older Americans over 65 are poor. Young children are especially impacted by the effects of poverty, often leading to life-long disadvantage. Poverty's impacts on young children are mediated by parenting. Family income affects parenting directly and through material hardship, including food insecurity, residential instability, inadequacy of medical care, serious financial difficulties, and the inability to pay monthly bills. The negative effects of low family income and increased material hardship are associated with increased parenting stress (including increased maternal depression and marital discord), decreased investment in children, and decreased positive parenting. Investment in children includes educational toys, books, high-quality early childhood care and education, as well as parent activities with the child outside the home and provision of extracurricular activities. In turn, these negative effects on parenting and provision of resources for the child lead to decreased cognitive skills (eg, reading and math) and decreased social-emotional competence (including problems with self-regulation, executive function, and increased externalizing behaviors) in the child.[15,16]

The differences in developmental outcomes for poor children and nonpoor children start early. Differences in language development can be observed almost as soon as expressive language begins, and by 2 or 3 years of age, these differences are marked.[17] These differences are directly related to the quantity and quality of the language that children are exposed to, primarily from their parents. By the time poor children start school, on average, their reading and math skills trail those who are at higher income, and many are never able to catch up.[18,19] Overall, poor children have higher rates of learning disabilities, serious emotional and behavioral difficulties, grade repetitions, and receipt of early intervention and special education services; their high school dropout rates are 1.5 to 2.5 the rates of nonpoor children.[20] There is growing evidence from studies of the Earned Income Tax Credit, Canada's National Child Benefit, welfare reform experiments, and natural experiments (eg, comparing Native American and non–Native American families when Native American families received distributions from casino profits) that increasing family income and decreasing poverty meaningfully improve developmental and academic outcomes in poor children.[16,20] In addition, exposure to concentrated neighborhood poverty further worsens the developmental, behavioral, and academic outcomes of poor children, and it may also lead to worse outcomes as children move through adolescence into adulthood.[20]

Recent studies have documented structural changes in the brain related to poverty. Children in poor families have been shown to have reduced volumes in the frontal and temporal cortices as well as the hippocampus. These are key areas of the brain necessary for school readiness and academic achievement and are associated with the development of executive function, language, and memory. It has been shown that brain volumes in the frontal and temporal cortices explain 15% to 20% of the difference in academic achievement test scores between poor and nonpoor children.[21] Parental income and education have also been shown to be related to the surface areas of the frontal, temporal, and parietal cortices of children, and these findings are strongest in those living below the federal poverty level.[22] Early childhood adversity and toxic stress is also more likely to be experienced by children growing up in poverty, and therefore, the disruption of brain architecture associated with toxic stress is another feature of poor children's development.[23] Other studies have documented increased cortisol levels in children living in poverty, with higher levels related to the duration of the poverty. A 2016 AAP technical report on the adverse effects of child poverty delineates these and other mediators of the negative effects of poverty on child development, behavior, mental health, and academic performance.[24]

In summary, children living in poverty receive fewer resources and less environmental stimulation for the normal progression of the child's cognitive, language, and social-emotional development, as well as school readiness/academic achievement. Children living in poverty also experience a high level of stress that is toxic to their brain's development and behavior. To a large degree, especially for young children, these impacts are mediated by parenting. Parenting may be less nurturing and positive in many poor households due to increased parenting stress related to low income and material hardship. For older children and adolescents, exposure to neighborhoods with concentrated poverty and inferior schools further worsens their outcomes.

Interventions to ameliorate the impact of poverty on children, as well as to decrease the number of children in poverty, as outlined in the AAP policy statement on poverty and child health,[25] include both advocacy for maintaining and strengthening government supports for poor families (eg, the Earned Income Tax Credit, the Supplemental Nutrition Assistance Program, and maternal-child home visiting programs), and screening and referral in the pediatric medical home for child developmental, behavioral, and mental health problems as well as for maternal depression. Importantly, the AAP also recommends screening and referral for risk factors for material hardship (often referred to as the social determinants of health) and supports early literacy and positive parenting programs integrated into the pediatric medical home.[25]

Parental Depression/Substance Abuse/Mental Health Issues and Family Systems

Behavioral health challenges are common in American families. According to the National Institute of Mental Health, 6.7% of American adults experienced at least 1 major depressive episode of 2 weeks or longer in 2015.[26] This figure is even higher in new mothers. According to the Centers for Disease Control and Prevention (CDC), in 2012, 11.5% of US mothers giving birth reported having postpartum depression (PPD) symptoms. Factors associated with the highest rates of PPD symptoms were: (1) being a teenage mother; (2) being of Native American or Asian Pacific Islander race/ethnicity; (3) having ≤12 years of education; (4) being unmarried; (5) being a smoker; (6) having experienced ≥3 life stresses in the year before birth; (7) giving birth to a low birth weight term infant or to multiple births (eg, twins, triplets); and (8) having an infant who required neonatal intensive care.[27]

Many studies have documented a higher prevalence of psychiatric disorders in children of depressed than in those of nondepressed parents. The risk for psychiatric disorders may be particularly high in children of low-income depressed mothers.[28] Exposure to both intimate partner violence and depression before age 3 years is associated with preschool-aged onset of attention-deficit/hyperactivity disorder (ADHD), and early exposure to parental depression is associated with preschoolers being prescribed psychotropic medication.[29] A 30-year study of 2 generations of individuals at high versus low risk for depression found that the biological offspring with 2 previous generations affected with major depression were at highest risk for major depression.[30]

Prospective research has shown that lower income and lower maternal education are associated with more behavioral concerns in children. Adjustment for maternal smoking, depressive symptoms, and alcohol use have been shown to attenuate the associations between socioeconomic status and child behavior problems by 25% to 50%.[31] This effect may be mediated through family functioning, maternal sensitivity and differential sensitivity to social adversities within populations of children, and it may be guided by epigenetic mechanisms.[32,33] This work also demonstrates that social disparities in women's health conditions may help shape the likelihood of behavior problems in subsequent generations. Improved public health services for disadvantaged women across the life course may address their own health needs and thereby reduce social disparities in the well-being and health of their children.

The prevalence of behavioral or emotional disorders in American children is 11% to 20%.[34] Developmental and behavioral disorders are now the top 5 chronic conditions causing functional impairment in children.[35] However, the ability of pediatric health care professionals to identify developmental-behavioral problems in primary care, on the basis of clinical judgment alone without the aid of a standardized measure, has low sensitivity (14% to 54%).[36]

Primary pediatric health care professionals play a key role in performing ongoing surveillance of families with these known sociodemographic risk factors and in referring for early intervention and resources to mitigate long-term sequelae. The AAP has clinical reports on incorporating postpartum depression screening into pediatric practice and on promoting optimal development through implementation of behavioral and emotional screening in practice.[12, 34] These reports outline how pediatric practices, as medical homes, can establish systems and overcome barriers so that they can implement behavioral, emotional, and postpartum depression screening. They also help practices identify community resources for the treatment of depressed mothers, support parent-child relationships, and address the social-emotional needs of children.[12,34] The Centers for Medicare & Medicaid Services have recently recognized the importance of this type of screening by allowing state Medicaid agencies to cover maternal depression screening as part of well-child visits. States must also cover any medically necessary treatment for the child as part of their Early and Periodic Screening, Diagnosis, and Treatment (EPSDT) benefit. In addition to covering this screening for Medicaid-eligible mothers, states may cover maternal depression screening for non-Medicaid-eligible mothers during well-child visits. States may also cover treatment for the mother when both the child and the mother are present, when treatment focuses on the effects of the mother's condition on the child, and when services are provided for the direct benefit of the child.[37]

Foster Care and Adoption

The research on ACEs demonstrates that child abuse and neglect can have a profound impact on the development of a child. When children are removed from their homes due to abuse or neglect, it is important to realize that this placement can potentially be another negative stressor for the child. Children are often separated from family, friends, neighborhoods, and schools. Half of foster children experience more than 1 foster care placement. Plans for reunification or adoption are often uncertain with no clear timeline in place. These stresses can all affect a child's behavior and development.[38]

Children in foster care have higher rates of mental health issues, developmental delays, and learning problems compared to peers. Up to 25% of young children in foster care have a developmental delay, up to 25% of teenagers in foster care have posttraumatic stress disorder, and 80% of adolescents aging out of the foster care system have a mental health diagnosis.[9] Over 40% of foster children receive special education services, and their rates of acute and chronic illness are also increased.[38]

Central to a child's social and emotional development is his or her ability to form a secure attachment to a stable, caring, responsive adult. The presence of a stable adult who provides unconditional love and acceptance is critical to helping a child overcome past abuse and neglect. The age and developmental level of a child at foster placement, as well as the quality of care he or she receives, will contribute to the emotional consequences of abuse and placement. Multiple foster care placements can further disrupt a child's ability to form secure attachments.[39]

The primary pediatric health care professional should keep in mind the effects that foster care placement have on a child and provide supports to both the child and the child's foster parents. By educating foster and adoptive parents about the effects of toxic stress on a child's learning, behavior, and health, the professional can encourage understanding of maladaptive and frustrating behaviors. A child may benefit from referral to trauma- informed counseling services, such as Parent-Child Interaction Therapy or Trauma Focused Cognitive Behavioral Therapy.[9]

Cultural and Community Factors

Cultural diversity in children and families is reflected in their traditions, languages, customs, beliefs, health practices, and social interactions.[40,41] This diversity exists within our communities, though communities may differ in other ways as well. For example, they can also vary in socioeconomic status, health status, academic attainment, and ethnic diversity. These differences have the potential to lead to a multitude of advantages or disadvantages and can result in disparities in child health and well-being. Communities with strong cultural bonds can also exhibit strong social capital, providing individuals with connections to their neighbors, supportive social networks, and a sense of trust and safety.[41] Strong communities may also provide a child with protective opportunities and resources, including libraries and parks, social networks, religious establishments, quality schools, and quality child care. However, for families that must frequently relocate due to economic strife, this sense of community and the social support it provides is relatively nonexistent.

Quality schools can provide children with supportive adult and peer relationships, predictable structure, a consistent environment, and a safe atmosphere that promotes self-expression.[42] They have been shown to improve children's social behavior, thereby decreasing rates of future criminal activity.[41] Quality early childhood education and child care programs improve children's cognitive and social-emotional development and long-term academic achievement. They result in increased earning and tax revenues, decreased reliance on social services, improved health behaviors and outcomes, and a more skilled workforce, with increased earnings and productivity potentially stopping the cycle of poverty.[43]

Sadly, violence is a widespread cultural influence on child development across the world today. Children experience acts of violence in the form of war, terrorism, unsafe neighborhoods, and abuse within the household.[42] As a result, children can lose their sense of trust and may become insecure, withdrawn, depressed, or anxious. Others externalize and act out with disruptive behaviors, irritability, and participation in risky behaviors.[41] Thus, the opportunity to develop positive relationships and social skills is thwarted. Exposure to violence can also lead to more physical symptoms, including loss of appetite, weight loss, poor growth, and fatigue due to sleep disturbance.[41] Indeed, those exposed to violence as children are likely to have adverse health outcomes of all kinds by adulthood.[44]

With the advent of screen-based technology (television, movies, video games, computers, tablets, smartphones, and the Internet) and its increasing availability, many children are spending hours a day with possible exposure to violence and sexual or other inappropriate content. A multitude of large studies demonstrate a correlation between excessive screen time and negative social-emotional development, decreased sleep, obesity, aggression, and academic underachievement in children.[41] Increased screen time is typically associated with less time for physical activity, for making friends or interacting with family, for development of academic skills, and for reading and creative play. However, some recent evidence has shown that limited use of interactive educational and prosocial programs, especially when viewed and discussed with caring adults, can be associated with improved cognitive, literacy, and social development in young children.[45] The AAP has developed a toolkit aimed at helping families and providers understand and communicate the impact of media on children's lives. It also provides tips on managing time spent with various media types by children of all ages by developing media plans.[46]

Cultural and community factors are key elements of the social determinants of health that impact child health and well-being from birth onward. In order to successfully care for children and their families, pediatric health care professionals must keep all aspects of these environmental factors in mind. The more we understand the delicate balance and intricate meshwork that these factors add to the equation, the more we will be able to recognize and implement effective ways to improve child development and behavior.

Prenatal and Postnatal Environmental Exposures

In addition to the psychosocial and cultural aspects of the environment that influence brain development, it is also important to note the effect of other environmental exposures on child development and behavior. There are multiple prenatal (eg, maternal malnutrition; congenital infections; prenatal exposure to cigarette smoke, alcohol, recreational drugs, or prescription medications) and postnatal (eg, malnutrition; meningoencephalitis; postnatal exposure to secondhand smoke, heavy metals, pesticides, or nonpesticide organic pollutants; exposure to cancer chemotherapy or radiation) environmental exposures that can also influence child development and behavior. These exposures have been shown to cause neuronal apoptosis, alter neuronal proliferation and migration, interfere with synaptogenesis, synaptic pruning, and myelination, and alter the methylation pattern of the epigenome.[47] It is also important to note that children at highest risk for ACEs and toxic stress are in double jeopardy, as they are also often at the highest risk for exposure to these environmental toxicants.

Potential Resilience Factors That Can Buffer Adversity

Though a great many environmental factors can contribute to adverse outcomes, some children are able to mitigate these effects through a trait called resilience. Resilience has been an area of research for many years. It is universally defined as one's ability to successfully adapt, positively transform, and return to baseline despite surrounding stressors and adversity. Resilient children "work well, play well, love well, and expect well."[48] Although the capacity for resilience is believed to be innate, its maturation may either be nurtured or hindered by various environmental factors.

What exactly are resilient qualities? Primarily 5 key characteristics have been described: social competence, problem-solving skills, critical consciousness, autonomy, and sense of meaning or purpose.[48,49]

Social competence encompasses the ability to obtain positive responses from others, to adapt, to empathize, to effectively communicate, and to develop a sense of humor. A sense of humor allows children to laugh at themselves or situations and view things from a different perspective. As a whole, this describes prosocial behavior, which leads to the development of positive relationships, including early friendships.[48,49]

Problem-solving skills allow one to plan and to be resourceful. Children with good problem-solving skills can think critically, abstractly, reflectively, and flexibly. These children can then formulate various solutions in both social and cognitive contexts.

This leads to perhaps the most pivotal skill, critical consciousness, or the awareness of surrounding oppression and the creation of ways to overcome it.[48,49]

Autonomy is a reflection of a strong sense of self-identity. This allows the child to think and act independently. Autonomous children may adaptively distance or separate themselves from a dysfunctional environment. As a result, they can develop internal control, a sense of task mastery, and a sense of self-efficacy.[48,49]

A **sense of meaning or purpose** creates belief in a positive future. This is provided through goals, educational aspirations, motivation, persistence, hopefulness, optimism, and spiritual connectedness. A sense of purpose is believed to be a major predictor of positive outcome. Children with a strong sense of purpose focus on fulfilling future gratification rather than the immediate gratification provided by risky behaviors.

So how does a child develop these resilient qualities? Positive influences that buffer a child's risk are deemed as "protective factors." Some protective factors are naturally acquired such as good health, being female, and having an easy temperament.[50] Other protective factors are found within the child's environment provided through his or her family, school, and community. Protective factors fall into 3 common themes: caring and supportive relationships, positive and high expectations, and meaningful participation.[48,49,51] An overlay of these protective factors at critical points in a child's development both spark and maintain the qualities needed for lifelong resilience.

A stable, loving and affectionate relationship, even if from only 1 parent, is the most critical protective familial factor. This relationship initiates and fuels a child's sense of basic trust, which is a critical early component of human development and attachment. Additionally, a child with a parent who sets high expectations and provides reasonable structure, discipline, household responsibilities, and rules achieves greater academic success with fewer behavioral problems.[48,49] Other familial protective factors include a smaller family unit, older maternal age, 2-parent families, stimulating home environments, stable parental employment, adequate income, and adequate housing.[50]

Community protective factors mirror those of the family. Most important is an adult role model or mentor who provides a consistent, positive adult relationship. Peer acceptance and positive relationships are also important sources of social support for children. These external relationships are particularly key because they may be able to mitigate any deficits in nurturing caregiver relationships within the home.[48,49] Other protective community factors include access to social networks and resources, supportive after-school programs, safe neighborhoods, access to quality health care, and access to quality child care and schools. Quality child care and after-school programs allow parents to maintain employment, and this in turn stabilizes their income.[50]

Consistent availability of these protective factors is the key to a child's success in the face of trauma or adversity. The daunting number of adversities described in this chapter that affect children all over the world on a daily basis cannot, unfortunately, be quickly eradicated or erased. However, as challenging as these difficulties may seem, they can often be offset by protective factors. Therefore, effective preventive measures and trauma informed interventions must be identified and implemented in order to mitigate the deleterious long-term consequences that childhood adversities can lead to across the life course.

The AAP has defined resilience as "the process by which the child moves through a traumatic event, utilizing various protective factors for support, and returning to 'baseline' in terms of an emotional and physiologic response to the stressor."[52] In partnership with the Center for the Study of Social Policy, the AAP has adopted the Strengthening Families Approach.[52] This defines the pediatric health care professional's role in strengthening each of 5 protective factors in partnership with families: parental resilience, knowledge of parenting and child development, social connections, concrete support in times of need, and children's social and emotional competence. It provides action steps for supporting families and responding to trauma, as well as information about how pediatricians are addressing this work across the United States.[53]

Evidence-based Interventions to Address Lack of Optimal Environmental Stimulation

It can be discouraging to read about how many negative environmental factors can influence a child's development, behavior, and life course trajectory. Though the problems faced by many children are complex, pediatric health care professionals should know what kind of guidance they can provide to help address the lack of optimal environmental stimulation. Evidence-based interventions are available to help enhance early childhood development, and pediatric health care professionals should take steps to make themselves aware of such interventions. In addition, the science informing these interventions is applicable to all young children and families. Interventions reflecting these principles should be integrated into pediatric preventive care and health promotion utilizing a public health approach.

Reach Out and Read

It is widely known that reading with young children promotes early language development and early literacy skills. In 2014, the AAP issued a policy statement expressing that literacy promotion is an essential component of primary care.[54] Reach Out and Read is an evidence-based program that promotes literacy during pediatric visits. Physicians and other staff are trained to speak with parents about the importance of reading out loud to their child, and each child is provided with a book at well-child visits from 6 months to 5 years of age. There are now more than 5,000 Reach Out and Read sites nationwide, serving 4.7 million children annually. Numerous studies conducted on the Reach Out and Read model have shown that children who participate in Reach Out and Read have higher receptive and expressive language scores. Studies have also shown that parents read more frequently to their children and are more likely to report reading as an enjoyable activity than parents of children not involved in Reach Out and Read.[55] Most of these intervention studies have been conducted with children at risk due to economic disadvantage. However, data supporting the conclusion that children read to early are more ready for school at kindergarten entry is universal. The real power of this intervention may be due to its starting in a parent's lap, and so, in addition to fostering a love of books and reading, it can also nurture the parent-child relationship. The most recent AAP policy on pediatric literacy promotion recommends that parents begin reading together with their infants as soon after birth as is feasible.[54]

High-Quality Early Education and Child Care

Participation in high-quality, early childhood programs has great potential to positively affect the development of a child, including his or her social, emotional, and cognitive development. Primary pediatric health care professionals can help educate families about the importance and availability of these high-quality programs.[56] Since its start in 1965 as part of President Lyndon B. Johnson's War on Poverty legislation, Head Start programs have provided services to more than 32 million low-income children. This federally funded preschool program promotes school readiness and also provides health and social services. Head Start programs positively impact children's development through their experiences in high-quality, early childhood education.[57]

Research has shown the substantive benefit of high-quality preschool programs. Such research includes the High/Scope Perry Preschool Study, in which 128 low-income, African American children from 1962 to 1967 in Ypsilanti, Michigan, were randomized to receive either a high-quality 2-year preschool program or no preschool. The preschoolers were taught by teachers with bachelor's degrees, there was a low student-to-teacher ratio, and teachers also provided weekly home visits. Follow-up of study participants has now been completed through age 40 years, showing positive benefits over the lifespan. Individuals who received the preschool program had higher scores on school achievement and literacy tests, were more likely to graduate from high school, were more likely to be employed, had higher income, and were less likely to be arrested than those who did not receive this high-quality, early education program.[58]

The Abecedarian program was a prospective randomized trial, conducted from 1972 through 1977, in which 111 infants from high-risk families in North Carolina were randomized to either the treatment or control group. In the treatment group, the children attended a full-time, high-quality child care center starting at an average age of 4.4 months and continued for 5 years. Children in the control group received a variety of care options, including parental care and other child care centers. These children have also been followed into adulthood. Children in the treatment group had better academic performance and were more likely to enroll in college. They also had higher IQ scores, and this gain in cognitive scores persisted into adulthood, though both groups saw a progressive decline in scores after early childhood.[59] At follow-up at age 30 years, adults from the treatment group were 4.6 times more likely to have earned college degrees.[60]

The Chicago Longitudinal Study followed children who were enrolled for preschool and kindergarten at federally funded Child-Parent Centers (CPC). A CPC expansion program provided services for grades 1 through 3. The CPC programs focused on comprehensive services, including nutrition and health, parent involvement, and literacy skills. Follow-up of preschool program participants at age 20 years showed improved high school graduation rates, less grade retention, lower rates of special education services, and lower rates of juvenile arrests than those not enrolled in the CPC programs.[61] Participation in the CPC expansion program showed greater benefit than participation in preschool/kindergarten alone, including higher reading achievement, decreased grade retention, and lower rates of special education services.[62]

Taken as a whole, these studies demonstrate the power of high-quality early childhood education with a community-building component to improve the life course of disadvantaged children. These data compelled Nobel laureate economist James Heckman and developmental-behavioral pediatrician Jack Shonkoff to write, "The most effective strategy for strengthening the future workforce, both economically and neurobiologically, and improving its quality of life is to invest in the environment of disadvantaged children during the early childhood years." In fact, they predicted a 15% return on investment for this intervention.[63]

Maternal and Child Home-Visiting Programs

Home-visiting programs provide voluntary, family-focused, and strength-based services to high-risk pregnant women and families with young children. These programs aim to address poverty and to support health and parenting.[64] The programs provide a variety of services, such as education regarding child development and information about healthy living and parenting skills. Since 2010, the Maternal, Infant, and Early Childhood Home Visiting Program (MIECHV) has been a federally funded, home-visiting program administered by the Department of Health and Human Services.[65] Funding is provided to states to focus on high-needs communities, such as those with high rates of child poverty, substance abuse, or child maltreatment. This funding supports a variety of home-visiting programs, including Early Head Start, Family Check-Up, Healthy Families America, Nurse Family Partnership, Healthy Steps, and Parents as Teachers.

Home-visiting programs are designed to improve outcomes in benchmark domains, such as child and maternal health, child development and school readiness, family economic self-sufficiency, and positive parenting practices. They have been found to reduce child maltreatment, to reduce family violence and crime, and to improve linkages and referrals to community resources.[66] Though the home-visiting programs have similar goals, how each program is designed and delivered differs. For example, Nurse Family Partnership enrolls at-risk, first-time young mothers before 28 weeks' gestation and supports them with regular nurse visits until their child is 2 years old, while Healthy Families America will work with families with more than 1 child. The AAP has supported home-visiting programs for some time and encourages pediatric health care professionals to become familiar with the home-visiting programs available in their areas and to refer families to these programs as early as possible.[65,67]

Positive Parenting Programs

Parents frequently turn to their primary pediatric health care professionals for advice on child-rearing and how to deal with troubling problem behaviors. For parents of children with behavioral diagnoses, such as oppositional defiant disorder or ADHD, even more questions can arise. It is helpful for the primary pediatric health care professionals to know that evidence-based parent training programs are available to help families build skills to successfully manage their children's behavior. Parent training programs draw upon family systems theory, social learning theory, and operant conditioning. The parent-child interaction is targeted, and parents are taught how to reinforce desirable behaviors in their children through the use of positive reinforcement, coaching, and other methods.[68] Evidence-based parent training programs available to families include The Incredible Years, Triple-P Positive Parenting Program, and Parent-Child Interaction Therapy.[69-71] These programs may be integrated into the pediatric medical home or may require referral.

The Incredible Years has programs available for parents, teachers, and children. The parent component is delivered in multiple sessions in a group format, led by a trained facilitator, and involves video vignettes, role-playing, discussion with other parents, and home practice. The Incredible Years uses a parenting pyramid where the foundation of parenting involves playing, listening, talking, providing positive attention, praise, and empathy, in order to first foster the parent-child relationship and promote the child's social-emotional health. Parents must first become comfortable with these positive parenting principles before moving up the pyramid and learning about rewards, limit setting, ignoring, redirections, and consequences. Only at the very top of the pyramid does one utilize time-out techniques and consequences.[72]

The Triple-P Positive Parenting program was developed in Australia and has been used in 25 countries and translated into 19 languages. Triple-P has a range of services from online courses to small groups. Specialized programs have also been developed for specific populations including children with disabilities and families going through divorce.

During another evidence-based program, Parent-Child Interaction Therapy, the therapist watches the parent and child interact from behind a mirrored glass. The therapist coaches the parent in specific parenting skills using a "bug in the ear."[71]

Research shows that these positive parent training programs result in a decrease in problem behaviors.[66,73,74] Despite the availability and research supporting these programs, most children with behavioral difficulties do not receive evidence-based care.[66] It is useful for primary pediatric health care professionals to become familiar with the programs available in their areas.

While these parenting programs address parenting in the context of identified child behavior problems or parent-child-interaction challenges, the Video Interaction Project (VIP) is designed to extend the Reach Out and Read model as a primary prevention intervention to improve and support parenting in poor and low-income families before problems arise. VIP is integrated into the pediatric primary care visit and has a considerable evidence base regarding positive results in improved parenting and enhanced child development. VIP starts at birth and includes an interaction with a child development specialist at scheduled well-child visits. The intervention, provided while the parent is waiting to see the pediatric health care professional, includes provision of toys and books, as well as a guided review of a videotaped interaction between the parent and child. The videotape review provides positive feedback for the parent's actions, discussion of the child's response, and suggestions for further parent-child interactions.[75,76]

The gold standard for addressing children's behavior challenges are these evidence-based programs promoting positive parenting. However, it is also important for pediatric health care professionals to be aware of more freely available programs that utilize the science behind these evidence-based positive parenting programs. Many of these are now Web based or available as free apps.

One example is **Text4baby.org,** which is a public-private partnership sponsored by the Health Resources and Services Administration and Johnson & Johnson, Inc. Mothers can enroll online at no cost during pregnancy or by entering their child's birthday, and they will receive weekly texts in English or Spanish with health-promoting information keyed to their gestation or their child's age. Text messages are free for those who have pay-as-you-go or prepaid cell phones from most major companies.

VROOM **(www.joinvroom.org)** is sponsored by the Bezos Family Foundation and has both a Web site and a free app that delivers child development promoting games to parents and caregivers that are keyed to the child's birth date. Each activity and tool briefly discusses the science behind each fun, brain-building moment. The curriculum was developed by an impressive cast of neuroscience and child development experts, is written in simple English, and also provides a brief rationale for each activity or baby game. The app also supplies badges as incentives for parent participation similar to the rewards provided to users of fitness apps. Child care providers are also encouraged to enroll in this messaging.

The early childhood advocacy group, Zero to Three **(www.zerotothree.org)** also has many free educational programs for caregivers of young children. These include videos, podcasts, and a free monthly electronic newsletter with information on ways to promote an infant's and toddler's development based on his or her age.

The CDC has a campaign called Learn the Signs. Act Early. **(www.cdc.gov/ncbddd/actearly/freematerials.html)** which provides a host of free materials for new parents. These include a Milestone Tracker app, a Milestones Moments booklet, a growth chart, developmental checklists, 2 children's books, and tips for parents about what to do when they have a concern, and how to talk with their doctor. Most materials are in English and Spanish, and some are also in Korean and Vietnamese.

Another important source of information on promoting healthy child development is the AAP Web site, **HealthyChildren.org**. This Web site was developed for parents and caregivers and aligns with all AAP policies and standards in the information provided. It links parents, caregivers, and child advocates to other AAP resources, including toolkits and advocacy resources.

Conclusion

The newborn's brain has 100 million neurons with 50 trillion synapses. During early childhood, these synapses proliferate, and those that are used are selectively strengthened while those connections that are neglected are pruned. This process continues into adolescence and young adulthood in the prefrontal cortex. A child's brain development is highly sensitive to environmental factors. Parenting is the first critical environmental factor influencing early brain and child development. By developing strong and nurturing relationships, parents foster secure attachment, as well as their child's healthy cognitive and social-emotional development. Parenting may be supported by intensive programs, such as maternal-child home visiting, or by positive parenting programs that are integrated into pediatric primary care or accessed through referral.

Quality child care and early education is the next level of environmental influence, which can promote school readiness. A child's community can also influence that child's development, behavior, and academic success. Strong communities exhibit strong social capital, as well as opportunities and resources that are both concrete and philosophical, supporting the child's developmental progress. Cultural traditions, customs, and beliefs, as well as exposure to screen-based technologies, can also impact a child's developmental trajectory.

Evidence informs us that environmental factors play a critical role in both child development and brain development. Early childhood adversity and toxic stress can be particularly harmful, causing disruption of the brain's developing architecture and resulting in negative impacts on memory, cognitive ability, self-regulation, and behavioral responses. These responses to toxic stress can lead to poor educational and health outcomes across the life course.

Poverty is a particularly potent, harmful influence on child development and behavior. This is driven by poverty's effect on parenting as well as on material hardship potentially threatening the ability of parents to meet their children's basic needs for food, clothing, and shelter. Related parenting stress can lead to decreased emotional availability of parents. Poor children are also more likely to experience a high level of stress that is toxic.

Placement in foster care, usually due to child abuse and neglect, is often psychologically traumatic for the child, as was the abuse or neglect leading to the placement. Rates of developmental and mental health diagnoses are extremely high in foster children, including posttraumatic stress disorder, developmental delays, and learning problems.

Foster children's experiences can lead to difficulties in forming secure attachments to adult caregivers, and multiple foster care placements further exacerbate this problem.

Resilience in the child may mitigate the impact of negative environmental factors. Resilience includes the key characteristics of social competence, problem-solving skills, critical consciousness of the surrounding environment, a sense of autonomy, and belief in a positive future. Although resilience is believed to be innate, its maturation may be either nurtured or hindered by environmental factors. Protective influences include caring and supportive relationships (most importantly with parents), parental high expectations and support of academic success, and community protective factors, such as strong social networks, safe neighborhoods, and high-quality child care, preschools, and schools.

Pediatricians and other pediatric health care professionals have a critically important role to play in optimizing environmental influences on child development and behavior. This role includes:

- Promoting positive parenting as part of the medical home through individual counseling, integrating parenting programs, and referring families to evidence-based programs and evidence-informed resources
- Screening for developmental and behavioral problems as well as material hardship and ensuring that families get the services they need
- Monitoring families for signs of parental stress, especially maternal depression, and looking for the early warning signs of child abuse and neglect
- Connecting families to high-quality child care and preschool and to maternal-child–home-visiting programs, if needed
- Advocating for funding of programs that ameliorate negative environmental influences on families
- Helping parents to understand the importance of the child's social-emotional development and work with families to provide the stable, loving, and nurturing environment that all children need to thrive

The policies, advocacy tools, and infrastructure of the AAP are readily available to all pediatric health care professionals to assist in this important work.

References

1. American Academy of Pediatrics. Early Brain and Child Development toolkit. American Academy of Pediatrics Web site. https://www.aap.org/ebcd. Published 2014. Accessed January 16, 2018
2. Center on the Developing Child. *The Science of Early Childhood Development*. (InBrief) Center on the Developing Child Web site. http://developingchild.harvard.edu/resources/inbrief-science-of-ecd/. Published 2007. Accessed January 16, 2018
3. Luby JL, Barch DM, Belden A, et al. Maternal support in early childhood predicts larger hippocampal volumes at school age. *Proc Natl Acad Sci U S A*. 2012;109(8):2854–2859
4. Shonkoff JP, Garner AS, American Academy of Pediatrics Committee on Psychosocial Aspects of Child and Family Health, Committee on Early Childhood, Adoption, and Dependent Care, and Section on Developmental and Behavioral Pediatrics. The lifelong effects of early childhood adversity and toxic stress. *Pediatrics*. 2012;129(1):e232–e246

5. Flores G, American Academy of Pediatrics Committee on Pediatric Research. Racial and ethnic disparities in the health and health care of children. *Pediatrics.* 2010;125(4):e979–e1020

6. Compas BE. Psychobiological processes of stress and coping: implications for resilience in children and adolescents—comments on the papers of Romeo & McEwen and Fisher et al. *Ann N Y Acad Sci.* 2006;1094:226–234

7. Gunnar M, Quevedo K. The neurobiology of stress and development. *Annu Rev Psychol.* 2007;58:145–173

8. McEwen BS. Physiology and neurobiology of stress and adaptation: central role of the brain. *Physiol Rev.* 2007;87(3):873–904

9. American Academy of Pediatrics. *Helping Foster and Adoptive Families Cope With Trauma: A Guide for Pediatricians.* American Academy of Pediatrics Web site. www.aap.org/traumaguide. Published 2016. Accessed January 16, 2018

10. Felitti VJ, Anda RF, Nordenberg D, et al. Relationship of childhood abuse and household dysfunction to many of the leading causes of death in adults. The Adverse Childhood Experiences (ACE) Study. *Am J Prev Med.* 1998;14(4):245–258

11. Garner AS, Shonkoff JP, American Academy of Pediatrics Committee on Psychosocial Aspects of Child and Family Health, Committee on Early Childhood, Adoption, and Dependent Care, Section on Developmental and Behavioral Pediatrics. Early childhood adversity, toxic stress, and the role of the pediatrician: translating developmental science into lifelong health. *Pediatrics.* 2012;129(1):e224–e231. Reaffirmed July 2016

12. Earls MF, American Academy of Pediatrics Committee on Psychosocial Aspects of Child and Family Health. Incorporating recognition and management of perinatal and postpartum depression into pediatric practice. *Pediatrics.* 2010;126(5):1032–1039. Reaffirmed December 2014

13. Centers for Disease Control and Prevention. The ACE Pyramid. Mechanisms by which adverse childhood experiences influence health and well-being throughout the lifespan. Centers for Disease Control and Prevention Web site. https://www.cdc.gov/violenceprevention/acestudy/about.html. Accessed January 16, 2018

14. Proctor BD, Semega JL, Kollar MA. *Income and Poverty in the United States: 2015.* Washington, DC: Government Printing Office; 2016

15. Gershoff ET, Aber JL, Raver CC, Lennon MC. Income is not enough: incorporating material hardship into models of income associations with parenting and child development. *Child Dev.* 2007;78(1):70–95

16. Yoshikawa H, Aber JL, Beardslee WR. The effects of poverty on the mental, emotional, and behavioral health of children and youth: implications for prevention. *Am Psychol.* 2012;67(4):272–284

17. Hart B, Risley TR. *Meaningful Differences in the Everyday Experience of Young American Children.* Baltimore, MD: Paul H. Brookes Publishing Co.; 1995

18. Bradbury B, Corak M, Waldfogel J, Washbrook E. *Too Many Children Left Behind: The U.S. Achievement Gap in Comparative Perspective.* New York, NY: Russell Sage Foundation; 2015

19. Heckman JJ. Skill formation and the economics of investing in disadvantaged children. *Science.* 2006;312(5782):1900–1902

20. Chaudry A, Wimer C. Poverty is not just an indicator: the relationship between income, poverty, and child well-being. *Acad Pediatr.* 2016;16(3 Suppl):S23–S29

21. Hair NL, Hanson JL, Wolfe BL, Pollak SD. Association of child poverty, brain development, and academic achievement. *JAMA Pediatr.* 2015;169(9):822–829

22. Noble KG, Houston SM, Brito NH, et al. Family income, parental education and brain structure in children and adolescents. *Nat Neurosci.* 2015;18(5):773–778

23. Blair C, Raver CC. Poverty, stress, and brain development: new directions for prevention and intervention. *Am Pediatr.* 2016;16(3 Suppl):S30–S36

24. Pascoe JM, Wood DL, Duffee JH, Kuo A, American Academy of Pediatrics Committee on Psychosocial Aspects of Child and Family Health, Council on Community Pediatrics. Mediators and adverse effects of child poverty in the United States. *Pediatrics.* 2016;137(4):e20160340

25. American Academy of Pediatrics Council on Community Pediatrics. Poverty and child health in the United States. *Pediatrics.* 2016;137(4):e20160339

26. National Institute of Mental Health. Major depression among adults. National Institutes of Health, National Institute of Mental Health Web site. https://www.nimh.nih.gov/health/statistics/prevalence/major-depression-among-adults.shtml. Accessed January 16, 2018

27. Ko JY, Rockhill KM, Tong VT, Morrow B, Farr SL. Trends in postpartum depressive symptoms—27 states, 2004, 2008, and 2012. *MMWR Morb Mortal Wkly Rep.* 2017;66(6):153–158

28. Feder A, Alonso A, Tang M, et al. Children of low-income depressed mothers: psychiatric disorders and social adjustment. *Depress Anxiety.* 2009;26(6):513–520

29. Bauer NS, Gilbert AL, Carroll AE, Downs SM. Associations of early exposure to intimate partner violence and parental depression with subsequent mental health outcomes. *JAMA Pediatr.* 2013;167(4):341–347

30. Weissman MM, Berry OO, Warner V, et al. A 30-year study of 3 generations at high risk and low risk for depression. *JAMA Psychiatry.* 2016;73(9):970–977

31. Kahn RS, Wilson K, Wise PH. Intergenerational health disparities: socioeconomic status, women's health conditions, and child behavior problems. *Public Health Rep.* 2005;120(4):399–408

32. Parade SH, Armstrong LM, Dickstein S, Seifer R. Family context moderates the association of maternal postpartum depression and stability of infant temperament. *Child Dev.* July 14 2017 doi: 10.1111/cdev.12895

33. Boyce WT. Epigenomic susceptibility to the social world: plausible paths to a "newest morbidity." *Acad Pediatr.* 2017;17(6):600–606

34. Weitzman C, Wegner L, American Academy of Pediatrics Section on Developmental and Behavioral Pediatrics, Committee on Psychosocial Aspects of Child and Family Health, Council on Early Childhood, Society for Developmental and Behavioral Pediatrics. Promoting optimal development: screening for behavioral and emotional problems. *Pediatrics.* 2015;135(2):384–395

35. Slomski A. Chronic mental health issues in children now loom larger than physical problems. *JAMA.* 2012;308(3):223–225

36. Sheldrick RC, Merchant S, Perrin EC. Identification of developmental-behavioral problems in primary care: a systematic review. *Pediatrics.* 2011;128(2):356–363

37. Wachino V. Maternal depression screening and treatment: a critical role for Medicaid in the care of mothers and children [Informational Bulletin]. https://www.medicaid.gov/federal-policy-guidance/downloads/cib051116.pdf. Published May 11, 2016. Accessed January 16, 2018

38. Forkey H, Szilagyi M. Foster care and healing from complex childhood trauma. *Pediatr Clin North Am.* 2014;61(5):1059–1072

39. American Academy of Pediatrics Committee on Early Childhood and Adoption and Dependent Care. Developmental issues for young children in foster care. *Pediatrics.* 2000;106(5):1145–1150

40. Chen X. Culture and early socio-emotional development. In: Tremblay RE, Boivin M, Peters RDeV, eds. *Encyclopedia on Early Childhood Development.* Centre of Excellence for Early Childhood Development and Strategic Knowledge Cluster on Early Child Development; 2009

41. Institute of Medicine. Children's health, the nation's wealth: assessing and improving child health. In: *Little Things Count: Evaluating Children's Health.* Washington, DC; Oxford: National Academies; Oxford Publicity Partnership; 2004:53–87

42. Seefeldt C, Castle S, Falconer RC. Factors affecting social development. In: *Social Studies for the Preschool/Primary Child.* Boston, MA: Pearson; 2014

43. Heckman J. *The Heckman Equation.* https://heckmanequation.org/the-heckman-equation/. Accessed January 16, 2018

44. Centers for Disease Control and Prevention. *Adverse Childhood Experiences (ACEs).* https://www.cdc.gov/violenceprevention/acestudy/. Accessed January 16, 2018

45. American Academy of Pediatrics Council on Communications and Media. Media and young minds. *Pediatrics.* 2016;138(5):e20162591

46. American Academy of Pediatrics. *Media and Children Communication Toolkit.* https://www.aap.org/en-us/advocacy-and-policy/aap-health-initiatives/pages/media-and-children.aspx. Accessed January 16, 2018

47. Lanphear BP. The impact of toxins on the developing brain. *Annu Rev Public Health.* 2015;36:211–230

48. Benard B. *Fostering Resiliency in Kids: Protective Factors in the Family, School, and Community.* Western Regional Center for Drug-Free Schools and Communities, Northwest Regional Educational Laboratory. Washington, DC: US Department of Education; August 1991

49. Benard B. *Fostering Resilience in Children.* ERIC Digest. ED 386327. Urbana, IL: ERIC Clearinghouse on Elementary and Early Childhood Education; 1995

50. Benzies K, Mychasiuk R. Fostering family resiliency: a review of the key protective factors. *Child Fam Soc Work.* 2009;14(1):103–114

51. Centers for Disease Control and Prevention. *Youth Violence: Risk and Protective Factors.* https://www.cdc.gov/violenceprevention/youthviolence/riskprotectivefactors.html. Page last updated June 23, 2017. Accessed January 16, 2018

52. American Academy of Pediatrics. *Promoting Resilience.* https://www.aap.org/en-us/advocacy-and-policy/aap-health-initiatives/resilience/Pages/Promoting-Resilience.aspx. Accessed January 16, 2018

53. Center for the Study of Social Policy, American Academy of Pediatrics. *Promoting Children's Health and Resiliency: A Strengthening Families Approach.* https://www.aap.org/en-us/Documents/resilience_messaging-at-the-intersections.pdf. Accessed January 16, 2018

54. American Academy of Pediatrics Council on Early Childhood. Literacy promotion: an essential component of primary care pediatric practice. *Pediatrics.* 2014;134(2):404–409

55. Zuckerman B. Promoting early literacy in pediatric practice: twenty years of Reach Out and Read. *Pediatrics.* 2009;124(6):1660–1665

56. American Academy of Pediatrics Committee on Early Childhood, Adoption, and Dependent Care. Quality early education and child care from birth to kindergarten. *Pediatrics.* 2005;115(1):187–191

57. US Department of Health and Human Services, Administration for Children and Families. *Head Start Impact Study Final Report: January 2010.* https://www.acf.hhs.gov/sites/default/files/opre/hs_impact_study_final.pdf. Accessed January 16, 2018

58. Schweinhart LJ. *The High/Scope Perry Preschool Study Through Age 40: Summary, Conclusions, and Frequently Asked Questions.* Ypsilanati, MI: High/Scopes Press; 2004. http://www.peelearlyyears.com/pdf/Research/INTERNATIONAL%20Early%20Years/Perry%20Project.pdf. Accessed January 16, 2018

59. Campbell F, Pungello E, Miller-Johnson S, Burchinal M, Ramey C. The development of cognitive and academic abilities: growth curves from an early childhood educational experiment. *Dev Psychol.* 2001;37(2):231–242

60. Campbell FA, Pungello EP, Burchinal M, et al. Adult outcomes as a function of an early childhood educational program: an Abecedarian Project follow-up. *Dev Psychol.* 2012;48(4):1033–1043

61. Reynolds AJ, Temple JA, Robertson DL, Mann EA. Long-term effects of an early childhood intervention on educational achievement and juvenile arrest: a 15-year follow-up of low-income children in public schools. *JAMA.* 2001;285(18):2339–2346

62. Reynolds A, Temple J. Extended early childhood intervention and school achievement: age thirteen findings from the Chicago longitudinal study. *Child Dev.* 1998;69(1):231–246

63. Knudsen EI, Heckman JJ, Cameron JL, Shonkoff JP. Economic, neurobiological, and behavioral perspectives on building America's future workforce. *Proc Natl Acad Sci USA* 2006;103(27):10155-10162

64. Minkovitz CS, O'Neill KMG, Duggan AK. Home visiting: a service strategy to reduce poverty and mitigate its consequences. *Acad Pediatr.* 2016;16(3 Suppl):S105–S111

65. Health Resources and Services Administration. *Maternal and Child Health.* https://mchb.hrsa.gov/maternal-child-health-initiatives/home-visiting-overview. Accessed January 16, 2018

66. Avellar S, Paulsell D, Sama-Miller E, Del Grosso P, Akers L, Kleinman R. *Home Visiting Evidence of Effectiveness Review: Executive Summary. January 2016.* Washington, DC: Office of Planning, Research and Evaluation, Administration for Children and Families, US Department of Health and Human Services; 2016

67. American Academy of Pediatrics Council on Child and Adolescent Health. The role of home-visitation programs in improving health outcomes for children and families. *Pediatrics.* 1998;101(3):486–489

68. Kaehler LA, Jacobs M, Jones DJ. Distilling common history and practice elements to inform dissemination: Hanf-Model BPT programs as an example. *Clin Child Fam Psychol Rev.* 2016;19(3):236–258

69. Leijten P, Gardner F, Landau S, et al. Research review: harnessing the power of individual participant data in a meta-analysis of the benefits and harms of the Incredible Years parenting program. *J Child Psychol Psychiatry.* 2017 July 11. doi:10.1111/jcpp.12781 [Epub ahead of print]

70. Sanders MR, Kirby JN, Tellegen CL, Day JJ. The Triple P-Positive Parenting Program: a systematic review and meta-analysis. *Clin Psychol Rev.* 2014 Jun;34(4):337–357

71. Thomas R, Abell B, Webb HJ, Avdagic E, Zimmer-Gembeck MJ. Parent-Child Interaction Therapy: a meta-analysis. *Pediatrics.* 2017:140(3):pii:e20170352

72. Webster-Stratton C. *The Incredible Years: A Trouble-Shooting Guide for Parents of Children Aged 3–8.* Toronto, Ontario, Canada: Umbrella Press; 2003

73. Menting AT, Orobio de Castro B, Matthys W. Effectiveness of the Incredible Years parent training to modify disruptive and prosocial child behavior: a meta-analytic review. *Clin Psychol Rev.* 2013;33(8):901–913

74. Barlow J, Stewart-Brown S. Behavior problems and group-based parent education programs. *J Dev Behav Pediatr.* 2000;21(5):356–370

75. Mendelsohn AL, Huberman HS, Berkule SB, Brockmeyer CA, Morrow LM, Dreyer BP. Primary care strategies for promoting parent-child interactions and school readiness in at-risk families: the Bellevue Project for Early Language, Literacy, and Education Success. *Arch Pediatr Adolesc Med.* 2011;165(1):33–41

76. Cates CB, Weisleder A, Mendelsohn AL. Mitigating the effects of family poverty on early child development through parenting interventions in primary care. *Acad Pediatr.* 2016;16(3 Suppl):S112–S120

CHAPTER 4

Biological Influences on Child Development and Behavior and Medical Evaluation of Children With Developmental-Behavioral Disorders

Austin A. Larson, MD

Ellen R. Elias, MD, FAAP, FACMG

Once a child has been identified as having a developmental-behavioral disorder, the initial evaluation will characterize the descriptive nature of the developmental disorder as well as attempt to determine the underlying etiology (see Chapter 11, Making Developmental-Behavioral Diagnoses). This chapter will discuss the primary pediatric health care professional's clinical evaluation including medical history, physical examination, and diagnostic medical testing with a focus on those aspects of the evaluation that may be most helpful in the determination of an etiological diagnosis underlying the descriptive developmental-behavioral disorder. Specific examples of disorders will be provided that best illustrate important concepts in the biological basis of disorders of development and behavior.

There are multiple reasons to diagnose the underlying etiology of a developmental-behavioral disorder rather than to simply characterize the descriptive nature of the disorder. The most important justification for determining an etiological diagnosis is to identify disorders that are treatable and for which timely intervention may improve the natural history of the disorder. Interventions may include pharmaceutical treatment, dietary modifications, or surveillance for known medical complications. Second, identification of a specific diagnosis may end the diagnostic odyssey, resolving detrimental uncertainty and anxiety for the family and preventing costly and invasive testing in the future. A specific diagnosis may also provide access to additional support services, to a community of similarly affected families, and to opportunities for participation in research. Third, medical professionals are likely to be able to provide a more accurate medical prognosis if the underlying etiology of the developmental disorder is known. Last, if a specific genetic etiology is identified, then genetic counseling can be provided to the family at risk for recurrence in future pregnancies within the nuclear or extended family.

Classical twin studies have shown that intelligence within the normal range is a heritable trait, likely as a function of the cumulative effect of many genetic variants that each have a small effect size. The focus of this chapter will not be the biological determinants of development and behavior that are prevalent in the population and of individually small effect size such as those identified using genome wide association studies in large cohorts.

Rather, the focus will be on those rare determinants of development that have a large effect size and that may be identifiable as a discrete etiological diagnosis with clinically available testing or careful history taking and physical examination.

History

Family History

Pedigree analysis is a well-established technique that can provide clues to the underlying etiology of developmental-behavioral disorders. A thorough analysis of the pedigree will include brief medical histories of the parents, siblings, grandparents, aunts, uncles, and cousins of the child being evaluated, as well as determination of the ethnic background of the family and a specific inquiry into whether the parents of the child are consanguineous. While consanguineous unions are rare in the United States, there are areas of the world in which recent shared ancestry of the two parents is the norm.[1] The presence of consanguinity would increase the likelihood that a developmental-behavioral disorder is the result of a recessive genetic condition. Similarly, even in the absence of consanguinity, if both parents are members of the same ethnic group, then the likelihood of recessive genetic disease is increased. Known founder effects in specific populations may allow the clinician to focus the diagnostic evaluation on those conditions. For example, the carrier status for Tay-Sachs, Canavan, and Niemann-Pick type A diseases are increased in the Ashkenazi Jewish population. There are multiple recessive genetic etiologies of developmental-behavioral disorders that are much more prevalent among the Amish and other endogamous religious communities. The absence of recent or remote shared ancestry between parents should not be considered reassuring against the possibility of a genetic diagnosis; it would simply moderately reduce the likelihood of a recessive genetic condition.

It is important to note that the specific presentation of a disorder may differ between a child with a specific developmental-behavioral disorder and previously affected generations in the family, a phenomenon known as variable expression. One relatively common genetic disorder that exemplifies variable expression is neurofibromatosis type 1 (NF1). While over 90% of those with NF1 will have the characteristic skin findings of café-au-lait macules and intertriginous freckling, about half will have learning disabilities and smaller percentages will have autism and intellectual disability.[2] This demonstrates the importance of a broad family history that addresses conditions beyond the realms of development and behavior.

Fragile X syndrome is another example of a condition with variable findings in the family history. In the case of fragile X, the unusual family history is due to genetic anticipation. The disorder is caused by an unstable trinucleotide repeat in the gene *FMR1*. The trinucleotide repeat may lengthen when inherited through the maternal germ line and result in more severe manifestations after the expansion, a circumstance called anticipation. Additionally, *FMR1* is on the X chromosome, meaning that males with a mutation are hemizygous (have only that allele of the gene) whereas females are

45

Chapter 4: Biological Influences on Child Development and Behavior and Medical Evaluation of
Children With Developmental-Behavioral Disorders

heterozygous (have a second normal allele of the gene). Thus, a boy with significant developmental delay due to *FMR1* trinucleotide repeat expansion may have a mother with premature ovarian insufficiency but normal cognition due to a smaller repeat expansion in the gene (a premutation). Male and female premutation carriers (eg the maternal grandfather) may develop the fragile X–associated tremor and ataxia syndrome (FXTAS), an adult-onset movement disorder that does not manifest with developmental delays in childhood.[3] For male patients with developmental delay, specific inquiry about the health and development of the maternal uncles and great-uncles is indicated to assess for fragile X and other causes of X-linked intellectual disability. For fragile X, like NF1, a family history of conditions other than atypical behavior and development may provide clues to the etiological diagnosis for the patient.

Families affected by mitochondrial disorders may also have pedigrees with distinctive characteristics. Mitochondrial DNA (mtDNA) is inherited exclusively from the mother, and specific attention to the health history of matrilineal relatives may reveal indications of mtDNA-mediated disease. Rather than the typical two copies of each gene encoded by nuclear DNA that are present, each cell will typically have thousands of copies of mtDNA. Mutations in mtDNA are not homozygous or heterozygous, but rather are present at levels of heteroplasmy that vary from zero to 100% (known as homoplasmy). The levels of heteroplasmy may vary between different tissues in the body and may change dramatically from generation to generation. A child presenting with developmental delay due to mitochondrial encephalomyopathy, lactic acidosis and stroke-like episodes (MELAS) due to high levels of heteroplasmy for the m.3243A>G mutation in mtDNA may have matrilineal relatives with normal development but who are affected by diabetes, hearing loss, or migraine headaches due to lower levels of heteroplasmy for the same mutation.[4]

The absence of a significant family history of illness should not be considered reassuring against the possibility of a genetic disease being the etiology of the developmental-behavioral disorder. Most patients with a recessively inherited condition will not have any affected family members, especially outside of endogamous communities. With extensive use of whole exome trio testing in recent years, it has become apparent that a significant proportion of genetic disease results from *de novo* mutations in the child being studied (proband) and not inherited mutations.

Conception

Specific questions about the conception of a child presenting with developmental delay may provide important information about an etiological diagnosis. A history of multiple miscarriages for the child's mother may indicate that she or her partner could be a carrier for a balanced chromosomal translocation. Such chromosomal anomalies are present in about 5% of couples with recurrent miscarriages.[5] A balanced translocation typically results in a normal gene complement and normal development for that individual. However, the chromosomes may become imbalanced in the germ cells, and the resulting conceptus may not be viable or may result in a child with gene dosage abnormalities that cause developmental delay. Recurrent miscarriage could also indicate the presence of a thrombophilic disorder for the mother. Thrombophilic disorders in either the mother or the fetus are a risk factor for ischemic stroke in the perinatal period that may lead to developmental delays.[6]

Use of assisted reproductive techniques such as in vitro fertilization (IVF) is not thought to result in significantly increased levels of developmental-behavioral disorders overall. However, there is likely an increased risk of disorders resulting from abnormal imprinting of DNA.[7] Imprinting is the process of altering DNA methylation and other epigenetic factors that govern the expression of genes. A relevant example of an epigenetic disorder is Angelman syndrome, which results in severe developmental delay due to DNA methylation abnormalities that prevent expression of the maternal allele of the gene *UBE3A*. Children with Angelman syndrome have a characteristically happy demeanor with frequent laughing and smiling. Ataxia and tremulousness are prominent and epilepsy is frequently present.

Gestation

The fetal environment is a critical determinant of the future health and development of a child. The presence of diabetes in the mother during gestation increases the risk for structural brain anomalies and other malformations, and it also appears to more subtly impair development for those children born to mothers with diabetes.[8,9] Maternal undernutrition resulting in a small-for-gestational-age child is also clearly correlated with poorer developmental outcomes.[10]

Maternal use of recreational drugs during gestation is linked to abnormal development in the child. Maternal alcohol use may result in a broad spectrum of manifestations from mild behavioral concerns to children with severe growth restriction and multiple congenital anomalies, depending on the quantity of alcohol consumption and the timing in gestation.[11] Evaluation of the effects of gestational exposure to cocaine, marijuana, opiates, and other drugs of abuse is ongoing, and a diverse range of behavioral, developmental, and morphological abnormalities have been linked to different agents.[12] In utero prescription drug exposure may also impact development and should be documented in a developmental history. The teratogenic effects of warfarin, phenytoin, valproate, retinoic acid, and other prescription drugs are well recognized and may have characteristic findings on physical examination.

Prenatal infections can significantly alter the developmental trajectory of a child. Vaccination of the population against varicella and rubella has reduced the number of fetuses exposed to these infections, though prenatal cytomegalovirus (CMV) infection remains a major cause of developmental delays in children. Roughly 1 in 150 children will have congenital CMV infection, and about 10% of infected infants will have clinical manifestations of the infection. Developmental delays are present in about two-thirds of the affected children, hearing loss in one-third, and visual impairment in about one-third.[13] Recently, prenatal Zika virus infection has been associated with microcephaly and developmental delays in affected children. The ultimate burden on the population of this newly recognized congenital infection remains to be seen.[14]

47

Chapter 4: Biological Influences on Child Development and Behavior and Medical Evaluation of Children With Developmental-Behavioral Disorders

In some rare cases, maternal medical concerns during pregnancy may be an indication that the fetus is affected by a specific disorder. For example, acute fatty liver of pregnancy is far more common among women carrying a fetus affected by long chain 3-hydroxyacyl-CoA dehydrogenase deficiency (LCHAD), a fatty acid oxidation disorder.

The Perinatal Period

The majority of parents can report the birth weights and gestational ages of their children to clinicians, and many are aware of the Apgar scores that their children were assigned at delivery. These readily available pieces of data are a critical component of a developmental history. There is extensive literature on the developmental outcomes of children born prematurely, with more significant developmental delays in those children born earlier in gestation and at lower birth weight.[15] Children born prematurely are at significantly higher risk for abnormalities on neuroimaging (such as hydrocephalus or periventricular leukomalacia) as well as other conditions associated with prematurity such as chronic lung disease.[16] While there are likely many causes of adverse developmental outcomes among premature infants, recent research has found that there are characteristic epigenetic alterations associated with premature birth, raising the possibility that there are persistent abnormalities of gene expression throughout life.[17] It should be noted that advances in the care of premature infants mean that developmental outcomes after premature birth are improving with time and that current premature infants likely have a better prognosis than infants born with the same degree of prematurity in previous decades. The literature on development after premature birth should be interpreted through this lens.

Apgar scoring, a systematic tool for assessing the status and response to resuscitation of neonates in the minutes after delivery, has been in use for decades, and lower Apgar scores at 5 minutes or longer have been consistently correlated with increased relative risk for poorer developmental outcomes later in life.[18] However, most infants with low Apgar scores will not develop neurodevelopmental disability.[18] The Apgar score is only one component of an assessment that an encephalopathic neonate has suffered a hypoxic-ischemic injury in the peripartum period. Laboratory testing for multisystem organ dysfunction, electroencephalography, and brain imaging should be employed when hypoxic injury is suspected, and it has prognostic significance for developmental outcomes; for example, normal brain MRI scans convey a better prognosis and deep gray matter injury conveys a worse prognosis than injury limited to the cortex.[19] Therapeutic hypothermia and high-dose erythropoietin appear to significantly improve the prognosis after perinatal hypoxic-ischemic brain injury, and the specific interventions that were employed in the neonatal period should also be documented if possible.[20]

Medical History

Children with chronic medical conditions are known to be at risk for developmental delays. Congenital heart disease is a common condition affecting nearly 1% of the population, with about 1 in 300 individuals requiring a surgical repair in childhood. The congenital heart malformation itself may be causative of developmental delay due to impaired cerebral blood flow and oxygen delivery. Alternatively, many common genetic syndromes have both congenital heart disease and developmental delays as manifestations, including Down syndrome, Turner syndrome, Noonan syndrome, Williams syndrome, and the 22q11 deletion syndrome. Guidelines have been developed for appropriate developmental screening and interventions for children with congenital heart disease.[21] Other chronic illnesses also impact development, such as the developmental delays seen in survivors of childhood cancers due to the effects of chemotherapy and radiation of the brain.[22] Sickle cell disease is the most prevalent genetic disease in the African American population of the United States. Affected individuals may suffer cerebral infarctions that cause developmental delays.[23]

Acute illnesses and accidents also have developmental consequences. Infections of the central nervous system, such as herpes simplex encephalitis or group B strep meningitis, result in developmental disorders in a significant proportion of affected children.[24] Traumatic brain injuries due to traffic accidents, falls, or abuse are a common occurrence for children, affecting up to 3% of all children. More severe acute brain injuries are associated with a larger impact on cognition later in life, with persistent developmental delays noted many years after initial injuries.[25]

Dietary and Nutritional History

Inquiry into the diet of a child with developmental delays may provide important clues to the etiology of the disorder and potential treatment. Children with autism spectrum disorder may have very restrictive diets, resulting in micronutrient deficiencies that have secondary consequences for development and for general health. Malnutrition resulting in stunted growth has a clear impact on developmental outcome, and primary pediatric health care professionals should ask about the food security of a family if there are growth concerns. Causality may also run in the opposite direction: Developmental disorders may significantly impair the nutritional status of a child in the case of neurological dysfunction resulting in
aspiration or dysphagia.[26]

Specific dietary patterns could be indicative of an inborn error of metabolism. Ornithine carbamoyltransferase (OCT) deficiency is a disorder of the urea cycle resulting in hyperammonemia. There is a wide spectrum of severity for this disorder, from fatal neonatal encephalopathy to individuals that remain asymptomatic into adulthood. This is particularly true for females because the causative gene is on the X chromosome, so females with a mutation are mosaic for one functional copy of the gene. Some individuals with OCT deficiency may have chronic mild hyperammonemia resulting in developmental delays without overt episodes of significant encephalopathy. A characteristic dietary history in an individual with OCT deficiency is either avoidance of dietary protein sources, such as meat, or transient mild encephalopathy after protein intake.[27]

49

Chapter 4: Biological Influences on Child Development and Behavior and Medical Evaluation of
Children With Developmental-Behavioral Disorders

Developmental Trajectory

In addition to documentation of the current level of development, attention should be
paid to the skills of a patient relative to the typically developing child throughout the
lifespan via a comprehensive developmental history (see Chapter 10, Developmental
Evaluation). Determining the developmental trajectory can be an important diagnostic
clue in determining an etiological diagnosis. A child with a developmental quotient of
50 through infancy and childhood would have a different set of diagnostic considerations
than a child with typical development followed by a plateau in skills and subsequent
developmental regression. The age of onset, speed of progression, and developmental
domains most affected by regression may be characteristic of specific diagnoses.

Many boys with X-linked adrenoleukodystrophy (X-ALD; a disorder of peroxisomal fatty
acid metabolism) will have typical development for the first several years of life followed
by subtle behavioral concerns and then by relatively rapid cognitive decline and fatal
progressive demyelinating neurodegenerative disease. If recognized early in the course
of the disease, bone marrow transplantation will halt the progression of the demyelinating process. Many boys will have a family history of adrenomyeloneuropathy (AMN)
in male and female relatives. AMN is an adult-onset progressive disease of the spinal
cord resulting in spasticity, abnormal gait, paresthesias, and bowel and bladder dysfunction. Other conditions that may present with typical development early in life followed
by behavioral concerns and subsequent progressive neurological signs and symptoms
include the lysosomal storage disorders Sanfilippo, Niemann-Pick C, and neuronal ceroid
lipofuscinosis.[28] Duchenne muscular dystrophy in boys is characterized by near normal
early gross motor development with plateauing and then progressive loss of strength
in childhood.

Mitochondrial diseases may result in stepwise developmental regression in the setting of
fasting or acute illnesses. Childhood-onset mitochondrial diseases that primarily affect
the central nervous system are referred to as Leigh syndrome, if the characteristic findings of bilateral basal ganglia or brainstem involvement are present on MRI of the brain.
Leigh syndrome may result from mutations in more than 75 different genes encoded by
nuclear DNA in addition to mutations of mtDNA.[29]

Rett syndrome is an X-linked dominant disorder that typically occurs due to *de novo*
mutations of the gene *MECP2*, which encodes a DNA-binding protein that alters the
expression of other genes important in neurological development. The typical developmental trajectory of females with Rett syndrome is one of apparently normal development over the first year of life, followed by rapid developmental regression, and then
followed by subsequent stability with severe developmental delays. Girls with Rett
syndrome may receive a diagnosis of autism and may have abnormal breathing
patterns, seizures, acquired microcephaly, and frequent hand-wringing movements.

In some cases, the finding that one developmental stream is significantly impaired out
of proportion to other areas may be a diagnostic clue. In the case of prominent gross
motor delay, a physician may consider diagnostic evaluation for spinal muscular atrophy

or muscular dystrophy. Inborn errors of metabolism affecting creatine synthesis and transport characteristically result in severe language delays disproportionate to delays in other areas of development.

Physical Examination

Growth Parameters

A universal and objective component of the medical developmental assessment is documentation of height, weight, and head circumference. Evaluation of the pattern of abnormalities noted on anthropomorphic measurements and their changes over time can guide providers to an etiological diagnosis.

A wide array of genetic etiologies of developmental delay may present with concomitant short stature, including Noonan syndrome. Noonan is one of the most prevalent genetic conditions in the population, present in up to 1 per 1,000 individuals. It results from heterozygous mutations in genes that disrupt the Ras intracellular signaling pathway, most commonly in the gene *PTPN11*. The mutations may be *de novo* but may also be inherited from an affected parent as an autosomal dominant trait with a 50% recurrence risk. Characteristic features of Noonan syndrome include short stature, characteristic facial features, mild developmental delays, as well as cardiomyopathy and valvular heart disease. Diagnosis of Noonan allows for a specific care plan to be enacted, including use of growth hormone, monitoring of heart disease, and assessment for associated bleeding diathesis.[30]

Several genetic disorders are associated with both tall stature and developmental delay. Klinefelter syndrome results from the presence of a 47,XXY chromosomal complement. Affected boys are likely to have language-based learning disabilities, small testes, and taller stature. Klinefelter is quite common, with up to 1 in 500 males affected.[31] Sotos syndrome results from heterozygous *de novo* mutations of the gene *NSD1*, which modifies histones to alter the transcription of other genes. Affected individuals typically have both tall stature and enlarged head circumference, as well as developmental delays and distinctive facial appearance.[32]

Enlarged head circumference (macrocephaly) may be present with both genetic and non-genetic etiologies of developmental delay. Hydrocephalus may be congenital or acquired, as in the case of premature infants with intraventricular hemorrhage. It may be isolated or associated with other anomalies, such as spinal dysraphisms. Fragile X syndrome, previously discussed, typically results in enlarged head circumference in affected males. Developmental regression in the setting of macrocephaly is seen in Alexander disease, which results from mutations in the gene *GFAP*, encoding a component of the cytoskeleton of neural cells. Up to 10% of patients with either developmental delay or autism and macrocephaly have mutations in the gene *PTEN*, which encodes a protein regulating cell growth and division.[33] A genetic diagnosis of children with *PTEN* mutations is of critical importance because of the high risk for breast, uterine, and thyroid cancers in individuals with *PTEN* mutations. Sequencing of this gene is indicated for all significantly macrocephalic patients with autism or developmental delay. If a *PTEN* mutation is found in the

51

Chapter 4: Biological Influences on Child Development and Behavior and Medical Evaluation of
Children With Developmental-Behavioral Disorders

child, parental testing is indicated, as an otherwise healthy, cognitively normal parent who possesses the same *PTEN* mutation has an increased cancer predisposition.

Microcephaly is a common finding among children with developmental delays and, like macrocephaly, may be either congenital or acquired. Microcephaly may be the sequela of a hypoxic or other injury in infancy. In that case, head circumference early in life is likely to be normal, with the circumference progressively dropping with respect to the average for age. This pattern of acquired microcephaly may also be seen in Rett syndrome. Patients with Angelman syndrome are also likely to have microcephaly. It is important to assess the head circumference in relation to height, as the relationship between the two percentiles may have diagnostic value. For example, patients with achondroplasia have both relative macrocephaly in comparison to height and absolute macrocephaly. Children with Sotos syndrome have tall stature and macrocephaly, whereas those with *PTEN* mutations have macrocephaly but typical stature.

Dysmorphology

Dysmorphology is the practice of identifying unusual physical features for the purpose of determining an etiological diagnosis. Standardized terminology has been developed for consistent description of features and is available at https://elementsofmorphology.nih.gov. The classic example of a syndrome with easily recognized dysmorphic features is Down syndrome. The characteristic features of Down syndrome are so well known that the clinical diagnosis is often made in the neonatal period, if it is not previously known due to prenatal testing. The exception may be the rare patients with mosaic trisomy 21, who have subtler dysmorphisms and less severe developmental delays. Dysmorphisms that are prevalent in Down syndrome include epicanthal folds, short palpebral fissures, midface hypoplasia, brachycephaly, short neck, single transverse palmar creases, and brachydactyly. The facial features of Noonan syndrome can also be quite characteristic, with ocular hypertelorism, ptosis, and low-set ears with posterior rotation in a patient with short stature (see Figure 4.1).

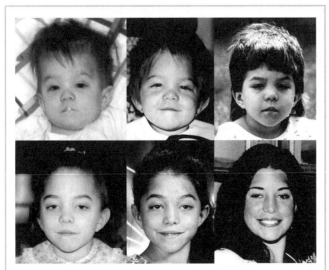

Figure 4.1. Characteristic facial features of Noonan syndrome in a patient at ages 4 months, 1, 2, 5, 9 and 21 years of age.

Reproduced with permission from Romano AA, Allanson JE, Dahlgren J, et al. Noonan syndrome: clinical features, diagnosis, and management guidelines. *Pediatrics*. 2010;126(4):746–759.

Assessment of the facial features is the typical starting point of a dysmorphology examination, but it is important to assess the morphology of the rest of the body as well. Smith-Lemli-Opitz syndrome is an inborn error of cholesterol metabolism resulting in developmental delays and dysmorphic features. Many patients may have ptosis, epicanthal folds, an upturned nose, microcephaly, and congenital heart defects, but less severely affected patients may lack these findings. Two characteristic dysmorphisms are often missed on examination: Affected males have abnormal genitals with hypospadias, cryptorchidism, or bifid scrotum, and most patients have syndactyly of the second and third toes. Without assessment of the morphology of the genitals and feet, the diagnosis may be missed.[34] Small testes may be the diagnostic finding on physical examination for Klinefelter syndrome, and macroorchidism may be noted in a postpubertal male with fragile X syndrome. The dysmorphology examination can play an important role in the decision regarding whether genetic testing is indicated for a patient with developmental delays. The yield of genetic testing is significantly higher for those patients with dysmorphic features.[35]

Neurological Examination

During the developmental assessment, the presence of abnormal findings on neurological examination can guide the medical evaluation. The presence of hypertonia and brisk reflexes indicates injury to the pyramidal tracts, as is often seen in cerebral palsy. Low muscle tone with age-appropriate cognitive skills should spur evaluation for spinal muscular atrophy and muscular dystrophies. Unlike some other muscular dystrophies, boys with Duchenne muscular dystrophy will typically have some speech and cognitive delays. Boys with this X-linked disorder typically come to medical attention due to mildly delayed early gross motor milestones. They will typically achieve ambulation, but they then become progressively weaker and lose the ability to ambulate by the early teens. Hypotonia can also be a feature of inborn errors of metabolism, including peroxisomal disorders and mitochondrial disorders.

Ataxia may be a prominent component of congenital disorders of glycosylation (CDGs), a group of inborn errors of metabolism resulting from dysfunctional incorporation of sugars onto proteins and fats. Other examination findings for the most common CDGs, caused by mutations in the gene *PMM2*, include hypotonia, developmental delay, internal strabismus, and subcutaneous lipodystrophy resulting in inverted nipples.[36] Dystonia or chorea indicate basal ganglia injury, as can be seen with some types of cerebral palsy, and it is also a common component of Leigh syndrome caused by mitochondrial disease.

Dermatological Examination

Careful assessment of the skin may reveal diagnostic clues in a patient with developmental delays. In Sturge-Weber syndrome, capillary malformations of the trigeminal distribution on the face indicate intracranial vascular malformations that can result in seizures and developmental delays. Sturge-Weber results from somatic mosaicism for a gain-of-function mutation of the growth-promoting gene *GNAQ* within the blood vessels. Findings of axillary freckling and café-au-lait macules may be diagnostic for

53

Chapter 4: Biological Influences on Child Development and Behavior and Medical Evaluation of Children With Developmental-Behavioral Disorders

neurofibromatosis type 1 (NF1). While IQ is typically normal in NF1, many patients have learning disabilities and may initially present for developmental assessment rather than for dermatological or other findings. Patients with tuberous sclerosis often have hypomelanotic macules of the skin that are more apparent using ultraviolet illumination (the Wood's lamp). They may also have angiofibromas of the face and nail beds. Autism, developmental delays, and epilepsy are all highly prevalent in patients with tuberous sclerosis.

Abdominal Examination

Assessment for hepatomegaly and splenomegaly are particularly important in children with developmental plateauing or regression. Many lysosomal storage disorders with developmental manifestations will also result in abdominal organomegaly. These include Gaucher disease, Niemann-Pick disease (types A/B and C), mucopolysaccharidoses (apart from Sanfilippo), and cholesterol ester storage disease. Patients with mucopolysaccharidosis I and II (Hunter and Hurler syndromes) have other distinctive physical examination features in addition to organomegaly. There is a characteristic facial appearance with macrocephaly, full lips, enlarged maxilla, and depressed nasal bridge. They also have skeletal abnormalities with the inability to extend the fingers fully and short stature.

Medical Evaluation

Newborn Screening

Newborn screening has been employed for many decades in the United States, and it has dramatically altered the natural history of some diseases. The specifics of the testing employed for the newborn screen differ slightly depending on the state in which a child is born, and these have changed significantly over time. Most (but not all) conditions on the Recommended Uniform Screening Panel (RUSP; determined by the Department of Health and Human Services) are covered in all states, and some states have added additional conditions that are not on the RUSP. Questions about the specific panel of diseases that were included at the time of a child's birth can be directed to a local geneticist or to the state laboratory. Generally, most disorders of amino acid and fatty acid metabolism, most organic acidemias, galactosemia, and biotinidase deficiency are included on the screen.[37]

Phenylketonuria (PKU) was a common cause of intellectual disability prior to the advent of newborn screening. With early identification, appropriate dietary management, and strict adherence to treatment, patients with PKU now have normal cognitive outcomes. Similarly, newborn screening for congenital hypothyroidism and for congenital hearing loss has significantly decreased the number of children in the population with potentially preventable developmental delays. Since many primary pediatric health care professionals are no longer familiar with the untreated phenotypes of these diseases, it is important to verify that the newborn screen was done and the state in which testing was done.

Assessment of Hearing and Vision

Hearing testing has been included on newborn screening because congenital deafness is a prevalent and modifiable cause of speech delay. In some cases, later-onset hearing loss can be a cause of developmental delays and should always be tested in appropriate circumstances given the availability of speech therapy, sign language, hearing aids, and cochlear implants as effective interventions. Alternatively, hearing loss may be a diagnostic clue to the etiological diagnosis underlying developmental delay. Examples of diagnoses that feature both developmental delay and hearing loss include CHARGE syndrome, mitochondrial diseases, peroxisomal disorders, Kabuki syndrome, and many others.

Formal ophthalmological examination with a dilated retinal examination is an important diagnostic tool for the developmentally delayed child. Some ophthalmological findings can be quite specific to the underlying diagnosis. Detection of cataracts may spur diagnostic evaluation for cerebrotendinous xanthomatosis, a disorder of cholesterol metabolism with effective pharmaceutical treatment. The finding of retinitis pigmentosa is associated with mitochondrial diseases, Bardet-Biedl syndrome, some disorders of glycosylation, and other diagnoses.

Imaging

The reported diagnostic yield of neuroimaging in the evaluation of a child with developmental delays varies widely depending on the specific population being studied and the method of ascertaining patients for inclusion in the analysis. For example, one study found a 7.5% diagnostic yield for magnetic resonance imaging (MRI) in children with developmental delay overall but a 28% diagnostic yield in children with developmental delay plus developmental regression, epilepsy, microcephaly, macrocephaly, or focal findings on neurological examination.[38] Some general principles have been reproducible in the literature on this topic: The likelihood of abnormal findings on neuroimaging is higher with MRI than with computed tomography (CT), and the diagnostic yield is higher with more severe developmental delay than with milder delays. The yield of imaging is higher in the setting of macrocephaly, microcephaly, or epilepsy, or with focal findings on neurological examination. Given these considerations, each primary pediatric health care professional must determine the appropriate application of neuroimaging in his or her specific practice setting. One consideration that may alter the risk/benefit calculation for the test is the need for general anesthesia for many young children and older children with developmental delays to undergo MRI.[39]

In some patients, MRI findings may be very helpful to guide the diagnostic evaluation, as in the case of leukodystrophy (abnormal signal of the white matter). If a confluent pattern of posterior leukodystrophy is identified, then X-ALD is a specific concern. Conversely, confluent leukodystrophy of the anterior white matter is concerning for Alexander disease. Bilateral abnormal signal of the basal ganglia, midbrain, brainstem, or cerebellum may indicate Leigh syndrome and high suspicion for mitochondrial disease.[40] Some institutions have access to magnetic resonance spectroscopy (MRS) to evaluate the relative concentration of specific metabolites in the brain. Elevated lactate

55

Chapter 4: Biological Influences on Child Development and Behavior and Medical Evaluation of Children With Developmental-Behavioral Disorders

on MRS can be seen in the setting of mitochondrial disorders and other defects of energy metabolism. The absence of creatine on MRS indicates a disorder of creatine synthesis or transport.

Genetic Testing

The availability of genetic services is widely variable by institution and by geographic location; hence the standard practice for genetic testing as part of a developmental evaluation will differ. The American Academy of Pediatrics (AAP) has recently published updated recommendations for genetic evaluation of children with developmental delays to incorporate current testing technologies (see Figure 4.2).[39] If a specific diagnosis is identified with comprehensive history and physical examination, then targeted testing for that disorder should be initiated. It is important to understand the genetic mechanisms responsible for the suspected disorder prior to testing. For example, Angelman syndrome may be caused by methylation abnormalities, sequence abnormalities, or deletion of the gene *UBE3A;* the different genetic mechanisms require different testing modalities to identify them. The ordering primary pediatric health care professional must have the knowledge that methylation testing has significantly higher diagnostic yield for Angelman syndrome than gene sequencing, in order to obtain appropriate testing. Similarly, trinucleotide repeat analysis of *FMR1* has dramatically higher diagnostic yield, and requires different methods, than assessment for sequence abnormalities or deletions of the gene.

If there is not suspicion for one specific diagnosis after the history and physical examination of a child with developmental delays, then trinucleotide repeat testing for fragile X syndrome and chromosome microarray analysis are indicated. Microarray is an untargeted test that will assess for copy number variants (CNVs) throughout the genome. Some CNVs, such as the common deletion at chromosome 22q11, are clearly pathogenic and result in well-defined clinical syndromes. Formerly known as DiGeorge syndrome, 22q11 deletion syndrome commonly causes mild developmental delay, congenital heart disease, abnormalities of the palate, hypoparathyroidism, and immunodeficiency due to hypoplasia of the thymus. Other causes of developmental delay that may be identified on microarray include Williams syndrome (7q11 deletion), Prader-Willi syndrome (paternally inherited 15q11 deletion), and Smith-Magenis syndrome (17p11 deletion).

In addition to the aforementioned recurrent deletions that are mediated by repetitive DNA, any other deletion that is above the resolution of detection for the specific microarray ordered will be compared to databases of known CNVs in the population, and if sufficiently rare, it will be reported by the lab to the ordering clinician as a potentially significant finding. Prior to obtaining the microarray, parents should be aware that the results may be ambiguous—neither clearly benign nor clearly pathogenic—and that parental follow-up testing may be required to further evaluate ambiguous CNVs. Occasionally, incidental but clearly pathogenic findings may occur, such as detection of the deletion of a tumor suppressor gene that would convey increased cancer risk. Lastly, most clinically available microarrays in current use will detect and report consanguinity between the parents of a child. Providers should obtain informed consent from the parents by reviewing the potential results of a microarray prior to obtaining the test.

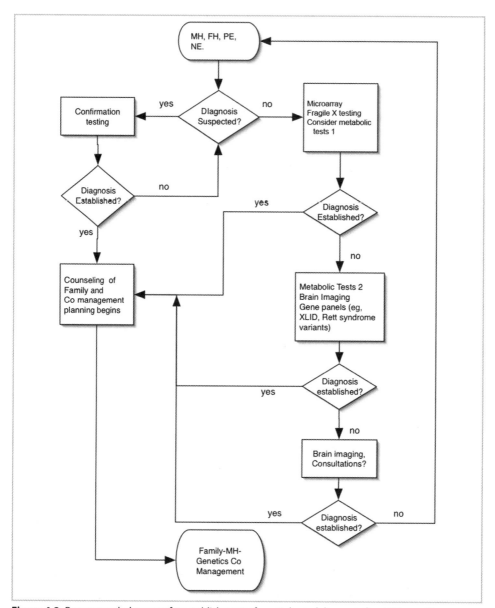

Figure 4.2. Recommended process for establishment of an etiological diagnosis for children with developmental delay.

Abbreviations: MH, medical history; FH, family history; PE, physical examination; NE, neurological examination; XLID, x-linked intellectual disability.

Reproduced with permission from Moeschler JB, Shevell M, Committee on Genetics. Comprehensive evaluation of the child with intellectual disability or global developmental delays. *Pediatrics*. 2014;134(3):e903–e918.

57

Chapter 4: Biological Influences on Child Development and Behavior and Medical Evaluation of
Children With Developmental-Behavioral Disorders

As the cost of sequencing declines with technological improvement, larger gene panels have come into common use and are being used earlier in the diagnostic evaluation of patients with developmental delays. Examples of commonly used gene panels include those for patients with epilepsy, X-linked intellectual disability, and Noonan syndrome. Whole exome trio—sequencing of the entire coding region of all genes for the affected individual as well as both parents—is increasingly prevalent in the diagnostic evaluation of patients with developmental delays, though clinical availability varies widely in different practice settings. Exome trio is the highest-yield test in the setting of a patient with developmental delays but without features of a specific recognizable syndrome. Despite the breadth of the test, clinicians should be aware that it will not detect deletions, methylation abnormalities, noncoding DNA variants, trinucleotide repeats, or mosaic genetic changes that do not include the cells containing the DNA that was sequenced. The issues that should be discussed in order to obtain informed consent for untargeted sequencing tests are similar to those that arise for microarray but with higher likelihood of ambiguous and incidental findings. See Table 4.1 for a comparison between different genetic tests.

Table 4.1. Clinically available diagnostic tests for genetic etiologies of developmental delay.		
Test	**Indication**	**Limitations**
Chromosomal microarray	Untargeted testing for deletions and duplications of genetic material genome-wide	Does not detect sequence changes or other genetic mechanisms; does not detect small deletions below the spatial resolution of the microarray; some risk of incidental or ambiguous findings
Single gene sequencing	Identification of sequence alterations in a specific gene	Low diagnostic yield unless there is suspicion for a specific disorder based on clinical evaluation; does not detect deletions, duplications, or other genetic mechanisms
Next-generation sequencing gene panel	Identification of sequence alterations in a group of genes with the same clinical presentation	Diagnostic yield depends on the clinical indication; detects only sequence alterations and not other genetic mechanisms
Whole exome sequencing	Untargeted testing for sequence changes throughout the protein-coding regions of the genome	Will not detect deletions, duplications, trinucleotide repeats, methylation abnormalities, regulatory sequence alterations, or some mosaic mutations; high risk of incidental or ambiguous findings; diagnostic yield is significantly higher with samples from both biological parents
Trinucleotide repeat expansion testing	Detection of a nucleotide repeat expansion in or near a specific gene	Targeted test: similar limitations to single gene sequencing
Methylation testing	Detection of a methylation abnormality at a specific genomic location	Targeted test: similar limitations to single gene sequencing
Metabolic testing	Detection of inborn errors of metabolism	Results may be dependent on physiological state of the patient; artefactual elevations with poor specimen handling

Metabolic Testing

The AAP Committee on Genetics recommends that clinicians conducting a diagnostic evaluation for patients with developmental delays consider obtaining metabolic testing in patients without a specifically recognized syndrome.[39] One reason to include metabolic testing as part of the evaluation is that many inborn errors of metabolism have specific treatment or management strategies. The reported diagnostic yield of metabolic testing in the setting of developmental delay is 1% to 5%, depending on how patients are ascertained and which tests are included in the panel. While there is some overlap between metabolic testing obtained for the indication of developmental delay and the newborn screening panel, it is important to remember that many inborn errors of metabolism are not covered by newborn screening. For the disorders that are covered, the newborn screen is optimized for the population as a whole and not for the individual patient with known developmental delays.

Tests included in the AAP recommendations for patients with developmental delays are serum amino acids, homocysteine, and acylcarnitine profiles, as well as urine organic acids, creatine metabolites, purines, pyrimidines, mucopolysaccharides, and oligosaccharides.[39] Additional testing that can be considered and has been discussed in other publications on the metabolic evaluation of patients with developmental delays include lactate, ammonia, copper, ceruloplasmin, cholestanol, 7-dehydrocholesterol, very long chain fatty acids, congenital disorders of glycosylation, and other tests.[41] Many of the listed metabolic tests will have results that differ depending on the physiological state of the patient (fed or fasted) and may have artefactual abnormal results with inappropriate specimen handling. Primary pediatric health care professionals conducting developmental assessments may wish to consult with a local metabolic genetics service to discuss the capabilities of the institutional laboratory and the appropriate ascertainment of patients for metabolic testing at the time of the assessment.

Conclusions

Many factors affect developmental outcome, including genetic, metabolic, infectious, and environmental exposures. A careful history, including prenatal, perinatal, early postnatal and childhood issues, and a detailed family history can provide important clues to determining etiologic factors causing developmental-behavioral disorders. A thorough physical examination is critical, with attention to subtle changes in facial features and limbs, as well as growth parameters.

Genetic testing has evolved significantly in recent years, with an improved ability to identify causative mutations and to make definitive diagnoses. Determining a clear diagnosis is now possible for many more patients with developmental-behavioral disorders than in previous decades. Identification of an etiological diagnosis can lead to tailored medical management and can improve developmental outcome in some cases. Having a better understanding of the underlying basis of the developmental-behavioral disorder also may help to clarify the prognosis, and it gives parents a better

59

Chapter 4: Biological Influences on Child Development and Behavior and Medical Evaluation of Children With Developmental-Behavioral Disorders

understanding of the recurrence risk in future pregnancies. With continued advances in genetic technology and better understanding of biological mechanisms, the coming years will bring yet more breadth and nuance to the understanding of the biological basis of developmental-behavioral disorders.

References

1. Bittles A. Consanguinity and its relevance to clinical genetics. *Clin Genet.* 2001;60(2):89–98
2. Lehtonen A, Howie E, Trump D, Huson SM. Behaviour in children with neurofibromatosis type 1: cognition, executive function, attention, emotion, and social competence. *Dev Med Child Neurol.* 2013;55(2):111–125
3. Garber KB, Visootsak J, Warren ST. Fragile X syndrome. *Eur J Hum Genet.* 2008;16(6):666–672
4. El-Hattab AW, Adesina AM, Jones J, Scaglia F. MELAS syndrome: Clinical manifestations, pathogenesis, and treatment options. *Mol Genet Metab.* 2015;116(1–2):4–12
5. Sugiura-Ogasawara M, Ozaki Y, Sato T, Suzumori N, Suzumori K. Poor prognosis of recurrent aborters with either maternal or paternal reciprocal translocations. *Fertil Steril.* 2004;81(2):367–373
6. Simchen MJ, Goldstein G, Lubetsky A, et al. Factor v Leiden and antiphospholipid antibodies in either mothers or infants increase the risk for perinatal arterial ischemic stroke. *Stroke.* 2009;40(1):65–70
7. Sutcliffe AG, Ludwig M. Outcome of assisted reproduction. *Lancet.* 2007;370(9584):351–359
8. Anderson JL, Waller DK, Canfield MA, Shaw GM, Watkins ML, Werler MM. Maternal obesity, gestational diabetes, and central nervous system birth defects. *Epidemiology.* 2005;16(1):87–92
9. Krakowiak P, Walker CK, Bremer AA, et al. Maternal metabolic conditions and risk for autism and other neurodevelopmental disorders. *Pediatrics.* 2012;129(5):e1121–e1128
10. Walker SP, Wachs TD, Gardner JM, et al. Child development: risk factors for adverse outcomes in developing countries. *Lancet.* 2007;369(9556):145–157
11. Riley EP, Infante MA, Warren KR. Fetal alcohol spectrum disorders: an overview. *Neuropsychol Rev.* 2011;21(2):73–80
12. Holbrook BD, Rayburn WF. Teratogenic risks from exposure to illicit drugs. *Obstet Gynecol Clin North Am.* 2014;41(2):229–239
13. Manicklal S, Emery VC, Lazzarotto T, Boppana SB, Gupta RK. The "silent" global burden of congenital cytomegalovirus. *Clin Microbiol Rev.* 2013;26(1):86–102
14. Mlakar J, Korva M, Tul N, et al. Zika virus associated with microcephaly. *N Engl J Med.* 2016;374(10):951–958
15. Bhutta AT, Cleves MA, Casey PH, Cradock MM, Anand KJS. Cognitive and behavioral outcomes of school-aged children who were born preterm: a meta-analysis. *JAMA.* 2002;288(6):728–737
16. Hutchinson EA, De Luca CR, Doyle LW, et al. School-age outcomes of extremely preterm or extremely low birth weight children. *Pediatrics.* 2013;131(4):e1053–e1061
17. Simpkin AJ, Suderman M, Gaunt TR, et al. Longitudinal analysis of DNA methylation associated with birth weight and gestational age. *Hum Mol Genet.* 2015;24(13):3752–3763
18. American Academy of Pediatrics Committee on Fetus and Newborn' American College of Obstetricians and Gynecologists Committee on Obstetric Practice, et al. The Apgar score. *Pediatrics.* 2015;136(4):819–822
19. Miller SP, Ramaswamy V, Michelson D, et al. Patterns of brain injury in term neonatal encephalopathy. *J Pediatr.* 2005;146(4):453–460
20. Wu YW, Mathur AM, Chang T, et al. High-dose erythropoietin and hypothermia for hypoxic-ischemic encephalopathy: a phase II trial. *Pediatrics.* 2016;137(6)
21. Marino BS, Lipkin PH, Newburger JW, et al. Neurodevelopmental outcomes in children with congenital heart disease: evaluation and management: a scientific statement from the American Heart Association. *Circulation.* 2012;126(9):1143–1172
22. Moore BD 3rd. Neurocognitive outcomes in survivors of childhood cancer. *J Pediatr Psychol.* 2005;30(1):51–63
23. Schatz J, Brown RT, Pascual JM, Hsu L, DeBaun MR. Poor school and cognitive functioning with silent cerebral infarcts and sickle cell disease. *Neurology.* 2001;56(8):1109–1111
24. Libster R, Edwards KM, Levent F, et al. Long-term outcomes of group B streptococcal meningitis. *Pediatrics.* 2012;130(1):e8–e15
25. Anderson V, Godfrey C, Rosenfeld JV, Catroppa C. Predictors of cognitive function and recovery 10 years after traumatic brain injury in young children. *Pediatrics.* 2012;129(2):e254–e261
26. Sullivan PB, Juszczak E, Lambert BR, Rose M, Ford-Adams ME, Johnson A. Impact of feeding problems on nutritional intake and growth: Oxford Feeding Study II. *Dev Med Child Neurol.* 2002;44(7):461–467

27. Lichter-Konecki U, Caldovic L, Morizono H, Simpson K. Ornithine transcarbamylase deficiency. In: Adam MP, Ardinger HH, Pagon RA, et al, eds. *GeneReviews*. Seattle, WA: University of Washington, Seattle; 2013

28. Walterfang M, Bonnot O, Mocellin R, Velakoulis D. The neuropsychiatry of inborn errors of metabolism. *J Inherit Metab Dis*. 2013;36(4):687–702

29. Lake NJ, Compton AG, Rahman S, Thorburn DR. Leigh syndrome: One disorder, more than 75 monogenic causes. *Ann Neurol*. 2016;79(2):190–203

30. Romano AA, Allanson JE, Dahlgren J, et al. Noonan syndrome: clinical features, diagnosis, and management guidelines. *Pediatrics*. 2010;126(4):746–759

31. Groth KA, Skakkebæk A, Høst C, Gravholt CH, Bojesen A. Klinefelter syndrome—a clinical update. *J Clin Endocrinol Metab*. 2013;98(1):20–30

32. Lane C, Milne E, Freeth M. Cognition and behaviour in Sotos syndrome: a systematic review. *PLoS One*. 2016;11(2):e0149189

33. Varga EA, Pastore M, Prior T, Herman GE, McBride KL. The prevalence of *PTEN* mutations in a clinical pediatric cohort with autism spectrum disorders, developmental delay, and macrocephaly. *Genet Med*. 2009;11(2):111–117

34. Bianconi SE, Cross JL, Wassif CA, Porter FD. Pathogenesis, epidemiology, diagnosis and clinical aspects of Smith-Lemli-Opitz syndrome. *Expert Opin Orphan Drugs*. 2015;3(3):267–280

35. Battaglia A, Doccini V, Bernardini L, et al. Confirmation of chromosomal microarray as a first-tier clinical diagnostic test for individuals with developmental delay, intellectual disability, autism spectrum disorders and dysmorphic features. *Eur J Paediatr Neurol*. 2013;17(6):589–599

36. Serrano M, de Diego V, Muchart J, et al. Phosphomannomutase deficiency (PMM2-CDG): ataxia and cerebellar assessment. *Orphanet J Rare Dis*. 2015;10:138

37. American College of Medical Genetics Newborn Screening Expert Group. Newborn screening: toward a uniform screening panel and system—executive summary. *Pediatrics*. 2006;117(5 Pt 2):S296–S307

38. Griffiths PD, Batty R, Warren D, et al. The use of MR imaging and spectroscopy of the brain inchildren investigated for developmental delay: What is the most appropriate imaging strategy? *Eur Radiol*. 2011;21(9):1820–1830

39. Moeschler JB, Shevell M, American Academy of Pediatrics Committee on Genetics. Comprehensive evaluation of the child with intellectual disability or global developmental delays. *Pediatrics*. 2014;134(3):e903–918

40. Schiffmann R, van der Knaap MS. Invited article: an MRI-based approach to the diagnosis of white matter disorders. *Neurology*. 2009;72(8):750–759

41. Sayson B, Popurs MA, Lafek M, et al. Retrospective analysis supports algorithm as efficient diagnostic approach to treatable intellectual developmental disabilities. *Mol Genet Metab*. 2015;115(1):1–9

CHAPTER 5

Interviewing and Counseling Children and Families

Prachi E. Shah, MD, MS

Julie Ribaudo, LMSW, IMH-E(IV)

> "*Don't walk in front of me; I may not follow. Don't walk behind me; I may not lead. Just walk beside me and be my friend* "
>
> Albert Camus (1913–1960)

The Pediatric Visit: An Opportunity to Build a Therapeutic Alliance and a Goal-Directed Partnership With Families

There is much wisdom from the French novelist, essayist, playwright, and Nobel Prize Laureate Albert Camus about what is needed to successfully interview and counsel families in the context of a pediatric visit. The primary pediatric health care professional need not dictate the agenda of the visit and "lead" the family according to a predetermined agenda. Nor should the health care professional limit the interview to the initial concerns that are expressed, without inquiring about and exploring other potential areas salient to child health and development that the family may not explicitly mention. Successful interviewing and counseling of families requires that the health care professional "walk with" a family and develop a therapeutic alliance with the child and caregivers based on mutual respect and the shared goal of optimizing the child's health and developmental-behavioral outcomes. This holistic, family-centered approach to patient care is most likely to be adopted into practice when this perspective is introduced early in medical training. Arguably, one of the most necessary skills to develop in residency training is the art of building a therapeutic alliance in the context of the patient encounter.[1] A healthy therapeutic alliance between a health care professional and a patient is thought to incorporate 3 main components: (1) agreement on goals that are the desired outcomes of the therapeutic process; (2) agreement on tasks that are the steps undertaken to achieve the goals; and (3) a bond between the health care professional and the patient built on shared values, such as trust, respect, genuineness, positive regard, and empathy.[2]

While many would agree that sensitive, empathic listening and building trust and respect are the foundation for building a therapeutic alliance, the reality is that a collaborative relationship between the primary pediatric health care professional and the patient evolves over time. If the ultimate goal is to build a therapeutic alliance in which the foundation is trust and respect, what is the first brick that should be laid? One possibility considers that perhaps the most important factor for building a therapeutic alliance between a health care professional and a family is the ability to collaboratively identify mutually agreed-upon goals for the health care professional's encounters with the family. This begins by uncovering the patient's goals for the encounter and by seeking the patient's and family's input on what may be done to achieve these goals. Rather than a problem-focused approach (eg, "What problem brings you in today?"), a goal-based approach begins the dialogue by asking the patient what his or her goals for the visit are, to which the health care professional can add and expand, and a goal-directed partnership can develop.

A mutual, goal-directed partnership between the pediatric health care professional and family is best achieved when pediatric care is continuous, comprehensive, family-centered, coordinated, compassionate, and culturally effective. This model is most successful when the health care professional is known to the child and family and when there is a partnership of mutual responsibility and trust between them.[3]

The characteristics of the ideal health care professional–family alliance are best captured in the model of the *medical home*. The *medical home* is a vision for how all individuals who are involved in the delivery of health care services can partner with their patients and their families to help them achieve their maximum potential. This vision of a comprehensive medical home is considered to be the standard of quality care for all children.[4] This vision posits that optimal care is provided in a system that fosters collaboration and cooperation among all members of the community in which the child and family live. In this model of the medical home, health care professionals can promote factors that foster resilience and inquire about factors that can confer developmental risk.[5,6]

The goal of the pediatric health supervision visit, according to the American Academy of Pediatrics, is to promote children's optimal growth and development.[7]

Because of the health care professional's regular and ongoing contact over time with infants, toddlers, and their families, the primary pediatric health care professional is well positioned to monitor and support early child development and behavior and optimize child health outcomes.[8] However, evidence suggests that the pediatric visit is an often underutilized opportunity to identify developmental and behavioral concerns and to provide anticipatory guidance to families. To better address developmental and behavioral concerns in the context of the primary care visit, the pediatric health supervision visit must be adapted to address this unmet need. The pediatric visit must provide an opportunity for the parent and health care professional to communicate about the issues that are most salient to childhood health, behavior, and development. To understand how to use this opportunity during the clinical visit, it is helpful to explore the content and meaning of dialogues between a family and pediatric health care professional that emerge in the context of the clinical interview.

Capturing Missed Opportunities: Optimizing the Pediatric Encounter

Creating a "Holding Environment" in the Context of the Pediatric Visit

The primary pediatric health care professional is well positioned to observe the nuances of the caregiving relationship, monitor early child development, identify difficulties, and offer support, guidance, and intervention when families struggle.[9] This "holistic health surveillance" occurring in the context of the pediatric health supervision visit is most successful when the parent feels heard, supported, and "beheld" in the context of the health care professional-patient encounter. Employing some general principles regarding interviewing and assessment is helpful to create an environment where the family can feel that their concerns are heard and respected. This involves building a therapeutic alliance with both the caregiver and the pediatric patient and viewing developmental and behavioral concerns though a culturally sensitive lens. This process is best achieved when the pediatric health care professional can provide a psychological "holding environment," in which parents feel safe articulating their fears, vulnerabilities, challenges, or concerns as parents.[10] The concept of the "holding environment" was first described by Donald Winnicott, a British pediatrician, psychiatrist, and psychoanalyst, as a means of articulating what infants need from their caregivers to feel safe and secure.[11] In Winnicott's "holding environment," the primary caregiver provides an environment of physical and psychological support, in which the infant can feel safe and develop a sense of self. In much the same way, the primary pediatric health care professional can create a supportive "holding environment" for parents, in which they feel a sense of safety, nurturance, support, and trust, and in which the health care professional can explore issues with the family that are most relevant to the child's and family's well-being.

Based on trust built of an ongoing caring relationship, the primary pediatric health care professional can comfortably ask important personal questions that shed light on the key resources for achieving each child's developmental potential. Because the health and well-being of children are intimately related to the parent's physical, emotional, and social health and social circumstances,[12] relevant areas of inquiry with parents may include their mood, family ties, work issues, perceived social support, social affiliations, child-care needs, health status, financial security, as well as conditions that can be toxic and maladaptive to the child's well-being.[13] Environmental toxins, such as air and water quality, as well as housing and food security are important areas to address as well. These conditions influence family dynamics, contribute to a child's health and growth, and as such, are essential domains for the primary pediatric health care professional to explore.[14]

The opportunity to identify problems begins when the clinician first inquires about positive developments within and between the child and family. Potential problems are further elucidated by discussing any concerns about their child's development and behavior. The clinical interview provides an ideal opportunity for the primary pediatric health care professional to enhance the relationships with patients and families, assess the emotional states of patients, and uncover clues that might point to psychosocial distress or disturbance within the family context. The clinical interview can serve as a tool for gathering information, providing an opportunity to form a therapeutic alliance with the family and serving as a means to influence behavior. Successful interviewing is maximized by using a developmental approach and some principles of family engagement and assessment.[15]

A potentially helpful framework to address parents' concerns and provide anticipatory guidance in the context of the pediatric encounter can be conceptualized by the mnemonic: SHARE.[16]

S *Set* the tone: Create a "holding environment" in the context of the pediatric visit. *Support* parent and child: Build a therapeutic alliance.

H *Hear* the parent's concerns about the child's behavior and development and the effects on family functioning through the use of some guided questions.

A *Address* specific risk factors for child development and family functioning. *Allow* parents to reflect how cultural traditions contribute to their expectations of child behavior and development.

R *Reflect* with parents on their experience of the child. *Reframe* the child's behavior and development in terms of the child's developmental level. *Revisit* the therapeutic goals set.

E *Empower* the parent and child by formulating an action plan to address the concerns voiced in the visit.

The Art of Interviewing

S Setting the Tone/Supporting the Parents and Child in the Pediatric Visit: Developing a Therapeutic Alliance

Creating a safe space and open environment to share the details that are most salient to child development and family functioning requires special attention to the nuances of the initial family encounter. Nurturing emotional development in children must begin with supporting and nurturing the parents in their roles as caregivers. As the family is the primary vehicle for children's early development, the family is the pediatric patient.[14] This alliance can begin by creating the time and space for parents and children to feel that they can voice their concerns. Some general principles regarding interviewing and counseling should be considered. Efficient communication requires unbroken attention. Privacy will increase the information shared during an interview and is especially important when sensitive psychosocial issues are being discussed. Equally important is explicitly addressing issues of confidentiality with patients and parents prior to clinical assessment and having adequate time to address the family's concerns. The primary pediatric health care professional has the added challenge of developing a therapeutic alliance with both the parent and the pediatric patient. This can be facilitated if an alliance can be forged with the child in a developmentally sensitive manner.

Infancy (0–1 year of age): In the period of infancy, the most primary developmental process is the development of a sense of trust in the child's caregiver and the world around him or her. The young infant is dependent on the caregiver for a sense of safety, security, and to help control and regulate emotions.[17]

In the first year of life, the "interview" of the child, or more accurately put, the assessment of the child, should take place in the presence of the caregiver, preferably, in the caregiver's arms if possible. A soft tone of voice and gentle handling of the infant are important means of helping the baby develop a sense of trust and comfort with the primary pediatric health care professional. Narrating to the infant what will happen in the context of the visit can help the infant and the caregiver feel more comfortable, as well as implicitly encouraging a more reticent parent to talk with the baby about the world and his or her experiences. A therapeutic alliance can be forged with both the infant and the caregiver when the caregiver's concerns are articulated and directed toward the infant during the assessment, "Your mommy wonders why you are so fussy at night. Is there something in your ears, in your tummy?"

Toddler Years (1–3 years of age): The hallmark of the toddler years is the desire for autonomy, stranger wariness, separation, and individuation. In the context of the health supervision visit, the toddler may seek to have more control and active participation in the health supervision visit. At the end of the first year of life, the infant has developed a framework of attachment to the primary caregiver based on his or her history of early experiences.[18] In this attachment relationship, the caregiver serves as both a "secure base" from whom the toddler can explore an unfamiliar environment and a "safe haven" to whom he or she can return when distressed.[19] Rapport can be built with the toddler by allowing and encouraging exploration, being sensitive to the toddler's needs for "emotional refueling" from the caregiver, and indulging the toddler's desire for autonomy and control, "First I will listen to your heart, then you can listen."

Preschool Years (3–6 years of age): Preschoolers are developmentally in Piaget's preoperational thinking stage. This developmental stage is characterized by egocentric and magical thinking. The preschool child has greater verbal and cognitive capacities than the infant and toddler but often views the world in a very concrete and self-oriented way. The preschooler may view illness as a punishment for certain behavior (eg, "My stomach hurts because I did not eat my vegetables last night") or may view illness as something that was caused by "magic." To engage the preschool child, it is often helpful to reassure the child that illness is not his or her fault or a result of "bad behavior." It can be helpful for the primary pediatric health care professional to probe with the child his or her understanding of why he or she does not feel well. The primary pediatric health care professional can further build rapport by engaging with the preoperational child in finding a solution: "What do you think we should do to help you feel better? Maybe we can give you some 'special medicine' to take away your earache."

School-aged Child: (7–12 years of age): The school-aged child is at a period of advancing verbal and cognitive development. The child's thinking is more logical, organized, and concrete, and the child is better able to understand cause and effect. Rapport with the school-aged child can be facilitated by inquiring about school, hobbies, and friends. The school-aged child can be more actively engaged in the clinical interview and can be directly queried about what his or her feelings, concerns, and goals are for the visit. The school-aged child can also be invited to assume a greater responsibility in the treatment process, "Now that you are such a big boy/girl, I need you to help your mom remember that you will need to take your medicine every day until it is all gone."

Adolescence: (13–21 years of age): Adolescence is a critical stage in development in which health behaviors, including those that will last a lifetime, are adopted.[20] Developmentally, the adolescent patient is in the process of gaining autonomy from the parents. This emerging autonomy can be respected by structuring the pediatric visit to include both time with the parent and adolescent together and time with the adolescent alone. Confidentiality and its limitations should be addressed and acknowledged before the parent leaves the room.[15] Building an alliance with the adolescent and caregiver can be facilitated if mutually agreed-upon therapeutic goals can be identified in the context of the visit and if both the adolescent and the caregiver are committed to achieving the desired change by working together toward the therapeutic goal.[21]

A successful therapeutic alliance between the primary pediatric health care professional, caregiver, and pediatric patient is best achieved when a partnership can be forged between the parents and the health care professionals caring for their children. This family-oriented approach incorporates the view that parents play an important role in the health and well-being of their children and is based on the following assumptions: (1) the parents know the children best and want the best for them, (2) each family is different and unique, and (3) a child's well-being is affected by the stress and coping of other family members.[22]

The pediatric encounter should be structured such that the parents' desires for the well-being of their child are acknowledged and addressed and that the parents can feel free to share with the primary pediatric health care professional those issues that are serving as a stress to the relationship. This can be facilitated through the careful use of guided, open-ended questions.

Facilitating a Dialogue

H Hear the Parent's Concerns About The Child's Behavior and Development and the Effects on Family Functioning

Parents often present to the pediatric visit with concerns about their child's health, development, or behavior. It has been suggested that nearly half of parents have concerns about their young child's behavior, speech, or social development,[23,24] but some parents are reluctant to share their concerns about developmental and behavioral issues with their pediatrician.[25-27] For some parents, societal and cultural beliefs influence what child behavior concerns they feel comfortable divulging to their primary pediatric health care professional and what concerns remain unshared.[25,28] To ensure that the parents' deepest concerns and needs are expressed and addressed, the pediatric health supervision visit must be adapted to address this aspect of the child's health. The pediatric health supervision visit must provide the opportunity for parents to tell their story and to express their perceptions about the strengths and vulnerabilities of their children and families.[29]

This can more readily occur when a therapeutic alliance built on trust and mutual respect has been established between the primary pediatric health care professional and the family. Problems, concerns, and beliefs that a family may present may differ radically from the attitudes and beliefs of the primary pediatric health care professional. To ensure that parents feel free to express their concerns honestly and openly, special attention must be placed on creating an interview environment of openness and acceptance. In an environment of "radical acceptance," the clinician actively welcomes all comments from parents and children in a nonjudgmental fashion and communicates a personal and professional commitment to openness during the interview, assessment, and treatment process.[30] In the spirit of this bidirectional openness, the parents and child may articulate deep underlying beliefs that may play an important role in a child's health and behavioral outcomes.

The interview can begin with very open-ended, general questions such as, "What is going on in your child's life? How has he been lately? Is there something specific that you would like us to focus on today?" This sets the agenda and the therapeutic goal toward which the visit can be directed. As is developmentally appropriate, this question can be addressed to the child, and his or her input on the goals for the visit can be incorporated as well. In addition to addressing the concerns that were explicitly articulated in the pediatric visit, the primary pediatric health care professional must also gently probe for areas of concern related to a child's development and behavior. Developmental and behavioral problems have been described as the "new morbidity" in pediatrics.[31,32]

Psychosocial concerns are more prevalent in pediatric primary care,[33] and the need to manage developmental, behavioral, and emotional concerns is increasing.[34] To probe more deeply into a parent's developmental or behavioral concerns about the child, the parent can be asked, "Do you have any questions or concerns about how your child is learning, developing, or behaving?" and "What is it like to take care of your child?" Exploration of the parents' opinions and concerns about their child's development and behavior is central to assessment; parental perceptions of the child and thoughts about caregiving have been shown to be especially predictive of the child's developmental and behavioral status and is a key to identifying children at risk for developmental or behavioral problems.[35,36] If a screening questionnaire was given prior to the pediatric patient encounter, often responses can guide the conversation and alert the health care professional to potential areas of concern.

When developmental or behavioral concerns are identified, it is often helpful to explore how the parent sees and views the child in light of these developmental and behavioral differences. What are the parents' perceptions of the child? What is the parents' understanding of the child's development and behavior? What are the parents' hopes and fears for the child? Exploration of these underlying issues often plays an important role in formulating a successful therapeutic intervention. It is also important to quantify how impairing is the child's behavior. Because there is often a reluctance to label a child's behavior as pathological, significant behavioral problems might be minimized or overlooked. A useful framework to help parents understand their child's behavior is to inquire how the child's behavior is affecting the family system and family functioning. If a child's behavior interferes with a parent's ability to maintain employment, maintain family routines, go out in public, or complete household chores, further evaluation may be warranted.[28]

In addition, the parents' perception of their child should be explored, as this perception influences parental behavior toward the child and affects the child's behavior toward the parent.[37] Do they convey a rich or more limited understanding of their child? The degree to which a parent seems to have a rich, flexible, and accurate understanding of the child is associated with variations in child outcomes.[38,39]

These parental perceptions of the child can provide valuable clues to the dynamics of the parent-child relationship and potential origins of behavioral disturbances.[40] Issues regarding a parent's perception of the child's behavior, and the impact of behavior on family functioning, can be explored with the caregiver using selected trigger questions to help elicit information that may be difficult for parents to talk about.[10] Asking a mix of the following questions, in an order that seems to match the priorities and concerns of the family, may be helpful:

- Does your child's behavior interfere with your ability to maintain family routines (eg, eating dinner together at home)?
- Does your child's behavior interfere with your ability to go out in public (eg, eating out at a restaurant, going to the grocery store)?
- Does your child's behavior keep you from getting things done at home (eg, doing chores at home, talking on the phone)?
- Has your child's behavior affected your ability to maintain employment (eg, because of a difficulty in maintaining child care)?

- How has your child's behavior affected your relationship with your spouse?
- Has your child's behavior affected his or her functioning at home, at school, or with his or her friends?
- Tell me what is most difficult about your child's behavior?
- Why do you think he or she does it?
- How does this behavior make you feel?
- Who does this behavior remind you of?
- What are your hopes for your child?
- What are your fears for your child?
- If you could pick 3 words to describe your child's personality, what would they be and why? Can you tell me of a recent incident that would help me understand why you chose [each word]?

Understanding the parents' perceptions of their child's behavior and hearing the parent's hopes and fears for their child are important pieces of information that can guide the therapeutic process. When a parent's deepest hopes and fears are freely expressed, the interventions can be targeted to actualize the parents' hopes and mitigate their fears. Parents who have difficulty empathizing with their child can be assisted by the primary pediatric health care professional's empathy for their struggles. In a two-generational approach to care, parents who do not have strong memories of having been cared for themselves can often use the feeling of concern for them to offer something different for their child.

> Nate and his mother, Liz, were seen for a routine 8-week visit. Following a brief but painful medical procedure, Nate was difficult to console. The pediatric health care professional noticed Liz's mixture of anxiety and embarrassment at Nate's distress and commented, "It is hard to see him so upset?" Liz replied, "My family thinks I spoil him and that's why he cries so much."

In this instance, the pediatric health care professional's empathy for the mother's distress could lead to a response that might appease the mother and offer a new model of responsivity. A validating comment such as "It is hard to go against what your family is telling you, but it sounds like you know that Nate needs you and you want to soothe him. That is just what he needs right now, so you are wise to listen to him" conveys to her the health care professional's concern for her and gives her permission to listen to her baby in a way that perhaps she did not experience as a child. Patterns of interaction developed in infancy and early childhood have been found to be intergenerationally transmitted, such that parents who were treated warmly and sensitively in early childhood tend to repeat the same style of caregiving with their own children. Conversely, harsh, punitive, or aggressive parenting has also been found to be transmitted from one generation to the next, particularly when a parent normalizes his or her own harsh treatment.[41,42]

Experiencing warm, empathic responses from a medical professional can offer a new model of relating, especially for parents whose behavior might tend to evoke judgment or recrimination from health care professionals.

Probing More Deeply

A Address Specific Risk Factors for Child Development and Family Functioning/ Allow Parents to Reflect How Cultural Traditions Contribute to Their Expectations of Child Behavior and Development

In addition to addressing the concerns that were brought up by the family in the context of the pediatric visit, it is important to inquire about specific risk factors for child developmental and behavioral problems. Divorce, marital discord, domestic violence, substance abuse, poverty, stress, perinatal mood or anxiety disorder, financial stresses, fears related to immigration status, tensions related to race and ethnicity, and a lack of social support are just a few of the struggles that affect today's families and impact the early parent-child relationship. In the context of the health supervision visit, primary pediatric health care professionals are well positioned to identify the negative impact of family-level adversities on child development. Furthermore, in the context of a family-centered pediatric medical home, the primary pediatric health care professional is also well poised to initiate interventions to optimize safety, stability, and nurturance in the caregiving relationship and to foster health, academic success, and child well-being.[43]

Relevant areas of inquiry with parents include their mood, family ties, work issues, perceived social support, social affiliations, child-care needs, health status, financial security, and neighborhood safety. These conditions influence the dynamic of the family and are foundational to supporting a child's health and growth.[44] Risk factors that affect the stability of the caregiving environment can manifest as child health and behavioral concerns[45,46] and can affect parenting practices.[47] The pediatric health supervision visit is a natural opportunity to inquire about the presence of risk factors that can challenge caregiving, including maternal depression, domestic violence, poverty, community violence, and parental discord, and to identify protective factors, including the presence of social and community support.

During the last decade, we have grown in our understanding of the detrimental effects of toxic stress and early childhood adversity on child health and well-being.[13,46,48,49] Toxic stress is described as the prolonged exposure to adverse childhood experiences (eg, child abuse or neglect, parental substance abuse, and maternal depression) in the absence of the buffering protection of a supportive, adult relationship.[48] Children exposed to such harsh conditions are at risk of developing stress-induced changes in the architecture of their developing brains that can have permanent effect on a multiplicity of functions, including stress regulation, skill acquisition, memory, and cognition.[13] The long-term health risks of the allostatic load of childhood stress are well established.[50]

Pediatric practices, with the deep regard communities have for them, are uniquely situated to identify and offer linkages to support.[44] Primary pediatric health care professionals who sensitively listen to and validate the experiences of feeling overwhelmed or numbed by the stresses that a parent identifies can lessen the severity of the stress. Some parents struggle with histories of unresolved adverse childhood experiences and often unwittingly recreate similar situations with their children.[51] Practitioners who are trained to sensitively ask about and respond to parental history of adversity can strengthen the relationship with a parent who may be working very hard to change behavioral patterns that were established in their distant past.[42,51]

In addition, special attention must be placed on the role of culture on parenting and child development and behavior. Cultural sensitivity implies an awareness of the influence of multiple factors that can shape the priorities and perspectives of individuals and families in society.[52] Culture can influence a parent's understanding and interpretation of child development and behavior[53] and can influence parenting practices.[54] The role of culture in families should be explored to better understand the issues that affect the health care of patients and their families.[55] For the pediatric patient, this can include, but is not limited to, the following: parenting philosophies, the influence of the American culture, parenting practices and discipline, religion and spirituality, and behavioral expectations. Some targeted questions to explore the role of culture in parenting are as follows:[54]

- Who do you live with?
- Whom do you trust to take care of your child?
- What are some important values that you want to teach your child?
- Do you want your child to keep your cultural traditions? In what way?
- Does spirituality and religion play a role in raising your children? How?
- How do you teach your child right from wrong?
- How do you discipline your child?
- Do you use any cultural or home remedies?
- What are some hopes and dreams that you have for your child?

Western practices of child rearing naturally inform a US-trained pediatric health care professional. When working with immigrant or families from non-Western societies, understanding the cultural lens through which the parents view child development and behavior can serve as an important framework in providing anticipatory guidance, feedback, and formulating a therapeutic plan with the family as well as avoiding offering culturally insensitive guidance that may serve to undermine the developing relationship with the family. Finally, refugee families, who have often come from unsafe situations, face particular challenges that can negatively affect parenting, including loss, trauma, and grief. In order to create a shared understanding of the parenting practices, more specific caregiving and context questions can be helpful. In addition to the questions noted above, the following are suggested:[56]

- How do you see your role in feeding your child?
- How do you show love to your child?
- How do you comfort your child?
- How has your move to the United States affected the way you show love to and respond to your child?
- Do you feel your parenting practices are respected in the United States?
- What barriers do you face? What supports do you need?
- What could we do to offer more support?

Providing Anticipatory Guidance and Feedback

R Reflect With Parents on Their Experience of the Child/Reframe Child Behavior and Development in Terms of the Child's Developmental Level /Revisit Therapeutic Goals Set

Once the family's concerns are identified in the pediatric interview and the appropriate assessment has been undertaken, it is important to provide feedback and anticipatory guidance to families. Anticipatory guidance is the provision of information to parents or children with an expected outcome being a change in parent or patient attitude or knowledge,[57] which can serve as the mechanism for strengthening a child's developmental potential.[58] The primary pediatric health care professional has the opportunity to support and encourage parents in the parenting role and help foster a sense of parental competence in the midst of challenging caregiving experiences. In the context of the supportive pediatric "holding environment," the primary pediatric health care professional can help the parent experience a sense of safety, nurturance, and support, and can address, acknowledge, and validate the parent's fears, anxieties, and experiences. In reflecting back to parents, the dialogue they have shared, (eg, *"What I hear you saying is . . ."; "It sounds like you are most concerned about . . ."*) the primary pediatric health care professional sends a very powerful message to the parent: *"I have heard your concerns, and I am with you in this process."* When a parent is assured that his or her fears and concerns are heard and recognized, it then becomes easier to offer another perspective of the child's behavior, perhaps informed by the child's developmental level: *"I wonder, when your child hits you because he is frustrated, it is because he does not have the words to tell you how he is feeling, so he communicates his feelings to you the only way he knows how, with his body instead of with his words."* Such interventions promote parental reflective functioning,[59] which is defined as the capacity to be aware of one's own emotions and to imagine the thoughts and feelings of another; it informs the process by which parents intuit the needs of young children. Parents with a history of having been maltreated who demonstrate higher levels of reflective functioning show stronger capacity to inhibit negative responses to children, thus protecting their child from intergenerationally transmitted trauma and maltreatment.[51]

Undoubtedly, there will be times when the primary pediatric health care professional and the parent have differences in philosophies, perspectives, and even in management strategies. At times, parents may even be resistant and difficult to engage. This is when it is helpful to revisit the initial therapeutic goals that were mutually agreed upon at the beginning of the visit. Often, the parent, child, and pediatric health care professional can find common ground and a therapeutic alliance by joining together to actualize the expressed hopes, (eg, *"I want us to have a better relationship.")* and prevent the spoken fears, (eg, *"I don't want him to get into drugs or a bad group of friends.")* When there are areas of ideological difference, the parents and health care professional can connect at the level of their shared desire to optimize the health and development of the pediatric patient. In an open and supportive bidirectional communication, the primary pediatric health care professional can engage in an open and nonthreatening dialogue with the parent about what can be done to foster and optimize the child's health, developmental, and behavioral outcomes.

Steps for the Future

E Empower the Parent and Child: Formulating an Action Plan to Address Concerns

One of the most powerful strategies a primary pediatric health care professional can offer a family experiencing challenges is to highlight the family's strengths and identify their capacity to achieve the therapeutic goals set. In the context of this family-centered approach, the parents and child are viewed as partners in the treatment process in hopes of facilitating family empowerment.[60] This family-centered approach to addressing developmental and behavioral concerns should address the needs of the whole family and should address the needs of the child in the context of the caregiving environment. Child behavior problems cannot be divorced from the experiences of the immediate caregiving environment,[61,62] and interventions to address child behavior concerns should address the needs of the family unit as a whole. These interventions should include such strategies as expanding social supports, utilizing family strengths, individualizing resources, and delivering services consistent with the family's cultural values and beliefs.[60] However, it has been posited that the most important element for treatment success is related to a family's ability to feel a sense of empowerment and locus of control over the presenting problem. By empowering families to develop possible solutions to problems or needs, the primary pediatric health care professional is not only helping with the current situation but is also helping the family to develop skills to solve future problems independently. In this approach, the primary pediatric health care professional involves the family as an active collaborator in finding a solution to the problem presented. The primary pediatric health care professional, through thoughtful and empathic interviewing, seeks out the treatment goals of the family as they present for evaluation and then actively seeks their input and alliance in formulating a treatment goal.[1]

In creating this health care professional–family alliance, the family members become active participants in identifying and implementing a solution to the identified concerns. Family empowerment has been demonstrated to be an important factor in child behavioral outcomes. When children and families were included in the decision-making process and were provided services that were sensitive to their unique needs, values, and strengths, parents reported improvement in their child's behavior and a greater confidence in their ability to handle behavioral concerns in the future.[60]

To foster the parents' feeling of empowerment and competence in the parenting role, it is important that the parents experience a sense of support and connectedness in their caregiving roles. This can occur through connecting the family with other supports and services available in the community (see Chapter 25: Social and Community Services for Children With Developmental Disabilities and/or Behavioral Disorders and Their Families). Supporting the needs of the child and family as part of a seamless continuum has been captured by the concept of contextual pediatrics or the idea that developmental support and guidance to families cannot be provided in isolation: Pediatric health care must be integrated into the framework of other community services.[63] The changing face of pediatric health care calls for a greater emphasis on collaborating with community partners such as teachers, child-care providers, early intervention specialists, etc., to optimize family functioning and child health.[44] This framework recognizes that early childhood health is an essential antecedent of health across the life span. Although the primary pediatric health care professional screens for social-emotional concerns in the context of the health supervision visit, collaborations with community partners to initiate preventive interventions early are critical to shaping a healthy childhood and reducing future health disparities. An interdisciplinary, cross-agency commitment to fostering healthy emotional development is necessary to provide the supportive, responsive, care that children need in all of the environments in which they live, grow, and develop. Because of the relationship primary pediatric health care professionals have with children and their families, they are well poised to identify maladaptive threats to child health and development, including the sequelae of poverty, environmental pollution, toxic stress, and other social determinants of health.[64,65] By the virtue of their holistic training, primary pediatric health care professionals understand the profound and enduring effects of poverty and environmental disadvantage on the health and well-being of children[66] and, using their authority as medical professionals, are well positioned to effect organizational change in the lives of children and their families. Pediatric advocacy is best operationalized in partnership with community-based organizations, business leaders, philanthropists, and policymakers[66,67] and can address a broad range of topics relevant to child health and family well-being including neighborhood adversity,[67] food insecurity, and the role of medical-legal partnerships.[68]

Conclusion

Given the frequent contact a primary pediatric health care professional has with families, there is a natural opportunity for primary pediatric health care professionals to talk with families about development, behavior, and psychosocial issues. The primary pediatric health care professional has the opportunity to optimize developmental, behavioral, and social-emotional development by being attentive to the quality of the family environment in which the child lives, by being attuned to risk factors in the caregiving environment, and by providing support and interventions to empower families when vulnerabilities are identified. By partnering with other childhood resources in the community, the primary pediatric health care professional can foster the health and well-being of the family and optimize the health and development of children across their lifespans.

References

1. Cheng, MKS. New approaches for creating the therapeutic alliance: solution-focused interviewing, motivational interviewing, and the medication interest model. *Psychiatr Clin North Am.* 2007;30(2):157–166
2. Bordin, ES. The generalizability of the psychoanalytic concept of the working alliance. *Psychother Theory Res Pract.* 1979;16:252–260
3. American Academy of Pediatrics Medical Home Initiatives for Children With Special Health Care Needs Project Advisory Committee. The medical home. *Pediatrics.* 2002;110:184–186. Reaffirmed May 2008
4. McAllister JW, Cooley WC, Van Cleave J, Boudreau AA, Kuhlthau K. Medical home transformation in pediatric primary care—what drives change? *Ann Fam Med.* 2013;11(1 suppl):S90–S98
5. McAllister JW, Presler E, Cooley WC. Practice-based care coordination: a medical home essential. *Pediatrics.* 2007;120:e723–e733
6. American Academy of Pediatrics Committee on Psychosocial Aspects of Child and Family Health and Task Force on Mental Health. Policy statement—The future of pediatrics: mental health competencies for pediatric primary care. *Pediatrics.* 2009;124(1):410–421
7. American Academy of Pediatrics Committee on Standards of Child Health Care. *Standards of Child Health Care,* 2nd ed. Evanston, IL: American Academy of Pediatrics; 1972
8. Boreman CD, Thomsgard MC, Fernandez SA, Coury DL. Resident training in developmental/behavioral pediatrics: where do we stand? *Clin Pediatr (Phila).* 2007;46:135–145
9. Shah PE, Muzik M, Rosenblum KL. Optimizing the early parent-child relationship: windows of opportunity for parents and pediatricians. *Curr Probl Pediatr Adolesc Health Care.* 2011;41:183–187
10. Shah P. Pediatric primary care: an opportunity to optimize attachment. *Zero to Three.* 2007;27(3):12–19
11. Winnicott DW. *Through Paediatrics to Psycho-Analysis.* New York, NY: Basic Books, Inc.; 1975
12. Schor EL, American Academy of Pediatrics Task Force on the Family. Family pediatrics: report of the Task Force on the Family. *Pediatrics.* 2003;111(6 Pt 2):1541–1571
13. Garner AS, Shonkoff JP, American Academy of Pediatrics Committee on Psychosocial Aspects of Child and Family Health, Committee on Early Childhood, Adoption and Dependent Care, Section on Developmental and Behavioral Pediatrics. Early childhood adversity, toxic stress, and the role of the pediatrician: translating developmental science into lifelong health. *Pediatrics.* 2002;129(1):e224–e231
14. Gorski P. Contemporary pediatric practice: in support of infant mental health (imaging and imagining). *Infant Ment Health J.* 2001;22:188–200
15. Gleason MM, Shah PE, Boris NW. Assessment and interviewing. In: Kliegman RM, Behrman RE, Jenson HB, Stanton BF, eds. *Nelson Textbook of Pediatrics.* 18th ed. Philadelphia, PA: WB Saunders; 2007:101–105
16. Shah PE. Interviewing and counseling children and families. In: *American Academy of Pediatrics Developmental and Behavioral Pediatrics.* Voigt RG, Macias MM, Myers SM, eds. 1st ed. Elk Grove Village, IL: American Academy of Pediatrics; 2010:23–36
17. Sroufe LA, Egeland B, Carlson EA, Collins WA. *The Development of the Person: The Minnesota Study of Risk and Adaptation.* New York, NY: Guilford Press; 2005
18. Ainsworth MDS, Blehar MC, Waters E, Wall, S. *Patterns of Attachment: A Psychological Study of the Strange Situation.* Hillsdale, NJ: Lawrence Erlbaum; 1978

19. Marvin R, Cooper G, Hoffman K, Powell B. The Circle of Security Project: attachment-based intervention with caregiver-preschool child dyads. *Attach Hum Dev.* 2002;4:107–124

20. Sawyer SM, Afifi RA, Bearinger LH, et al. Adolescence: a foundation for future health. *Lancet.* 2012;379: 1630–1640

21. DiGiuseppe R, Linscott J, Jilton R. Developing the therapeutic alliance in child—adolescent psychotherapy. *Applied and Preventive Psychology.* 1996;5:85–100

22. Macnab AJ, Richards J, Green G. Family-oriented care during pediatric inter-hospital transport. *Patient Educ Couns.* 1999;36:247–257

23. Halfon N, Inkelas M. Optimizing the Health and Development of Children. *JAMA.* 2003;290:3136–3138

24. Halfon N, Hochstein M, Sareen H, et al. Barriers to the provision of developmental assessment during pediatric health supervision. In: *Pediatric Academic Societies Meeting.* Baltimore, MD: American Academy of Pediatrics; 2001. Periodic Survey #46

25. Horwitz SM, Leaf PJ, Leventhal JM. Identification of psychosocial problems in pediatric primary care: do family attitudes make a difference? *Arch Pediatr Adolesc Med.* 1998;152:367–371

26. Horwitz SM, Gary LC, Briggs-Gowan MJ, Carter AS. Do needs drive services use in young children? *Pediatrics.* 2003;112:1373–1378

27. Horwitz SM, Leaf PJ, Leventhal JM, Forsyth B, Speechley KN. Identification and management of psychosocial and developmental problems in community-based, primary care pediatric practices. *Pediatrics.* 1992;89:480–485

28. Carter A, Briggs-Gowan, MJ, Davis NO. Assessment of young children's social-emotional development and psychopathology: recent advances and recommendations for practice. *J Child Psychol Psychiatry.* 2004;45:109–134

29. Stein MT, Plonsky C, Zuckerman B. Reformatting the 9 month health supervision visit to enhance developmental, behavioral and family concerns. *J Dev Behav Pediatr.* 26(1):56–60

30. Sommers-Flanagan J, Sommers-Flanagan R. Our favorite tips for interviewing couples and families. *Psychiatr Clin North Am.* 2007;30(2):275–281

31. Committee on Psychosocial Aspects of Child and Family Health. The pediatrician and the "New Morbidity." *Pediatrics.* 1993;92:731–733

32. American Academy of Pediatrics Council on.Children With Disabilities. Developmental surveillance and screening of infants and young children. *Pediatrics.* 2001;108:192–196

33. Cooper S, Valleley RJ, Polaha J, Begeny J, Evans JH. Running out of time: physician management of behavioral health concerns in rural pediatric primary care. *Pediatrics.* 2006;118(1): e132–e138

34. Leslie LK, Sarah R, Palfrey JS,; Behrman, R. Child health care in changing times. *Pediatrics.* 1998;101(4 pt 2):746–752

35. Glascoe FP, Dworkin PH. The role of parents in the detection of developmental and behavioral problems. *Pediatrics.* 1995;95(6):829–836

36. Bogin J. Enhancing developmental services in primary care: the Help Me Grow experience. *J Dev Behav Pediatr.* 2006;27(1 Suppl):S8–S12

37. Stern-Bruschweiler N, Stern DN. A model for conceptualizing the role of the mother's representational world in various mother-infant therapies. *Infant Ment Health J.* 1989;10:142–156

38. Zeanah CH, Benoit D. Clinical applications of a parent perception interview in infant mental health. *Child Adolesc Psychiatr Clin N Am.* 1995;4(3):539–554

39. Zeanah CH. Mother's representations of their infants are concordant with infant attachment classifications. *Developmental Issues in Psychiatry and Psychology* 1994;1:9–18

40. Zeanah CH, Jr, ed. *Handbook of Infant Mental Health,* Zeanah H. Jr., ed. 2nd ed. New York, NY: Guilford Press; 2000

41. Belsky J, Jaffee SR, Sligo J, Woodward L, Silva PA. Intergenerational transmission of warm-sensitive-stimulating parenting: A prospective study of mothers and fathers of 3-year-olds. *Child Dev.* 2005;76:384–396

42. Fraiberg S, Adelson E, Shapiro V. Ghosts in the nursery: a psychoanalytic approach to the problems of impaired infant-mother relationships. *J Am Acad Child Psychiatry.* 1975;14:387–421

43. Garner AS, Forkey H, Szilagyi M. Translating developmental science to address childhood adversity. *Acad Pediatr.* 2015;15:493–502

44. Mistry KB, Minkovitz CS, Riley AW, et al. A new framework for childhood health promotion: the role of policies and programs in building capacity and foundations of early childhood health. *Am J Public Health.* 2012;102:1688–96

45. Larson K, Russ SA, Crall JJ, Halfon N. Influence of multiple social risks on children's health. *Pediatrics.* 2008;121:337–344

46. Shonkoff JP, Richter L, van der Gaag J, Bhutta ZA. An integrated scientific framework for child survival and early childhood development. *Pediatrics.* 2012;129:e460–e472

47. McLearn KT, Minkovitz CS, Strobino DS, Marks E, Hou W. The timing of maternal depressive symptoms and mothers' parenting practices with young children: implications for pediatric practice. *Pediatrics.* 2006;118:e174–e182

48. Shonkoff JP, Garner AS. The lifelong effects of early childhood adversity and toxic stress. *Pediatrics.* 2012;129:e232–e46

49. Shonkoff JP. Building a new biodevelopmental framework to guide the future of early childhood policy. *Child Dev.* 2010;81:357–67

50. Felitti VJ, Anda RF, Nordenberg D, et al. Relationship of childhood abuse and household dysfunction to many of the leading causes of death in adults. The Adverse Childhood Experiences (ACE) Study. *Am J Prev Med.* 1998;14:245–58

51. Ensink K, Normandin L, Plamondon A, Berthelot N, Fonagy P. Intergenerational pathways from reflective functioning to infant attachment through parenting. *Canadian Journal of Behavioural Science/Revue canadienne des sciences du comportement.* 2016;48:9

52. Dennis RE, Giangreco MF. Creating conversation: reflections on cultural sensitivity in family interviewing. *Exceptional Children.* 1996;63(1):103–116

53. Gidwani P, Opitz G, Perrin JM. Mother's views on hyperactivity: a cross cultural perspective. *J Dev Behav Pediatr.* 2006;27:121–125

54. McEvoy M, Lee C, O'Neill A, Groisman A, Roberts-Butelman K, Dinghra K, Porder, K. Are there universal parenting concepts among culturally diverse families in an inner-city pediatric clinic? *J Pediatr Health Care.* 2005;19:142–150

55. Flores G, Association of Medical Pediatric Department Chairs, Inc. Providing culturally competent pediatrics care: integrating pediatricians, institutions, families, and communities in the process. *J Pediatr.* 2003;143(1):1–2

56. Mawani FN. Sharing attachment across cultures. *IMPrint, Newsletter of Infant Mental Health Promotion Project (IMP).* 2001–2002;32:1–5]

57. Dworkin PH. Promoting development through child health services Introduction to the Help Me Grow roundtable. *J Dev Behav Pediatr.* 2006;27:S2–S4

58. Brazelton TB. Anticipatory guidance. *Pediatr Clin North Am.* 1975;22:533–544

59. Fonagy P, Target M. Attachment and reflective function: their role in self-organization. *Dev Psychopathol.* 1997;9(4):679–700

60. Graves KN, Shelton TL. Family empowerment as a mediator between family-centered systems of care and changes in child functioning: identifying an important mechanism of change. *J Child Fam Stud.* 2007;16(4):556–566

61. Sameroff A. A unified theory of development: a dialectic integration of nature and nurture. *Child Dev.* 2010;81:6–22

62. Sameroff AJ, Fiese BH. Models of development and developmental risk. In: Zeanah C, Jr., ed. *Handbook of Infant Mental Health.* 2nd ed. New York, NY: Guilford Press; 2000:3–19

63. Green, M. No child is an island: contextual pediatrics and the "new" health supervision. *Pediatr Clin North Am.* 1995;42:79–87

64. American Academy of Pediatrics Council on Community Pediatrics. Poverty and child health in the United States. *Pediatrics.* 2016;137(4):pii:e20160339

65. Kuo AA, Shetgiri R, Guerrero AD, et al. A public health approach to pediatric residency education: responding to social determinants of health. *J Grad Med Educ.* 2011;3:217–23

66. Plax K, Donnelly J, Federico SG, Brock, L, Kaczorowski JM. An essential role for pediatricians: becoming child poverty change agents for a lifetime. *Acad Pediatr.* 2016;16:S147–S154

67. Henize AW, Beck AF, Klein MD, Adams M, Kahn RS. A road map to address the social determinants of health through community collaboration. *Pediatrics.* 2015;136:e993–e1001

68. Gilbert AL, Downs SM. Medical legal partnership and health informatics impacting child health: interprofessional innovations. *J Interprof Care.* 2015;29:564–569

CHAPTER 6

Early Intervention

Jennifer K. Poon, MD, FAAP

David O. Childers Jr, MD, FAAP

Primary pediatric health care professionals are tasked with assisting the promotion and optimization of child development. Facilitation of optimal development is one of the key roles not only for primary care pediatricians but also for pediatric subspecialists and other primary care professionals who care for children. The American Academy of Pediatrics (AAP) Council on Children With Disabilities provides guidance for primary pediatric health care professionals through the policy statement, "Role of the Medical Home in Family-Centered Early Intervention Services."[1] This policy statement states that various federal and state statutes mandate that community-based, coordinated, multidisciplinary, family-centered early intervention programs (EIPs) be established, and primary pediatric health care professionals, in close collaboration with families and the early intervention (EI) team, should assume a proactive role in ensuring that at-risk children receive appropriate clinical and developmental EI services.[1] Thus, when concerns are elicited through developmental surveillance or screening, primary pediatric health care professionals should refer their patients to local EIPs. (See also Chapter 9, Developmental and Behavioral Surveillance and Screening Within the Medical Home.) EIPs exist to benefit development in children from birth to 36 months of age who have an existing developmental disability or delay, or who are at risk for developmental delay.

What Is Early Intervention?

EIPs strive to improve developmental outcomes for children who exhibit or are at high risk for developmental delays. They are based on evidence that much of early brain development is experience-dependent and that developmental trajectories can potentially be improved by appropriate and EI. Aims of specific programs may include teaching parents about infant development and how to enhance developmental stimulation, helping parents understand their infant's behavioral cues, acknowledging and addressing sources of parental stress, enhancing the parent-child relationship, or providing developmental therapies (eg, physical therapy, occupational therapy).

EIPs are mandated by federal law and available in every county in all 50 states, as well as the District of Columbia. These programs provide a system of family-centered services to help children who are experiencing developmental delays or who have a medical diagnosis that carries a high risk for developmental delay (eg, genetic disorders such as Down syndrome, very-low-birth-weight preterm infants). EI services were first mandated in 1986 by an amendment to the 1975 Education for All Handicapped Children Act. Over time, the Education for All Handicapped Children Act was reauthorized and renamed the Individuals with Disabilities Education Act (IDEA), and the guidelines for EI services are listed under Part C, the "Grants for Infants and Families Program" of IDEA; thus, EI is often times referred to as Part C. Currently, EI services are mandated to meet the needs of any child from birth through 36 months of age who has delays in one or more of the following areas:

- Cognitive
- Physical (gross motor, fine motor, vision, and hearing)
- Communication
- Social or emotional
- Adaptive
- Children referred to Children's Protective Services who are detained based on concerns of neglect and/or abuse (mandated referral under the Child Abuse Protection Act)

A state may choose to continue Part C services beyond age 3 years; however, those services will cease at the age when the child is eligible to enter kindergarten or elementary school. Parents must be informed of the differences between services provided under Part C and preschool services provided under Part B of IDEA.

Part C of IDEA awards grant funding to support comprehensive, coordinated care among different disciplines and agencies to eligible infants and toddlers from birth to 36 months of age. While Part C provides guidelines for eligibility criteria, each state determines what at-risk conditions and diagnoses are eligible. IDEA was reauthorized in 2004 (IDEA 2004) to include additional criteria for development of early identification and referral programs, development of Individualized Family Service Plans (IFSP). It also strengthened the requirement for provision of services in natural environments and established the Interagency Coordination Council (ICC). The ICC, which exists to ensure and advise proper implementation of Part C, is a statewide interagency system that is multidisciplinary and includes parents.

Under the IDEA, a family must be offered, at no cost to the family, a developmental eligibility assessment within 45 days of the request for evaluation. If the child is determined to be eligible for EI services, the intervention services may be offered at no cost to the family, billed to the family's medical insurance, or supported by family co-pays (participation fees), as determined by each state. By federal statute, available services must include[1]

- Early identification, screening, and assessment services
- Care coordination services

- Medical services (only for diagnostic or evaluation purposes)
- Family training, counseling, and home visits
- Special instruction (provided by early EI specialists)
- Speech-language therapy
- Audiology services
- Occupational and physical therapy
- Psychological services
- Health services that are necessary to enable the infant or toddler to benefit from other EI services
- Social work services
- Vision services
- Assistive technology devices and services
- Transportation, language interpretation services, and other related costs that are necessary to enable a child and family to receive other services

The Evidence for Early Intervention

EI has been shown to improve parent-child interactions, help parents modify their behavior in response to their child's needs, provide support for families, reduce parental stress, and help families learn strategies for effectively advocating for their children.[2] In terms of altering the developmental trajectory, EI has been shown to be quantitatively most successful in children with mild versus severe delays, in children at environmental risk (eg, low socioeconomic status, barriers to appropriate developmental stimulation at home or child care, toxic stress) versus neurobiological risk (genetic syndromes, structural brain anomalies) for developmental delay, and in children at risk for developmental disability versus in children with known disability.[3] Neurocognitive research has shown that there are optimal periods of brain development in which learning is most efficient.[1] Intervention that is well planned and provided as early as possible can improve the functional outcome and quality of life for all children with developmental delays or those who are at risk for developmental delays and their families.[4-6] Intervention services provided during the preschool years have the potential to provide the greatest benefit to children and their families in minimizing developmental and behavioral problems for children at risk. They also serve to maximize the child's functional potential and prevent secondary social, emotional, or behavioral problems at later stages of development, and they provide support to families in caring for their children at home.[4-6]

Shonkoff and Hauser-Cram conducted a meta-analysis of 31 studies of EI for families of children with disabilities less than 3 years of age.[7] They found that EI services were effective in the promotion of developmental progress, but children classified as "developmentally delayed" made greater cognitive gains than those who were found to have more severe cognitive disabilities, and children with motor disabilities were found to make the least gains. Well-defined EI curricula were shown to have greater effects on child development, as opposed to programs with less structure. A high level of parental involvement and interventions that pair the child and parent together during service delivery proved to be the most effective characteristics of EI programs.

While EI may serve a variety of types and severity of conditions with different intensity and types of services, studies have shown that there are short- and long-term improvements in cognitive outcomes, social-emotional function, as well as helping parent-child interactions with a supportive environment for the household.[2,8-13] Overall, the literature supports that EI programs that focus on the family unit are more effective than those programs that are solely focused on the child. While children with severe developmental disabilities living in very stimulating home environments make the least quantitative gains through EI services, these services still foster a more comfortable and developmentally appropriate interaction between the parent and child with a disability (preventing secondary social, emotional, or behavioral impairments), enhance the ability of parents to care for their child with a severe disability at home, and improve functional outcomes. For families with children with severe disabilities, the provision of EI services can also be a critical component of long-term acceptance, knowing that intervention programming was implemented.[13]

Contemporary research has shown that some of the most profound impacts of EI are not only on the child but also on the parents and family units related to the child. The National Early Intervention Longitudinal Study (NEILS) found that families who participated in EI reported positive family outcomes at completion and felt that they were better off as a result of it.[2,14] Furthermore, they felt competent in their roles as parents, as well as in their collaborative roles with professionals. Most were positive about their child's future.[14] The NEILS also identified some challenges, such as parents feeling less competent in handling their child's behavior versus handling other basic needs, and parents reported less chance for participation in community activities (eg, religious, school, and social events) versus the strong support received from their own family and friends.

Environmental risk factors can clearly have a negative impact on child development, and this potential negative impact can be prevented or ameliorated through EI.[15,16] The Abecedarian Project[17] demonstrated the benefits of EI in children from low-income, multirisk families. This study found that on average, those who received EI had higher cognitive test scores, higher achievement scores in reading and math, more years of education, a higher likelihood of attending a 4-year college, and lower likelihood of becoming teenage parents. In 2016, the AAP policy statement, "Poverty and Child Health in the United States," highlighted the effects of poverty as a contributor to child health disparities and tasked primary pediatric health care professionals with helping to ameliorate the adverse effects of poverty through both community practice and advocacy.[18] Unfortunately, while it is most effective in children at environmental risk, many EI programs fail to qualify children at environmental risk for EI services, if they are not also exhibiting a large enough quantitative delay in their development.

The Primary Pediatric Health Care Professional's Role

The primary pediatric health care professional plays a key role in identifying developmental concerns. Routine pediatric health supervision visits are crucial times when a child's development should be reviewed with the family. In 2006, the AAP published a policy statement regarding surveillance and screening for developmental problems (see Chapter 9, Developmental and Behavioral Surveillance and Screening Within the Medical Home).[19] Developmental surveillance should be conducted at every well-child visit, and the components of surveillance include

- Eliciting parental concerns about development and behavior
- Recognizing protective and risk factors for developmental delay (eg, prematurity or poverty)
- Obtaining and recording a developmental history
- Making accurate direct observations of the child
- Documenting findings based on this process

Developmental screening using a standardized screening instrument should occur at the 9-, 18-, and 30-month well-child visits. If concerns about development or behavior are identified by developmental surveillance or screening, a referral to the family's local EI program should be made. While identifying a possible developmental delay can begin an uncomfortable conversation, waiting/monitoring is not the recommended course. Primary pediatric health care professionals should explain their concerns to families; this provides an opportunity for a bidirectional conversation not only about the child's development but also about the family's viewpoints and expectations, which may be useful information to share with the EI team.[20] Additionally, most research has shown that families are highly satisfied with their involvement in EIPs, which should boost primary pediatric health care professionals' confidence in making referrals for EI services.[4–6,12,21–24] EI services that are able to combine child-focused educational activities with strengthening of the parent-child relationship are most effective.[25] Families of children with disabilities face significant challenges, and family support is an essential component of EI for these families.

From a practice standpoint, a method for referral tracking helps facilitate a timely evaluation.[26] Furthermore, when referring a patient to EI, it may be wise to obtain family permission to communicate with the EI program, so that the provider is aware of the evaluation results and the EI program is aware of the medical history. While developmental screening tools help to identify children at risk for a possible developmental disorder, they do not yield a diagnosis. Fortunately, a specific diagnosis (such as autism spectrum disorder, intellectual disability, or cerebral palsy) is not necessary for an EI referral, and waiting for a diagnostic evaluation only prolongs access to services. However, along with the EI referral, primary pediatric health care professionals are responsible for pursuing a developmental diagnosis and underlying medical etiology, either within the medical home or through subspecialty consultation (see Chapter 4, Biological Influences on Child Development and Behavior and Medical Evaluation of Children with Developmental-Behavioral Disorders, and Chapter 11, Making Developmental-Behavioral Diagnoses).

Primary pediatric health care professionals should be familiar with the referral process for EI in their state. States have different names for their EIPs, and the agencies providing EI services vary from state to state. Each state has its specific eligibility criteria for qualification for receipt of EI services and fee structure to fund EI services. While guidelines exist as to who may be eligible, there is variability among states regarding eligible diagnoses, and there is even variability in the definition of developmental delay across states (eg, use of percent delay versus standard deviation or a combination).[27] Currently, 22 state-specific, numerical definitions for EI eligibility exist in the United States. As mentioned earlier, each state must provide the initial assessment at no cost to families. Thereafter costs are state dependent, and primary pediatric health care professionals should be aware of the costs of their state's programs for families.

Studies have found that in children without established medical diagnoses, EI referral rates were lower for conditions such as speech delay and parental concern.[28] As previously mentioned, there is not a prerequisite to have an established medical diagnosis for a referral to EI. If a concern is raised by developmental surveillance or screening, primary pediatric health care professionals should promptly refer to their local EI. More information about individual state EI programs can be found through the Early Childhood Technical Assistance Center's Web site: **http://ectacenter.org/contact/ ptccoord.asp.**

Once a referral is made to EI, the program will contact the family to arrange for an evaluation to establish eligibility. Participation by families in EI is not mandatory, and the evaluation and services are contingent upon family approval.

What Is an IFSP?

After a child is referred to be evaluated by his or her local EIP, a standardized assessment instrument evaluating development in at least 5 domains (cognitive, physical, communication, social or emotional, adaptive), administered by 2 different disciplines, is mandated. Furthermore, there is an assessment of the family's resources, priorities, and concerns, to identify the support and resources needed. Following this assessment, if eligibility is determined, the EI staff and family meet as a team to develop an IFSP that documents the specific plan for how the EIP will address both the delays and concerns identified during standardized assessment and the parental concerns and goals.

An IFSP is essentially analogous to the Individualized Education Program (IEP) for children receiving IDEA Part B special educational services. It is referred to as a family service plan because of the family-centered focus of EI, and the interventions are delivered in the "most natural environment" of the home or child-care setting.

The guidelines for IFSPs vary from state to state, but the IFSP is a legal contract, and generally, an IFSP comprises the following:

- An objective description of the child's current development in all domains
- Family and caregiver resources, priorities, and concerns
- Expected measureable results or outcomes
- Specific services to be received
- The natural environment in which the services will be delivered
- The projected timeline for service initiation, frequency, and duration
- An identified service coordinator who is responsible for implementing the plan and coordinating with others
- Steps to help with transition to public school services at 36 months of age

Parental consent is required before the provision of EI services. The IFSP should be reviewed periodically by the multidisciplinary team to review whether the current needs are being met. The plan is evaluated yearly and modified as appropriate. The IFSP presents an opportunity for primary pediatric health care professionals to work with families and other professionals in care coordination.[29]

EI services are optimally provided in the "most natural environment," meaning either the child's home or child-care program, obviating the need for the family to travel to center-based services. By implementing interventions in the most natural setting and with a caregiver training component, the interventions can be carried out continuously and integrated into the daily routine, resulting in an immersion model that both increases stimuli to the child's developing brain and enhances parent-child interactions. Parent education is known to be an important component of EI, as most of a child's opportunities to practice developmental skills occur within the context of daily routines. Parents can be taught how to adapt the child's play environment to provide opportunities for active learning. Clinic-based therapies are not necessarily advantageous over home-based services, and EI programs aim to provide services within the child's natural environment. Having a well-defined curriculum is another characteristic of EI programs associated with greater effectiveness.[7]

After services are initiated, collaboration between the primary pediatric health care professional and the EI program is essential. This includes the exchange of information among the EI team, parents, and the medical home. For example, with the parents' permission, the EI team should keep the primary pediatric health care professional informed of specific therapy goals, objectives, and progress, while the primary pediatric health care professional should keep the intervention team and parents aware of new diagnoses or changes in the child's medical condition. Elements of the role of primary pediatric health care professionals in being a member of the collaborative EI team include[30]

- Communication: avoiding medical jargon and formal terminology, two-way conversation
- Commitment: demonstrating dedication to children and their families

- Equality: valuing all members' contributions, especially the family who facilitates much of the team's functions
- Skills: competence; willingness to learn and keep up to date
- Trust: reliable, safe, and discreet relationships
- Respect: being courteous and providing person-centered care rather than treating a medical diagnosis or label

Patient- and family-centered care coordination was highlighted by the AAP in a 2014 policy statement.[29] This statement encouraged primary pediatric health care professionals to facilitate care coordination, as this action optimizes quality and cost outcomes. Some of the recommendations that can be applied to caring for families enrolled in EI include

- Empowering families with knowledge and skills
- Ensuring needs are met through formal assessment, teams, and tracking
- Involving the family throughout the process
- Utilizing health information technology systems
- Providing care coordination across settings with comanagement
- Education of other health professionals who are stakeholders (eg, extended providers, staff, and trainees)

In addition to providing services in "the most natural environment," IDEA also provides a model with an early interventionist (or early childhood special educator) or other primary therapist who receives consultation from other disciplines as indicated. Most EI services are not directed toward a rehabilitation model (which is designed to provide one-on-one therapy between a therapist and a child to reacquire lost skills), but rather toward a habilitative model—early interventionists providing families and other caregivers a framework of developmentally stimulating experiences for the child to acquire developmental milestones—such that intervention can occur on a continuous basis throughout the day.

Primary pediatric health care professionals are often called on to prescribe the frequency of specific habilitative therapies (speech, occupational, or physical) that supplement the services provided by early childhood special educators.[31] Unfortunately, there is not a strong evidence base in the medical literature to guide health care professionals in this endeavor. While speech, occupational, and physical therapies clearly improve the developmental trajectory when employed in rehabilitative settings (such as in children who need to relearn previously acquired skills following a head injury), evidence to support the ability of these therapeutic modalities to clearly alter developmental trajectories in habilitative settings is less clear, although many studies have focused on scores on standardized developmental measures rather than on functional outcomes.[32,33] The most important concept for therapeutic intervention is that therapeutic goals need to be worked on both informally and formally throughout daily activities across settings, rather than being limited to the short therapy session. In this model, it is the parent or primary caregiver who becomes the true therapist and who generalizes the specific therapy across settings. This model requires a buy-in from both parents and therapists. Simplistically, a child may not need a speech therapist to start to talk or point; however, parents may require the services of the therapist to learn to engage their child in regular activities throughout the day and to establish a milieu to encourage the child's generalization of the specific goals of therapy. This model of parents as primary therapists is supported by results of the Early Intervention Collaborative Study, which showed that mother-child interaction was a key predictor of change in both child developmental outcomes and parent well-being beyond the type of disability experienced by the child. [7,34] In this study, family relations also predicted change in children's social skills.[34] Unfortunately, this consultative, family-centered model is not the historical approach to therapy; rather, the direct service model—therapist with child—is the model most therapists are trained in and what most parents expect. Primary pediatric health care professionals should assume an educational role with the family in explaining the importance of generalizing therapeutic goals and activities across settings. The results of the Early Intervention Collaborative Study showed that, despite the great variability of child and family function and of the types and extent of services offered, most young children in EIPs improved in many domains of functioning.[1,34]

At a systems level, primary pediatric health care professionals are at the forefront of identifying issues that need advocacy, such as advocating for appropriate and equal access to EI services for all eligible children. Furthermore, work may be done through state AAP chapters, as well as participating in local and state interagency coordination councils. Participation in these councils provides a medical perspective to the group members, who may include representative from state Medicaid programs, state welfare agencies, and other stakeholders.

Conclusion

Studies of EI have provided evidence to demonstrate positive impact upon individual children, as well as upon their families and caregivers. Furthermore, there are societal benefits, which may include reducing the economic burden through improved functional outcomes; reduced long-term social, emotional, or behavioral impairments; or a decreased need for special education services. Primary pediatric health care professionals, through their developmental surveillance and screening efforts, are thus most critical for identifying developmental and behavioral concerns and referring to EI services as early as possible to optimize outcomes for children and their families.

References

1. American Academy of Pediatrics Council on Children With Disabilities, Duby JC. Role of the medical home in family-centered early intervention services. *Pediatrics*. 2007;120(5):1153–1158

2. Bailey DB Jr, Hebbeler K, Spiker D, et al. Thirty-six-month outcomes for families of children who have disabilities and participated in early intervention. *Pediatrics*. 2005;116(6):1346–1352

3. Lipkin PH, Schertz M. Early intervention and its efficacy. In: Accardo PJ, ed. *Capute & Accardo's Neurodevelopmental Disabilities in Infancy and Childhood*. 3rd ed. Baltimore, MD: Paul H. Brookes Publishing; 2008:519–551

4. Shore R. *Rethinking the Brain: New Insights into Early Development*. New York, NY: Families and Work Institute; 1997

5. Wynder EL. Introduction to the report on the conference on the "critical" period of brain development. *Prev Med*. 1998;27(2):166–167

6. National Research Council (United States) and Institute of Medicine (United States) Committee on Integrating the Science of Early Childhood Development, Shonkoff JP, Phillips DA, eds. *From Neurons to Neighborhoods: The Science of Early Childhood Development*. Washington, DC: National Academies Press; 2000

7. Shonkoff JP, Hauser-Cram P. Early intervention for disabled infants and their families: a quantitative analysis. *Pediatrics*. 1987;80(5):650–658

8. Majnemer A. Benefits of early intervention for children with developmental disabilities. *Semin Pediatr Neurol*. 1998;5(1):62–69

9. Bennett FC, Guralnick MJ. Effectiveness of developmental intervention in the first five years of life. *Pediatr Clin North Am*. 1991;38(6):1513–1528

10. Berlin LJ, Brooks-Gunn J, McCarton C, McCormick MC. The effectiveness of early intervention: examining risk factors and pathways to enhanced development. *Prev Med*. 1998;27(2):238–245

11. Guralnick MJ. Early intervention for children with intellectual disabilities: current knowledge and future prospects. *J Appl Res Intellect Disabil*. 2005;18(4):313–324

12. Ramey CT, Bryant DM, Wasik BH, et al. Infant Health and Development Program for low birth weight, premature infants: program elements, family participation, and child intelligence. *Pediatrics*. 1992; 89(3):454–465

13. McCarton CM, Brooks-Gunn J, Wallace IF, et al. Results at age 8 years of early intervention for low-birth-weight premature infants. The Infant Health and Development Program. *JAMA*. 1997;277(2):126–132

14. Hebbeler K, Spiker D, Bailey D, et al. *Early Intervention for Infants and Toddlers With Disabilities and Their Families: Participants, Services, and Outcomes*. Menlo Park, CA: SRI International; 2007

15. Glascoe FP, Leew S. Parenting behaviors, perceptions, and psychosocial risk: impacts on young children's development. *Pediatrics*. 2010;125(2):313–319

16. Sameroff AJ, Seifer R, Barocas R, Zax M, Greenspan S. Intelligence quotient scores of 4-year-old children: social-environmental risk factors. *Pediatrics*. 1987;79(3):343–350

17. Campbell FA, Ramey CT, Pungello E, Sparling J, Miller-Johnson S. Early childhood education: young adult outcomes from the Abecedarian Project. *Appl Dev Sci*. 2002;6(1):42–57

18. American Academy of Pediatrics Council on Community Pediatrics. Poverty and child health in the United States. *Pediatrics*. 2016;137(4):e20160339

19. American Academy of Pediatrics Council on Children With Disabilities, Section on Developmental and Behavioral Pediatrics, Bright Futures Steering Committee, Medical Home Initiatives for Children With Special Health Needs Project Advisory Committee. Identifying infants and young children with developmental disorders in the medical home: an algorithm for developmental surveillance and screening. *Pediatrics*. 2006;118(1):405–420

20. Adams RC, Tapia C, American Academy of Pediatrics Council on Children With Disabilities. Early intervention, IDEA Part C Services, and the medical home: collaboration for best practice and best outcomes. *Pediatrics*. 2013;132(4):e1073–e1088

21. Brooks-Gunn J, McCarton CM, Casey PH, et al. Early intervention in low-birth-weight premature infants: Results through age 5 years from the Infant Health and Development Program. *JAMA*. 1994;272(16):1257–1262

22. Black JE. How a child builds its brain: some lessons from animal studies of neural plasticity. *Prev Med*. 1998;27(2):168–171

23. Ramey CT, Ramey SL. Early intervention: optimizing development for children with disabilities and risk conditions. In: Wolraich ML, ed. *Disorders of Development and Learning*. 3rd ed. Ontario, Canada BC: Decker; 2003:89–99

24. Bailey DB, Hebbeler K, Scarborough A, Spiker D, Mallik S. First experiences with early intervention: a national perspective. *Pediatrics*. 2004;113(4):887–896

25. Hollomon HA, Scott KG. Influence of birth weight on educational outcomes at age 9: the Miami site of the Infant Health and Development Program. *J Dev Behav Pediatr*. 1998;19(6):404–410

26. King TM, Tandon SD, Macias MM, et al. Implementing developmental screening and referrals: lessons learned from a national project. *Pediatrics*. 2010;125(2):350–360

27. Rose L, Herzig LD, Hussey-Gardner B. Early intervention and the role of pediatricians. *Pediatr Rev*. 2014;35(1):e1–e10

28. Silverstein M, Sand N, Glascoe FP, et al. Pediatrician practices regarding referral to early intervention services: is an established diagnosis important? *Ambul Pediatr*. 2006;6(2):105–109

29. American Academy of Pediatrics Council on Children With Disabilities and Medical Home Implementation Project Advisory Committee. Patient- and family-centered care coordination: a framework for integrating care for children and youth across multiple systems. *Pediatrics*. 2014;133(5):e1451–e1460

30. Blue-Banning M, Summers JA, Frankland HC, Nelson LL, Beegle G. Dimensions of family and professional partnerships: constructive guidelines for collaboration. *Except Child*. 2004;70(2):167–184

31. Michaud LJ, American Academy of Pediatrics Committee on Children With Disabilities. Prescribing therapy services for children with motor disabilities. *Pediatrics*. 2004;113(6):1836–1838

32. Palmer FB, Shapiro BK, Wachtel RC, et al. The effects of physical therapy on cerebral palsy. *N Engl J Med*. 1988;318(13):803–808

33. Law J, Garrett Z, Nye C. Speech and language therapy interventions for children with primary speech and language delay or disorder. *Cochrane Database Syst Rev*. 2003(3):CD004110

34. Hauser-Cram P, Warfield ME, Shonkoff JP, et al. Children with disabilities: a longitudinal study of child development and parent well-being. *Monogr Soc Res Child Dev*. 2001;66(3):i–viii, 1–114, 115–126

CHAPTER 7

Basics of Child Behavior and Primary Care Management of Common Behavioral Problems

Nathan J. Blum, MD, FAAP

Mary E. Pipan, MD, FAAP

Introduction

Behavioral and emotional concerns are among the most common reasons that children are seen by primary pediatric health care professionals. Epidemiological studies show that 11% to 20% of children meet criteria for a behavioral or emotional disorder.[1] Parents also raise concerns and seek intervention for problematic behaviors that do not reach the diagnostic threshold of a specific disorder but are nonetheless distressing to the child or family. To help these children and families, primary pediatric health care professionals must assess the nature and severity of the problem in order to decide whether to intervene in the office or to refer to a behavioral health specialist. Sometimes families only require reassurance and a sympathetic ear. Other times, contributing factors can be readily identified and remedied. This chapter presents a brief overview of why behavioral and emotional problems occur, how to assess the problem, and factors to consider in deciding to intervene or to refer to a behavioral health specialist. Principles of behavior management for primary pediatric health care professionals will then be outlined so that families can be given effective advice and appropriate behaviors can be proactively promoted. Finally, interventions for some common behavioral problems will be reviewed.

Assessment of Behavioral Problems in Children

Screening for Behavior Problems

Screening to ensure that a child's physical and behavioral health support optimal growth and development is one of many goals of a pediatric health supervision visit. While some parents will directly raise concerns about their child's behavior, others hesitate to do so, in part because they are not sure whether troublesome behaviors are within the range of normal, and in part because society often places responsibility for misbehavior on parental management. Medical professionals may hesitate to ask about behavioral concerns when they do not see such concerns as part of their scope of practice, if they lack the time, tools, or knowledge to screen and gather information efficiently, or if they lack the skill set to effectively intervene. When problems require referral to a behavioral health specialist, many communities have a dearth of effective resources, and many resources for less severe behavior problems are not covered by insurance.[2] Thus, the US health care system does not reliably identify or treat behavioral and emotional concerns and disorders.[1]

The use of standardized behavioral screening tools is one strategy to efficiently improve detection of behavioral and emotional problems in primary care. The Pediatric Symptom Checklist (PSC) is a 35-item parent-report scale that has been demonstrated to improve detection of behavioral and emotional problems in children from 4 to 15 years of age.[3] It is available online at **http://www.massgeneral.org/psychiatry/services/psc_online.aspx.** Parents can complete the PSC in 5 to 10 minutes, and it can be scored in less than 5 minutes. Recently, an abbreviated 17-item version (PSC-17) has been reported to be an even more efficient behavioral screening measure, although it may miss children with anxiety disorders.[4] For younger children, the Brief Infant-Toddler Social and Emotional Assessment (BITSEA)[5] or Ages & Stages Questionnaires: Social-Emotional, 2nd Edition (ASQ:SE-2)[6] are brief behavioral screening tools appropriate for use in primary care.

Defining the Problem

Once a behavioral concern is identified, the primary pediatric health care professional needs to obtain a description of what is happening, including the antecedents (what happens before the behavior), a description of the behavior, and the consequences (what happens after the behavior). This is often referred to as the ABCs of the behavior. Knowing the antecedents will help identify what triggers the behavior, such as whether it occurs only in certain settings (eg, school or home) or with certain caregivers. A complete description of the behavior will identify its intensity, duration, and frequency. This will allow the clinician to determine whether the behavior is outside the range of typical for a child of that age or developmental level and whether it potentially threatens the safety of the child or others. The consequences will include how parents (or others) respond to the behavior, which may help identify responses that are increasing the likelihood of the behavior continuing to occur (reinforcing the behavior). Primary pediatric health care professionals will also want to know when the behavior started and the impact the behavior is having on the child and family.

Behaviors that occur at high frequency, high intensity, and in the presence of multiple caretakers or in multiple environments are more suggestive of a behavioral or emotional disorder.[7] Behaviors that are of new onset may represent a new stage in a child's development, but they may be a result of pain or discomfort or a reaction to trauma, stress, or a change in family circumstances. All of this information will help clinicians determine whether a problem can be managed in primary care or needs referral for additional assessment and treatment. Families are more likely to listen to advice to pursue such resources when primary pediatric health care professionals express empathy for the challenges the child's behaviors present and confidence that, with help, the behaviors can improve.

Understanding the Problem

Understanding why a problem behavior is occurring is key to providing effective intervention. This involves careful identification of contributing factors intrinsic to the child, the environment, and the circumstances within which the behavior occurs. Factors to consider include the child's age and developmental level, the child's temperament or personality, and the possibility of behavioral, developmental, emotional, or physical disorders.

Age and Development: Behavior reflects a child's ability to interpret and respond to the world around him or her. Thus, a 2-year-old responds very differently to an adverse situation than a 4-year-old. A 2-year-old may tantrum, whereas a 4-year-old might ask why. A 4-year-old may be acting like a 2-year-old because his or her development is delayed and at a 2-year-old level. Children with developmental disorders, including speech and language disorders, learning disabilities, intellectual disabilities, and social and emotional impairments (eg, in autism spectrum disorder) have an increased frequency of behavioral and emotional disorders.

Temperament: Children vary in how they approach and respond to different situations. Some children are not upset easily, while others have a low threshold for frustration, and relatively small triggers may result in large reactions. Some children go with the flow, transition well, and take changes in stride. Others have more difficulty shifting gears and need predictability in order to function well. Some children are able to pay attention and persevere in tasks until finished. Others get distracted by new projects and may need prodding to finish what they started. These differences in behavioral tendencies reflect variations in temperament. Temperament traits are in part inherited and in part born of experience.[8] The different dimensions along which one sees variability in these behavioral tendencies is the subject of ongoing debate, but one frequently used model describes 9 dimensions along which these differences can be observed: adaptability, regularity, activity, intensity, persistence, approach/withdrawal (to new situations), sensitivity to sensory stimuli, mood, and distractibility.[9] Certain temperament characteristics tend to be associated with an increased likelihood of difficult behaviors, particularly low adaptability, high intensity, low regularity, withdrawal in new situations, and negative mood. Helping parents to appreciate their child's temperament and adjust their approach to better match the child's temperament can minimize behavior problems and decrease parental tendency to feel like they are to blame for their child's behaviors.[9]

Modeling and Learning: A key component of a child's environment involves the child's exposure to role models and teaching. Children learn through imitation of others. Imitation of simple motor movements starts in infancy. As children get older, they imitate more complex social and communicative behaviors. A child's misbehavior may be due to lack of experience and/or opportunity to practice appropriate behavior. Another factor could be a child's indiscriminate imitation of others (eg, a child imitating a parent's adult language or imitating behavior from videos with inappropriate content). When inappropriate behavior results from inappropriate role models or skill deficits, interventions will need to provide exposure to appropriate role models and to teach the desired skill.

Setting Variables: Circumstances that make children (and adults) more irritable—that is, lower their thresholds for getting upset or frustrated—are referred to as setting variables. Commonly these include situations in which the child experiences fatigue, hunger, stress, overstimulation, boredom, pain, or illness. When misbehavior occurs primarily in these situations, the goal of intervention will be either to avoid these situations or to help a child cope more effectively in them. For example, if a child's behavior deteriorates when the child is tired, ensuring an adequate amount and quality of sleep may be the primary intervention needed in addressing the problem. This may require a behavioral intervention, but if one obtains a history of loud snoring, pauses or gasps during sleep, and daytime sleepiness, discussing obstructive sleep apnea as a cause for the behavior problems may be the most important step in managing the problem. When a problem behavior occurs in the context of a setting variable, addressing this variable will often be more effective than a behavioral intervention.

Antecedents (Triggers): Antecedents are events that occur directly before the behavior that trigger the behavior. Knowing a child's triggers will help the clinician decide whether to focus on changing parents' responses to behavior once it occurs, avoiding or modifying the antecedents, or both. Among the most common triggers of misbehavior include the child being told, "no," "don't," or "stop" (restricted access); the child seeking attention; and the child being told to do something he or she does not want to do (task demands). Although interventions in these situations will typically involve counseling parents to change their response to the problem behavior, modifying antecedents may also be an important option to consider. For example, if the child's behavior is triggered by seeking attention, it is important to assess the frequency with which the child is receiving positive adult attention. If the frequency of positive attention is low, then increasing the frequency of this type of attention may be very effective in decreasing problem behaviors. How parents give instructions (discussed later) is another important antecedent to consider. For many triggers, the most effective interventions will emphasize **proactive, preventative strategies** such as avoiding the trigger, providing support to help the child manage the situation better, or teaching skills that help relieve frustration, manage emotion, or help the child problem solve. For example, when a child is triggered by transitions, changes in routine, or changes in what the child expects, parents can provide the child with warnings, a visual schedule, or a countdown to successfully reduce misbehavior. These are common strategies for children with an inflexible temperament. Children who tend to be anxious, or have high sensitivity to certain sensory inputs, may be triggered by fear or sensory experiences. For children with high levels of sensory sensitivity, even ordinary sensory inputs (eg, bright lights, noise from the vacuum cleaner) can cause an aversion like nails grating on a chalkboard does for many people. In this situation, the focus of intervention will likely be a combination of avoidance of triggers and gradual desensitization (see discussion of fearful/anxious behaviors under Common Behavioral Syndromes).

Consequences (Responses to Behavior): Before intervention, the primary pediatric health care professional must know how the parents understand the behavior, how the parents have been responding to the behavior, and what attempts they have made to change the behavior. The parents' understanding of the behavior may be influenced by family, community, or cultural factors, all of which the clinician will need to consider when counseling the family. When a problem behavior occurs repeatedly, it is very likely that the response to the behavior reinforces it. Any response to a behavior (regardless of the intent of the response) that maintains or increases the frequency of the behavior is referred to as a reinforcer. The persistence of misbehavior often results from caregivers inadvertently reinforcing the problem behaviors. For example, when a child frequently tantrums when told "no," it is likely that the parents are giving in frequently enough that the child is not sure whether no really means no. Parental attention, even negative attention such as yelling in response to the child's misbehavior, is another common reinforcer of problem behaviors.

Knowing how parents respond to their child's behavior will help the primary pediatric health care professional determine whether these responses are helping the child learn appropriate behavior or are safely and effectively discouraging misbehavior. Asking how parents respond to their child's challenging behavior takes both empathy and a trusting relationship, so parents do not feel blamed for the problem behavior. Parents must perceive that they and their primary care clinician are both working toward a common goal: helping the child learn how to function to the best of his or her ability in their social and cultural milieu to become a happy, successful young adult.

When assessing parents' past attempts to change problem behavior, it is very important to have parents describe what happens and not just name the procedure they used. Parents may have tried to ignore a specific behavior, but they may have done this only inconsistently or for brief periods. Other parents may have tried to reward appropriate behavior, but the child rarely, if ever, earned the rewards. These parents believe that they have tried ignoring or rewarding as behavioral change strategies, but as will be described later in this chapter, they have not followed these strategies effectively.

When to Refer: A parent's gratitude for behavioral advice that works can be very rewarding to pediatric health care professionals, but some families will require more time and guidance than can be provided in a primary care visit. This may occur when the behavioral difficulty is a sign of child psychopathology and/or family stress or discord. Factors to consider when deciding whether to refer a child are included in Box 7.1. If these factors are present, the primary pediatric health care professional should consider referral to a behavioral therapist, developmental-behavioral pediatrician, child psychiatrist, psychologist, school guidance counselor, parenting class, or a community mental health agency. Primary pediatric health care professionals should provide families some guidance as to the services they should expect and follow up with the family to ask whether these services have been helpful.

Box 7.1. Factors That Make It More Difficult to Change Behavior

- ► Problem behaviors are pervasive across time, persons, and settings.
- ► Problem behaviors cause severe disruption at home, school, or community.
- ► Problem behaviors threaten the safety of the child or others.
- ► Previous attempts to change the behavior have failed (particularly if previous attempts were well executed).
- ► Problem behaviors occur in the context of multiple psychosocial stressors.
- ► Parents do not agree on behavior management strategies.

Principles of Behavior Management

Behavior management starts with gaining an understanding of the behavior, which then guides the next step: changing behavior. The focus of behavioral change should be on encouraging the desired behavior, as well as discouraging the undesired behavior. Behavioral intervention occurs on several different levels, depending on the particular problem and situation (Table 7.1). Antecedent modification refers to changing the factors that trigger the problem in order to prevent the problem behavior from occurring. Giving instructions communicates how we want the child to behave. Finally, consequence modification refers to changing how the caregivers respond to both problem and desired behaviors.

Modifying Antecedents

One method for modifying antecedents is to alter the child's physical environment. Childproofing, for example, removes access to hazards, decreasing the likelihood that the child might play with hazardous materials. Tantrums in a toy store can be reduced by limiting the time spent shopping or not going to a store when the child is tired or hungry. Aggressive behavior noted after the child plays fighting video games can be reduced by removing the child's access to such games. Placing a high latch on a door decreases the likelihood of a young child escaping.

Antecedent modification may include teaching skills needed for alternative behaviors that accomplish the same goal. Misbehaviors that occur because of frustration often require these interventions. For example, teaching effective communication skills through sign language or picture exchange communication would be part of the behavioral plan for a child who gets frustrated because of difficulty with language. Similarly, if a child's misbehavior is related to frustration with handwriting, obtain-ing occupational therapy and teaching computer keyboard skills might be useful interventions.

Another means of antecedent control is to ensure that appropriate behavior is modeled by the child's peers and other adults. As discussed earlier, one of the most important ways that children learn behavior is through imitation.[10] In order to use modeling to change behavior, parents need to be mindful of the behavior they want their child to display and to display such behavior themselves. For example, for a child who gets explosively angry, the appropriate behavior to model would be a calm response when upset and using words

Table 7.1. Examples of Antecedent and Consequence Modification for Different Triggers		
Trigger	**Antecedent Modification**	**Consequence Modification**
Restricted access (being told "no," "you can't," "stop," "don't," etc)	Remove forbidden items from environment (eg, childproofing). Clearly state rules for access (eg, first you do "X," then you get to do "Y"). Distract the child to another activity prior to the child gaining access to what is forbidden.	Consistently enforce rules. Allow access for appropriate behavior. Remove child from situation. Ignore misbehavior while persisting in denying access.
Need or desire for attention	Play with child with frequent positive comments on their play. Spend time with child without distractions from work, phone, computer, TV, etc. Plan family activities. Have someone available to engage child when caregiver is busy.	Increase frequency of attention for appropriate behavior. Ignore misbehavior meant to get attention. Institute time-out for certain attention-seeking misbehavior. Avoid inadvertent attention to minor misbehavior.
Task demands (that a child does not want to do)	After gaining the child's attention, clearly explain to the child, or show them, what is expected. Clearly state what will happen when the task is accomplished (first … then …). Clearly state what will happen if the child does not comply (eg, use a single warning).	Follow through on task demands. Carry out warnings that are made when task not completed.
Difficulty with task demands or communication	Alter task demand if difficulty is too high; provide breaks. Help child before frustration occurs. Model the behavior desired. Provide low-stress time for practicing skill. Show the child in pictures the sequence of tasks expected. Augment communication with sign language, pictures, etc.	Reward efforts for successful task completion. Follow nonpreferred tasks with preferred tasks. Provide help when request for help is made appropriately.
Transitions, change in routine, or change in what child expects	Create visual schedules. Prepare the child for changes and transitions. Establish routines. Teach skills related to flexibility.	Calmly persist with change while ignoring inappropriate behavior. Praise successful transitions. Schedule nonpreferred activities before preferred activities.
Provocation by sibling or peer	Monitor interactions. Teach appropriate interactions. Find activities both enjoy.	Pay attention when siblings are interacting well. Institute time-out or other punishment (eg, toy is removed) for both participants.
Fear or aversive sensory stimulus	Avoid fearful or adverse stimulus. Expose gradually.	Reward successful adaptation to exposure. Respond to appropriate requests for breaks or escape.

to relay the problem rather than behavior. Getting angry and yelling back at the child models the undesired behavior. For a child who is very anxious, a parent needs to model calm, confident reassurance.

Children who are exposed to inappropriate behavior often imitate that behavior. Most children are quick learners; that is, within their ability, they can model new behavior even after only a brief exposure—a parent's curse word is repeated by the child, or a wrestling hero's move is tried on a peer. When children display inappropriate adult behavior, such as sexualized behavior or threats of violence, one must also explore where such behavior has been witnessed. Such behavior may have been directly experienced in the home environment, at a babysitter's or child care, or indirectly through TV, videos, or the Internet.

Parents can modify antecedents by changing their expectations of their child's behavior based on their understanding of their child's developmental abilities, temperament, learning differences, and physiological and behavioral health status. For example, parents of a very active child may give the child "movement breaks" throughout a meal instead of expecting the child to sit quietly for the duration of the whole meal. Parents may minimize demands when a child is tired or stressed. Parents of older children may give them more responsibility and allow more participation in family decision-making.

Giving Instructions

A child's behavior can be shaped through the instructions the child is given. Helping parents give instructions more effectively is an important part of behavioral counseling.[11] Effective instruction starts with gaining the child's attention. This sounds obvious, but too often parents try to engage their child when the child is doing something else. If a parent yells, "It's time for dinner!" from the kitchen when the child is absorbed in a video game in the basement, it is likely that the child is selectively attending to the video game and not the parents' instruction. Both the parent and child get rapidly exasperated if the parent sees the child as making an active decision to disobey. Such exasperation can be avoided if the parent first makes eye contact or receives verbal assurance that the child is listening before giving the instruction.

Instructions to alter or engage in a specific behavior need to be given in simple language that fits the comprehension abilities of the child. In general, the number of words used in the instruction should not be longer than the typical length of the child's sentences. This does not mean that parents should always talk to the child in short sentences, but simplifying language when directing the child's behavior helps the child understand what is expected. Instructions should also be given as firm statements and not as a question, unless the instruction is a choice ("It's time to clean up." versus "Can we clean up now?"). A "firm" voice (or "sergeant" voice) helps the child differentiate a parent's directive from a choice.

Instructions that specify the desired behavior are more likely to be followed than general commands or "don't" instructions. "Behave" is less likely to be successful than

"Come sit by Mommy." Saying "Walk." is better than "Stop running." Minimizing "don't" instructions often requires parents to ignore minor misbehavior and redirect the child to what they want him or her to do.

Finally, successful instruction requires that the parent follow through with the instruction. Figure 7.1 illustrates a protocol to help parents follow through consistently with instructions to a child. After getting the child's attention, the parent issues the instruction or directive followed by 5 to 10 seconds of silence. The period of silence is to allow the child to process the instruction. If the child listens, the parent could notice and sometimes provide a reinforcer (next section). If the child does not listen, the parent should reissue the instruction with a warning ("If you don't put your shoes on now, the TV is getting turned off."). If the child listens, the parent notices. If the child does not comply, the parent carries out the warning, and if the instruction was to complete a task, the parent reissues the directive. Children who do not comply unless the parent repeats the instruction multiple times or threatens them are likely playing the odds that a parent will drop the demand. From experience, they have learned that the likelihood a parent will follow through on a demand increases once a threat is issued, or once a parent's voice reaches a certain angry pitch. Once a child learns that a parent is more consistent with follow through, warnings will not be needed as often in the future.

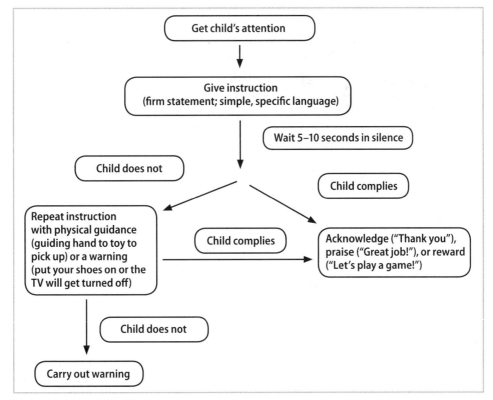

Figure 7.1. Giving instructions.

If a child does not follow an instruction because he or she did does not understand the instruction, a different approach is needed. In this case, parents can reissue the instruction with physical guidance, with a prompt, or by modeling the behavior.

If a child is chronically oppositional, parents may need to practice this sequence with only a few instructions a day, and start with instructions with which the child is likely to comply. Success with these instructions will help bolster the parent's confidence and teach the child that compliance will be recognized with praise and adult attention. This will facilitate success with harder directives later.

Manipulating Consequences

Behavioral change can be augmented by altering the consequences of behavior; that is, changing the rewards or punishments that occur as a consequence of the behavior. Rewards are more effective behavioral interventions than are punishments. Therefore, a child needs to succeed at meeting parents' expectations most of the time. Initially this may require adults to change or lower expectations (an antecedent modification) to more easily achievable goals, which then can be altered as the child and parent become more successful.

To be effective, reinforcing consequences need to have a positive value for the child and punishing consequences a negative value. They also need to be acceptable to the caregivers, affordable, and available. Attention (eg, praise) has a positive value for most children. Table 7.2 gives a list of suggested reinforcers. Withdrawal of attention (a time-out, discussed later in the chapter) has an aversive value to most children. The value of reinforcers is otherwise quite individual and will vary over time.

Table 7.2. Types of Reinforcers	
Reinforcer	**Examples**
Social attention	Praise, comments, reprimands (negative attention is still attention), playing games, reading books, pat on the back, hair tousling
Tangibles	Treats, stickers, objects, and toys
Privileges	Computer or television time, play activities with parent, later bedtime or curfew, car on the weekend, greater independence
Tokens (that can be exchanged for reinforcers or privileges)	Money, stickers, checkmarks earned for good behavior that can be turned in for backup reinforcers (eg, 3 stickers = ice cream with grandpa on Friday). This allows more immediacy of the reinforcer and more choice (and thus maximizes value) for the child earning the reward.
Negative reinforcement (escape or avoidance)	Breaks from chores, break from homework

Both reinforcing and punishing consequences are most effective if they immediately follow the behavior. This is especially important for younger children and for children with developmental-behavioral disorders. For example, if a child repeatedly says Mom to no avail, and then kicks Mom, followed by Mom asking "What do you want?", the behavior being reinforced is the kicking, not calling Mom's name; eventually the child will preferentially kick to get attention. As children become older, reinforcers or punishments can be more delayed (eg, bedtime behavior rewarded with breakfast treat or school misbehavior punished by restriction of electronic games at home).

Rewards that a child earns frequently may lose their efficacy over time (satiation). They also will not be effective if a child has unlimited access regardless of behavior. Thus, parents need to be able to restrict access to reinforcers in order for them to be effective. To avoid this satiation, reinforcers need to be varied across time.

Reinforcers and punishments are more effective if caregivers are careful to specify the behavior that is being rewarded or punished. For example, telling a child "Good job." without reference to what that refers to will not be as effective as telling the child, "I like the way you got yourself dressed this morning, and you did all your buttons! Good job!" Initially, when trying to increase desired behaviors, the reinforcer should be provided each time the desired behavior occurs. As the desired behavior becomes more frequent, the reinforcer should be provided only intermittently. Intermittent reinforcement is very effective at getting behaviors to persist across time.

Many behavioral expectations of children are not single-event behaviors but require compliance across time (eg, sitting still, staying by the cart in the grocery store, or keeping one's seatbelt buckled). To reinforce these behaviors, parents should reinforce periodically throughout the period of the expected behavior. A parent may be advised to bring special treats and small rewards (eg, stickers) to use at regular intervals during these types of activities.

If a child engages in an undesired behavior, a parent can ignore or punish the undesired behavior. Ignoring the undesired behavior may seem counterintuitive to parents. However, undesired behavior is often being reinforced by parental attention as described previously. When the undesired behavior is no longer reinforced, the frequency of the behavior decreases over time. This process is termed *extinction*. Clinicians counseling parents to use extinction as a behavior change strategy should warn families about the *extinction burst,* a term that describes the fact that often the behavior may worsen before it improves. For example, if a child has learned that tantrums are an effective means of getting a candy bar, the first few times the parent refuses to give the child a candy bar, the child's tantrum may be longer or louder than it ever was before. Only after this fails on a few occasions will the child learn that the tantrums will no longer be reinforced, and the frequency of the tantrums will decrease.

Punishment is a planned consequence to a behavior by the caregiver that decreases the frequency of that behavior. Punishment does not teach desired behaviors but may be a necessary component of behavior management plans for undesired behaviors that cannot be ignored, such as behaviors that are a danger to self or others, or the destruction of property. For more minor behaviors, warnings can be applied prior to the actual punishment. The success of punishment is defined as whether the behavior reduces in frequency over time, not by the child's distress by the punishment itself. Children may appear nonchalant or even be insolent ("You're not the boss of me!"). Parents need to ignore these distracting behaviors and calmly apply a punishment consistently across time before deciding whether it works or not.

One of the most frequently recommended punishment strategies for children is time-out from positive reinforcement (referred to as time-out from here on). Time-out is defined as the contingent withdrawal of social attention and activities for a specified time. A time-out is usually implemented by having a child sit in a chair, stand in the corner, or go to his or her room for a brief period (1 to 5 minutes). During this time, no one talks to the child, makes eye contact with the child, nor is in physical contact with the child. Time-out is a well-studied and effective punishment procedure, but many families have difficulty administering it correctly. Pitfalls of time-out include not specifying the behavior being punished, lecturing the child while the child is in time-out, or placing the child in time-out in a location where he or she has access to attention and fun activities. This can be a problem with a room time-out if there is a TV, computer, or video games in the room. Another problem can be that some children do not stay in time-out. It may be that the time-out is too long. A time-out for hyperactive or younger children who have difficulty staying in one place for more than a few seconds can be as short as 20 to 30 seconds. Until a child is aware of how time passes, 2 minutes would be the maximum time needed. It may be helpful to use a timer so that the child can see the passage of time and prevent the child from arguing with the parents about how much time has passed. Once a child knows the difference between 1 minute and 5 minutes (around 5 years), longer periods may be appropriate depending on the infraction. If the child does leave the time-out before time is up, he or she should be escorted back with minimal attention from the parent.

Other punishment strategies are listed in Table 7.3. Although corporal or physical punishment (eg, spanking) continues to be commonly used, it is not recommended. Corporal punishment models behavior that would be inappropriate for the child to demonstrate with peers and adults, and it has been found to have negative effects on parent-child relationships, child development and behavior, and child and adult mental health across cultures.[12,13] Although most people in the United States would agree that not all forms of corporal punishment are child abuse, most child abuse starts as corporal punishment.[13] For these reasons, practitioners should discourage parents from using corporal punishment and should emphasize the proactive and positive approaches described earlier in the chapter.

Behavior management counseling based on understanding the child factors, settings, expectations, and consequences that influence the behavior will often be successful. One-size-fits-all advice is generally neither rewarding nor successful.

Table 7.3. Types of Punishment	
Punishment	**Description**
Time-out	Contingent withdrawal of social attention and activities for a brief period.
Verbal reprimand	Brief instruction to change behavior.
Privilege withdrawal	Not allowing the child to engage in a fun activity for a brief period.
Response cost	Usually used in conjunction with a reward system in which the child can earn tokens for appropriate behavior and lose tokens for inappropriate behavior. If the child is losing more tokens than they are earning, it will not be effective.
Grounding	This is a specific type of privilege withdrawal in which the child is required to stay at home and not interact with friends for a specified period.
Job grounding	The child is grounded as just defined until he or she completes a specific task or chore. The length of the grounding is determined by when the child completes the task.
Natural consequences	Allowing the child to experience the consequences of a poor choice as opposed to fighting with the child about it; works well for activities such as getting cold when not wearing a coat but not for behaviors with more serious potential consequences.

Common Behavioral Syndromes

Infant Crying/Colic

The time infants spend crying progressively increases to a mean of approximately 2.5 hours per day during the second month of life and decreases progressively thereafter. When otherwise healthy infants cry intensely for an excessive duration, they are often referred to as having colic. The amount of crying required for a diagnosis of colic is not agreed on, but in research studies, more than 3 hours a day for more than 3 days per week is a frequently used definition.

The diagnosis of colic requires that the child be otherwise healthy and feeding well. Thus physical problems that can cause excessive crying must be excluded. Acute disorders that should be considered in a crying infant include conditions such as infections, corneal abrasion, glaucoma, skull or long-bone fracture, incarcerated hernia, supraventricular tachycardia, intussusception, midgut volvulus, and a hair tourniquet on a digit.[14] A number of chronic conditions have been proposed to be the cause of infant colic, including cow's milk allergy, lactose intolerance, constipation, and gastroesophageal reflux. Although in any one case, these problems are potential causes of crying, no well-designed study has suggested that these are common causes of excessive crying, and controlled studies using interventions targeting these problems in infants with colic have not been found to be effective for most infants.[15] Recently, there have been studies of treatment with *Lactobacillus*-containing probiotics with mixed results.[16]

Infants with excessive crying have been found to have differences in temperament from those who cry less. Perhaps, not surprisingly, parents tend to rate these infants as more intense and more difficult to soothe (less easily distracted). However, these temperament characteristics of infants with excessive crying are also supported by independent observations. For example, independent observers of infants undergoing a physical examination rated infants with colic as crying more intensely and being more difficult to console.[17] Infants with more persistent crying differ from those with less crying in that they have a higher crying-to-fussing ratio (suggesting greater intensity), and infants with colic have been found to be less likely to soothe in response to an orally administered sucrose solution than were infants without colic.[18]

Management of colic involves empathizing with parents about the stress and frustration colicky babies cause and reassuring them that their child is healthy. Helping parents to understand their infant's temperament traits can allow them to better understand the infant's crying and remain calm despite the crying. Parents should be counseled that crying is the infant's way of communicating that there is something that the infant wants, but it is not necessarily a sign of pain or illness. Parents usually think of some things that an infant might want, such as to be played with, fed, or have a diaper changed. However, parents may not think of the crying as a sign of the need to be quietly held, the need for nonnutritive sucking, or the need to be left alone to sleep.[19] Furthermore, parents need to understand that these infants are more difficult to soothe, and thus, even when the parent is providing what the infant wants, it may take many minutes before the infant stops crying. If parents rapidly change from one activity to another in futile attempts to soothe the infant, they may stop providing the infant with what he or she wants before the infant communicates to the parent that it is what he or she wants by stopping the crying.

Bedtime Resistance/Night Wakings

Sleep occurs in cycles that typically last about 60 minutes in babies, gradually increasing to 90 minutes in older children and adolescents. During the cycles, the child goes from light non-REM (rapid eye movement) sleep (described as Stage 1 and Stage 2 sleep) to deep non-REM sleep (Stage 3 and Stage 4 sleep) or into REM sleep. Most deep non-REM sleep occurs in the first third of the night, and most REM sleep occurs in the second half of the night.[19] Individuals wake briefly between sleep cycles but tend not to be aware of this, as they rapidly go into the next sleep cycle. During the first year of life, average total daily sleep time decreases from about 16 hours a day in newborns to 13 hours a day at 1 year of age, with further decreases to about 9 to 10 hours per day during the elementary school–age years.[20]

Falling asleep is facilitated by a calming and familiar environment and a consistent bedtime routine occurring at around the same time each night. Children need to learn to put themselves to sleep. Many associate different activities or objects with falling asleep (sleep associations). Younger children may have a favorite blanket or a stuffed animal or may fall asleep being rocked or nursed. Older children may have a favorite pillow or something they think about when they go to sleep. When these sleep associations are not available, initiating sleep may be more difficult for the child. In most children with night wakings, the problem is not actually the waking, but rather trouble falling back asleep because a sleep association is no longer present.[22] For example, a parent lying down next to a child to get the child to fall asleep may be problematic because the parent is not present when the child wakes between sleep cycles during the night. In addition, infants should not have soft objects in the crib and should not sleep in the same bed as an adult due to the increased risk of sudden unexpected infant death.[21] Other common problematic sleep associations include having an infant fall asleep while being rocked or nursed. Sometimes the parent is not part of the sleep association, but may be needed to help with a sleep association. For example, an infant may fall asleep sucking on a pacifier, but if the pacifier falls out of the child's mouth, the child may need the parent to put the pacifier back in the mouth during the night. Night wakings can be managed by teaching the child to fall asleep without the problematic sleep association. This often results in bedtime resistance, which should be managed as described subsequently.

If a child is having trouble falling asleep, primary pediatric health care professionals should assess whether principles of good sleep hygiene are being maintained (Box 7.2). A regular morning wake-up time, consistent nap time and length, and a positive, calming bedtime routine followed by a consistent bedtime are particularly important. When unclear, it is helpful for parents to complete a 1- to 2-week sleep diary focusing on whether the expected time of sleep is consistent with the child's physiological needs or tendencies. Trying to get a child to sleep when he or she is not tired or to sleep past the time the biological clock awakens the child is not likely to be successful. This may happen if parents do not understand the rapid decrease in the need for sleep during the infancy and toddler years or if the child has delayed sleep phase syndrome, which is characterized by a delay in initiation of sleep in relation to the desired sleep-wake times but an adequate total amount of sleep. In children with delayed sleep phase, one should slowly (in 10 to 15 minute increments) move the bedtime and morning wake-up times earlier. In addition, low doses of melatonin (1 to 5 mg/night) given 3 to 4 hours before the usual bedtime can be helpful.[23]

Some children will resist going to bed at an appropriate bedtime because they have difficulty with parental limits or because they are being required to learn to fall asleep in the absence of an established sleep association. In this situation, parents often have to let children cry until they fall asleep.[24] After a few nights, most

Box 7.2. Good Sleep Hygiene

ENVIRONMENT
- Dark (no more than a night-light)
- Quiet
- Comfortably cool

SCHEDULE
- Regular morning wake-up time
- Consistent nap length
- Regular bedtime

ACTIVITIES AROUND BEDTIME
- Child put into bed drowsy, but still awake
- No frightening TV or stories before bed
- No vigorous physical exercise in the hour before bed
- Consistent and soothing bedtime routine
- Avoid meals or hunger around bedtime

infants and toddlers will learn to fall asleep on their own, but the protests the first couple of nights can be dramatic and prolonged. Ignoring the tantrums is difficult for many parents, but if parents are going to check, they should briefly and calmly reassure the child that it is time for sleep and leave without touching the child. They should resist reintroducing the sleep association (eg, lying down with the child), as this would just teach the child that tantrums are effective in getting what he or she wants.

Breath-holding Spells

Breath-holding spells are involuntary (reflexive) events. Typically they occur in response to an event that causes anger, frustration, fear, or minor injury. The child cries, becomes apneic at the end of exhaling, and then becomes pale or cyanotic.

The child may lose consciousness and have a brief convulsion. Breath-holding spells usually begin between 3 and 18 months of age and may occur infrequently or multiple times a day. It is rare for breath-holding spells to persist beyond 7 years of age.[25] Breath-holding spells are thought to be caused by dysregulation of the autonomic nervous system.

Children with breath-holding spells should have hemoglobin and iron studies performed, as these spells have been associated with anemia and iron deficiency. If the history is typical, no further medical evaluation is needed. When the history is not clear, an electroencephalogram may be helpful in distinguishing breath-holding spells from seizures. If a child is pale and loses consciousness, an electrocardiogram should be obtained to distinguish the spells from conditions associated with cardiac arrhythmias, such as long QT syndrome. In infants, one should consider the possibility of gastroesophageal reflux resulting in apnea. In very rare cases, breath-holding spells have been associated with brainstem dysfunction caused by tumors or Arnold-Chiari malformations.

In most cases, treatment primarily involves demystification and reassurance that even if the child loses consciousness, he or she will start to breathe again without intervention. Parents should be cautioned to avoid allowing breath-holding spells to prevent them from setting limits, even if the limits provoke the spells. If children learn that emotional outbursts prevent parents from setting firm limits, the frequency of the outburst and the associated breath-holding spells are likely to increase.

If the child is anemic, he or she should be treated with iron, as this will decrease the frequency of breath-holding spells in many children. Although much less well investigated, treatment with iron has also been reported to decrease the frequency of breath-holding spells in children who are not anemic.[26] Thus, if the breath-holding spells are severe, treatment with iron could be considered.

Fearful/Anxious Behaviors

Fear and anxiety are both part of the typical human experience. Each is necessary to alert us to real dangers. However, for some, the severity of the fear response, and the inability to regulate emotions once aroused, can lead to an inordinate amount of time and energy spent upset or worrying. Formal treatment is suggested when fears and anxiety interfere with sleep, daily activities, social functioning, or academics. Initial treatment consists of cognitive-behavioral approaches. Studies of cognitive-behavioral therapy for anxiety in children have shown it to be effective in greater that 50% of cases.[27]

Cognitive-behavior therapy (CBT) helps children identify their anxious thoughts and challenge these thoughts through both learning about the stimulus causing anxiety and stepwise exposure to the stimulus from the least frightening element of a stimulus or situation to the entire stimulus or situation. Relaxation techniques are often taught to help regulate emotional arousal. A schedule for daily practice is set up, and rewards may be used for successfully tolerating the exposure.[28] For example, if a child is afraid of cats, he or she might learn about cats as loving pets; during stepwise exposure the child might first be shown pictures of cats, followed by being in the room with a cat, then petting a cat someone else is holding, and eventually holding and petting the cat. An increase in the use of active coping strategies as required during exposure to the stimulus is the best predictor of improvement during anxiety treatment.[29]

Medications for anxiety are considered when cognitive-behavior therapy is not possible or effective. Selective serotonin reuptake inhibitors (SSRIs) and selective serotonin-norepinephrine reuptake inhibitors (SNRIs) have been shown to decrease anxiety in children, with a moderate effect size.[30] Small doses of SSRIs or SNRIs can be effective, and the dose should be increased slowly to minimize side effects. Children on SSRIs or SNRIs should be monitored for suicidal ideation, which may occur in a small percentage of children on these medications. Benzodiazepines may be prescribed for children with anxiety related to a medical procedure but are not usually used on a regular basis because of their potential for negative effects on cognition and dependence.

Repetitive Behaviors and Habits

Repetitive behaviors are part of normal child development. Body rocking, head banging, or digit- sucking occur in most infants during the first year of life.[31] Usually these behaviors decrease in frequency during the toddler and preschool years, but occasionally they persist even into adulthood. Repetitive behaviors may help children modulate their level of arousal. They can serve a self-calming function during anxiety-provoking situations and a self-stimulating function during periods of low arousal. Repetitive behaviors may be viewed as problematic when they cause tissue damage or subjective distress for the child. Distress for the parent alone would not usually be a reason to treat repetitive behaviors.

Repetitive behaviors represent a diverse group of behaviors that include body rocking, digit-sucking, head-banging, nail-biting, hair-pulling (trichotillomania), tics, and Tourette disorder. Of these, thumb-sucking is the behavior most frequently addressed by primary pediatric health care professionals and is the behavior that will be focused on in this section. Thumb-sucking is usually harmless in infants and young children, but it can cause problems when it persists at high frequency after 4 to 6 years of age. Some of the most frequent sequelae involve dental problems, such as an anterior open bite, decreased alveolar bone growth, mucosal trauma, and even altered growth of the facial bones. Thumb- or digit-sucking is a common cause of paronychia in children, and it may be associated with an increased incidence of accidental ingestion. Rarely, deformities of the fingers and thumb may occur. Thumb-sucking is associated with stigma among both adults and peers. Peers view children who suck their thumbs as less desirable playmates.[32]

Treatment of thumb-sucking should be considered in children older than 4 to 6 years. However, if the thumb-sucking occurs infrequently (eg, only at night) or only as a temporary response to a stressor, treatment is not usually indicated. Treatment is indicated if thumb-sucking causes dental problems, digital malformations, or distress to the child. If thumb-sucking has resulted in significant negative reactions from the parents, a moratorium on parental comments on the thumb-sucking should precede any other treatment. This reduces tension between the parent and child and may decrease the sucking if it had been reinforced by parental attention. If other sources of stress or anxiety are thought to be related to the thumb-sucking, a plan to manage these stressors should be developed before the sucking is treated. Treatments are most effective when the child is a willing partner in the process.

Praise for not sucking the thumb in combination with use of a device to remind the child not to suck is the most common treatment. A variety of devices have been used from bandages on the thumb to a thumb splint. Aversive taste treatments use a spicy hot commercially available substance applied to the thumb nail to remind children not to suck their thumbs. Intraoral appliances inserted by dentists that block the child from thumb-sucking can be used. All of these treatments can be problematic if the child is not motivated to stop the thumb-sucking. The digital appliances can be removed by the child, and the intraoral devices can be bent or broken by children who want to continue to thumb-suck.

Conclusion

Primary pediatric health care professionals will encounter many parents who are concerned about their child's behavior. Often, an understanding of child physiological and temperamental factors contributing to the behavior, along with an assessment of the settings in which the behavior occurs, events preceding the behavior, and consequences of the behavior, will enable practitioners to provide advice to parents that will facilitate successful management of their child's behavior. Occasionally this assessment will reveal that the behaviors are severely disruptive, dangerous, pervasive, or occurring in the context of multiple psychosocial stressors. In these situations, referral to a behavioral health professional should be considered.

Resources

Web Sites
Parenting Essentials and Positive Parenting Tips from the Centers for Disease Control and Prevention
https://www.cdc.gov/parents/essentials/index.html
https://www.cdc.gov/ncbddd/childdevelopment/positiveparenting/index.html

Healthy Children.org from the American Academy of Pediatrics
https://www.healthychildren.org

Caring for Kids from the Canadian Pediatric Society
http://www.caringforkids.cps.ca/

The Incredible Years Parenting Program
www.incredibleyears.com

Triple P Positive Parenting Program
http://www.triplep.net/glo-en/home/

Books
Forehand R, Long N. *Parenting the Strong-Willed Child: The Clinically Proven Five-Week Program for Parents of Two- to Six-Year-Olds.* 3rd ed. New York, NY: McGraw Hill Education; 2010

Phelan TW. *1-2-3 Magic: Effective Discipline for Children 2–12.* 6th ed. Naperville, IL: Sourcebooks; 2010

Barkley RA, Benton CM. *Your Defiant Child: Eight Steps to Better Behavior.* 2nd ed. New York, NY: Guilford Press; 2013

Greene RW. *The Explosive Child: A New Approach for Understanding and Parenting Easily Frustrated, Chronically Inflexible Children.* 5th ed. New York, NY: Harper Paperbacks; 2014

Ginsburg KR, Ginsburg I, Ginsburg T. *Raising Kids to Thrive: Balancing Love With Expectations and Protection With Trust.* Elk Grove Village, IL: American Academy of Pediatrics; 2015

References
1. Weitzman C, Wegner L, American Academy of Pediatrics Section on Developmental and Behavioral Pediatrics, et al. Promoting optimal development: screening for behavioral and emotional problems. *Pediatrics.* 2015;135(2):384–395
2. Perrin E, Stancin T. A continuing dilemma: whether and how to screen for concerns about children's behavior. *Pediatr Rev.* 2002;23(8):264–276
3. Jellinek MS, Murphy JM, Little M, et al. Use of the Pediatric Symptom Checklist to screen for psychosocial problems in pediatric primary care: a national feasibility study. *Arch Pediatr Adolesc Med.* 1999;153(3):254–260
4. Gardner W, Lucas A, Kolko DJ, Campo JV. Comparison of the PSC-17 and alternative mental health screens in an at-risk primary care sample. *J Am Acad Child Adolesc Psychiatry.* 2007;46(5):611–618

5. Briggs-Gowan MJ, Carter AS, Irwin JR, Wachtel K, Cicchetti DV. Brief infant toddler social emotional assessment: screening for social-emotional problems and delays in competence. *J Pediatr Psychol.* 2004;29(2):143–155

6. Squires J, Bricker D, Heo K, Twombly E. Identification of social-emotional problems in young children using a parent-completed screening measure. *Early Child Res Q.* 2001;16:405–419

7. Wakschlag LS, Briggs-Gowan MJ, Carter AS, et al. A developmental framework for distinguishing disruptive behaviors from normative misbehavior in preschool children. *J Child Psychol Psychiatry.* 2007;48(10):976–987

8. Saudino KJ. Behavioral genetics and child temperament. *J Dev Behav Pediatr.* 2005;26(3):214–223

9. Carey WB. Teaching parents about infant temperament. *Pediatrics.* 1998;102(5 suppl E):1311–1316

10. Bandura A. *Principles of Behavior Modification.* New York, NY: Holt, Rinehart and Winston, Inc.; 1969

11. Forehand RL, McMahon RJ. *Helping the Noncompliant Child: A Clinician's Guide to Parent Training.* New York, NY: Guilford Press; 1981

12. MacKenzie MJ, Nicklas E, Waldfogel J, Brooks-Gunn J. Spanking and child development across the first decade of life. *Pediatrics.* 2013;132(5):e1118–e1125

13. Durant JE. Physical punishment, culture, and rights: current issues for professionals. *J Dev Behav Pediatr.* 2008;29(1):55–66

14. Herman M, Le A. The crying infant. *Emerg Med Clin North Am.* 2007;25(4):1137–1159

15. Lucassen P. Colic in infants. *BMJ Clin Evid.* 2010Feb 5; 2010:pii 0309

16. Xu M, Wang J, Wang N, et al. The efficacy and safety of the probiotic bacterium *Lactobacillus reuteri* DSM 17938 for infantile colic: a meta-analysis of randomized controlled trials. *PLoS One.* 2015;28(10):e0141445

17. White BP, Gunnar MR, Larson MC, Donzella B, Barr RG. Behavioral and physiologic responsivity, sleep, and patterns of daily cortisol production in infants with and without colic. *Child Dev.* 2000;71(4):862–877

18. Barr RG, Young SN, Wright JH, Gravel R, Alkawaf R. Differential calming responses to sucrose taste in crying infants with and without colic. *Pediatrics.* 1999;103(5):e68

19. Taubman B. Parental counseling compared with elimination of cow's milk or soy milk protein for the treatment of infant colic syndrome: a randomized trial. *Pediatrics.* 1988;81(6):756–761

20. Galland BC, Yaylor BJ, Elder DE, Herbison P. Normal sleep patterns in infants and young children: a systematic review of observational studies. *Sleep Med Rev.* 2012;16(3):213–222

21. American Academy of Pediatrics Task Force on Sudden Infant Death Syndrome. SIDS and other sleep-related infant deaths: updated 2016 recommendations for a safe infant sleeping environment. *Pediatrics.* 2016;138(5):e20162938

22. Meltzer LJ, Mindell JA. Sleep and sleep disorders in children and adolescents. *Psychiatr Clin North Am.* 2006;29(4):1059–1076

23. Bruni O, Alonso-Alconada D, Besag F, et al. Current role of melatonin in pediatric neurology: clinical recommendation. *Eur J Paediatr Neurol.* 2015;19(2):122–133

24. Mindell JA. Empirically supported treatments in pediatric psychology: bedtime refusal and night wakings in young children. *J Pediatr Psychol.* 1999;24(6):465–481

25. DiMario FJ Jr. Prospective study of children with cyanotic and pallid breath-holding spells. *Pediatrics.* 2001;107(2):265–269

26. Zehetner AA, Orr N, Buckmaster A, Williams K, Wheeler DM. Iron supplementation for breath-holding attacks in children. *Cochrane Database Syst Rev.* 2010;12(5): CD008132

27. James A, Soler A, Weatherall R. Cognitive behavioural therapy for anxiety disorders in children and adolescents. *Cochrane Database Syst Rev.* 2005;19;(4):CD004690

28. Silverman WK, Kurtines WM. *Anxiety and Phobic Disorders, A Pragmatic Approach.* New York, NY: Plenum Press; 1996

29. Kendall PC, Cummings CM, Narayanan MK, Birmaher B, Piacentini J, et al. Mediators of change in the child/adolescent anxiety multimodal treatment study. *J Consult Clin Psychol.* 2016;84(1):1–14

30. Strawn JR, Welge JA, Wehry AM, Keeshin B, Rynn MA. Efficacy and tolerability of antidepressants in pediatric anxiety disorders: a systematic review and meta-analysis. *Depress Anxiety.* 2015;32(3):149–157

31. Kravitz H, Boehm JJ. Rhythmic habit patterns in infancy: their sequence, age of onset, and frequency. *Child Dev.* 1971;42(2):399–413

32. Friman PC, McPherson KM, Warzak WJ, Evans J. Influence of thumb sucking on peer social acceptance in first-grade children. *Pediatrics.* 1993;91(4):784–786

CHAPTER 8

Development and Disorders of Feeding, Sleep, and Elimination

Marie Reilly, MD

Alison Schonwald, MD, FAAP

Feeding

Milestones

Exclusive breastfeeding is recommended by the American Academy of Pediatrics (AAP) for about the first 6 months of a child's life. Readiness skills indicate when to offer solids in addition to breast milk (Box 8.1).

Box 8.1. Readiness Skills for Solids

> ▷ Does the infant hold his or her head up while sitting in a supportive chair?
> ▷ Does he or she watch adults' eating behavior?
> ▷ Does he or she reach for food on other people's plates?
> ▷ Is he or she opening his or her mouth when food is coming?
> ▷ Can he or she move food from a spoon to his or her mouth then his or her throat?
> ▷ Has the child reached twice the birth weight?

Mastering the ability to eat solid foods requires oromotor control and reduction in sensitivity to touch around the mouth and lips. Infants first exposed to food textures after 9 months of age are more likely to have feeding difficulty and be experienced as fussy eaters. First foods can be mashed or pureed meat, a single grain, fruit, or vegetable; one new food should be offered every 2 to 3 days, so caregivers can monitor for reactions. Within a few months, the infant should be eating a variety of food groups.

Finger feeding requires an infant to sit independently (expected at around 6 months of age) and to have a pincer grasp (expected at around 9 months of age). Small pieces of soft food that are easy to pick up and swallow include noodles, banana, scrambled egg, tofu, sweet potato, avocado, or ripe pear. From early on, anticipatory guidance can promote healthy eating behaviors for the developing child (Table 8.1).

By 19 to 24 months of age, from 20% to 60% of toddlers are described as picky eaters.[1] Picky eaters have strong preferences about food groups and/or preparation, agree to a limited variety of options, and often impact mealtime harmony for their families.[2] Food preference results from a combination of genetics, exposures, feeding context,

Table 8.1. Anticipatory Guidance	
Action	**Rationale**
Regularly scheduled time-limited meals	Prevents grazing; maintains schedule
Low-calorie snacks	Opportunity to develop hunger and satiety and develop preference for healthy eating
Neutral, distraction-free environment	Limits conflict, keeps focus on eating
Allow children to play with food, tolerate mess	Uses typical developmental learning; maintains positive environment
Provide the same food for all family members	Expands variety of food texture, flavor, and parents model healthy food choices
Small portions, easy to bite or grasp	Encourages autonomy
Encourage self-feeding	Encourages autonomy

Adapted with permission from Phalen JA. Managing feeding problems and feeding disorders. *Pediatr Rev.* 2013;34(12):552.

and associated physical and social consequences.[3] Clinicians can educate parents of young children about their ability to encourage healthy eating to impact lifelong health.[4] However, picky eating itself is common, and children who are growing and developing well need not be referred to a specialist unless there is excessive family distress.

Feeding and Eating Disorders

Feeding disorders occur in only 3% to 5% of children. In contrast to picky eating, true feeding disorders are characterized by significantly impaired physical health or psychosocial function. Feeding disorders are more common (up to 80%) in children with developmental disabilities, such as cerebral palsy, autism spectrum disorder, intellectual disability, and other chronic medical conditions (40% to 70%); they are also associated with gastrointestinal disorders (including gastroesophageal reflux and constipation) and craniofacial abnormalities.

The feeding and eating disorders described in the *Diagnostic and Statistical Manual of Mental Disorders,* Fifth Edition (*DSM-5*)[5] include pica, rumination disorder, avoidant/restrictive food intake disorder, anorexia nervosa (AN), bulimia nervosa (BN), and binge eating disorder (BED). Primary pediatric health care professionals may see many children diagnosed with the avoidant/restrictive food intake disorder (ARFID), which replaces the previous diagnosis of "feeding disorder of infancy or early childhood." It no longer requires onset before 6 years of age. Avoidant/restrictive food intake disorder therefore captures both children and adolescents. Initial studies characterize affected children as often having picky eating since early childhood, along with generalized anxiety and/or gastrointestinal symptoms and/or fears of eating related to vomiting, choking, or food allergies.[6]

Anorexia nervosa, BN, and BED typically present in adolescence. A final diagnosis of "other specified feeding or eating disorder" (OSFED) includes 5 disorders: AN, BN of low frequency and/or limited duration, BED of low frequency and/or limited duration, purging disorder, and night eating syndrome. Unspecified feeding or eating disorder (UFED) is warranted for patients not meeting more specific diagnostic criteria.

Evaluation

Assessment always begins with a careful history (perinatal, developmental, feeding, medical, family, and social history), dietary assessment, and physical examination (including growth parameters over time). Medical conditions (eg, dysphagia and aspiration), environmental factors, and cultural practices must be explored and addressed when appropriate. Details about mealtime activities and behaviors should be elicited, and ideally, the clinician should observe a live or videotaped feeding interaction. Organic and behavioral red flags are listed in Box 8.2. Investigation routinely includes complete blood counts, full biochemistry panel, thyroid function tests, urinalysis and culture,[7] and celiac serology. Referral to a speech and language pathologist and/or occupational therapist is indicated with suspicion of oral motor delay and oropharyngeal dysphagia. A dietitian might evaluate caloric and nutritional intake. Gastroenterologists and developmental-behavioral pediatricians might evaluate (and co-manage) contributing causes. Inpatient hospitalization is warranted only for the most difficult cases.

Box 8.2. Red Flags in the Evaluation of Feeding Concerns

Mealtime Behavior	Signs and Symptoms
Prolonged meal	Dysphagia
Disruptive and stressful mealtimes	Aspiration
Dependent feeding	Appearance of pain with feeding
Nocturnal eating	Vomiting and diarrhea
Failure to advance textures	Developmental disability
Forceful, intrusive feeding	Chronic cardiorespiratory symptoms
Abrupt cessation after trigger event	Failure to thrive
Anticipatory gagging	

Adapted with permission from Kerzner B, Milano K, MacLean WC, et al. A practical approach to classifying and managing feeding difficulties. *Pediatrics*. 2015;135(2):346.

Treatment

Behavioral interventions start with anticipatory guidance in the medical home. If office-based counseling is not successful, referral to an expert in behavioral treatment is indicated. Pica rarely requires surgical removal of ingested contents. Subsequently, for pica, RD, and ARFID, behavioral treatment with a specialist is indicated. Milder cases are often treated successfully with a nutritionist or registered dietitian. Some children will require referral to a psychologist, speech pathologist, and/or occupational therapist with specific expertise in treating children with feeding disorders. Overall, limited randomized controlled trials exist to guide treatment, but behavioral intervention is the principal method for more involved cases and is backed by a preponderance of evidence suggesting positive outcomes. Behavioral methods often used include relaxation to reduce arousal, desensitization, and positive reinforcement. Treatment is ideally multidisciplinary, with a primary focus on responding to hunger and satiety with patience and encouragement within developmentally appropriate expectations. Treatment is typically outpatient, can be individual or group, and must include a caregiver component. Calorie concentration and off-label use of appetite-enhancing medication may take place while or after behavior and context are addressed; nonoral methods of feeding, such as temporary nasogastric tube use, should occur only after multidisciplinary treatment has been unsuccessful in the context of nutritional compromise. Inpatient therapy is indicated only for those most severely involved. Follow-up focuses on anthropomorphic trajectory.

Sleep

Typical Development

Quality sleep is important to a child's overall growth and development. Decreased sleep can negatively impact children's emotional, behavioral, and cognitive functioning. Disrupted sleep can impact not only the child's overall functioning, but that of his or her family as well. Primary pediatric health care professionals therefore have the opportunity to have a significant impact on the lives of children and their families by providing age-appropriate anticipatory guidance, as well as screening for and managing common pediatric sleep issues.

As a first step, it is helpful to be familiar with the necessary amount of time a typical child should sleep each day; a child's sleep requirement varies with age. Sleep recommendations vary, as listed in Figure 8.1.

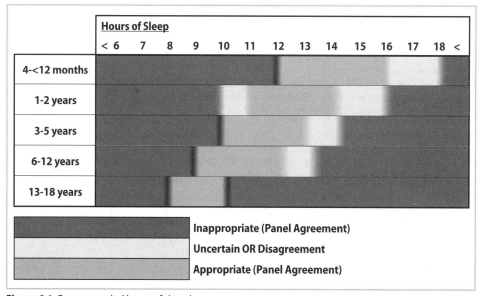

Figure 8.1. Recommended hours of sleep by age group.

Republished with permission of American Academy of Sleep Medicine, from Paruthi S, Brooks LJ, D'Ambrosio C, et al. Consensus Statement of the American Academy of Sleep Medicine on the recommended amount of sleep for healthy children: methodology and discussion. *J Clin Sleep Med.* 2016;12(11):1549-1561; permission conveyed through Copyright Clearance Center, Inc.

Anticipatory guidance around sleep and the identification of sleep problems are an important component of well-child care. Allen et al[8] proposed use of the mnemonic, ABCs of SLEEPING, as a tool for primary pediatric health care professionals to identify sleep problems and to counsel patients and families regarding healthy sleep. The mnemonic is as follows:

ABCs: Age-appropriate **B**edtimes and wake-times with **C**onsistency of

S Schedules and routines

L Location

E Exercise and diet

E No Electronics in the bedroom or before bed

P Positivity

I Independence when falling asleep

N Needs of child met during the day

G Equal Great Sleep

Sleep recommendations, and the level of empirical support for these recommendations, are summarized in Table 8.2.[8]

Sleep Disorders

The prevalence of sleep problems presenting in the primary care setting varies widely depending on the method of data collection (parent report versus primary care provider report versus record review). Overall, primary pediatric health care professionals estimate that sleep challenges occur in approximately 20% of children aged 6 months to 4 years.[9] However, primary pediatric health care professionals may underestimate sleep problems in older children and adolescents and underdiagnose sleep disorders.

The following describes the most common disorders of sleep development encountered in pediatrics:

1. **Sleep terrors/night terrors:** Sleep terrors are nighttime arousals that occur during nonrapid eye movement (NREM) sleep. Because NREM sleep occurs earlier in sleep, sleep terrors do as well. Sleep terrors present as episodes of abrupt terror associated with an alarming vocalization and signs of autonomic arousal in children typically between the ages of 2 and 12 years. Children who experience night terrors are confused during the episode (often not recognizing their parents), are difficult to console, and cannot recall the episode afterward. As a result, families are more distressed by sleep terrors than the child is.

Table 8.2. Sleep Recommendations and Level of Support		
Recommendation	**Clinicians Should Ask About**	**Level of Support**
Age-appropriate bedtimes and wake-times with consistency	Timing and regularity	Strong support for ensuring that children nap, go to bed, and wake up at times that allow them to obtain age-appropriate amounts of sleep
		Moderate support for bedtimes no later than 9:00 pm
		Moderate support for maintaining a regular sleep schedule
		Insufficient support that sleep schedules should not vary more than 30–60 minutes
Schedules and routines	Daily routines, Bedtime routines	Strong support for establishing bedtime routines
		Insufficient support for wake time routines
		Insufficient support for consistency in daytime routines
Location	Quiet, Comforts, Ambient light	Limited support for children's rooms needing to be dark
		Limited support for quiet bedrooms
		Equivocal support for avoiding sounds as children go to sleep
		Equivocal support for children needing their own bedroom
		Insufficient support for children having a comfortable bed in a familiar bedroom
Exercise and diet	Timing of activity, Amount of activity, Caffeine, Eating before bed, Sugar	Limited support for limiting caffeine consumption
		Limited support for maintaining a healthy, balanced diet
		Limited support for children not going to bed hungry or not consuming a large meal before bedtime
		Equivocal support for engaging in daily physical activity
		Insufficient support for not eating too much close to bedtime
		Non-support for avoiding exercise within 1–4 hours of bedtime
No electronics in the bedroom or before bed	Television, Media, Computers	Strong support for limiting access to electronics during and after bedtime by removing them from children's bedrooms
Positivity	Family conflict, Emotional environment, Relaxation, Parent-child conflict	Moderate support for establishing a positive atmosphere in the child's living environment
		Limited support for parents maintaining a positive attitude toward sleep
		Limited support for children being relaxed and calm before bed
		Limited support for children avoiding fun, exciting, or frustrating activities before bed
Independence when falling asleep	Parental presence, Sleep associations	Strong support for children learning to settle in their own bed, without their parents to avoid dependence on parental presence to fall asleep or after night wakings
Needs of child met during the day	Attachment; Emotional needs	Moderate support for ensuring children's emotional needs are met during the day
		Insufficient support for ensuring that children's physiological needs are met during the day

Adapted from Allen SL, Howlett MD, Coulombe JA, Corkum PV. ABCs of SLEEPING: a review of the evidence behind pediatric sleep recommendations. *Sleep Med Rev.* 2016;29:1–14, with permission from Elsevier.

Potential factors that may be linked to both sleep terrors and sleepwalking include: sleep deprivation, stress, obstructive sleep apnea syndrome (OSAS), restless legs syndrome (RLS), and sleeping in unfamiliar settings.[10] Children who experience sleep terrors often have a family history of sleep terrors as well.

Aside from screening for sleep disorders like OSAS and RLS, management of sleep terrors primarily focuses on counseling families. However, in the case of *nightly* sleep terrors, scheduled awakenings 15 to 30 minutes before the time at which episodes typically occur may be helpful for 2- to 4-week periods that can be repeated as needed. If sleep terrors persist, low-dose clonazepam (0.125–0.5 mg at bedtime) for 3 to 6 months, with a slow taper, may be helpful. Common side effects of clonazepam include drowsiness, ataxia, and behavioral problems.[11]

2. **Somnambulism:** Somnambulism, or sleepwalking, is also an arousal disorder that occurs during NREM sleep. Again, because NREM sleep occurs earlier in sleep, sleepwalking does as well. Sleepwalking behaviors are quite variable and can include walking, running, as well as complex tasks out of the bed. When others attempt to intervene or redirect the sleepwalker, the individual may be inappropriate or unresponsive.

The diagnosis of sleepwalking is made by parent/caregiver history, as individuals have partial to complete amnesia of sleepwalking episodes. Key components of the history, in addition to those just described, include the recurrent nature of these episodes of incomplete awakening, as well as limited to no associated dream imagery.

Given the potential for some children who sleepwalk to leave the home during an episode, safety considerations are a key component of overall management (Box 8.3).

Box 8.3. Safety Considerations for Sleep Walkers

> ▶ Place alarms or bells on doors and windows.
> ▶ Remove potentially dangerous items from the child's room and common pathways.
> ▶ Have child sleep on mattress on first floor.

If sleepwalking persists, clinicians can consider low-dose clonazepam at bedtime for a period of 3 to 6 months, followed by a slow taper.

3. **Obstructive Sleep Apnea Syndrome:** Obstructive sleep apnea syndrome is a sleep disorder commonly resulting from upper airway obstruction that causes partial to complete airway obstruction during sleep. These periods of obstruction cause increased respiratory effort, disrupted sleep, and alterations in gas exchange.

Greater than 95% of cases of OSAS are caused by structural airway obstruction, with the small remainder resulting from neurological causes. The prevalence of OSAS in children from 2 to 8 years of age is between 1% and 5%. This peak incidence period may be due to the relative size of the tonsils and/or adenoids in comparison to the upper airway at this time in development.

The pathophysiology of OSAS is not completely known; however, factors that decrease upper airway size or increase upper airway collapsibility increase the likelihood of OSAS.[12] These can include adenotonsillar hypertrophy, obesity, craniofacial abnormalities, and inflammatory causes like rhinosinusitis. When caring for children with Down syndrome, providers should ask regularly about symptoms of OSAS. In addition, all children with Down syndrome should complete a sleep study by 4 years of age.

At night, individuals with OSAS present with snoring, witnessed apnea, gasping or snorting, mouth breathing, restless sleep, sleepwalking, night terrors, diaphoresis, frequent awakenings, nocturnal enuresis, unusual sleep position, and/or paradoxical chest wall movement. These individuals may present with daytime sleepiness, difficulty waking, headaches, hyponasal speech, inattention, hyperactivity, impulsivity, irritability, depression, and/or aggression.

The gold standard for diagnosis of OSAS is nocturnal in-lab polysomnography. Treatment options for OSAS fall into the broad categories of surgery (eg, tonsillectomy/adenoidectomy), medications (eg, topical nasal glucocorticoids), and positive airway pressure. Positive airway pressure is indicated when a child experiences persistent OSAS symptoms despite adenotonsillectomy, in the setting of minimal adenotonsillar tissue, or when surgery is contraindicated.

Untreated OSAS can have a variety of consequences ranging from cardiovascular (increased susceptibility to pulmonary hypertension and right heart failure in severe cases) to impaired cognitive and behavioral functioning (attention-deficit/hyperactivity disorder [ADHD]-like symptoms, learning challenges) to metabolic effects (fatty liver disease, dyslipidemia).

4. **Restless Legs Syndrome:** Restless legs syndrome is a condition that is characterized by the urge to move one's legs or by an unpleasant feeling described by some children as pain, difficulty getting comfortable, or a "creepy crawly" sensation. These unpleasant sensations are relieved by movement or distraction. Children with RLS experience these sensations during *both* the day and night; however they can become more notable at nighttime. As such, approximately 85% of children with RLS experience sleep disturbance.

Although the pathophysiology of RLS is not completely known, genetic factors as well as the dopamine pathway are thought to contribute to RLS. It is important for clinicians to note that low iron status also is a risk factor for RLS. Iron plays a role in dopamine synthesis, myelin synthesis, energy production, and neurotransmitter systems that may contribute to RLS.[13] Recognizing the role of iron in RLS is important, as it provides a potential source of intervention. Serum ferritin levels are found to be low in more than 80% of children with RLS.

The diagnosis of RLS is made through a focused history (see Box 8.4 for criteria). Once diagnosed, serum ferritin levels should be obtained. There is some disagreement among experts regarding a threshold for a low ferritin. Some suggest iron supplementation for a ferritin level below 50 mcg/L, while others suggest a cutoff of 75 mcg/L. Children with low ferritin levels should be treated with 2 mg/kg to 4 mg/kg of elemental iron up to twice a day (but check for maximum dosing, to avoid overdosing children with obesity). In 3 months, symptoms should be reassessed and serum ferritin rechecked. However, providers should recall that ferritin is an acute-phase reactant and may be artifactually elevated by inflammation or infection.

Box 8.4. Criteria for Restless Legs Syndrome

- ▶ Urge to move the legs; usually accompanied by, or thought to be caused by, uncomfortable and unpleasant sensations in the legs.
- ▶ Symptoms begin or worsen during periods of rest or inactivity.
- ▶ Symptoms are partially or totally relieved by movement.
- ▶ Symptoms occur exclusively or predominantly in the evening or night.

Other management options for RLS include massage, warm baths, socks or compression stockings, and avoidance of potentially exacerbating factors, such as decreased sleep and caffeine. There are no medications currently approved for use in children with RLS, although dopaminergic agents and gabapentin are approved for adults.

5. **Narcolepsy:** Narcolepsy is a rare sleep disorder that occurs with an estimated prevalence between 0.025% and 0.4% across all ages. Individuals with narcolepsy can experience cataplexy (a medical condition in which strong emotion or laughter causes a person to suffer sudden physical collapse though remaining conscious), hypnagogic hallucinations (just before sleep and may be accompanied by sleep paralysis), hypnopompic hallucinations (considered as part of a dream by the subject and can be accompanied by feelings of difficulty breathing and muscle tightness), sleep paralysis, and/or very fragmented sleep. For many individuals, symptoms first emerge during childhood. The first presenting sign of narcolepsy is usually excessive daytime sleepiness. These daily periods of the irrepressible need to sleep or daytime lapses into sleep significantly impact multiple areas of the individual's life, including behavior, mood, and social functioning. Individuals with narcolepsy can also experience weight gain of unclear origin.

The diagnosis of narcolepsy is made based on a history of daily periods of irrepressible need to sleep or daytime lapses into sleep for at least 3 months. Further diagnostic criteria include cataplexy, a mean sleep latency of less than or equal to 8 minutes, and 2 or more sleep-onset rapid eye movement periods on a multiple sleep latency test. Performing human leukocyte antigen (HLA) studies and obtaining cerebrospinal fluid (CSF) hypocretin-1 levels can be considered in some cases.[14]

Nonpharmacological options for narcolepsy management include consistent sleep-wake schedules, regular naps, exercise, and accommodations such as preferential seating and avoidance of cataplexy-inducing activities. Pharmacological options approved in adults include stimulant medications used to treat ADHD, as well: modafinil and armodafinil.

Evaluation

As illustrated, history taking is a key component in the diagnosis of many sleep disorders. A focused history should consider aspects of sleep hygiene, as well some of the more concerning signs and symptoms associated with the conditions described herein. An alternative to the ABCs of SLEEPING is the BEARS mnemonic, which can also be used to guide a sleep history. The mnemonic is as follows:

B Bedtime resistance or sleep-onset delay

E Excessive daytime sleepiness

A Awakenings at night

R Regularity, patterns, and duration of sleep

S Snoring and other symptoms

Physical examination focuses on attributes contributing to the suspected sleep disorder:

- Obstructive sleep apnea syndrome: obesity, failure to thrive, hyponasal speech, tonsillar crowding, mouth breathing, adenoid facies (long and narrow face, low tongue placement, narrow upper jaw, steep mandible, and open anterior bite)
- Restless legs syndrome: pallor
- Narcolepsy: sleepiness in the office, precocious puberty features, absent tendon reflexes during an episode of cataplexy[10]

Primary Versus Specialty Care

Despite the frequency of sleep-related concerns among children, there are a limited number of pediatric sleep medicine providers in the United States. Further, these providers tend to be located in urban settings. As a result, many primary pediatric health care professionals find themselves managing sleep difficulties and disorders in their patients. Primary pediatric health care professionals can accurately diagnose and effectively manage sleep difficulties, as well as sleep disorders such as sleep terrors, sleepwalking, and RLS; however, further diagnostic evaluation and treatment is required for a child with suspected and then confirmed OSAS (via sleep medicine, otolaryngology, or pulmonary specialists), depending on the region and accessibility. Finally, given the diagnostic testing associated with suspected narcolepsy, children with this condition will likely be best served by a subspecialty provider.

Sleep Medications

It is helpful for primary pediatric health care professionals to be familiar with pharmacological options for children who experience poor sleep (Table 8.3). There is little evidence to guide pharmacological decision-making, and there are currently no medications for sleep problems in children that have been approved by the US Food and Drug Administration.

Table 8.3. Sleep Medications				
Drug Category	**Example**	**Use/Indication**	**Suggested Dosing**	**Side Effects**
Antihistamines	Diphenhydramine Hydroxyzine	Insomnia	Diphenhydramine 0.5 mg/kg up to 25 mg (25–50 mg in adults) Hydroxyzine 0.5 mg/lb	Drowsiness Palpitations Restlessness
Alpha Agonists	Clonidine Guanfacine	Insomnia (particularly in children with ADHD) Nightmares (in adults with PTSD)	Clonidine 0.05–0.1 mg starting dose Guanfacine 0.5 mg (titrate no higher than 4 mg/day)	Orthostatic hypotension Bradycardia Arrhythmia
Benzodiazepines	Clonazepam	Parasomnias (night terrors, somnambulism) Insomnia	Clonazepam 0.125–0.5 mg at bedtime	Ataxia Behavior problems Dizziness
Nonbenzodiazepine Benzodiazepine Receptor Agonists	Zolpidem Eszopiclone	Insomnia	Zolpidem 0.25 mg/kg	Headache Dizziness Dysgeusia
Antidepressants	Trazodone Amitriptyline Mirtazapine Nefazodone	Insomnia	Trazodone 25–50 mg Amitriptyline 5 mg starting dose (should not exceed 50 mg)	Priapism Weight gain Xerostomia
Melatonin	Melatonin	Insomnia	0.05 mg/kg given 1–2 hours before desired bedtime	Headache Confusion Fragmented sleep
Melatonin Receptor Agonists	Ramelteon Tasimelteon	Insomnia	Reported efficacy at 2–8 mg	Dizziness Nausea Headache

Abbreviations: ADHD, attention-deficit/hyperactivity disorder; PTSD, posttraumatic stress disorder.

Derived from Troester MM, Pelavo R. Pediatric sleep pharmacology: a primer. *Semin Pediatr Neurol*. 2015;22(2):135–147; Owens JA, Rosen CL, Mindell JA, Kirchner HL. Use of pharmacotherapy for insomnia in child psychiatric practice: a national survey. *Sleep Med*. 2010;11(7):692–700; and Hintze JP, Paruthi S. Sleep in the pediatric population. *Sleep Med Clinics*. 2016;11(1):91–103.

Elimination

Toilet Training and Continence
– Typical Developmental Milestones

Toilet training is a complex milestone requiring integration and coordination of multiple developmental skills, demanding competence in fine and gross motor, language, and social domains. Not accomplishing the task of toilet training can have financial, social, and educational consequences: failing to become toilet trained as expected can likewise generate startling levels of family distress. While some children appear to "train themselves overnight," other children take a slower course. Regardless of a child's path, he or she must have acquired all necessary links in the toilet training chain.

Kaerts et al[15] identified 21 separate skills (and the age range when they develop) necessary for continence (Table 8.4). The more commonly discussed "major" readiness signs of toilet training are highlighted within the table that follows. The age ranges listed suggest that truly independent toilet training is developmentally unattainable prior to about 2 years of age. "Elimination Communication" or "Assisted Infant Toilet Training" achieves dryness, but as a result of a parent carefully reading a toddler's cues and placing the child over the toilet to urinate or defecate; this method can keep children clean and dry, but requires a caregiver partner to achieve.[16]

In the United States, the average age of toilet training has increased over the years. In the 1980s, children were trained on average by 24 to 27 months of age. By the 1990s, this increased to 35 to 39 months of age. Overall, girls are toilet trained 2 to 3 months earlier than are boys.

Table 8.4. Developmental Skills Required for Independent Toilet Training			
Developmental Skill	**Age Attained (months)**	**Developmental Skill**	**Age Attained (months)**
Imitates	2–25	Has an interest in potty training	12–28
Sits steadily	4–16	Has increased bladder capacity	12–32
Walks	8–18	Completes tasks alone	12–36
Picks up small objects	9–18	Asks for the potty	12–35
Says "no"	9–24	Wants to be clean	18–24
Controls pelvic muscles	9–24	Wants to wear grownup clothes	18–24
Follows simple command	9–26	Pulls clothes on and off	18–36
Expresses a need to go	9–16	Has no overnight bowel movement	21–26
Enjoys putting things into containers	10–26	Puts things where they belong	22–27
Is aware of bladder sensation	12–24	Sits on potty for 5–10 minutes	25–33
Understands potty words	12–26		

Derived from Kaerts N, Van Hal G, Vermandel A, Wyandaele JJ. Readiness signs used to define the proper moment to start toilet training: a review of the literature. *Neurourol Urodyn.* 2012;31(4):437–440.

There is no evidence for a best toilet training strategy. The AAP supports the child-centered approach, while others prefer the adult-guided toilet-train-in-a-day option (Table 8.5). The latter, more intensive method can include verbal reprimands, with some studies reporting hitting, temper tantrums, and avoidance behavior developing as a consequence. Pediatric health care professionals often favor the child-centered approach, as it accounts for variations in child temperament and the developmental norm of toddlers and preschoolers seeking autonomy via mastery and control of their world, aspects absent from the more directive toilet training method.[17]

Table 8.5. Approaches to Toilet Training	
Child-Centered Approach	**Toilet-Train-in-a-Day Approach**
Weeks to months	One to 2 days
Identify child's interest and readiness	Adult-determined starting time
Introduce a potty chair	Demonstrate with a doll
Encourage additional steps with positive reinforcement	Remain in one room, give large amounts of fluids, frequent reminders and dryness checks every 3 to 5 minutes; positive reinforcement of successes
Acknowledge accidents without reprimand	Verbally reprimand accident, take responsibility to change into dry pants

Anticipatory Guidance

Clinicians generally review readiness signs of toilet training during well-child visits, starting at 18 to 24 months. Suggested questions are listed in Table 8.6. Rather than recommending a best age to initiate toilet training, a child's readiness, sex, family stressors, and cultural norms should be considered.

Table 8.6. Suggested Questions to Ascertain Toilet Training Readiness	
Readiness Assessment Questions	**Readiness Skill**
Is he or she dry for 2 hours at a time?	Increased bladder capacity
Does he or she know the toilet words of your family (eg, poop, poo, caca, doody, pee, pee-pee, etc.)?	Understand potty words
Does he or she watch caregivers in the bathroom?	Interest in toilet training
Can he or she get undressed independently?	Pull clothes on and off

Children who are difficult to toilet train are more likely to be constipated, to have difficult temperamental traits, or to have developmental delays compared to peers trained more easily.[18] When toilet training fails to progress, primary pediatric health care professionals need to determine what obstacles may play a role before making recommendations for the family to follow (Figure 8.2). In all scenarios, the contributing factor of constipation needs to be considered.

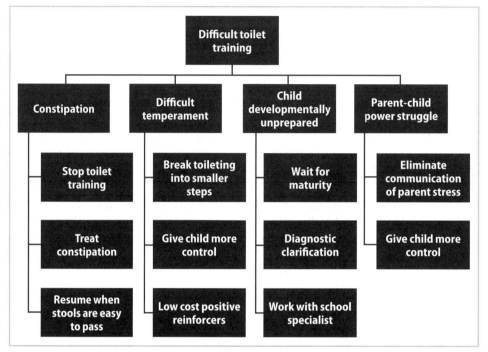

Figure 8.2. Considerations when there is difficulty with toilet training.

Enuresis and Encopresis
– Typical Development Versus Disordered Development

By 2 years of age, 30% of typical children sense bladder fullness and by 4 years of age, all typical children should sense the urge to void.[19] As a result, by 4 years of age, the majority of typically developing children are able to use the bathroom independently.[20] When a child's development deviates from this expected pattern, both child and family functioning can be negatively affected. For example, children who experience fecal incontinence are at increased risk of peer rejection, stigmatization, and bullying.[21] Families also describe their child's incontinence as a significant stressor. Given this, it is important for primary pediatric health care professionals to be prepared to diagnose, manage, and provide parental guidance regarding elimination disorders.

– Elimination Disorders

Enuresis refers to the repeated passage of urine into bed or clothes, whether involuntary or intentional, in a child whose developmental level is at least 5 years of age.[5] Children with enuresis experience episodes of incontinence at least twice a week, for a period of at least 3 consecutive months, and experience clinically significant distress or impairment in important areas of functioning.[5]

Enuresis can be specified as diurnal (passage of urine during waking hours), nocturnal (passage of urine only during nighttime sleep), or combined nocturnal-diurnal.[5] In addition, it is important to note whether the enuresis is primary (child was not previously continent) or secondary (child was continent for at least 6 months), as this can inform the differential diagnosis.

Fecal incontinence or *encopresis* refers to the repeated passage of feces into inappropriate places, whether involuntary or intentional, in a child whose developmental level is at least 4 years of age.[5] Children with encopresis experience episodes of incontinence at least once a month, for a period of at least 3 months.[5] This behavior is not attributable to the physiological effects of a substance, such as laxatives, or another medical condition, except through a mechanism involving constipation.[5]

A child with primary fecal incontinence has never been successfully toilet trained, whereas a child with secondary fecal incontinence has been toilet trained and now experiences incontinence. Again, clarifying this distinction is important to understanding etiology and determining a treatment plan.

– Evaluation and Management
Urinary Incontinence
History: A targeted history can be sufficient to determine diagnosis and eliminate the need for further testing. It is important to ask about the presence of lower urinary tract symptoms, as this can help determine etiology (Box 8.5) and management. Lower urinary tract symptoms include increased/decreased voiding frequency, urgency, hesitancy, straining, weak stream, intermittency, holding maneuvers, a feeling of incomplete emptying, postmicturition dribble, and genital/lower abdominal pain. A comprehensive history should also address drinking habits, bowel symptoms, previous treatments, family and child response to incontinence, as well as triggering events, abuse, or trauma. If a child experiences symptoms at night only, providers should ask about snoring, apnea, seizures, or parasomnias.

Box 8.5. Causes of Urinary Incontinence

> Spinal cord lesions: tethered cord, spina bifida

> Peripheral neuropathies: trauma, diabetes mellitus

> Anatomical abnormalities: ectopic ureter, posterior urethral valves, urethral stenosis or diverticula, labial adhesions, and urethral trauma

> Excessive urine production: diabetes mellitus, diabetes insipidus, sickle cell disease, volume overload, and diuretic use

> Bladder wall irritability: bacteria, viruses, calciuria

> Constipation

> Emotional stress: PTSD, sexual abuse, and major life changes

> Functional voiding disorders: overactive bladder/urge incontinence, giggle incontinence, underactive bladder, Hinman syndrome, and voiding postponement

Abbreviation: PTSD, posttraumatic stress disorder.

Derived from Nasir R, Schonwald A. Urinary function and enuresis. *Developmental-Behavioral Pediatrics.* 4th ed. Philadelphia, PA: Saunders/Elsevier; 2009:602–609.

Physical Examination: Abdominal examination should include palpation for organomegaly, bladder distension, and stool burden. The lower back should be examined for cutaneous manifestations of spinal dysraphism. Similarly, a neurological examination should include assessment of lower extremity strength, gait, deep tendon reflexes, and sacral reflexes, including anal wink and cremasteric reflex in boys. Inspection of the genital area may indicate anatomical abnormalities. Primary pediatric health care professionals should also be alert to signs of sexual or physical abuse.

Diagnostic Studies: Children presenting with diurnal incontinence should have a urinalysis to rule out glucosuria, renal concentrating defects, or signs of a urinary tract infection, which, if present, indicate the need for a urine culture.

Management: The management of daytime enuresis focuses on education regarding lower urinary tract function, regular voiding habits, correct voiding posture, and fluid intake. Bladder diaries can also be used. Treatment of constipation can also alleviate urinary incontinence. Behavioral approaches can include scheduled voids, sticker charts for bathroom visits, and positive reinforcement. It is also important to manage family stress by educating parents that incontinence is involuntary and that the child should not be punished.

Children who continue to experience diurnal urinary incontinence despite the above may benefit from medication management with an anticholinergic agent, such as oxybutynin.[22,23] If symptoms persist despite pharmacotherapy, these children would benefit from referral to a pediatric urologist for further evaluation.

The management of nocturnal enuresis begins with treatment of daytime urinary incontinence and constipation. Parent and child guidance should focus on the importance of regular daytime voids, appropriate fluid intake, and emptying the bladder before bed.

A 2013 Cochrane review of behavioral interventions for nocturnal enuresis found that simple behavioral interventions (reward systems such as star charts for dry nights, lifting and waking the child at night to urinate, bladder training, and fluid restriction) were superior to no active treatment, but inferior to alarm therapy and some drug therapy.[24] Alarm therapy can be curative in 60% of children, but it is highly dependent on the motivation of the child and family.

Effective use of an enuresis alarm includes the use of the following recommendations (Table 8.7 and Box 8.6):

Table 8.7. Recommendations for Effective Use of Enuresis Alarms	
Ownership	The child should be encouraged to take ownership of the alarm and its correct use. The child should be reminded that the alarm will not work unless he or she listens for it and responds to it quickly. The child should hook up the alarm system solo. The child should also trigger the alarm a few times by touching the sensor with a wet finger and then practice getting up to go to the bathroom, as he or she would at night.
Nightlight or Flashlight	A light source should be available so that the child can see what he or she is doing when the alarm sounds.
Pep Talk	The child should prepare and practice to "beat the buzzer" and wake up when his or her bladder is full, before becoming wet. If the buzzer does go off, the child should try to wake up and stop urinating as soon as possible.
Once Awake	Once awake, the child should turn off the alarm, go to the bathroom, and urinate. Then, the child should change into dry underwear and pajamas, reconnect the alarm, and place a dry towel over any wet spots in bed.
Calendar	In the morning, the child should mark on the calendar whether he or she was dry (no alarm), whether there was a wet spot (awoke after the alarm sounded), or whether he or she was wet (did not get up).
Patience	Children and families should be counseled to use the alarm every night until a 3- to 4-week period of dryness is reached. This can take a few months to achieve.

Adapted from Schmitt BD. *Your Child's Health: Pediatric Guide for Parents*. New York, NY: Bantam Books; 1987

Box 8.6. A Self-Awakening Program

GO TO BED BEFORE EMPTYING YOUR BLADDER

Practice these steps 3 times:

- ▸ Lie down with your eyes closed.
- ▸ Pretend it's the middle of the night and your bladder is full.
- ▸ Pretend your bladder is starting to ache.
- ▸ Pretend your bladder is trying to wake you up and is saying, "Get up before it's too late!"
- ▸ Run to the bathroom and urinate a small amount.
- ▸ Lie down again.

On the third practice run, empty your bladder

- ▸ Remind yourself to get up like this if you need to urinate during the night.

Adapted from Schmitt BD. *Your Child's Health: Pediatric Guide for Parents*. New York, NY: Bantam Books; 1987

Medication options for persistent nocturnal enuresis include desmopressin and imipramine. The starting dose of desmopressin is 0.2 mg, with the possibility of increasing to 0.4 mg.[25] Providers should be aware that excessive fluid intake before or after a desmopressin dose can lead to water intoxication, hyponatremia, and convulsions.[25] While many patients respond to desmopressin, the recurrence risk after completion of desmopressin treatment remains high.[25] The starting dose of imipramine is 25–50 mg at bedtime.[25] Experts recommend reevaluating after one month; if symptoms are under good control, providers should then taper imipramine to the lowest effective dose.[25] Experts also recommend a 2-week trial off imipramine every 3 months in order to assess for persistence of enuresis.[25]

Fecal Incontinence

History: In the majority of cases, a thorough history and physical examination are sufficient to identify both fecal incontinence and its underlying cause. As fecal incontinence can be a multifactorial condition, it is important to obtain a comprehensive history in order to clarify contributing factors and identify opportunities for intervention. Key elements of the history include frequency of symptoms, consistency and size of bowel movements (BMs), ease of passage, volume of incontinence (ie, full evacuation of stool or smearing/staining), timing of incontinence, and previous treatments. The history should also address diet, individual or family history of conditions that can contribute to constipation (Box 8.7) and/or fecal incontinence (Table 8.8), and a social history, including abuse, trauma, or stressors.

Primary pediatric health care professionals should also ask about urinary incontinence when assessing a child with fecal incontinence, as a large stool burden can exert pressure on the bladder, resulting in bladder spasms and involuntary emptying. In addition, girls who experience fecal incontinence are at particular risk of urinary tract infections.

Box 8.7. Rome III Criteria for Functional Constipation

Must include 2 or more of the following occurring at least once per week for a minimum of 1 month with insufficient criteria for a diagnosis of irritable bowel syndrome. These symptoms also cannot be better explained by an alternative medical condition.

1. Two or fewer defecations in the toilet per week in a child of a developmental age of at least 4 years
2. At least one episode of fecal incontinence per week
3. History of retentive posturing or excessive volitional stool retention
4. History of painful or hard bowel movements
5. Presence of a large fecal mass in the rectum
6. History of large-diameter stools that can obstruct the toilet

Adapted from Hyams JS, Di Lorenzo C, Saps M. Childhood functional gastrointestinal disorders: child/adolescent. *Gastroenterology.* 2016;150(6):1456–1468, with permission from Elsevier.

Table 8.8. Other Causes of Fecal Incontinence	
Category	**Etiology**
Malformations	Anal stenosis, partial imperforate anus
Neurogenic	Occult spinal dysraphism, tethered cord, or tumor
Endocrine-metabolic	Multiple endocrine neoplasia III, thyroid disorder, or electrolyte imbalance
Neuromuscular	Muscular dystrophy or Hirschsprung disease
Medications	Laxatives
Sexual abuse	
Diarrheal disease	Celiac disease

Derived from Weissman L, Bridgemohan C. Bowel function, toileting, encopresis. In: Carey WB, Crocker AC, Coleman WL, Elias ER, Feldman HM, eds. *Developmental-Behavioral Pediatrics*. 4th ed. Philadelphia, PA: Saunders/Elsevier; 2009:610–618.

Physical Examination: The physical examination of a child with fecal incontinence begins with assessment of growth parameters, possible dysmorphisms, and the parent-child interaction. The latter can provide clues regarding treatment approaches and the need for parental guidance and education regarding fecal incontinence. Abdominal examination may indicate signs of constipation, including fullness, distension, or palpable stool. The lower back should be examined for cutaneous manifestations of spinal dysraphism. The neurological examination should include assessment of lower extremity strength, gait, deep tendon reflexes, and sacral reflexes, including anal wink and cremasteric reflex in boys. A digital rectal examination may be difficult to conduct during the first visit but should be conducted during the course of treatment, as it can provide information regarding sphincter tone, rectal content, and possible Hirschsprung disease, if examination results in subsequent explosive stool. As always, primary pediatric health care professionals should be alert to signs of physical or sexual abuse.

Diagnostic Studies: Fecal incontinence is a clinical diagnosis and does not require obtaining an abdominal radiograph or laboratory studies.

Pathophysiology: Constipation-associated fecal incontinence often begins when children withhold stool, causing it to accumulate and harden in the colon. Progressive stool retention results in gradual rectal and colonic dilation that inhibits contraction and propulsion by the rectal musculature. This gradual dilation can also stretch local nerve fibers, causing difficulty controlling the external anal sphincter and decreased recognition of the urge to stool. As a result, semiliquid stool can leak around preexisting stool, thereby causing fecal incontinence.

Management: Management of fecal incontinence begins with parent and child education regarding the pathophysiology of fecal incontinence. A key point to emphasize is that the child cannot control these episodes and should not be punished for them. Dietary counseling (eg, high-fiber foods) and intervention may also be helpful in preventing constipation.

Children with constipation benefit from medication management to promote the passage of soft, regular stools. Many children with significant constipation require a complete bowel cleanout in which they take higher doses of softeners or laxatives for a short time in order to pass retained stool. This cleanout period is then followed by maintenance dosing. The authors recommend against the routine use of enemas in young children.

Behavioral approaches to treat fecal incontinence include scheduled toilet sitting times, which serve to promote evacuation of stool and increase the child's level of comfort with using the toilet. Sitting times last only a few minutes and can be timed to occur approximately 20 to 30 minutes after a meal in order to take advantage of the gastro-colic reflex. Scheduled sitting times with foot support can also be helpful in minimizing parent-child struggles related to using the toilet. It is important that the child be motivated to participate in the behavioral plan. Younger children may enjoy earning stickers on a sticker chart for engaging in sitting times. Older children may also enjoy stickers but can also be offered the opportunity to earn desired items or special time with a parent.

– Primary Versus Specialty Care

Most children with enuresis and encopresis can be managed successfully by their primary pediatric health care professional. Children who do not respond to enuresis interventions at first may benefit from a treatment break lasting a few months. However, if enuresis persists, these children would benefit from referral to a pediatric urologist, in order to clarify the anatomy and function of the lower urinary tract.

Fecal incontinence can also be managed effectively in the primary care office setting by utilizing the medical, educational, and behavioral strategies outlined earlier. However, primary pediatric health care providers may want to refer to a behavioral health professional, based on the child's presentation. Fecal incontinence tends to be a relapsing and remitting condition that requires sustained treatment over the course of months. Limited family adherence to comprehensive treatment plans can also influence outcomes. It is important for primary pediatric health care professionals to be aware of these concepts and to be able to counsel children and families accordingly. Children with truly refractory encopresis would benefit from consideration of additional causes of constipation, laboratory evaluation, and/or referral to a pediatric gastroenterologist.

Suggested Resources

Feeding

Kelly N, Shank L, Bakalar J, Tanofsky-Kraff M. Pediatric feeding and eating disorders: current state of diagnosis and treatment. *Curr Psychiatry Rep.* 2014;16(5):446

Kerzner B, Milano K, MacLean WC Jr, et al. A practical approach to classifying and managing feeding difficulties. *Pediatrics.* 2015;135(2):344–353

Lukens CT, Silverman AH. Systematic review of psychological interventions for pediatric feeding problems. *J Pediatr Psychol.* 2014;39(8):903–917

Phalen JA. Managing feeding problems and feeding disorders. *Pediatr Rev.* 2013;34(12):549–557

Romano C, Hartman C, Privitera C, Cardile S, Shamir R. Current topics in the diagnosis and management of the pediatric non organic feeding disorders (NOFEDs). *Clin Nutr.* 2015;34(2):195–200

Sleep

Owens JA. Sleep and sleep disorders in children. In: Carey WB, Crocker AC, Coleman WL, Elias ER, Feldman HM, eds. *Developmental-Behavioral Pediatrics.* 4th ed. Philadelphia, PA: Saunders/Elsevier; 2009:619–627

Hintze, JP, Paruthi S. Sleep in the pediatric population. *Sleep Med Clin.* 2016;11(1):91–103

Hirshkowitz M, Whiton K, Albert SM, et al. National Sleep Foundation's sleep time duration recommendations: methodology and results summary. *Sleep Health.* 2015; 1(1):40–43

Honaker SM, Meltzer LJ. Sleep in pediatric primary care: a review of the literature. *Sleep Med Rev.* 2016;25:31–39

Li, Z, Celestin J, Lockey RF. Pediatric sleep apnea syndrome: an update. *J Allergy Clin Immuno Pract.* 2016;4(5):852–861

Mindell JA, Owens JA. *Clinical Guide to Pediatric Sleep Diagnosis and Management of Sleep Problems.* Philadelphia, PA: Wolters Kluwer Health; 2010

Troester MM, Pelayo R. Pediatric sleep pharmacology: a primer. *Semin Pediatr Neurol.* 22(2);2015:135–47

Elimination

Toilet Training and Continence

Howell D, Wysocki K, Steiner MJ. Toilet training. *Pediatr Rev.* 2010;31(6):262–263

Schonwald A, Rappaport L. Toilet training. In: Shweder RA, ed. *The Child: An Encyclopedic Companion.* Chicago, IL: University of Chicago Press; 2009

Enuresis and Encopresis

Weissman L, Bridgemohan C. Bowel function, toileting, encopresis. In: Carey WB, Crocker AC, Coleman WL, Elias ER, Feldman HM, eds. *Developmental-Behavioral Pediatrics.* 4th ed. Philadelphia, PA: Saunders/Elsevier; 2009:610–618

Nasir R, Schonwald A. Urinary function and enuresis. *Developmental-Behavioral Pediatrics.* 4th ed. Philadelphia, PA: Saunders/Elsevier; 2009:602–609

Hyams JS, Di Lorenzo C, Saps M. Childhood functional gastrointestinal disorders: child/adolescent. *Gastroenterology.* 2016;150(6):1456–1468

Maternik M, Krzeminska K, Zurowska A. The management of childhood urinary incontinence. *Pediatr Nephrol.* 2014;30(1):41–50

References

1. Carruth BR, Ziegler PJ, Gordon A, Barr SI. Prevalence of picky eaters among infants and toddlers and their caregivers' decisions about offering a new food. *J Am Diet Assoc.* 2004;104(1 Suppl 1):S57–S64

2. Micali N, Simonoff, E, Elberling H, et al. Eating patterns in a population-based sample of children aged 5 to 7 years: association with psychopathology and parentally perceived impairment. *J Dev Behav Pediatr.* 2011;32(8):572–580

3. Shim JE, Kim J, Mathai RA, STRONG Kids Research Team. Associations of infant feeding practices and picky eating behaviors of preschool children. *J Am Diet Assoc.* 2011;111(9):1363–1368

4. Lytle LA, Seifert S, Greenstein J, McGovern P. How do children's eating patterns and food choices change over time? Results from a cohort study. *Am J Health Promot.* 2000;14(4):222–228

5. American Psychiatric Association. *Diagnostic and Statistical Manual of Mental Disorders.* 5th ed. Arlington, VA: American Psychiatric Association; 2013

6. Fisher MM, Rosen DS, Ornstein RM, et al. Characteristics of avoidant/restrictive food intake disorder in children and adolescents: a "new disorder" in DSM-5. *J Adolesc Health.* 2014;55(1):49–52

7. Romano C, Hartman C, Privitera C, Cardile S, Shamir R. Current topics in the diagnosis and management of the pediatric non organic feeding disorders (NOFEDs). *Clin Nutr.* 2015;34(2):195–200

8. Allen SL, Howlett MD, Coulombe JA, Corkum PV. ABCs of SLEEPING: a review of the evidence behind pediatric sleep practice recommendations. *Sleep Med Rev.* 2016;29:1–14

9. Honaker SM, Meltzer LJ. Sleep in pediatric primary care: a review of the literature. *Sleep Med Rev.* 2016;25:31–39

10. Hintze, JP, Paruthi S. Sleep in the pediatric population. *Sleep Med Clin.* 2016;11(1):91–103

11. Provini F, Tinuper P, Bisulli F, Lugaresi E. Arousal disorders. *Sleep Med.* 2011;12(Suppl 2):S22–26

12. Li, Z, Celestin J, Lockey RF. Pediatric sleep apnea syndrome: an update. *J Allergy Clin Immunol Pract.* 2016;4(5):852–861

13. Burhans MS, Dailey C, Beard Z, Wiesinger J. Iron deficiency: differential effects on monoamine transporters. *Nutr Neurosci.* 2005;8(1):31–38

14. Ferber RA. *Solve Your Child's Sleep Problems.* New York, NY: Touchstone; 2006

15. Kaerts N, Van Hal G, Vermandel A, Wyndaele JJ. Readiness signs used to define the proper moment to start toilet training: a review of the literature. *Neurourol Urodyn.* 2012;31(4):437–40

16. Howell DM, Wysocki K, Steiner MJ. Toilet training. *Pediatr Rev.* 2010;31(6):262–263

17. Vermandel A, Van Kampen M, Van Gorp C, Wyndaele JJ. How to toilet train healthy children? A review of the literature. *Neurourol Urodyn.* 2008;27(3):162–166

18. Schonwald A, Sherritt L, Stadtler A, Bridgemohan C. Factors associated with difficult toilet training. *Pediatrics.* 2004;13(6):1753–1757

19. Jansson UB, Hanson M, Sillen U. Voiding pattern and acquisition of bladder control from birth to age 6 years–a longitudinal study. *J Urol.* 2005;174(1):289–293

20. Scharf RJ, Scharf GJ, Stroustrup A. Developmental milestones. *Pediatr Rev.* 2016;37(1):25–38

21. Rajindrajith S, Devanarayana NM, Benninga MA. Review article: faecal incontinence in children: epidemiology, pathophysiology, clinical evaluation and management. *Ailment Pharmacol Ther.* 2012;37(1):37–48

22. Austin PF, Ferguson G, Yan Y, et al. Combination therapy with desmopressin and an anticholinergic medication for nonresponders to desmopressin for monosymptomatic nocturnal enuresis: a randomized, double-blind placebo-controlled trial. *Pediatrics.* 2008;122(5):1027–1032

23. Nevéus T, Läckgren G, Tuvemo T, Olsson U, Stenberg A. Desmopressin resistant enuresis: pathogenetic and therapeutic considerations. *J Urol.* 1999;162(6):2136–2140

24. Caldwell PH, Nankivell G, Sureshkumar P. Simple behavioural interventions for nocturnal enuresis in children. *Cochrane Database Syst Rev.* 2013;19(7):CD003637

25. Maternik M, Krzeminska K, Zurowska A. The management of childhood urinary incontinence. *Pediatr Nephrol.* 2015;30(1):41–50

CHAPTER 9

Developmental and Behavioral Surveillance and Screening Within the Medical Home

Michelle M. Macias, MD, FAAP

Paul H. Lipkin, MD, FAAP

Developmental disabilities and behavioral disorders are among the most common health conditions present in children, with current prevalence estimates suggesting a frequency of approximately 15% or 1 in 6 children in the United States,[1] with a profound effect on the children's health and functional status when compared to unaffected peers.[2] Intellectual disability (ID) affects 1 in 150 children,[1] while autism spectrum disorder (ASD) has been most recently identified in 1 in 68 children.[3] Cerebral palsy (CP), the most common severe motor disability, affects nearly 3 per 1,000 or 1 in 345 children.[4] The more common and lower-severity disorders, such as attention-deficit/hyperactivity disorder (ADHD)[5] or the speech and language disorders,[6] can each affect as many as 1 in 10 children. Behavioral and emotional disorders affect as many as 23% of children in the United States, with approximately 6% described as serious.[7] Given the frequency of these disorders and the evidence-based benefits of early developmental and medical interventions for many of these conditions, the first task for primary pediatric health care professionals in the management of affected children is early and appropriate identification of these disorders through developmental surveillance and screening. Given their lifelong impact and needs associated with developmental or behavioral disorders, primary pediatric health care professionals need to establish medical homes for affected children and youth from which care is initiated, coordinated, and monitored, and with which families can form a reliable alliance for information, support, and advocacy from the time of diagnosis through the transition to adulthood.[8] As part of establishing the medical home, the primary pediatric health care professional should also develop a system of care coordination tied to local community-based health, developmental, and educational professionals for collaborative management of the special needs of the child.

Developmental surveillance and screening are critical functions of a family-centered medical home. The child who fails developmental screening and who is identified with a developmental disorder on developmental evaluation (eg, CP, ID, ASD, or a milder condition such as a speech-language disorder or motor coordination disorder) should be designated as a child with special health care needs within their medical home.[9-11] It is now clear that a child with special health care needs who receives care in a family-centered medical home can experience improvements in the use of services, health status, satisfaction, access to care, communication, systems of care, family functioning, and family impact and cost.[12]

The surveillance and screening for developmental and behavioral disorders follows the same principles used in other health conditions managed within the medical home. Pediatric health surveillance occurs at every well-child visit through routine performance of the health history and physical examination by the primary pediatric health care professional. In contrast, health screening involves the administration of a low-cost, brief, standardized laboratory test by health assistants at an age-determined visit, with interpretation of the results of screening and treatment initiation performed by the medical staff. In the example of a case of anemia, signs or symptoms, such as tachycardia, pallor, or fatigue, may be noted by surveillance at a routine visit. Screening for anemia, on the other hand, is performed routinely by laboratory testing at the newborn visit (to rule out sickle cell anemia), 12 months of age (to rule out iron deficiency or hereditary anemias), and adolescence (to rule out iron deficiency anemia in menstruating females).[13] When a concern for anemia is identified by surveillance or screening, the health care professional will pursue further evaluation. Such methods are similarly incorporated into developmental surveillance and screening, as recommended in the American Academy of Pediatrics (AAP) clinical report on these practices (Box 9.1).[14]

Box 9.1. American Academy of Pediatrics Key Recommendations on Developmental Surveillance and Screening[14]

- ▶ Perform developmental surveillance for the child at every health supervision visit throughout childhood and ensure that such surveillance looks at the child in full. Vigilant surveillance should be performed at the 4- and 5-year visits to identify concerns not previously noted that may be of importance upon initiation of elementary school.

- ▶ Administer a standardized developmental screening tool for all children at the 9-, 18-, and 30-month visits.

- ▶ Administer a standardized developmental screening tool for those whose surveillance yields concerns about delayed or disordered development, including those with concerns seen at the 4- or 5-year visit.

- ▶ Administer a standardized ASD screening tool for children at the 18- and 24-month visits and at any time for those whose surveillance yields concerns about delayed or disordered social development.

- ▶ Undertake a medical diagnostic evaluation of a child when development is concerning, to identify an underlying etiology and to provide related counseling and treatment. Testing to be considered includes hearing evaluation, vision screening, laboratory testing—including genetic testing—and brain imaging.

- ▶ Schedule early return visits for continued close surveillance of children whose surveillance raises concerns that are not confirmed by a developmental screening tool.

- ▶ Refer the child in whom screening results are concerning to early intervention and early childhood programs.

- ▶ Refer the child who has positive screening results for further developmental evaluation in order to identify a specific developmental disorder.

- ▶ Document all surveillance, screening, evaluation, and referral activities in the child's health record.

As currently defined by the AAP, *developmental screening* is the administration of a brief standardized tool for the identification of children at risk of a developmental disorder. It is administered at specific ages, based on known patterns of development. In contrast, *developmental surveillance* is defined as a flexible, longitudinal, continuous, and cumulative process that is aimed at identifying children who may have developmental problems and is performed at every well-child visit. Six key components are grounded in the history and the observation of the child: (1) eliciting and attending to the parents' concerns about their child's development; (2) documenting and maintaining a developmental history; (3) making accurate observations of the child; (4) identifying risk and protective factors; (5) maintaining an accurate record of documenting the process and findings; and (6) sharing and obtaining opinions and findings with other professionals, such as child care providers, home visitors, preschool teachers, and developmental therapists, especially when concerns arise. As in the example of anemia, when a child is identified by screening or surveillance as high risk for a developmental disorder, the health care professional performs (see Chapter 10: Developmental Evaluation) or refers the child for more detailed evaluation. The *developmental evaluation,* like the evaluation of the child with anemia, is aimed at identifying the specific developmental disorder or disorders affecting the child (see Chapter 11: Making Developmental-Behavioral Diagnoses). When coupled with further medical evaluation of the child, both a specific developmental disorder and related medical etiology and/or associated medical conditions can be identified (see Chapter 4, Biological Influences on Child Development and Behavior and Medical Evaluation of Children With Developmental-Behavioral Disorders), and a program of treatment and care management, such as referral for early intervention services (see Chapter 6, Early Intervention), can be initiated.

Developmental Surveillance

Over past decades, the pediatric practice dedicated to the identification of developmental problems has been rooted in a practice now defined as developmental surveillance. Traditionally, primary pediatric health care professionals have performed informal developmental monitoring through a review of developmental milestones with the parent at pediatric health supervision visits. The health care professional has typically coupled this history with the child's medical history of known risk factors for developmental problems and observations of the child's skills and interactions at the visit. While often referred to in the past as screening, such practice is now referred to as *developmental surveillance,* in concert with other concepts of health surveillance. First so named by Paul Dworkin in 1988, *developmental surveillance* remains a mainstay in the early identification of children affected by developmental disorders.[15] As now defined by the AAP, it is distinct from developmental screening.[14] Developmental surveillance is performed at each pediatric health supervision visit. It is composed of several key historical and observational components: (1) inquiry about developmental concerns, (2) developmental history, (3) identification of historical risk and protective factors, and (4) observation of a child's development during the physical examination and visit (Box 9.2).

Box 9.2. Components of Developmental Surveillance

▶ History
- Parental developmental concerns
- Developmental history: milestone achievement, with identification of abnormal patterns
  - Delay
  - Dissociation
  - Deviancy or deviation
  - Regression
- Medical and family historical risk factor identification, including social determinants of health
- Protective factor identification (also including social determinants)

▶ Developmental observation
- Gross and fine motor skills
- Speech, language, and social engagement
- Spontaneous and responsive behavior
- Related neurological function on physical examination

Medical History

The history obtained from the family is a powerful tool in the process of developmental surveillance. Parental concerns about their child's development can be an important predictor of developmental problems and are therefore a key area of inquiry during the pediatric health supervision visit.[16-18] The history obtained from the parent should also consider significant family biological and psychosocial risk factors, such as other family members with genetic, developmental, or behavioral disorders. The family history may reveal a pedigree of developmental disorders like that seen in X-linked disorders, such as fragile X syndrome or Duchenne muscular dystrophy. Patterns of language disorders can be seen in families of children with ASD. The milder learning disorders and ADHD are also known to have strong familial components, often noted by academic underachievement in family members. A family history of substance abuse is also of note due to concerns of a child's prenatal exposure, parental underachievement, and the social and environmental risks posed.

Similarly, the child's medical history may contain known factors for increased risk for developmental disability. The child born preterm or with perinatal complications is at known risk for a wide range of developmental disabilities from CP and sensory impairments to learning, attention, and intellectual disorders. A history of neurological problems, such as seizures or traumatic brain injury, also places a child at higher risk for associated neurodevelopmental disorders. A child with congenital anomalies, including complex congenital heart disease, may also have underlying neurodevelopmental disorders identifiable through surveillance. Abnormal growth patterns, including failure to thrive, overgrowth, macrocephaly, or microcephaly, also suggest higher risk.

Finally, the history should include a thorough social history considering social determinants of health to identify psychosocial and socioeconomic factors within the family and community that may place a child at increased risk for developmental delay.

Developmental History

The developmental history is classically obtained through the tracking of a child's attainment of key developmental markers, commonly referred to as milestones, throughout childhood. The milestones can be classified into 4 skill areas: gross motor, fine motor, verbal language (expressive and receptive), and social language and self-help (see Table 9.1). Milestone tracking and review may reveal known patterns of timing, order, or sequence seen in developmental disorders.[19,20] *Delay* is the most widely known pattern of atypical development. With developmental delay, the child acquires skills in the typical sequence but at a slower rate. It may occur within a single stream or across several developmental streams. *Dissociation* is noted when a child's development is delayed in one stream and not another. Such patterns can help distinguish developmental disabilities. For example, a child with a language disorder would have a delay in verbal language, while acquiring gross or fine motor skills consistent with age norms. *Deviancy* or *deviation* occurs when a child achieves milestones out of the usual sequence within a stream of development, such as when a child crawls before sitting, as seen in some types of CP, or uses words before their meaning is understood, a pattern commonly seen in autism. Echolalia, or the repetition of words or phrases, may be seen briefly in typical development. However, it represents deviant development when it occurs in place of interactive speech and language or when it occurs for a prolonged period. *Regression* is the least common but most concerning pattern. It typically presents with a child losing milestones, but it can more subtly be recognized when a child stops acquiring new developmental skills or has a slowing in the rate of developmental progress over time; it is seen in metabolic disorders, such as X-linked adrenoleukodystrophy; neurogenetic syndromes, such as Rett syndrome or Duchenne muscular dystrophy; and is frequently reported in children with ASD.

While obtaining a history of developmental milestone acquisition, primary pediatric health care professionals can calculate a child's rate of developmental progress with use of the developmental quotient (DQ). The DQ is calculated by dividing the child's developmental or best milestone age (DA) by the child's chronological age (CA) (DQ = DA/CA × 100). A DQ of 100 represents the mean or average rate of development, while a DQ below 70 is approximately 2 standard deviations below the mean and suggests a significant delay that requires further evaluation. For example, a child with a motor DQ of 70 or less may have CP or other motor disability. A DQ below 70 for language milestones strongly implies a language or intellectual disability.

Table 9.1. Developmental Milestones for Developmental Surveillance at Preventive Care Visits[a]

Age	Social Language and Self-help	Verbal Language (Expressive and Receptive)	Gross Motor	Fine Motor
Newborn–1 week	Makes brief eye contact with adult when held	Cries with discomfort Calms to adult voice	Reflexively moves arms and legs Turns head to side when on stomach	Holds fingers closed Grasps reflexively
1 month	Calms when picked up or spoken to Looks briefly at objects	Alerts to unexpected sound Makes brief short vowel sounds	Holds chin up in prone	Holds fingers more open at rest
2 months	Smiles responsively (ie, social smile)	Vocalizes with simple cooing	Lifts head and chest in prone	Opens and shuts hands
4 months	Laughs aloud	Turns to voice Vocalizes with extended cooing	Rolls over prone to supine Supports on elbows and wrists in prone	Keeps hands unfisted Plays with fingers in midline Grasps object
6 months	Pats or smiles at reflection Begins to turn when name called	Babbles	Rolls over supine to prone Sits briefly without support	Reaches for objects and transfers Rakes small object with 4 fingers Bangs small object on surface
9 months[b]	Uses basic gestures (holds arms out to be picked up, waves "bye-bye") Looks for dropped objects Picks up food with fingers and eats it Turns when name called	Says "Dada" or "Mama" nonspecifically	Sits well without support Pulls to stand Transitions well between sitting and lying Balances on hands and knees Crawls	Picks up small object with 3 fingers and thumb Releases objects intentionally Bangs objects together
12 months	Looks for hidden objects Imitates new gestures	Says "Dada" or "Mama" specifically Uses 1 word other than Mama, Dada, or personal names Follows a verbal command that includes a gesture	Takes first independent steps Stands without support	Drops object in a cup Picks up small object with 2-finger pincer grasp
15 months	Imitates scribbling Drinks from cup with little spilling Points to ask for something or to get help	Uses 3 words other than names Speaks in jargon Follows a verbal command without a gesture	Squats to pick up objects Climbs onto furniture Begins to run	Makes mark with crayon Drops object in and takes object out of a container

Table 9.1. Developmental Milestones for Developmental Surveillance at Preventive Care Visits[a] *(continued)*

Age	Social Language and Self-help	Verbal Language (Expressive and Receptive)	Gross Motor	Fine Motor
18 months[b,c]	Engages with others for play Helps dress and undress self Points to pictures in book Points to object of interest to draw attention to it Turns and looks at adult if something new happens Begins to scoop with spoon	Uses 6–10 words other than names Identifies at least 2 body parts	Walks up with 2 feet per step with hand held Sits in small chair Carries toy while walking	Scribbles spontaneously Throws small ball a few feet while standing
2 years[c]	Plays alongside other children (parallel) Takes off some clothing Scoops well with spoon	Uses 50 words Combines 2 words into short phrase or sentence Follows 2-step command Uses words that are 50% intelligible to strangers	Kicks ball Jumps off ground with 2 feet Runs with coordination	Stacks objects Turns book pages Uses hands to turn objects (eg, knobs, toys, and lids)
2½ years[b]	Urinates in a potty or toilet Engages in pretend or imitative play Spears food with fork	Uses pronouns correctly	Begins to walk up steps alternating feet Runs well without falling	Grasps crayon with thumb and fingers instead of fist Catches large balls
3 years	Enters bathroom and urinates by self Plays in cooperation and shares Puts on coat, jacket, or shirt by self Engages in beginning imaginative play Eats independently	Uses 3-word sentences Uses words that are 75% intelligible to strangers Understands simple prepositions (eg, *on, under*)	Pedals tricycle Climbs on and off couch or chair Jumps forward	Draws a single circle Draws a person with head and 1 other body part Cuts with child scissors

Table 9.1. Developmental Milestones for Developmental Surveillance at Preventive Care Visits[a] *(continued)*

Age	Social Language and Self-help	Verbal Language (Expressive and Receptive)	Gross Motor	Fine Motor
4 years	Enters bathroom and has bowel movement by self Brushes teeth Dresses and undresses without much help Engages in well-developed imaginative play	Uses 4-word sentences Uses words that are 100% intelligible to strangers	Climbs stairs alternating feet without support Skips on 1 foot	Draws a person with at least 3 body parts Draws simple cross Unbuttons and buttons medium-sized buttons Grasps pencil with thumb and fingers instead of fist

[a] Developmental milestones are intended for discussion with parents for the purposes of surveillance of a child's developmental progress and for developmental promotion for the child. They are not intended or validated for use as a developmental screening test in the pediatric medical home or in early childhood day care or educational settings. Milestones are also commonly used for instructional purposes on early child development for pediatric and child development professional trainees.

These milestones generally represent the mean or average age of performance of these skills when available. When not available, the milestones offered are based on review and consensus from multiple measures as noted.

[b] It is recommended that a standardized developmental test be performed at these visits.

[c] It is recommended that a standardized autism screening test be performed at these visits.

Sources: Capute AJ, Shapiro BK, Palmer FB, Ross A, Wachtel RC. Normal gross motor development: the influences of race, sex and socio-economic status. *Dev Med Child Neurol.* 1985;27(5)635–643; Accardo PJ, Capute AJ. *The Capute Scales: Cognitive Adaptive Test/Clinical Linguistic and Auditory Milestone Scale (CAT/CLAMS).* Baltimore, MD: Paul H. Brooks Publishing Co; 2005; Beery KE, Buktenica NA, Beery NA. *The Beery-Buktenica Developmental Test of Visual-Motor Integration, Sixth Edition (BEERY VMI).* San Antonio, TX: Pearson Education Inc; 2010; Schum TR, Kolb TM, McAuliffe TL, Simms MD, Underhill RL, Lewis M. Sequential acquisition of toilet-training skills: a descriptive study of gender and age differences in normal children. *Pediatrics.* 2002;109(3):E48; Oller JW Jr, Oller SD, Oller SN. *Milestones: Normal Speech and Language Development Across the Lifespan.* 2nd ed. San Diego, CA: Plural Publishing Inc; 2012; Robins DL, Casagrande K, Barton M, Chen CM, Dumont-Mathieu T, Fein D. *Validation of the Modified Checklist for Autism in Toddlers, Revised with Follow-Up (M-CHAT-R/F). Pediatrics.* 2014;133(1):37–45; Aylward GP. *Bayley Infant Neurodevelopmental Screener.* San Antonio, TX: The Psychological Corporation; 1995; Squires J, Bricker D. *Ages & Stages Questionnaires, Third Edition (ASQ-3): A Parent-Completed Child Monitoring System.* Baltimore, MD: Paul H. Brookes Publishing Co; 2009; and Bly L. Motor Skills Acquisition Checklist. Psychological Corporation; 2000.

Suggested citation: Lipkin P, Macias M. Developmental milestones for developmental surveillance at preventive care visits. In: Hagan JF, Shaw JS, Duncan PM, eds. *Bright Futures: Guidelines for Health Supervision of Infants, Children, and Adolescents.* 4th ed. Elk Grove Village, IL: American Academy of Pediatrics; 2017.

Developmental Observation

Observation during the course of the preventive care visit may also demonstrate that the child has an abnormal pattern of development. Problems in movement or posture may be seen while the child sits with the parent or when placed on the examination table. Associated neurological abnormalities, such as increased or decreased muscle tone, should be considered when this is observed. Difficulties with interpersonal engagement or eye contact with the parent may also be noted during the course of the visit. The young child is often reticent during the visit, limiting one's ability to observe the child's speech and language skills. However, a speaking child's pattern of communication may provide insight into the child's development in this area.

Implementation of each of these components of developmental surveillance at each health supervision visit can identify the child with developmental concerns and a possible developmental disorder. When the primary pediatric health care professional identifies a concern, these findings should be documented in the paper or electronic medical record for ongoing tracking of these issues. In addition, formal developmental screening or referral for developmental evaluation should be completed to verify these concerns. Such screening or evaluation may need to be completed at a separate visit based on time demands at the preventive care visit. When a typical pattern of development and no concerns are identified during surveillance, the primary pediatric health care professional can make recommendations for specific developmental stimulation activities for the child and parent. Whether the child is noted to have concerns and risks or has typical development, child and parent activities should be promoted based on simple age-specific developmental goals. Working in conjunction with the family and health care professional within the medical home, developmental care plans can be developed to encourage optimal developmental stimulation as a component of family-centered care. The parent of the sitting child can be encouraged to provide opportunities for standing-based play. The parents of the child with limited word use or recognition can be instructed in the benefits of vocabulary development through reading picture books. The timing of subsequent visits with ongoing surveillance should be determined at the conclusion of the preventive care visit. When a child has a typical pattern of development, the usual periodicity schedule can be followed. If there are concerns about the child, however, subsequent visits for surveillance or screening should be planned earlier. At all of these follow-up visits, the child's attainment of the promoted skills should be reassessed.

Behavioral Surveillance and Screening

As in the AAP statement on developmental surveillance and screening,[14] the universal health care concepts of surveillance and screening that are critical components of the medical home can also be incorporated into the early identification of behavior disorders. The 2015 AAP Clinical *Report Promoting Optimal Development: Screening for Behavioral and Emotional Problems* provides detailed information on this topic and contains a comprehensive list of screening tools.[21] Surveillance for behavioral and emotional problems is recommended at all health supervision visits, with use of a formal behavioral screen when surveillance reveals concerns.[21]

Medical History

Parents' concerns about their child's behavior and social skills have been important in the identification of significant problems in the child, particularly in children older than 4 years.[22] The family and social histories may also reveal areas of concern. A child's behavior issues may be tied to known familial mental health problems, such as anxiety disorders, mood disorders, or ADHD. Exposure to environmental, familial, and psychosocial risk factors disproportionately affects behavioral and emotional development.[21] There has been increasing recognition of the effect of "toxic stress" on the developing child.[23,24] Regular surveillance is recommended regarding family psychosocial risk factors and adverse childhood experiences (ACEs) leading to toxic stress, including maternal depression, poverty, substance abuse, and/or family disorganization[23,25] (see Chapter 3, Environmental Influences on Child Development and Behavior).

Behavior History

The behavior history obtained during surveillance is more typically symptom based, rather than milestone based, as in developmental surveillance. The primary pediatric health care professional should inquire about the child's relationships and engagement with parents, siblings, and other familiar persons, other children (particularly same-aged peers), and unfamiliar children and adults. Inquiry should be made about the child's behavior during daily living activities, including eating, sleeping, and playing. Concern about problems with compliance, tantrums, attention, activity level, impulsivity, and aggression should be elicited. A history of unusual patterns of behavior may also be reported. Examples include repetitive speech or play, excessive preoccupation with objects or specific ideas, unusual visual gaze, hand-flapping, or potentially self-injurious hand-biting or face-slapping.

Behavior Observation

During the preventive care visit, the primary pediatric health care professional should observe the child's engagement and communication with the parent or caregiver in the office. Impulsivity, decreased attention span, or increased activity level suggest attention problems. Observed tantrums and oppositionality should be considered in the context of the child's age and the history provided by the family. The unusual behavior problems described earlier should elicit further evaluation when directly observed in the medical office setting. As with developmental surveillance, the primary pediatric health care professional should pursue screening or further evaluation when concerns about behavior are identified through behavioral surveillance. In addition, counseling around behavior management and discipline is a critical component of a family-centered care plan derived from the family and professional partnership contained within the medical home (see Chapter 7, Basics of Child Behavior and Primary Care Pediatric Management of Common Behavioral Problems). If the patterns of behavior are typical for the child's age, counseling on typical behavior patterns and their management should be offered. The parents of a child with stranger or separation anxiety can learn techniques of anticipation and consolation. Discipline methods for management of mild tantrums or oppositionality, such as time-out techniques, can also be included in a behavioral care plan. Interactive child and parent activities and child play should be promoted.[26,27] As with developmental surveillance, subsequent visits should be arranged based on behavioral issues noted. Early follow-up should be arranged when there are specific concerns identified. If no improvement is noted at follow-up, an early intervention referral should be considered.

Developmental Screening

In the pursuit of the early identification of developmental disorders, the primary pediatric health care professional is charged with developmental screening periodically during early childhood. Such screening involves the administration of a brief and standardized test in the medical home and is similar to screening of other health conditions. It differs from developmental surveillance in several key features. First, developmental (and behavioral) screening involves use of a formal, standardized test with known reliability, validity, sensitivity, and specificity (Boxes 9.3, 9.4, and 9.5). Second, given its implicit time demand and cost, screening is not employed at every pediatric health supervision visit, as is surveillance. Instead, it is administered at ages based on key times for identification of developmental disorders. Third, as in other health care screening, the developmental screening test is typically ordered and interpreted by the clinician but may be administered by associated health care staff, while surveillance is usually performed directly by the primary pediatric health care professional in the course of the preventive care visit. Like surveillance, screening identifies children at high risk of a developmental disorder. Scoring of screening tests typically is categorical, with assignment of a child into a risk category—such as no risk, suspect, or high risk—rather than a numeric score. Those with scores in the suspect category are typically followed by additional surveillance or screening, while those at highest risk are in need of more detailed developmental evaluation and medical testing for the determination of a diagnosis and treatment needs.

The AAP currently recommends formal developmental screening at 9 months, 18 months, and 30 months of age during the first 3 years of life, as well as at any time that the parent or primary pediatric health care professional has concerns about appropriate development[14] (Table 9.2). In addition, vigilant surveillance is recommended at the 4- and 5-year preventive care visits before a child enters elementary school, in order to identify concerns not previously noted, with screening performed when a concern is observed. Screening specifically for ASD is also recommended at the 18-month visit and again at the 24-month visit.[28,29]

Age of Visit, months	Critical Developmental Streams Screened	Common Developmental Disorders Identified
Table 9.2. Developmental Screening Visits in the American Academy of Pediatrics Periodicity Schedule[13,14,30]		
9	Vision, hearing, gross motor, fine motor, receptive language	Visual impairment, deafness and hearing loss, cerebral palsy, and other neuromotor disorders
18	Gross motor, fine motor, verbal language (expressive and receptive), social language	Cerebral palsy (mild to moderate), mild neuromotor or neuromuscular disorder, autism spectrum disorder, language disorders, intellectual disability
30	Verbal language (expressive and receptive), social language, behavior	Language disorders, autism spectrum disorder, intellectual and other learning disabilities, attention disorders, disruptive behavior disorders

The ages for screening were selected based on times when key developmental problems can be identified and time available at each health supervision visit. Screening at the 9-month visit is aimed at identification of deafness and hearing loss not identified in newborn screening, visual disorders, and delays in motor development resulting from neuromotor disorders (eg, CP). At the 18-month visit, the clinician can identify milder motor problems, such as abnormalities of gait or coordination seen in mild CP, or early signs of neuromuscular disorders, such as the muscular dystrophies. In addition, this visit is critical for the early identification of autism spectrum, language, or intellectual disorders. The next screening visit is recommended at 30 months of age.[14] This visit is also centered on the development of language, social, or intellectual skills and may also identify ASD, intellectual disorders, or milder speech-language disorders. Children with neuromuscular disorders may also begin showing signs of motor or other developmental problems at this visit. Performance of screening at these early ages enables referral to local early intervention agencies for further evaluation and initiation of early intervention services[28] (see Chapter 6, Early Intervention) for those children who fail screening. Such early screening also allows early identification of related medical conditions, with associated early initiation of related medical treatments. The earlier services are initiated, the greater the likelihood for improved outcomes. Testing to be considered includes hearing evaluation, vision screening, laboratory testing, including genetic testing, and brain imaging (see Chapter 4, Biological Influences on Child Development and Behavior and Medical Evaluation of Children With Developmental-Behavioral Delays/Disorders).

Screening Tests

In performing developmental screening at these key visits, the primary pediatric health care professional must choose a screening test based on multiple factors (Box 9.3).

Box 9.3. Characteristics of Developmental and Behavioral Screening Tests Used in Test Selection

TEST PROPERTIES

▷ Reliability: the ability of a test to produce consistent results

▷ Predictive validity: the accuracy of a test to predict later test performance or development

▷ Sensitivity: the test's accuracy in the identification of delayed development or disability

▷ Specificity: the test's accuracy in the identification of children who are not delayed

▷ Standardization sample: the group of children whose test performance comprises the test norms; used for comparison to later individual child performance on the same test

▷ General screening test: a test that evaluates multiple areas of development

▷ Domain-specific screening test: a test that evaluates one area or domain of development (eg, motor or language)

▷ Disorder-specific screening test: a test aimed at identifying a specific developmental disorder (eg, autism)

IMPLEMENTATION PROPERTIES

▷ Completed by parent or administered by clinician

▷ Age range

▷ Administration time

▷ Languages available

▷ Test cost

Box 9.4. Common Current Developmental Screening Tests[14]

▷ General Developmental Screening
  – Parent Report
    • Ages and Stages Questionnaires (ASQ)
    • Parents' Evaluation of Developmental Status (PEDS)
    • Parents' Evaluation of Developmental Status: Developmental Milestones (PEDS:DM)
    • Survey of Well-Being of Young Children ([SWYC] initial validation, promising)
▷ Language Screening
  – Communication and Symbolic Behavior Scales Developmental Profile Infant-Toddler Checklist (CSBS DP ITC)
▷ Autism Spectrum Disorder Screening
  – Modified Checklist for Autism in Toddlers, Revised with Follow-Up (M-CHAT-R/F)
  – Social Communication Questionnaire (SCQ)
  – Early Screening for Autism and Communication Disorders ([ESAC] in development, promising)

Box 9.5. Common Current Behavioral Screening Tests[21]
(see also Chapter 12, Social/ Emotional Development and Disorders and Table 12.2, Screening and Assessment Tools)

GENERAL (BROADBAND) BEHAVIOR SCREENING

- ▶ Ages and Stages: Social-Emotional-2 (ASQ:SE-2; 2 m-6 y)
- ▶ Brief Infant-Toddler Social and Emotional Assessment ([BITSEA] 12–36 months)
- ▶ Eyberg Child Behavior Inventory (2–16 y)
- ▶ Pediatric Symptom Checklist (4–16 y)
- ▶ Strengths and Difficulties Questionnaire (3–17 y)
- ▶ Survey for Well-Being in Childhood

CONDITION-SPECIFIC (NARROW BAND) BEHAVIORAL SCREENING

Depression

- ▶ Patient Health Questionnaire-9
- ▶ Patient Health Questionnaire-2

Anxiety

- ▶ Generalized Anxiety Disorder 7-item (GAD-7) scale
- ▶ Screen for Child Anxiety Related Disorders ([SCARED] ≥8 years)

ADHD

- ▶ ADHD-IV Rating Scale (6–18 y)
- ▶ ADHD-IV Rating Scale (preschool; 3–5 y)
- ▶ Vanderbilt ADHD Diagnostic Rating Scales (4–18 y)

First, a screening test should be normed and standardized on a large sample of children and should meet appropriate standards in reliability, validity, sensitivity, and specificity. These test standards ensure that the test can accurately identify those children about whom there is a developmental concern, as well as distinguish them from those without a developmental concern. A good screening test should provide consistent results if administered by multiple testers (reliability). It should strike an appropriate balance in identification, minimizing both overidentification and overreferral of those without developmental problems and underidentification and underreferral of those with a true developmental disorder.[31,32] The predictive validity of a test is generally most useful for the clinician. If the test result is positive for a concern, positive predictive validity provides insight into what percentage of children with such a result are truly affected by a developmental disorder. Sensitivity measures the percentage of affected children identifiable with a test, while specificity reports the percentage of unaffected children testing negative. As such, these measures are most useful in public health and test development, frequently reported in the test manuals and in studies examining their validity. Sensitivity and specificity rates of 70% to 80% or a sum of both greater than 150 are commonly recommended for developmental screening tests.[32,33] Caution must be exercised, however, in interpreting these rates in developmental screening. While some measures are validated in the general pediatric setting, others have been performed on a known high-risk group, such as premature infants, or outside of a health care environment, such as in a child care or school setting. The measured outcome of developmental screening is risk for a developmental disorder rather than the confirmation of the presence of a specific developmental disorder. The clinical utility of these measures has also been questioned due to their instability, outcome verification bias, small sample sizes, test score bias with young children, and errors in selection and use of diagnostic tests.[34]

Other characteristics of the available screening tests should be considered by the clinician when selecting one for use in practice. The most common format for developmental screening tests is *general,* sometimes referred to as broadband, where multiple developmental domains are screened at each test administration; it is modeled after the first widely used screening test, the Denver Developmental Screening Test (DDST).[35,36] These tests cover a broad range of ages, typically infancy through early school age. This format offers the clinician economy of time and cost in the use of a single test for all children. Such screening tests are most often validated against other developmental tests. Commonly used tests at the present time include the Parents' Evaluation of Developmental Status (PEDS)[37] and the Ages and Stages Questionnaires (ASQs).[38] Alternatively, screening tests can be *domain-specific,* where the test screens a specific area of development (eg, language) for specific disorders (eg, language disorders).[39,40] While less widely used and validated, such screening tests may be useful for the identification of risk for specific developmental problems or disorders. Use of such tests requires that the clinician select a test appropriate to the specific age at screening. For example, at the 18-month visit, a test for language would be chosen. Finally, a screening test can be *disorder-specific* by screening for a known developmental disorder. This model is most similar to screening for other medical conditions, with the positive result measured against a defined developmental disorder. Currently, screening for ASD follows this model, with screening test results measured against criteria for autism or other pervasive developmental disorders.[41,42] Diagnosis-specific screening also requires appropriate timing for the screening test administration. In the case of autism screening, the AAP recommends such screening at 18 and 24 months.[14] The *Modified Checklist for Autism in Toddlers, Revised with Follow-Up (M-CHAT-R/F)* is widely used for this purpose and is available in the public domain.[42,43] At present, it is unclear which of these methodologies have the best potential for early identification of the developmental disorders, particularly given the wide array of screening tests available. However, current efforts in both general screening and autism screening may provide better knowledge of the best pathway to be taken in future screening.

Practical aspects of implementation may also guide the clinician in choice of instrument. The time required for test administration is important, as the primary pediatric health care professional fits the test into the pediatric health supervision visit. The AAP recommendations have specifically taken this concern into account by considering the time available at each preventive care visit and typically recommending that screening tests take less than 15 minutes to administer. Parent-completed developmental questionnaires allow screening to be performed in part outside of the clinic examination room, in the home, or in the medical office waiting area. They can then be scored by office staff or by the clinician, who can interpret the results, review them with the family, and make appropriate recommendations. In choosing a test, consideration must be given to languages available if a practice serves multilingual populations.

Many screening tests are now available for use in the pediatric health care setting, making the selection challenging for the clinician. When choosing, the clinician should consider the test's style and properties, as well as the population being screened and the office characteristics. The AAP has provided a table of available and acceptable screening tests in the policy statement on developmental screening.[14] Other practical guides are available on the Internet[44-46] and in the literature[45,47] for selecting developmental screening tests. See **https://www.aap.org/en-us/advocacy-and-policy/aap-health-initiatives/Screening/Pages/default.aspx**.

Implementation of Developmental Surveillance and Screening

In the AAP Periodic Survey of 2002, pediatricians reported high rates of developmental surveillance (up to 71%) but low rates of formal developmental screening using a standardized instrument (23%), with pediatricians voicing concerns regarding time limitations, lack of staff, and inadequate reimbursement for performance of screening.[48] In response, the 2006 AAP recommendations on developmental surveillance and screening aimed to create a practical guideline for implementation.[14] A clinical algorithm was created with the intent of clarifying the recommendations with a visual practice tool with electronic health record compatibility.[14] As illustrated in Figure 9.1 on pages 152 and 153, children identified with a developmental concern through developmental surveillance at any pediatric visit should undergo formal developmental screening for confirmation of the concern. When developmental screening is performed, either as part of preventive health care or in response to concerns identified through surveillance, a child will be found to have either a normal pattern of development or a pattern of concern for a developmental disorder. When typical development is seen, the child should be followed through the routine schedule of developmental surveillance and screening or through more frequent surveillance if concerns remain. When a concern is identified, further management strategies should be initiated by the primary pediatric health care professional (See the following section, Management of the Child With Developmental Concerns).

With the publication of the 2006 AAP guidelines on surveillance and screening, multiple national projects were initiated aimed at improving this practice. In 2009 and again in 2016, the AAP repeated its Periodic Survey of Fellows on this practice, noting major increases in pediatrician-reported rates of screening (48% in 2009, 63% in 2016).[49,50] Insights gained from the survey of pediatricians and the experiences of surveillance and screening implementation projects provide guidance for its practical implementation.[44,51-56] Successful implementation of developmental surveillance first requires that the medical home identify a clinician practice champion who can lead the office effort in creating a system for surveillance and screening. The first task for the clinical staff will be selecting an appropriate screening test for use at the 9-, 18-, and 30-month preventive care visits. In addition, for specific screening for ASD, an autism-specific screening test must be chosen for implementation at both the 18- and 24-month visits. Implementation projects have shown that developing an office system approach is critical, with medical office staff playing key roles in scheduling, test distribution and scoring, and referral and tracking of children identified in need of further evaluation and treatment. Standardized parent-completed screens have been widely adopted, with a decline in direct pediatric testing of development. Refer to Box 9.6 for additional details on key factors for successful implementation of developmental surveillance and screening.

Box 9.6. Key Strategies in Implementation of Developmental-Behavioral Surveillance and Screening[14,28]

SCREENING PROCEDURES

▷ Choose a screening tool.
  – Population served (parental education level, languages spoken)
  – Office staff skill level
  – Medical staff skill level
  – Test time and cost

▷ Train staff in patient visit flow changes and in screening tests used.

▷ Plan test distribution in advance.

▷ Consider need for readers and translators.

▷ Develop office and medical staff reminder systems for screening at targeted ages (9, 18, and 30 months).

▷ Train staff and use coding and billing practices appropriate to screening.

REFERRAL PROCEDURES

▷ Develop office system for referral of children to early intervention and community therapy programs.
  – See AAP Screening in Practices Initiative: Screening Technical Assistance & Resource (STAR) Center (https://www.aap.org/en-us/advocacy-and-policy/aap-health-initiatives/Screening/Pages/default.aspx)

▷ Establish working relationships with local community programs, services, and resources for assisting the child in need of special services or assistance.

▷ Identify network of medical consultants for medical evaluations.

▷ Identify resources and referral systems for further developmental evaluation.

MEDICAL HOME STRATEGIES

▷ Create tracking system for referrals.

▷ Create a practice registry and office system for chronic condition management and planning of children with developmental disorders and special health care needs.

▷ Ensure ongoing close developmental surveillance.

▷ Develop a chronic condition management/care plan.

▷ Deliver family-centered care, develop partnerships with families, and get regular feedback.

▷ Identify community resources for support services.
  – Parent-to-parent organizations
  – Government agencies
  – Advocacy groups

▷ Implement respite systems.

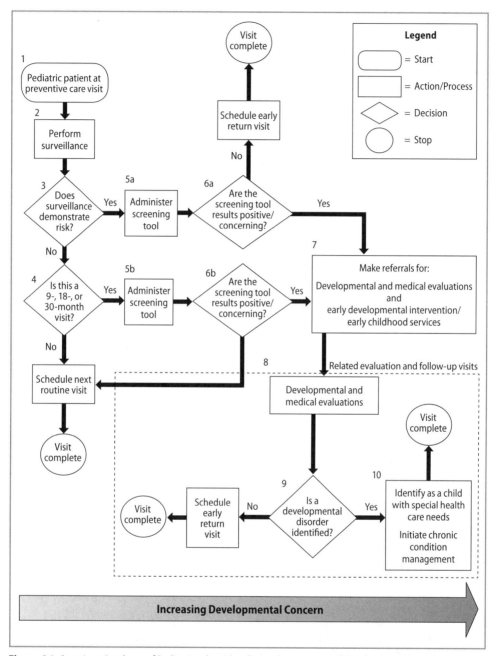

Figure 9.1. American Academy of Pediatrics algorithm for implementation of developmental surveillance and screening.[14]

Reproduced with permission from American Academy of Pediatrics Council on Children With Disabilities, Section on Developmental Behavioral Pediatrics, Bright Futures Steering Committee, Medical Home Initiatives for Children With Special Needs Project Advisory Committee. Identifying infants and young children with developmental disorders in the medical home: an algorithm for developmental surveillance and screening. *Pediatrics.* 2006;118(1):405–420.

Figure 9.1. American Academy of Pediatrics algorithm for implementation of developmental surveillance and screening.[14] *(continued)*

1. Pediatric patient at preventive care visit

Developmental concerns should be included as one of several health topics addressed at each pediatric preventive care visit throughout the first 5 years of life.

2. Perform surveillance

Developmental surveillance is a flexible, longitudinal, continuous, and cumulative process whereby knowledgeable health care professionals identify children who may have developmental problems. There are 5 components of development surveillance: eliciting and attending to the parents' concerns about their child's development, documenting and maintaining a developmental history, making accurate observations of the child, identifying the risk and protective factors, and maintaining an accurate record and documenting the process and findings.

3. Does surveillance demonstrate risk?

The concerns of both parents and child health professionals should be included in determining whether surveillance suggests the child may be at risk of developmental delay. If either parents or the child health professional expresses concern about the child's development, a developmental screening to address the concern specifically should be conducted.

4. Is this a 9-, 18-, or 30-month visit?

All children should receive developmental screening using a standardized test. In the absence of established risk factors or parental or provider concerns, a general developmental screen is recommended at the 9-, 18-, and 30-month visits. Additionally, autism-specific screening is recommended for all children at the 18-month visit.

5a and 5b. Administer screening tool

Developmental screening is the administration of a brief standardized tool aiding the identification of children at risk of a developmental disorder. Developmental screening that targets the area of concern is indicated whenever a problem is identified during developmental surveillance.

6a and 6b. Are the screening tool results positive/concerning?

When the results of the periodic screening tool are normal, the child health professional can inform the parents and continue with other aspects of the preventive visit. When a screening tool is administered as a result of concerns about development, an early return visit to provide additional developmental surveillance should be scheduled, even if the screening tool results do not indicate a risk of delay.

7. Make referrals for: Developmental and medical evaluations and early developmental intervention/early childhood stories

8. Developmental and medical evaluations

If screening results are concerning, the child should be scheduled for developmental and medical evaluations. **Developmental evaluation** is aimed at identifying the specific developmental disorder or disorders affecting the child. In addition to the developmental evaluation, a **medical diagnostic evaluation** to identify an underlying etiology should be undertaken. **Early developmental intervention/early childhood services** can be particularly valuable when a child is first identified to be at high risk of delayed development, because these programs often provide evaluation services and can offer other services to the child and family even before an evaluation is complete. Establishing an effective and efficient partnership with early childhood professionals is an important component of successful care coordination for children.

9. Is a developmental disorder identified?

If a developmental disorder is identified, the child should be identified as a child with special health care needs and chronic condition management should be initiated (see number 10). If a developmental disorder is not identified through medical and developmental evaluation, the child should be scheduled for an early return visit for further surveillance. More frequent visits, with particular attention paid to areas of concern, will allow the child to be promptly referred for further evaluation if any further evidence of delayed development or a specific disorder emerges.

10. Identify as a child with special health care needs; Initiate chronic condition management

When a child is discovered to have a significant developmental disorder, that child becomes a child with special health care needs, even if that child does not have a specific disease etiology identified. Such a child should be identified by the medical home for appropriate chronic condition management and regular monitoring and entered into the practice's children and youth with special health care needs registry.

Management of the Child With Developmental Concerns

When screening identifies or confirms a developmental concern in a child, the primary pediatric health care professional should initiate a series of simultaneous actions aimed at the identification and treatment of the child with a developmental disorder. These actions include: (1) a full developmental evaluation for diagnosis of a specific developmental disorder (see Chapter 10, Developmental Evaluation); (2) a medical evaluation for determination of etiology of the developmental concerns (see Chapter 4, Biological Influences on Child Development and Behavior and Medical Evaluation of Children with Developmental-Behavioral Disorders); (3) referral for therapeutic intervention to the local early intervention program (EIP), community therapy, or early childhood education providers (see Chapter 6, Early Intervention); and (4) initiation of a medical home program and chronic condition management for the child with special health care needs (see Chapter 25, Social and Community Services for Children With Developmental Disabilities and/or Behavioral Disorders and Their Families).

The developmental evaluation of a child who has been identified through screening is aimed at identifying a specific developmental disorder and can provide prognostic information and specific direction for therapeutic interventions. Pediatric subspecialists, such as neurodevelopmental or developmental-behavioral pediatricians or neurodevelopmental pediatric neurologists, can perform the developmental diagnostic evaluation, as can other early childhood professionals (eg, early childhood educators, child psychologists, speech-language pathologists, audiologists, physical therapists, or occupational therapists) in conjunction with the child's primary pediatric health care professional.

Given the shortage of subspecialists and the long waiting times at tertiary care developmental evaluation centers, a child's medical evaluation may be performed by the primary pediatric health care professional within the medical home. This medical evaluation is intended to determine underlying etiology and initiate related medical treatments. It should be a comprehensive medical evaluation, including review of the developmental and behavioral histories; review of newborn metabolic screening and growth charts; risk identification from the environmental, medical, family, and social histories; and a comprehensive physical examination. Vision screening and audiological evaluation should be performed when indicated. Laboratory investigation is also recommended for identification of specific developmental etiologies. Guidelines for such investigations are available from the AAP, American Academy of Neurology, Child Neurology Society, and the American College of Medical Genetics.[29,57–60] Typical laboratory tests considered include neuroimaging, DNA analysis for fragile X syndrome, and chromosomal microarray analyses (see Chapter 4, Biological Influences on Child Development and Behavior and Medical Evaluation of Children With Developmental-Behavioral Disorders).

The child whose developmental screening is of concern should also be referred for early intervention programming, which may include early childhood special education, physical therapy, speech-language therapy, occupational therapy, and/or behavioral therapy services, as appropriate. Such a referral can be made contemporaneously with initiation of the medical evaluation, as these services are not predicated on a diagnosis but instead are offered typically based on the presence of a significant developmental delay, deviancy, or regression. Services delivered through local EIPs may also include service coordination, social work services, assistance with transportation and related costs, family training, counseling, and home visits.[28,61] As reported previously, the AAP Developmental Surveillance and Screening Policy Implementation Project reported that a diverse sample of practices could successfully implement developmental screening as recommended by the AAP. Unfortunately, however, these practices reported that only 61% of children who failed screens were referred, that many practices struggled to track their referrals, and those that did track their referrals found that many families did not follow through with the recommended referrals. Thus, this study indicates that primary care practices are able to initiate developmental care through screening as recommended by the AAP, but barriers remain in terms of care coordination and monitoring for children who fail developmental screening.[53] In the 2016 Periodic Survey of Fellows, 97% of pediatricians reported making any direct referrals to early intervention, but they also reported referring only 59% of those found to be at risk for developmental delay/ASD on screening.[62] This suggests a gap between identification and referral practice that may result in delayed treatment services. This highlights the importance of discussing concerns and typical screening results as a way to initiate discussion around development and improve provider and family satisfaction and trust, so that when a concern does arise, families are more likely to follow through on recommendations for further evaluation and intervention.

As briefly reviewed early in this chapter, the child identified with a developmental disorder (eg, CP, ID, or ASD) should be designated as a child with special health care needs within a family-centered medical home.[9–11] Children with special health care needs who receive care in a medical home receive an improved quality of care, including improvements in the receipt of evidence-based care, minimized delays in receipt of appropriate health care, and improved health status and family functioning.[12,63] Providing a program of chronic condition management allows for regular health and developmental monitoring and proactive care. Such a program typically includes specialized condition-related office visits, written care plans (developed with families and recognizing and addressing specific family needs), explicit comanagement with medical specialists, appropriate patient education, and an effective system for monitoring and tracking. Community-based support services, such as respite care and advocacy organizations, may be helpful to the child and family, and parent-to-parent organizations (eg, Family Voices) and condition-specific organizations (eg, Autism Speaks, Autism Society of America, The Arc) offer further support, assistance, and information. It is useful and advantageous for offices to have readily available lists of these resources to distribute to families. Financial benefits are available for eligible children through supplemental social security income, public insurance, waiver programs, and state programs for children and youths with special health care needs.[64] (See Chapter 25, Social and Community Services for Children With Developmental Disabilities and/or Behavioral Disorders and Their Families.)

Behavioral Screening

A comprehensive system and algorithm for screening for behavior disorders similar to that of developmental screening has not yet been developed, but the developmental screening system generalizes well for the screening and identification of behavior concerns and related disorders. While the screening of development is focused most on early identification during the infancy and preschool years, a strategy for identification of school-age developmental disorders and behavior disorders requires extension into later childhood and adolescence. Key ages for behavioral screening have not been identified, but should be considered at the 30-month preventive care visit, the 4- or 5-year visit (prior to school entry), the 8-year visit (early elementary age), and other key ages during preadolescence and adolescence.

Several screening tests have been developed for behavioral screening. The Pediatric Symptom Checklist (PSC) is a 35-question checklist to be completed by the parent for children ages 4 to 16 years or by an adolescent in its Youth Report form.[65] They take 5 to 10 minutes to complete and are available in multiple languages. A summary score is derived. If it is above a defined score, further behavioral evaluation by a medical or mental health professional is recommended. While not diagnostic, the PSC has been identified in its screening role as useful for the identification of moderate to serious impairments in children's psychosocial functioning.

The Ages & Stages Questionnaires: Social-Emotional, 2nd Edition (ASQ:SE-2) is a parent-completed system for social-emotional screening of children from ages 3 to 60 months.[66] The ASQ:SE-2 specifically targets personal and social skills in self-regulation, compliance, communication, adaptive functioning, autonomy, affect, and interaction with people. It takes 10 to 15 minutes to complete and score and is available in English and Spanish. Children scoring above the predetermined cutoff scores are recommended for further behavioral evaluation.

The Brief Infant-Toddler Social and Emotional Assessment (BITSEA) is a 42-item, parent-completed screening test for children between 12 and 36 months of age.[67,68] It has a 31-item problem scale, assessing problems such as aggression, defiance, overactivity, negative emotionality, anxiety, and withdrawal. Its 11-item competence scale measures empathy, prosocial behavior, and compliance. Cutoff points based on scores below the 15th percentile are used to indicate higher risk for social or emotional problems.

The Strengths and Difficulties Questionnaire is a 25-item, parent-report form assessing emotional problems, conduct, hyperactivity and inattention, peer relationships, and prosocial behaviors. It is available in more than 50 languages and covers children ages 3 through 17 years.[69] Parent, teacher, and adolescent self-report forms are available. Specificity of 95% and sensitivity of 63% for psychiatric diagnoses have been reported, with particular strength around identification of conduct, hyperactivity, and depressive and anxiety disorders.

The National Institute for Children's Health Quality (NICHQ) Vanderbilt Assessment Scale, a component of the ADHD toolkit developed by the AAP and NICHQ, is a set of parent- and teacher-reported scales aimed at identifying psychiatric disorders in school-aged children ages 6 years and older, including ADHD, oppositional defiant disorder, conduct disorder, and anxiety and depression symptoms.[70,71] Associated school academic and behavioral performance are also screened. The parent scale consists of 55 questions and the teacher scale has 43 questions. They are available in English, French, and German. The scales require 10 to 15 minutes to complete and score.

As recommended with these screening tests, and in accordance with the algorithm for developmental screening, children showing behavioral concerns on screening should have further evaluation by a medical or mental health professional. Behavioral evaluation may be completed by primary pediatric health care professionals within the medical home or through referral to specialty physicians trained in such evaluation, including pediatric specialists in developmental-behavioral pediatrics, neurodevelopmental disabilities, adolescent medicine, and child and adolescent psychiatrists (see Chapter 7, Basics of Child Behavior and Primary Care Pediatric Management of Common Behavioral Problems; Chapter 12, Social/Emotional Development and Disorders; Chapter 18, ADHD; Chapter 21, Disruptive Behavior Disorders ; Chapter 22, Anxiety and Mood Disorders; and Chapter 23, Basics of Psychopharmacological Management). Other mental health professionals who may be available in the community include psychologists, psychiatric nurse practitioners, and social workers. Behavioral evaluations are aimed at determining a diagnosis and developing an effective treatment program of psychotherapeutic and/or psychopharmacological management. Comorbid medical or developmental disorders may be identified and may require additional medical or developmental evaluation. As with children with developmental disorders, medical home strategies directed at chronic condition management should be implemented in the primary care medical home for children with behavioral disorders.

Conclusion

With the high frequency of developmental and behavioral disorders in children, the primary pediatric health care professional is challenged to identify these problems in the course of providing health care to children in the context of a medical home. Through creation of a systematic and algorithmic approach based on the universal health care concepts of surveillance, screening, and evaluation, early identification has been shown to be feasible during the course of preventive health care. Routine developmental and behavioral surveillance allows for ongoing monitoring of a child's development, whether it is typical or not. Use of standardized, objective screening tests at discrete, defined ages provides further support toward this process, ensuring acceptable levels of sensitivity and specificity for distinguishing children with developmental or behavioral disorders from those without. The child with a developmental or behavioral concern identified through surveillance and screening can begin the process of diagnostic evaluation, both developmental and medical, with initiation of developmental, behavioral, and medical treatments targeting the identified conditions. Successful implementation of surveillance and screening is now achievable in the primary care medical home through the use of a clinician-guided, office system–based approach that is supportive of the child and the family. Both surveillance and screening are critical to identifying children with developmental and behavioral disorders as early as possible to intervene and improve outcomes. Continued advances in the practice of surveillance, screening test development, developmental and medical evaluation procedures, and developmental and medical treatments will further assist in the early identification and treatment of children with developmental or behavioral disorders.

American Academy of Pediatrics Policy Statements and Resources

American Academy of Pediatrics. *Caring for Children With Autism Spectrum Disorders: A Resource Toolkit for Clinicians.* 2nd ed. Elk Grove Village, IL: American Academy of Pediatrics; 2012

American Academy of Pediatrics Committee on Practice and Ambulatory Medicine, Bright Futures Periodicity Schedule Workgroup. 2017 recommendations for preventive pediatric health care. *Pediatrics.* 2017;139(4):e20170254

American Academy of Pediatrics Council on Early Childhood, Council on School Health. The pediatrician's role in optimizing school readiness. *Pediatrics.* 2016;138(3):e20162293

American Academy of Pediatrics Subcommittee on Attention-Deficit/Hyperactivity Disorder, Steering Committee on Quality Improvement and Management. ADHD: clinical practice guideline for the diagnosis, evaluation, and treatment of attention-deficit/hyperactivity disorder in children and adolescents. *Pediatrics.* 2011;128(5): 1007–1022

American Academy of Pediatrics Council on Children With Disabilities. Care coordination in the medical home: integrating health and related systems of care for children with special health care needs. *Pediatrics.* 2005;116(5):1238–1244

American Academy of Pediatrics Council on Children With Disabilities. Supplemental Security Income (SSI) for children and youth with disabilities. *Pediatrics.* 2009;124(6)1702–1708. Reaffirmed February 2015

Adams RC, Tapia C, American Academy of Pediatrics Council on Children With Disabilities. Early intervention, IDEA Part C services, and the medical home: collaboration for best practice and best outcomes. *Pediatrics.* 2013;132(4):e1073–1088. Reaffirmed September 2013

American Academy of Pediatrics Council on Children With Disabilities, Section on Developmental Behavioral Pediatrics, Bright Futures Steering Committee, Medical Home Initiatives for Children With Special Needs Project Advisory Committee. Identifying infants and young children with developmental disorders in the medical home: an algorithm for developmental surveillance and screening. *Pediatrics.* 2006;118(1):405–420. Reaffirmed August 2014

American Academy of Pediatrics, National Initiative for Children's Healthcare Quality. *ADHD: Caring for Children with ADHD: A Resource Toolkit for Clinicians.* 2nd ed. Elk Grove Village, IL: American Academy of Pediatrics; 2012

Garner AS, Shonkoff JP, Siegel BS, et al. Early childhood adversity, toxic stress, and the role of the pediatrician: translating developmental science into lifelong health. *Pediatrics.* 2012;129(1):e224–e231

Milteer RM, Ginsburg KR; American Academy of Pediatrics Council on Communications and Media, Committee on Psychosocial Aspects of Child and Family Health. The importance of play in promoting healthy child development and maintaining strong parent-child bond: focus on children in poverty. *Pediatrics.* 2012;129(1):e204–213

American Academy of Pediatrics Council on Community Pediatrics, Gitterman BA, Flanagan PJ, Cotton WH, et al. Poverty and child health in the United States. *Pediatrics.* 2016;137(4):e20160339

Glassy D, Romano J; American Academy of Pediatrics Committee on Early Childhood, Adoption, and Dependent Care. Selecting appropriate toys for young children: the pediatrician's role. *Pediatrics.* 2003;111(4 Pt 1):911–913. Reaffirmed May 2011

Hagan JF, Shaw JS, Duncan PM. *Bright Futures: Guidelines for Health Supervision of Infants, Children, and Adolescents.* 4th ed. Elk Grove Village, IL: American Academy of Pediatrics; 2017

Johnson CP, Myers SM, American Academy of Pediatrics Council on Children With Disabilities. Identification and evaluation of children with autism spectrum disorders. *Pediatrics.* 2007;120(5):1183–1215. Reaffirmed August 2014

Murphy NA, Carbone PS, American Academy of Pediatrics Council on Children With Disabilities. Parent-provider-community partnerships: optimizing outcomes for children with disabilities. *Pediatrics.* 2011;128(4):795–802

Noritz GH, Murphy NA, Neuromotor Screening Expert Panel. Motor delays: early identification and evaluation. *Pediatrics.* 2013;131(6):e2016–e2027. Published correction appears in *Pediatrics.* 2017;140(3):e20172081

Shonkoff JP, Garner AS, American Academy of Pediatrics Committee on Psychosocial Aspects of Child and Family Health; Committee on Early Childhood, Adoption and Dependent Care; Section on Developmental and Behavioral Pediatrics. The lifelong effects of early childhood adversity and toxic stress. *Pediatrics*. 2012;129(1):e232–e246. Reaffirmed July 2016

Weitzman C, Wegner L, American Academy of Pediatrics Section on Developmental and Behavioral Pediatrics, Committee on Psychosocial Aspects of Child and Family Health, Council on Early Childhood, Society for Developmental and Behavioral Pediatrics. Promoting optimal development: screening for behavioral and emotional problems. *Pediatrics*. 2015;135(2):384–395

Web Sites

The AAP Screening in Practices Initiative: Screening Technical Assistance & Resource (STAR) Center Web site includes information on screening tools, practice resources, family resources, a webinar series, and an e-learning course, **www.aap.org/screening**

The AAP Council on Children With Disabilities Web site includes a collection of resources on developmental surveillance and screening and incorporating into preventive services, **https://www.aap.org/en-us/about-the-aap/Committees-Councils-Sections/Council-on-Children-with-Disabilities/Pages/Surv-and-Screening.aspx**

The Developmental Surveillance and Screening Quality Improvement Toolkit includes resources and tools from a developmental surveillance and screening quality improvement project. It is geared toward AAP chapters, clinics, and practices interested in developing and implementing a quality improvement or maintenance of certification project on developmental surveillance and screening. See **https://www.aap.org/en-us/about-the-aap/Committees-Councils-Sections/Council-on-Children-with-Disabilities/Pages/Quality-Improvement-Toolkit.aspx**

Freely available developmental and behavioral screening and assessment tools are available from the AAP Section on Developmental and Behavioral Pediatrics Practice Tools Web site, **https://www.aap.org/en-us/about-the-aap/Committees-Councils-Sections/sodbp/Pages/qi-best-practices.aspx**

Birth to 5: Watch Me Thrive! is a coordinated federal effort to encourage healthy child development, universal developmental and behavioral screening for children, and support for the families and providers who care for them. See **http://www.acf.hhs.gov/programs/ecd/watch-me-thrive**

In addition to the milestone checklists and other materials you are already familiar with, the CDC's Learn the Signs: Act Early program also recently launched the iOS and Android version of an app titled "CDC's Milestone Tracker." This developmental surveillance resource is available for free download at **https://www.cdc.gov/ncbddd/actearly/milestones-app.html**. See **https://www.cdc.gov/ncbddd/actearly/index.html** for further information.

References

1. Boyle CA, Boulet S, Schieve LA, et al. Trends in the prevalence of developmental disabilities in US children, 1997–2008. *Pediatrics*. 2011;127(6):1034–1042

2. Boulet SL, Boyle CA, Schieve LA. Health care use and health and functional impact of developmental disabilities among US children, 1997–2005. *Arch Pediatr Adolesc Med*. 2009;163(1):19–26

3. Christensen DL, Baio J, Van Naarden Braun K, et al. Prevalence and characteristics of autism spectrum disorder among children aged 8 years—autism and developmental disabilities monitoring network, 11 sites, United States, 2012. *MMWR Surveill Summ*. 2016;65(3):1–23

4. Durkin MS, Benedict RE, Christensen D, et al. Prevalence of cerebral palsy among 8-year-old children in 2010 and preliminary evidence of trends in its relationship to low birthweight. *Paediatr Perinat Epidemiol*. 2016;30(5):496–510

5. Visser SN, Danielson ML, Bitsko RH, et al. Trends in the parent-report of health care provider-diagnosed and medicated attention-deficit/hyperactivity disorder: United States, 2003–2011. *J Am Acad Child Adolesc Psychiatry*. 2014;53(1):34–46. e32

6. Law J, Boyle J, Harris F, Harkness A, Nye C. Prevalence and natural history of primary speech and language delay: findings from a systematic review of the literature. *Int J Lang Commun Disord*. 2000;35:165–188

7. Simon AE, Pastor PN, Reuben CA, Huang LN, Goldstrom ID. Use of mental health services by children ages six to 11 with emotional or behavioral difficulties. *Psychiatr Serv*. 2015 Sep;66(9):930–937

8. Cooley WC. Providing a primary care medical home for children and youth with cerebral palsy. *Pediatrics*. 2004;114(4):1106–1113

9. McPherson M, Arango P, Fox H, et al. A new definition of children with special health care needs. *Pediatrics*. 1998;102(1):137–139

10. Lipkin PH, Alexander J, Cartwright JD, et al. Care coordination in the medical home: integrating health and related systems of care for children with special health care needs. *Pediatrics*. 2005;116(5):1238–1244

11. Cooley WC, McAllister JW. Building medical homes: improvement strategies in primary care for children with special health care needs. *Pediatrics*. 2004;113(suppl 4):1499–1506

12. Kuhlthau KA, Bloom S, Van Cleave J, et al. Evidence for family-centered care for children with special health care needs: a systematic review. *Acad Pediatr*. 2011;11(2):136–143. e138

13. American Academy of Pediatrics Committee on Practice and Ambulatory Medicine Bright Futures Steering Committee. Recommendations for preventive pediatric health care. *Pediatrics*. 2007;120(6):1376–1376

14. American Academy of Pediatrics Council on Children With Disabilities, Section on Developmental Behavioral Pediatrics, Bright Futures Steering Committee, Medical Home Initiatives for Children With Special Needs Project Advisory Committee. Identifying infants and young children with developmental disorders in the medical home: an algorithm for developmental surveillance and screening. *Pediatrics*. 2006;118(1):405–420

15. Dworkin PH. British and American recommendations for developmental monitoring: the role of surveillance. *Pediatrics*. 1989;84(6):1000–1010

16. Glascoe FP, Altemeier WA, MacLean WE. The importance of parents' concerns about their child's development. *Am J Dis Child*. 1989;143(8):955–958

17. Glascoe FP. Parents' concerns about children's development: prescreening technique or screening test? *Pediatrics*. 1997;99(4):522–528

18. Glascoe FP, Sandler H. Value of parents' estimates of children's developmental ages. *J Pediatr*. 1995;127(5):831–835

19. Capute AJ, Palmer FB. A pediatric overview of the spectrum of developmental disabilities. *J Dev Behav Pediatr*. 1980;1(2):66–69

20. Accardo PJ, Accardo JA, Capute AJ. A neurodevelopmental perspective on the continuum of developmental disabilities. In: Accardo PJ, ed. *Capute and Accardo's Neurodevelopmental Disabilities in Infancy and Childhood*. 3rd ed. Baltimore, MD: Paul H. Brookes Publishing Co.; 2008:3–26

21. Weitzman C, Wegner L. Promoting optimal development: screening for behavioral and emotional problems. *Pediatrics*. 2015;135(2):384–395

22. Glascoe FP. Parents' evaluation of developmental status: how well do parents' concerns identify children with behavioral and emotional problems? *Clin Pediatr (Phila)*. 2003;42(2):133–138

23. Garner AS, Shonkoff JP, Siegel BS, et al. Early childhood adversity, toxic stress, and the role of the pediatrician: translating developmental science into lifelong health. *Pediatrics*. 2012;129(1):e224-e231

24. Shonkoff JP, Garner AS, Siegel BS, et al. The lifelong effects of early childhood adversity and toxic stress. *Pediatrics*. 2012;129(1):e232-e246

25. Gitterman BA, Flanagan PJ, Cotton WH, et al. Poverty and child health in the United States. *Pediatrics*. 2016:peds. 2016–0339

26. Ginsburg KR. The importance of play in promoting healthy child development and maintaining strong parent-child bonds. *Pediatrics*. 2007;119(1):182–191

27. Glassy D, Romano J, American Academy of Pediatrics Committee on Early Childhood, Adoption, and Dependent Care. Selecting appropriate toys for young children: the pediatrician's role. *Pediatrics.* 2003;111(4):911–913

28. Duby J. Role of the medical home in family-centered early intervention services. *Pediatrics.* 2007;120(5):1153–1158

29. Johnson CP, Myers SM. Identification and evaluation of children with autism spectrum disorders. *Pediatrics.* 2007;120(5):1183–1215

30. Hagan JF, Shaw JS, Duncan PM, eds. *Bright Futures Guidelines for Health Supervision of Infants, Children, and Adolescents,* 4th ed. Elk Grove Village, IL: American Academy of Pediatrics; 2017

31. Grimes DA, Schulz KF. Uses and abuses of screening tests. *Lancet.* 2002;359(9309):881–884

32. Evans MI, Galen RS, Britt DW. Principles of screening. *Semin Perinatol.* 2005;29(6):364–366

33. Barnes KE. *Preschool screening: The measurement and prediction of children at-risk.* Charles C. Thomas Publisher; 1982

34. Camp BW. What the clinician really needs to know: questioning the clinical usefulness of sensitivity and specificity in studies of screening tests. *J Dev Behav Pediatr.* 2006;27(3):226–230

35. Frankenburg WK, Dodds JB. The Denver developmental screening test. *J Pediatr.* 1967;71(2):181–191

36. Frankenburg WK, Dodds J, Archer P, Shapiro H, Bresnick B. The Denver II: a major revision and restandardization of the Denver Developmental Screening Test. *Pediatrics.* 1992;89(1):91–97

37. Glascoe FP. *Parents' Evaluation of Developmental Status (PEDS).* Nolensville, TN: Ellsworth & Vandermeer Press, Ltd; 1997

38. Squires J, Bricker D, Twombly E, et al. *Ages & Stages Questionnaires, (ASQ-3): A Parent-Completed Child Monitoring System.* 3rd ed. Baltimore, MD: Paul H. Brookes Publishing Co.; 2009

39. Coplan J, Gleason JR. Test-retest and interobserver reliability of the Early Language Milestone Scale. *J Pediatr Health Care.* 1993;7(5):212–219

40. Belcher HM, Gittlesohn A, Capute AJ, Allen MC. Using the clinical linguistic and auditory milestone scale for developmental screening in high-risk preterm infants. *Clin Pediatr (Phila).* 1997;36(11):635–642

41. Dumont-Mathieu T, Fein D. Screening for autism in young children: the Modified Checklist for Autism in Toddlers (M-CHAT) and other measures. *Dev Disabil Res Rev.* 2005;11(3):253–262

42. Robins DL, Casagrande K, Barton M, Chen CA, Dumont-Mathieu T, Fein D. Validation of the Modified Checklist for Autism in Toddlers, revised with follow-up (M-CHAT-R/F). *Pediatrics.* 2014;133(1)

43. Chlebowski C, Robins DL, Barton ML, Fein D. Large-scale use of the modified checklist for autism in low-risk toddlers. *Pediatrics.* 2013;131(4):e1121–e1127

44. Maternal and Child Health Bureau. Boston Children's Hospital. Developmental Screening Tool Kit for Primary Care Providers. www.developmentalscreening.org. Accessed January 17, 2018

45. Drotar D, Stancin T, Dworkin PH, Sices L, Wood S. Selecting developmental surveillance and screening tools. *Pediatr Rev.* 2008;29(10):e52–e58

46. Centers for Disease Control and Prevention. Learn the signs. Act Early Program. Centers for Disease Control and Prevention Web site. www.cdc.gov/ActEarly. Accessed November 17, 2017

47. Rydz D, Shevell MI, Majnemer A, Oskoui M. Topical review: developmental screening. *J Child Neurol.* 2005;20(1):4–21

48. Sand N, Silverstein M, Glascoe FP, Gupta VB, Tonniges TP, O'Connor KG. Pediatricians' reported practices regarding developmental screening: do guidelines work? Do they help? *Pediatrics.* 2005;116(1):174–179

49. Radecki L, Sand-Loud N, O'Connor KG, Sharp S, Olson LM. Trends in the use of standardized tools for developmental screening in early childhood: 2002–2009. *Pediatrics.* 2011;128(1):14–19

50. Lipkin PH, Baer B, Macias MM, et al. Trends in standardized developmental screening: Results from national surveys of pediatricians, 2002–2016. Pediatric Academic Societies annual meeting; 2017; San Francisco, CA

51. Developmental Surveillance and Screening Policy Implementation Project (D-PIP). http://www.medicalhomeinfo.org/how/clinical_care/developmental_screening/d-pip/index.aspx

52. Earls MF, Hay SS. Setting the stage for success: implementation of developmental and behavioral screening and surveillance in primary care practice—the North Carolina Assuring Better Child Health and Development (ABCD) Project. *Pediatrics.* 2006;118(1):e183-e188

53. King TM, Tandon SD, Macias MM, et al. Implementing developmental screening and referrals: lessons learned from a national project. *Pediatrics.* 2010;125(2):350–360

54. Jimenez ME, Barg FK, Guevara JP, Gerdes M, Fiks AG. Barriers to evaluation for early intervention services: parent and early intervention employee perspectives. *Acad Pediatr.* 2012;12(6):551–557

55. Jimenez ME, Barg FK, Guevara JP, Gerdes M, Fiks AG. The impact of parental health literacy on the early intervention referral process. *J Health Care Poor Underserved.* 2013;24(3):1053–1062

56. Jimenez ME, Fiks AG, Shah LR, et al. Factors associated with early intervention referral and evaluation: a mixed methods analysis. *Acad Pediatr.* 2014;14(3):315–323

57. Schaefer GB, Mendelsohn NJ. Clinical genetics evaluation in identifying the etiology of autism spectrum disorders. *Genet Med.* 2008;10(4):301–305

58. Schaefer GB, Mendelsohn NJ, Practice P, Committee G. Clinical genetics evaluation in identifying the etiology of autism spectrum disorders: 2013 guideline revisions. *Genet Med.* 2013;15(5):399–407

59. Michelson DJ, Shevell MI, Sherr EH, Moeschler JB, Gropman AL, Ashwal S. Evidence report: genetic and metabolic testing on children with global developmental delay: report of the Quality Standards Subcommittee of the American Academy of Neurology and the Practice Committee of the Child Neurology Society. *Neurology.* 2011;77(17):1629–1635

60. Ashwal S, Russman B, Blasco P, et al. Practice parameter: diagnostic assessment of the child with cerebral palsy report of the Quality Standards Subcommittee of the American Academy of Neurology and the Practice Committee of the Child Neurology Society. *Neurology.* 2004;62(6):851–863

61. Lipkin P, Schertz M, Accardo P. Early intervention and its efficacy. In: Accardo PJ, ed. *Capute and Accardo's Neurodevelopmental Disabilities in Infancy and Childhood.* 3rd ed. Baltimore, MD: Paul H. Brookes Publishing Co.; 2008:519–552

62. Macias MM, Levy SL, Lipkin PH, et al. Referral Trends of Young Children Screened for Developmental Delay and Autism Spectrum Disorder: Results from National Surveys of Pediatricians, 2002-2016. Paper presented at: Pediatric Academic Societies Meeting; May 6–9, 2017; San Francisco, CA

63. Strickland BB, Jones JR, Newacheck PW, Bethell CD, Blumberg SJ, Kogan MD. Assessing systems quality in a changing health care environment: The 2009–10 National Survey of Children with Special Health Care Needs. *Matern Child Health J.* 2015;19(2):353–361

64. American Academy of Pediatrics Council on Children With Disabilities. Supplemental Security Income (SSI) for children and youth with disabilities. *Pediatrics.* 2009;124(6):1702–1708. Reaffirmed February 2015

65. Massachusetts General Hospital. Pediatric Symptom Checklist. Massachusetts General Hospital Web site. http://www.massgeneral.org/psychiatry/services/psc_home.aspx. Accessed December 16, 2017

66. Squires J, Bricker DD, Twombly E. *ASQ-SE-2 User's Guide.* Baltimore, MD: Paul H. Brookes Publishing Co.; 2015

67. Briggs-Gowan MJ, Carter AS, Irwin JR, Wachtel K, Cicchetti DV. The Brief Infant-Toddler Social and Emotional Assessment: screening for social-emotional problems and delays in competence. *J Pediatr Psychol.* 2004;29(2):143–155

68. Briggs-Gowan MJ, Carter AS. Social-emotional screening status in early childhood predicts elementary school outcomes. *Pediatrics.* 2008;121(5):957–962

69. Goodman R, Ford T, Simmons H, Gatward R, Meltzer H. Using the Strengths and Difficulties Questionnaire (SDQ) to screen for child psychiatric disorders in a community sample. *Br J Psychiatry.* 2000;177(6):534–539

70. Wolraich ML, Lambert W, Doffing MA, Bickman L, Simmons T, Worley K. Psychometric properties of the Vanderbilt ADHD diagnostic parent rating scale in a referred population. *J Pediatr Psychol.* 2003;28(8):559–568

71. American Academy of Pediatrics. *ADHD: Caring for Children With ADHD. A Resource Toolkit for Clinicians.* 2nd ed. Elk Grove Village, IL: American Academy of Pediatrics; 2012

CHAPTER 10

Developmental Evaluation

Mary L. O'Connor Leppert, MB, BCh, FAAP

The American Academy of Pediatrics (AAP) has established a policy for developmental surveillance and screening in the primary care setting that, when applied consistently, will identify children who are not meeting expected developmental milestones.[1] This policy statement recommends that children who are identified by screening as being at risk receive a developmental evaluation to confirm a developmental diagnosis, a medical evaluation to investigate the etiology of the developmental condition, and a referral to initiate early intervention services. The AAP policy statement specifies that pediatric subspecialists, such as neurodevelopmental pediatricians, developmental-behavioral pediatricians, child neurologists, pediatric physiatrists, or child psychiatrists, can perform the diagnostic developmental evaluation for children who fail screening. However, 1 in 6 children in the United States has a developmental disability, and the prevalence of autism spectrum disorder (ASD), attention-deficit/hyperactivity disorder (ADHD), and other developmental delays has been increasing over time.[2] Further, most child neurologists, child psychiatrists, and pediatric physiatrists do not routinely perform standardized developmental evaluations. While neurodevelopmental pediatricians and developmental-behavioral pediatricians do routinely perform such standardized developmental evaluations, of the 118,292 pediatricians currently certified by the American Board of Pediatrics, only 775 are board-certified in developmental-behavioral pediatrics and only 255 are board-certified in neurodevelopmental disabilities.[3] Thus, referral for subspecialty diagnostic evaluation is a futile proposition for the vast majority of children who fail screening.[4] Given this high prevalence of developmental-behavioral disorders, the scarcity of subspecialists to whom to refer, and the extremely long wait lists at tertiary care developmental centers, developmental evaluation needs to be considered as basic to primary care pediatric practice as are assessing and diagnosing asthma and other common chronic medical conditions encountered daily in pediatric practice.[4] Thus, it is important to note that the AAP policy statement does include a recommendation that a diagnostic developmental evaluation can be performed by early childhood professionals in conjunction with the child's primary pediatric health care professional. This chapter describes a neurodevelopmental evaluation process that primary pediatric health care professionals may consider adopting in cases of developmental screening failure in order to make developmental diagnoses within the medical home, rather than waiting for generally inaccessible subspecialty consultation. Through adoption of this process, primary pediatric health care professionals can contribute to both making a developmental diagnosis and attempting to establish a cause of the developmental disorder.

Principles of Development

Neurodevelopment is a complex, dynamic process that begins at birth and typically proceeds in a predictable sequence and at a predictable rate. The study of development has concentrated on the first years of life, as the observations of developmental markers in infants, toddlers, and preschoolers are rich in number and show little variability. Five areas, or "streams" of development (a term coined by Dr Arnold Capute to reflect the fluid or dynamic process of development) that have been consistently studied and are evaluated during developmental evaluations are gross motor, language, visual-motor problem-solving, social skills, and adaptive skills.[5] Each of these streams of development has milestones of expected achievements ascribed to specific ages. Milestones do not represent the process of development, but rather, they reflect the product of a developmental process. Defined milestones are the measure by which typical or atypical development is assessed.

Modern developmental evaluations are based largely on the pioneering work of Dr Arnold Gesell, who established the first norms of milestones in the 5 streams of development.[6] Gesell assiduously recorded the timing and sequence of normal development in infants and children. He found typical development to be an orderly, timed, and sequential process that occurs with such regularity that it is predictable.[6] The marvel of development, however, is not so much in the regularity of the acquisition of milestones within any given stream, but in the synchrony of development across streams.

In atypical development, the timing, order, or sequence of the acquisition of milestones is disturbed within a given stream or across several streams. The assessment of atypical development employs the principles of delay, deviation (or deviance), and dissociation. Developmental delay describes a phenomenon in which milestones within a given stream are attained in the typical sequence, but at a delayed rate. Delay can occur within a single stream or across several developmental streams. Deviance or deviation represents an uncustomary sequence of milestone attainment within a single stream of development. A child who is able to crawl before he or she is able to sit demonstrates deviation in gross motor skill attainment. Dissociation is a descriptive term that indicates differing rates of development across the 5 streams of development.

The developmental quotient (DQ) is a measure of the rate of development within a stream, and it is the metric by which delay is determined. The DQ represents the percentage of normal development within a given stream that is present at the time of testing. Using the age at which specific milestones are generally present, a functional age equivalent (AE) can be ascribed to a child's development. For example, a child whose best motor function is sitting unsupported has a functional age equivalent of 6 months (Box 10.1). The DQ is calculated by dividing the child's age equivalent within a given stream by his or her chronological age (CA). The DQ is arithmetically represented by DQ = AE/CA × 100. Developmental delay has traditionally been defined by a DQ of less than 70.

Box 10.1. Approximate Ages of Gross-Motor Milestones

> ▸ At **1 month** of age, the child can lift his or her head off the table in the prone position.

> ▸ At **2 months** of age, the child can lift his or her chest off the table in the prone position.

> ▸ At **3 months** of age, the child can lift him- or herself up to the elbows in the prone position.

> ▸ At **4 months** of age, the child can lift him- or herself up to the wrists in the prone position and can roll from the prone position to the supine position.

> ▸ At **5 months** of age, the child can roll from the supine position to the prone position and can sit with support.

> ▸ At **6 months** of age, the child sits alone.

> ▸ At **8 months** of age, the child comes up to a sitting position, crawls, and pulls him- or herself up to a standing position.

> ▸ At **9 months** of age, the child cruises.

> ▸ At **11 months** of age, the child walks with his or her hand held.

> ▸ At **12 months** of age, the child walks alone.

> ▸ At **15 months** of age, the child runs.

Derived from Capute AJ, Shapiro BK. The motor quotient: a method for the early detection of motor delay. *Am J Dis Child.* 1985;139(9):940–942.

The application of the DQ to determine delay within a single stream, or dissociation between streams, can imply diagnoses, which should be supported by historical and examination findings. A child with a gross motor DQ of 50, a history of delay in motor milestone acquisition, and abnormal findings on physical and neurological examination is consistent with a diagnosis of cerebral palsy. Delays in language and nonverbal/ visual-motor abilities, with DQs of 70 or less in both domains, place a child at risk for a diagnosis of intellectual disability. However, delayed language skills in the presence of age-appropriate nonverbal/visual-motor skills (dissociation) imply a diagnosis of a communication disorder. Unlike delay and dissociation, deviation is not used diagnostically. Rather, it is a finding that suggests atypical development within a single stream, and it should heighten the clinician's suspicions regarding underlying pathology. For example, identifying letters and reciting the alphabet while not using any words to communicate a request could suggest ASD (see Chapter 11, Making Developmental-Behavioral Diagnoses).

Developmental Milestones
– Gross Motor Milestones

Motor development is the easiest stream to observe because of the numerous achievements that occur within the first year of life. Newborns demonstrate little voluntary motor ability and are restricted by primitive (involuntary) reflexes. At birth, a newborn does not have enough motor control to lift his or her head when lying in a prone position. Over the first 4 months of life, neck and trunk tone are acquired in a cranial-caudal direction. By 1 month of age, an infant in a prone position should have enough neck tone to lift the head from the bed. By 2 months of age, with head and trunk tone, an infant can lift the head and chest off the bed. By 3 months, an infant can prop up on elbows, and by

4 months, on the wrists. After trunk tone is acquired, the ability to dissociate shoulder and hip movement enables derotative rolling at 4 to 5 months of age. By 6 months of age, trunk tone is sufficient to allow the child to be put into a sitting position and to maintain that position. Shortly after sitting, the child integrates trunk tone with the derotational abilities required for pivoting, allowing him or her to come into a sitting position independently at 8 months. Independent sitting gives way to the ability to assume a quadruped position, ultimately leading to reciprocal crawling and pulling to a stand at 8 months, walking with hands held at 11 months, and walking independently at 12 months[7] (Box 10.1).

In addition to a developmental history of acquisition of motor skills over time elicited from parents and/or caregivers and direct observation of current motor skills, the motor evaluation requires a standard neurological examination, including the observation of primitive reflexes and postural reactions. Abnormalities of tone, primitive reflexes, and postural reactions can mitigate the sequence and rate of motor development. The infant's neurological examination should include observation of the position the infant assumes at rest and the repertoire of spontaneous movement of the child in a supine resting position. Abnormal posture of the extremities, or a paucity of movement in one or more extremities, should increase the suspicions of the examiner. Flexor tone predominates in the newborn but diminishes over the first 4 months of life. However, normal infant flexor tone is symmetrical, and despite the flexion, there is a normal passive range of movement across all joints. The persistence of flexor tone past the newborn period, or the absence of flexor tone (generally signaling hypotonia) during the newborn period, can interfere with expected motor development. Asymmetry of tone and exaggerated tone (increased or decreased) are abnormal neurological findings, which are further evaluated with deep tendon reflexes and primitive reflexes.

Primitive reflexes are automated patterns of movement that are present in utero and persist until 3 to 6 months of life. Primitive reflexes are well described patterns that have qualitative and temporal characteristics that add valuable information to the classic neurological examination of infants. Classical primitive reflexes include the Moro, Galant, and Landau reflexes, as well as the asymmetrical tonic neck reflex (ATNR), the tonic labyrinthine reflex (TL), the positive support reflex, and the symmetrical tonic neck reflex (STNR). Each reflex may be observed in the spontaneous movement of the newborn or can be elicited by an examiner. The quality of the reflex, the ability or inability to suppress reflexes with repeated elicitations, and advancing age may precede or accompany motor delay and deviancy.[8] Primitive reflexes that persist past the first 6 months of age are atypical, and their presence is a useful marker in the detection of motor disorders. For purposes of delineating the clinical usefulness of the primitive reflexes, the ATNR and TL will be described.

The asymmetrical tonic neck reflex (ATNR) is a primitive reflex in which rotation of the head to either side causes extension of the extremities on the chin side and flexion of the extremities on the occipital side. In the typical infant, rotation of the head to one side will elicit an ATNR, but if the head is kept to one side, the flexion and extension patterns caused by the ATNR relax, and the extremities resume a neutral position. Similarly if the head is rotated to one side to elicit the ATNR, successive head rotations produce progressively diminished responses to the head turn. The ATNR is considered obligatory or exaggerated if the child maintains the flexion/extension pattern of the ATNR the entire time the head is turned to one side or if the child does not exhibit diminished response to the ATNR with subsequent repetitions. The tonic labyrinthine (TL) reflex may be elicited with the child in the supine position or in prone suspension. This reflex is produced with flexion and extension of the neck. When the neck is brought into flexion, the infant flexes all extremities, and when the neck is brought into extension, the infant extends all extremities and retracts the shoulders. Like the ATNR, the TL should not be exaggerated or obligatory and should not persist past 6 months of age. Obligatory or exaggerated responses are considered atypical and should be factored into the assessment of the motor examination.

Postural reactions are responses of equilibrium and protection that appear midway through the first year as the primitive reflexes disappear. Postural reactions allow for the development of functional movement while keeping the head and body upright and oriented. Postural reactions include the Landau reaction; head righting; derotative righting; upper and lower extremity parachutes; and anterior, lateral, and posterior propping (which are required for sitting). Unlike primitive reflexes, which arouse suspicion of motor disorder by their exaggerated or prolonged presence, postural reactions raise suspicion by their failure to appear at appropriate ages or by asymmetry of their appearance.

The motor evaluation, then, consists of the assessment of the motor age equivalent (gleaned from a combination of a developmental history elicited from parents and/or caregivers and direct professional observation), the motor DQ (calculated by using the motor age equivalent), the neurological examination, and the assessment of primitive reflexes and postural reactions. A motor DQ of less than 50 signifies considerable motor impairment, most commonly cerebral palsy. Motor quotients of 50 to 70 represent more mild motor delays, which are often based in hypotonia or motor coordination difficulties, and are frequently associated with delays or deviancies in other streams of development.

– Visual-Motor Problem-solving Milestones

The visual-motor problem-solving stream of development is a domain of nonverbal abilities that are dependent on cognitive function, visual capacity, and fine motor ability. Like gross motor skills, visual-motor and fine motor abilities are acquired in a timed and orderly pattern (Table 10.1). Visual-motor development dominates the first 4 months of life. In the first month of life, an infant will use eye movement and slight head turning for visual fixation and following to the midline. During the second month, visual pursuit uses eye and head movement that extends past the midline and in both vertical and horizontal planes. By the third month, the eyes and head can visually follow in a circle and a visual threat response can be elicited. By the fourth month, the eyes and head turning are coupled with directed upper extremity use.[9] The ability to visually attend and track provides targets for the upper extremity to engage.

Table 10.1. Visual-Motor Milestones	
Age (months)	**Milestone**
1	Visually fixes
2	Visually follows in horizontal and vertical plane
3	Visually follows in a circle Exhibits a visual threat
4	Hands unfisted
5	Hands come to midline Reaches for object Transfers from one hand to another
6	Picks up large object with a radial rake
8	Picks up small object with a radial rake
9	Picks up small object with immature pincer
11	Picks up small object with a mature pincer

Adapted from Accardo PJ, Caputo AJ. *The Caputo Scales: Cognitive Adaptive Test and Clinical Linguistic and Auditory Milestone Scale (CAT/CLAMS)*. Baltimore, MD: Paul H. Brookes Publishing Co.; 2005.

Upper extremity movement, like trunk tone, develops in a proximal to distal fashion, beginning with coarse movement originating at the shoulders at 5 months and advancing to a precise pincer movement of the forefinger and thumb at 11 months. At 4 months of age, the hands come together in midline. By 5 months, a child can reach up from the shoulders, grasp an object, and pull it towards himself or herself, as well as transfer an object from one hand to the other. At 6 months, a child in a sitting position can reach out in front of him or her and grasp an object presented within reach. Grasp develops in an ulnar to radial fashion. Initially, grasp requires support of the ulnar border of the hand and forearm on a surface to secure an object with a rake-like movement initiated by the index and middle finger, employing 3 fingers and a thumb. The radial rake gives way to the immature pincer grasp at 9 months, in which the child can pick up a pellet-sized object with an overhand movement using only the thumb, index, and middle fingers. The mature pincer grasp of an 11-month-old child employs only the index finger and thumb in an overhand movement that is precise.

Nonverbal problem-solving skills are the product of visual, fine motor, and intellectual abilities. Once the visual and fine motor milestones of the first year of life are acquired, cognition becomes the testable variable of the nonverbal domain. Parents typically are able to provide a history of gross motor and language skill acquisition, but a history of visual-motor problem-solving skills is more difficult to elicit. Thus, visual-motor problem-solving milestones must be demonstrated by the child in the developmental evaluation. Most standard instruments for evaluating visual-motor problem-solving skills employ test batteries modified from the early work of Arnold Gesell,[6] which was considerably shortened by Cattell[10] and further adapted by many authors over the next few decades. To be clinically useful, tests of nonverbal abilities for young children must provide age equivalents in order to quantify development using a developmental quotient.

Atypical visual-motor development can result from visual impairment, significant fine motor impairment, and/or intellectual disability. Impairments sufficient to preclude assessment are identified in the first few months of life in the case of visual impairments and in the latter half of the first year of life in the case of significant fine motor impairment. Occasionally, children demonstrate qualitatively poor fine motor abilities that do not prevent testing but that may slow or diminish the accuracy of movement, but the child should be credited if he/she shows the cognitive intent to perform the test item. In the absence of significant motor or visual impairments, delays in problem-solving skills are the result of cognitive or intellectual disability. Developmental deviance in problem-solving is observed in children with qualitatively poor fine motor skills (children with poor writing skills may be unable to perform age-appropriate graphomotor tasks but do well with other age-appropriate tasks) and in children with attentional deficits sufficient to interfere with task completion, despite the motor and cognitive capacity to perform at age-appropriate levels.

– Speech and Language Milestones

Language development is an intricate process by which an infant establishes a repository of words that becomes a vocabulary available for the understanding of verbally presented information and for communication. Typical language development requires the presence of adequate hearing, the cognitive ability to acquire vocabulary and build a word repository, the ability to attend to verbal information, and the desire to establish rapport with a speaker.[11] A child who has all the prerequisites of language development will gradually store vocabulary to which he or she is exposed. This stored lexicon also records the visual images, word patterns, and affective associations with which the vocabulary is learned. Over time, the stored lexicon is sufficient for the understanding of very complex communication. This understanding of linguistic cipher is referred to in development as receptive language, and it is measured by a few milestones in the first year of life and more plentiful milestones thereafter (Table 10.2).

Table 10.2. Receptive and Expressive Milestones		
Age (months)	**Receptive Milestone**	**Expressive Milestone**
1	Alerts to sound	
2	Social smile	
3		Coos
4	Orients to voice	Laughs
6		Babbles
8		Mama or Dada nonspecifically
10	Understands "No"	Mama and Dada specifically
12	Follows one step commands with a gesture	2-word vocabulary
18	Points to one picture Identifies >2 body parts	7- to 10-word vocabulary
21	Points to two pictures	20-word vocabulary, 2-word phrases
24	Follows 2-step commands	50-word vocabulary, 2-word sentences
30	Understands the concept of "1" Points to 7 pictures	Uses pronouns appropriately
36	Follows 2-step prepositional commands	250-word vocabulary Uses 3-word sentences

Adapted from Accardo PJ, Capute AJ. *The Capute Scales: Cognitive Adaptive Test and Clinical Linguistic and Auditory Milestone Scale (CAT/CLAMS)*. Baltimore, MD: Paul H. Brookes Publishing Co.; 2005.

Expressive language development is dependent on a rich word repository or receptive language skills from which information is drawn, as well as the neurological and oral motor skills to produce speech. Expressive language skills progress over the first 12 months of life, from guttural language from birth to 2 months to prelinguistic skills between 3 and 11 months.[9] Guttural language represents vocalizations that are largely physiological noises devoid of social significance, such as crying, burping, coughing, and yawning. The guttural phase of language is followed by the prelinguistic phase, in which there is a social intent to vocalize, albeit at a preword level. Prelinguistic skills begin with the social smile at 2 months and cooing at 3 months of age; these are followed by razzing, laughing, ah-gooing, and babbling. Babbling begins at 6 months of age as a string of hard consonants and vowel sounds: da-da-da-da and ba-ba-ba-ba, and progresses to da-da, which is used nonspecifically at 8 months. Discriminate use of "Dada" and "Mama" to identify the child's parents begins at 10 months of age and herald the beginning of the linguistic phase of development. The linguistic phase begins at about 11 months of age when the first identifiable word is uttered and grows exponentially over the next 2 years of life. Between 12 and 18 months of age, the child's vocabulary expands only to 7 to 10 words, but it swells to 50 words and 2-word sentences at 24 months and to 250 words and 3-word sentences by 36 months of age.

Atypical language development may be a primary disorder of language that occurs in the absence of an identifiable cause, or it may be a secondary disorder that occurs as a consequence of intellectual disability, hearing impairment, autism, or motor speech disorder. Language impairments include expressive, mixed receptive and expressive, and pragmatic disorders. Expressive language impairment is a failure to demonstrate age-appropriate verbal skills; it is manifest as limited single-word vocabulary, delayed connected-language use, or poor speech production (articulation, phonation, or fluency difficulties). Expressive language disorder assumes a delay in expressive language and a dissociation between the rate of expressive language and that of typical ability in receptive language and cognition. Speech production disorders affect the quality of verbalizations rather than the size of vocabulary or use of connected language. In the early linguistic phase, some children use word approximations in which they may drop the beginning or ending sound of a word ("bott" or "ottle" for bottle) or use sound substitutions ("bobble" for bottle) but are quite consistent and specific with word use. Word approximations, when employed specifically and consistently, should be counted when estimating the size of a child's vocabulary. Similarly, articulation deficits, phonological disorders, or speech fluency disorders (stuttering) affect the quality rather than the content of expressive language. An expressive language disorder should be suspected in a child who is not babbling or using gesture language by 12 months, not using single words by 16 months, or not using 2 word phrases by 24 months of age (Table 10.2).

Receptive language requires the ability to process and understand spoken language precisely and efficiently. Receptive language disorder represents impairment in comprehension that is unexpected given a child's cognitive ability, evidenced by a delay in receptive language and a dissociation between the delayed rate of language milestone acquisition and an age appropriate rate of nonverbal cognitive milestone acquisition. Receptive language skills are a prerequisite for learning expressive language skills. Therefore, when receptive language is delayed, there is co-occurring expressive language disorder or mixed receptive-expressive language disorder. Receptive and expressive language disorders generally present because of expressive language delay, but parents may also complain that their child does not seem to listen to or follow simple commands. There is a paucity of observed receptive language milestones in the first year of life, but a number of receptive milestones are defined in the second and third years, some of which may be demonstrated in the examination and some of which are credited by parental history.

Pragmatic language disorders can be conceptualized as inadequate understanding of communication at the nonword level. Pragmatic language is the ability to derive meaning from the tone or prosody of voice, rather than the word's meaning, and is required for understanding humor, sarcasm, idioms, and other verbal references that require drawing inference. Pragmatic skills also include the understanding of nonverbal communication such as facial expression, eye contact, and body language. Children with pragmatic language disorders appreciate only the pedantic meaning of utterances, thereby missing valuable nonverbal meanings of communication. Pragmatic language skill deficits manifest largely as social delays and are most often appreciated in children who are on the autism spectrum or who have a social (pragmatic) communication disorder. Pragmatic language skills are appreciated in the developmental evaluation but are formally tested by experienced speech-language pathologists.

– Social and Adaptive Milestones

The last two streams of development, social and adaptive skills, are different from the other developmental streams in that (1) they are dependent on motor, language, and cognitive abilities; (2) they are more subject to environmental and cultural influences; and (3) delays in social or adaptive skills do not directly infer diagnoses but provide further evidence for suspected diagnoses. Social skills require a combination of language and nonverbal problem-solving skills but are more heavily dependent on appropriate language, so much so that if language skills are delayed, social skills are also likely to be delayed. A child of 3 years of age is expected to have reciprocal play skills but may continue to engage in parallel play if language skills are delayed enough to interfere with reciprocal play. Learning to play reciprocally and to share require the language skills to establish the rules of playing fairly and the problem-solving skills to know, for example, that if there is only one toy, two children cannot each have it at once. Adaptive skills, or self-help skills, require both language and nonverbal skills but are most heavily dependent on nonverbal or problem-solving skills. Adaptive skills such as feeding, toileting, and dressing rely on adequate motor skills as well as cognitive ability. Adaptive skills are so dependent on cognition that delays in adaptive skill attainment must be documented for the diagnosis of intellectual disability, thereby affirming the diagnosis suspected by significant delays in language and nonverbal test measures. Delays in social skills may be seen in children with global cognitive delay or in children with normal cognition with communication disorders. Delays in social skills, coupled with dissociated delays or deviation in communication are most pronounced in children with ASD or social (pragmatic) communication disorders (see Chapter 11, Making Developmental-Behavioral Diagnoses).

Presentation of Developmental Disorders

The age at which children present for evaluation of developmental disorders varies with the stream of development in question, as well as the severity of the delay. In general, disorders of greater severity (but of lower prevalence) present at early ages and to medical professionals. Disorders of lesser severity (but of higher prevalence) present later and may present to nonmedical professionals (therapists or teachers). Sensory deficits, including hearing and vision impairment, are often detected in the first few months of life when a child does not respond to sound in the first months, turn to voice at 4 to 5 months, or fails to visually fix or follow in the first 3 months. Delays in language should always prompt the primary pediatric health care professional to refer for formal hearing evaluation, and delays in visual-motor problem-solving skills should always prompt a formal vision evaluation.

Motor deficits typically present in the second 6 months of life when children fail to sit, crawl, or pull up to stand. Walking is expected at 12 months, with 15 months accepted as the upper limit of normal variation. Children with motor DQs below 70 warrant a full neurodevelopmental evaluation with a developmental history, physical examination, neurological examination, and evaluation of other streams of development, even though motor delay can occur independent of delays in other domains. A motor DQ of less than 70 would include sitting at ages older than 8.5 months, crawling later than 11.5 months, and walking at later than 17 months. Motor developmental quotients of 50 or less are nearly pathognomonic of cerebral palsy, which presents at an average age of 12 months.[12] Delays in communication or cognition present at an average age of 27 to 32 months, most often due to failure to demonstrate the expected expressive language skills.[12] Social impairments and behavioral disorders present over a wide range of ages, again depending on the extent to which the disorder is impacting the child and/or his or her caregivers. Attention-deficit/hyperactivity disorder may present in preschool years because of concerns that activity levels or impulsivity preclude normal family function, jeopardize preschool or child-care placements, or compromise the child's safety. Attention deficits alone, however, often present later, when distractibility or poor concentration hinder academic success. Adaptive skill delays are not a common presenting complaint but are noted during the developmental history in children who present with other concerns. Disorders of learning generally do not present until school age, when children are put to the task of learning and are unsuccessful.

Neurodevelopmental Evaluation

History

The first step in neurodevelopmental evaluation, as in any other form of medical evaluation, is to obtain a thorough history including the presenting complaint and birth, medical, developmental, behavioral, educational, social, and family histories. The complete history offers clues to developmental diagnosis, provides evidence of the child's developmental trajectory, and uncovers historical risks for atypical development. The presenting complaint will define the stream of development that is the focus of parental concern, the age of the child when parents first became concerned, and the impact that the complaint is having on the child's function. Presenting complaints are typically focused: A child is not sitting or crawling on time or is not speaking enough or clearly. Occasionally, presenting complaints are curiously vague, for example, "My son is not like my other children" or "The teachers told me to have my son evaluated." In either case, a thorough assessment is required to assess the stream of development in question and also to look for lesser concerns in other streams of development, which may not have been appreciated by the family. It is imperative that the primary pediatric health care professional recognize that the presenting complaint may represent the tip of the iceberg, highlighting only a single component of a more extensive developmental disorder (see Chapter 11, Making Developmental-Behavioral Diagnoses).

– Birth History

Children with significant complications in their birth histories (prenatal, perinatal, or neonatal) should have their development monitored more closely from birth by their primary pediatric health care professional or by specified follow-up clinics (eg, the neonatal intensive care unit [NICU] or preterm follow-up clinics) because they are at higher risk for developmental disorders.

The birth history ascertains the maternal age and parity at the time of the child's gestation, paternal age, medical complications of pregnancy (bleeding, hypertension, gestational diabetes, clotting disorders, infections, and intrauterine exposures), complications identified by fetal evaluation (congenital heart disease, structural cerebral anomalies, neural tube defects, and genetic disorders), complications of labor and delivery, and neonatal conditions and complications. Intrauterine exposures to certain infections (varicella, herpes, toxoplasmosis, cytomegalovirus, or Zika virus) or to toxins (alcohol, tobacco, drugs of abuse, or specific groups of prescribed medications) exert effects on fetal development and put infants at risk for neurodevelopmental sequelae. Difficulties with parturition, including prolonged labor with fetal distress, neonatal depression, and premature delivery pose varying risks to immediate and long-term outcome. Infants born at ages younger than 37 weeks' gestation are considered premature and comprise 11.4% of the deliveries in the United States, with 1.4% of those children born weighing less than 1,500 grams.[13] The risk for developmental disorders, including cerebral palsy, intellectual disability, ASD, vision and hearing impairment, learning disability, and ADHD, are increased in the entire preterm population, but the risk of neurodevelopmental sequelae increases with decreasing gestational age and birth weight. Neonatal complications, including hypoxic-ischemic encephalopathy, hy perbilirubinemia, sepsis/meningitis, hypoglycemia, acidosis, seizures in the first 24 hours, intraventricular hemorrhage, periventricular leukomalacia, chronic lung disease, retinopathy of prematurity (ROP), and necrotizing enterocolitis compound the risk of early or difficult birth and contribute to the established risk for adverse developmental outcome.

– Medical History

Medical and surgical histories explore established and associated risk of serious infec- tions; head trauma; seizure disorders; chronic medical, metabolic, or endocrine dis- orders; and surgical procedures. The history of an acute illness, such as meningitis or a traumatic head injury, or a chronic illness, such as hypothyroidism, will establish a risk for developmental disorders that guides the primary pediatric health care profes- sional in the developmental evaluation and medical workup of a child with delays. Furthermore, the history can provide information that informs the pediatric health care professional of associated risks. The history of an uncomplicated submucosal cleft palate repair or a cardiac anomaly repair, for instance, may not directly influence developmental outcome but should remind the evaluator of possible genetic syndromes associated with midline defects and associated neurodevelopmental disorders.

– Family History

Varying types and degrees of risk are established by family history. The child being evaluated may be at increased risk for certain disorders due to ethnicity or family history of recurrent loss of pregnancy; diagnosed genetic, neurological, or psychiatric disorders; intellectual disabilities; speech or language delays; hearing or vision impairments; learn- ing disability; ADHD; or autism. Some aspects of family history are more relevant to the patient than others; for example, a history of hearing impairment diagnosed in an octo- genarian in the family contributes little of relevance to the child, whereas a family history of autism is of greater interest because of the evidence of a genetic basis to autism.[14]

– Developmental History

A careful developmental history offers an essential contribution to the neurodevelop- mental evaluation. Each stream of development should be reviewed to ascertain the age at which specific milestones were attained in order to formulate an estimate of past DQs within each stream, thereby approximating a relative rate of development over time. As an example, in a child who presents with motor delay, a history of rolling over at 8 months, sitting at 12 months, and crawling at 16 months provides retrospective evidence of a consistent motor DQ of 50 and infers a static rate of development, which implies continued delays over time. The estimation of developmental rates using the timing of prerequisite milestone achievement in comparison to DQs acquired during direct developmental evaluation offers powerful information about developmental trajectories within a given stream of development and thereby assists with prognos- tication. The patterns of milestone achievement are of profound importance to the assessment. The persistence of delay over time, or a static pattern of delay, suggests continued delay is likely, while a developmental plateau or a history of developmental regression requires special attention. A developmental plateau, in which a child fails to acquire new milestones after a previous pattern of steady milestone attainment, is seen most frequently in language development. The timing of the language plateau is informative; children with severe hearing impairment acquire language normally until they reach the babbling stage, then they fail to progress past babbling.[15] Also, as many as a third of children on the autism spectrum are reported to either plateau in language or lose previously achieved language and social skills between 18 and 30 months of age.[16]

Regression, or loss of previously achieved milestones, though fairly commonly reported in the language and social domains of children on the autism spectrum, may require extra consideration in the etiological workup. When regression includes motor or cognitive streams of development, a full neurological evaluation, including neuroimaging and laboratory studies, is warranted to rule out a degenerative disorder such as those that occur because of an inborn error of metabolism (see Chapter 4, Biological Influences on Child Development and Behavior and Medical Evaluation of Children with Developmental-Behavioral Disorders).

Behavioral and educational histories are important components of the developmental history, and they offer qualitative information about the child's function in his or her environment and reveal evidence of associated deficits. Behavioral disorders may be found in the areas of social behavior, noncompliance, aggression, attention, activity, stereotypic behavior, and self-injurious behavior. Atypical or immature play skills not explained by developmental level (parallel play at an age when symbolic or reciprocal play is expected), lack of desire to interact with other children, or awkwardness in or avoidance of social situations may be uncovered during the social history and direct the evaluator to further explore ASD, especially when social delay accompanies stereotypic behavior and language delays. Attention-deficit/hyperactivity disorder commonly co-occurs with developmental disorders that may be raised in the presenting complaint or during the initial observation of a child, but it is further explored by inquiring about attention, distractibility, impulsivity, and hyperactivity. Noncompliance and aggression, when present, should prompt the evaluator to determine whether these behaviors are secondary to frustration originating from language or cognitive demands that exceed the child's capability or if they represent primary behavior problems that require behavioral modification. Stereotypic behaviors may have a diverse presentation but are characterized by repetitive movements, such as hand flapping, spinning, jumping, or pacing, that occur with greater frequency in children with intellectual disabilities and ASD. Self-injurious behaviors also occur with increased frequency in children with intellectual disabilities and sensory deficits.

The educational history may reveal an existing Individualized Educational Program (IEP), with a determination of the educational handicapping condition used to qualify a child for services, the type of services, special educational instruction, or special classroom settings that a child may be provided. The IEP may also provide documentation of previous assessments for review. If no IEP meeting has been convened for a child who is exhibiting academic, functional, or behavioral challenges in the classroom, primary pediatric health care professionals may recommend such a meeting and request assessments that may help with both diagnostic clarification and service determination (see Chapter 20, Interpreting Psychoeducational Testing Reports, Individualized Family Service Plans [IFSP], and Individualized Education Program [IEP] Plans, and Chapter 25, Social and Community Services for Children With Developmental Disabilities and/or Behavioral Disorders and Their Families).

– Social History

Social history should evaluate the psychosocial and socioeconomic risks and the supports and services that the child receives within the family and the community. The assessment of psychosocial stressors that may impact the family and child, either directly or indirectly, include parental education and employment status; financial status; marital discord or separations; single-parent households; frequent moves; substance use or exposure; physical, sexual, or emotional abuse; members of the household with physical, developmental, or mental health disabilities or infirmities; and the quality of child care. Review of early intervention services that a child requires or is receiving must be appraised in light of the child's needs, the resources and stressors of the family, and the services available in the community.

Physical Examination

The physical examination includes an assessment of growth parameters, a general physical exam, and a neurological examination. Measurements of head circumference, height and weight at the time of the examination, as well historical growth of these parameters, can prove to be of diagnostic importance. Uniformly small growth (height, weight, and head circumference) may be explained by family history or known risks, such as prematurity, fetal alcohol exposure, or intrauterine infection, or it may alert a clinician to genetic disorders. Short stature with normal head circumference and weight also raises questions about familial stature, endocrine dysfunction, and genetic disorders. In a child with microcephaly (head circumference measurement under the 2nd percentile), evaluation of the trajectory of head measurements may provide etiological clues; a child microcephalic at birth may have been compromised by infection or a cerebral disruption in utero, while a child with a normal head circumference at birth, but progressively diminishing percentile measurements in the first few months of life, may have suffered a peripartum event. Diminishing head circumference measurements in the second half of the first year of life in girls brings suspicions of Rett syndrome, particularly if associated with loss of developmental skills and the onset of certain behaviors, such as hand wringing. Macrocephaly (head circumference greater than the 98th percentile) is associated with congenital hydrocephalus, acquired hydrocephalus, a number of genetic overgrowth syndromes, and metabolic syndromes such as Canavan disease, all of which carry risks of associated developmental disorders.

Tall and short stature must be considered first in light of familial growth patterns. If a child's height is two standard deviations below the mean and is discrepant from familial growth, etiological considerations include disorders of endocrine function, fetal exposures such as alcohol, or syndromes associated with short stature (chondrodysplasias).

If a child's height is two standard deviations above the mean and is discrepant from familial growth, etiologic considerations include Klinefelter, fragile X, and Marfan syndromes and overgrowth syndromes (height, weight, and head circumference are all two standard deviations above the mean), as in Simpson-Golabi-Behmel, Bannanyan-Riley-Ruvalcaba, and Sotos syndromes.

The general physical exam is expanded to include a search for markers or unusual features that may provide an indication of an underlying genetic disorder. Examination of the skin should note unusual hair distribution, neurocutaneous markers of neurofibromatosis (café-au-lait macules, unusual freckles), or with the assistance of a Wood's lamp, of tuberous sclerosis (hypopigmented patches, shagreen patches). Midline defects noted on general examination, such as cleft lip or palate (including submucosal clefts), cardiac defects, and genitourinary findings may be informative. Dysmorphic features of the head, face, ears, hairline, trunk, or extremities may be subtle but contribute to an overall constellation of features that might suggest a specific syndrome. It is important to be aware that most genetic syndromes are in fact a constellation of physical and neurobehavioral features—no single dysmorphism or neurobehavioral pattern is diagnostic, and no syndrome requires a complete constellation of features for diagnosis.

Neurological Examination

The neurological examination is critical to the complete evaluation, as it may provide explanation for motor findings, as in the case of the infant with motor delay or the older child with coordination difficulties. The neurological examination of the infant and young child must include a standard evaluation of cranial nerve function, tone, strength, and reflexes, as well as pathological, primitive and postural reflexes, and a thorough evaluation of motor function. In the ambulatory child, the quality of gait, functional movement (climbing stairs, rising from a sitting or squatting position), and fine motor movement quality impart additional information to the neurological examination. Finally, in older children who present with concerns regarding cognition, language, learning, or behavior, an examination for soft neurological signs adds to the standard neurological evaluation. Soft neurological signs, such as mild axial hypotonia, synkinesia, mirror movements, or overflow activity (which are observed when a child is asked to do specific repetitive hand movements or walk with a stressed gait and extraneous movement in a limb not involved in the motor action is observed), often accompany disorders of communication, learning disabilities, and ADHD.[17]

Neurodevelopmental Evaluation

Children who fail developmental screening require standardized developmental evaluation on a validated assessment tool. Developmental evaluation may be accomplished through the local early intervention program, the primary pediatric health care professional within the medical home, or by a subspecialist. There are advantages and disadvantages to each evaluation option; early intervention programs will determine eligibility for and provide services to those children who meet eligibility criteria, but they will not provide diagnoses. They also do not provide services to children who are delayed but not sufficiently delayed so as to meet criteria for intervention, and they do not investigate etiology of developmental disorders. Primary pediatric health care professionals who are willing to evaluate development in the medical home have the advantage of understanding their patient's historical risk and developmental, family, and psychosocial histories. Primary pediatric health care professionals can provide guidance for families with children who are delayed but who do not meet criteria for early intervention services, and they can deepen the trust of the family through shared decision-making. Primary pediatric health care professionals, however, may experience difficulty with the time, training, disrupted clinic flow, and payment that accompanies developmental evaluation in the medical home. Subspecialty referral is an option for primary pediatric health care professionals who face such barriers, but a shortage of subspecialists, long distances to attend subspecialty clinics, long waiting lists, and variable insurance coverage for subspecialty evaluations may all be barriers to subspecialty evaluation.

Regardless of the evaluator, the developmental evaluation should minimally include the history of developmental skill acquisition to date to establish patterns of developmental delay, a review of both neurobiological (prenatal, perinatal, and postnatal history, past medical history, family history, etc) and psychosocial (socioeconomic status, parental mental health, quality of child care, etc) historical risk factors for developmental delay, a general physical examination (focusing on dysmorphology and neurocutaneous features), a neurological examination, and direct observation and evaluation of development in all streams to confirm parental concerns, the rate of development established by the developmental history, or concerns raised by a failed screen. The use of a valid, standardized evaluation measure that can provide quantitative information about the rate of development, and therefore the presence and degree of delay within a single stream or the dissociation of developmental rates among streams, assists with the diagnostic formulation. Tests such as the Capute Scales[18] are brief, standardized developmental evaluation measures specifically designed for use in primary care pediatric practice.

Many developmental evaluation measures are designed for use by subspecialists or specific discipline experts, such as neuropsychologists or speech-language pathologists, and are therefore less applicable in primary care pediatric settings. However, a number of assessment tools are commercially available that range in scope from comprehensive evaluation measures that evaluate several domains of development to those that measure specific domain functions, such as articulation, receptive language, pragmatic skills, fine motor skills, or writing skills. Specific evaluation measures are chosen based on the age of the child being tested, the streams of development being explored, the psychometric properties of the test (validity, reliability, specificity, and sensitivity), the time required for test administration, and the preferences of the examiner. Ideal tests are expeditious, valid, and reliable measures that provide quantifiable results in a specific scope of evaluation and have good specificity and sensitivity. Often, comprehensive developmental evaluation requires the employment of a number of narrow-scope tools to verify information or to complement information gleaned on broad tests of development or from direct behavioral observation.

Estimation of cognitive ability is the first order of testing, as academic, language, social, adaptive, and behavioral findings are all assessed in relation to the child's cognitive potential. Measurement of intellectual capacity in the verbal (language) and nonverbal (visual-motor problem-solving) domains is imperative because by employing the principles of delay and dissociation, it will distinguish the child with intellectual disability from the child with age-appropriate nonverbal skills and a communication disorder. As concerns about language delay and global developmental delay become evident to parents in the second and third year of life, many of the developmental evaluation measures for early identification of children with such difficulties target children from birth to 3 years of age, some of which extend use to early elementary school years. The Capute Scales[18]; the Battelle Developmental Inventory, Second Edition (BDI-2)[19]; the Mullen Scales of Early Learning[20]; the Brigance Inventory of Early Development III (Brigance IED III)[21]; the Parents' Evaluation of Developmental Status: Developmental Milestones (PEDS:DM)[22]; and the Gesell Developmental Observation–Revised (GDO-R)[23] are all valid developmental assessment tools that measure language and visual motor skills in the infant, toddler, and preschooler, and they require varying degrees of expertise and time to administer. Several of these evaluation measures include additional streams of development including motor, self-help/adaptive, and social/emotional skills, in addition to language and visual-motor streams.

Additional standardized tools are available to measure communication and visual-motor or graphomotor skills in the older preschooler and early school-aged child. The Fluharty Preschool Speech and Language Screening Test, 2nd Edition[24]; the Clinical Evaluation of Language Fundamentals—Preschool (CELF-P)[25]; the Peabody Picture Vocabulary Test, Fourth Edition (PPVT-4)[26]; and the Expressive One-Word Picture Vocabulary Test[27] are practical, psychometrically sound measures of verbal capacity in children that produce quantifiable results. Additional measures of visual-motor or graphomotor skills in older preschoolers and young school-aged children include subtests from standardized tests, such as Gesell's figure drawing and block design,[28] the Goodenough (Draw-a-Person) Test,[29] and the Beery-Buktenica Developmental Test of Visual-Motor Integration. Specific nonverbal test measures used by subspecialists include the Leiter International Performance Scale, 3rd Edition[30]; the Raven Coloured Progressive Matrices[31]; and the Test of Nonverbal Intelligence-4.[32] Caution in the interpretation of nonverbal skills that rely largely on pencil and paper tasks is prudent, as children with even mild neuromotor disorders may have sufficient graphomotor impairment to cause the evaluator to underestimate a child's nonverbal abilities unless a battery of measures that do not require pencil and paper assessments is also engaged. Formal psychological measures of intelligence performed by a school psychologist will confirm the neurodevelopmental estimates of cognitive ability.

In the school-aged child referred for concerns about educational success, measures of academic achievement levels on standardized instruments, such as the Wide Range Achievement Test, Fourth Edition (WRAT-4)[33] or the Comprehensive Inventory of Basic Skills—Revised (CIBS-R),[34] are useful in elucidating academic underachievement and possible learning disabilities in reading decoding, reading comprehension, spelling, and arithmetic. Difficulties in written language and composition are common in children with language-based learning difficulties and may be evaluated using measures such as the Test of Written Language (TOWL).[35] In academic testing, it is essential to assess the time required for children to perform specific batteries of tests, as well as the quality of the work produced. Timed tests may alter performance, either by limiting the quantity of work accomplished or by limiting the quality of work, and thereby underestimate the capacity of the child to complete work at a higher level if given more time. The distinction between poor performance because of inadequate time to perform and poor performance because of inability to perform should not be overlooked, as the interventions for the two scenarios are very different—the slower, capable worker requires accommodations to succeed, while the child with specific learning disabilities needs remedial or supportive services in the academic setting.

Behavioral Evaluation

A number of challenges exist in the assessment of behavior in the child who fails screening. Parents may report behavior as primary, while behavior may be a manifestation or consequence of an underlying neurodevelopmental condition. Parents or teachers may report behaviors that are not evident in the child during the developmental evaluation. Further, anxious, inattentive, or hyperactive behavior may mitigate the validity of the neurodevelopmental evaluation results. A child with ADHD may demonstrate difficulties with attention during developmental or academic testing and may also show overt hyperactivity and impulsivity during the examination. Similarly, a child being assessed for early language delay, developmental delay, or concerns about ASD may display signs of autism, such as gaze avoidance, or may refuse to respond to verbal prompts because of underlying anxiety. Behavioral assessment requires a historical account of behavior, direct observation of behavior in the clinical setting, and developmental evaluation to rule out underlying neurodevelopmental diagnoses. The historical account of behavior may be enhanced by the use of specific behavioral rating scales in the medical home, as they offer relative quantification of severity and objective information from parents, teachers, or day care providers regarding the child in different social or academic environments. Behavioral rating scales should never be used as diagnostic tools; rather, they are measures that may assist in gathering information on symptoms of a suspected diagnosis.

Attention-deficit/hyperactivity disorder diagnosis requires an evaluation for coexisting developmental, behavioral, and mental health disorders, and evidence that ADHD symptoms cause impairment in more than one setting.[36] Attention-deficit/hyperactivity disorder rating scales for parent and teacher reporting, such as the National Institute for Children's Health Quality Vanderbilt Assessment Scales 2nd Edition[37] or the Conners Comprehensive Behavior Rating Scales[38] provide observations of the child in different settings. Attention-deficit/hyperactivity disorder rating scales are also very valuable as tools to measure differences in ADHD symptoms before and after interventions are initiated in order to gather comparative data on the efficacy of the intervention.

Children who fail autism screens may have autism rating scales completed as part of the neurodevelopmental evaluation, such as the Childhood Autism Rating Scale (CARS).[39] However, as with ADHD, these scales are not diagnostic, though they may add information to the diagnostic formulation.[40] Parent and/or caregiver completed autism rating scales include the Gilliam Autism Rating Scale, 3rd Edition,[41] and the Social Communication Questionnaire.[42] Despite the capacity to quantify degree of likelihood of ASD, these rating scales are quite subjective, and ultimately, a diagnosis of ASD is based on clinical information and direct observation rather than on rating scales.

Disorders such as anxiety or oppositional defiant disorder, which may contribute to ADHD or ASD features or may coexist with ADHD or ASD, may also be assessed with subtests of measures such as the National Institute for Children's Health Quality Vanderbilt Assessment Scales 2nd Edition[37] or the Conners Comprehensive Behavior Rating Scales,[38] while anxiety symptoms may be assessed by parents and older children on the Screen for Childhood Anxiety Related Emotional Disorders (SCARED) (see Chapter 21, Disruptive Behavior Disorders, and Chapter 22, Anxiety and Mood Disorders).[43]

Interpretation of Developmental Evaluation: Diagnoses

The principles of delay, dissociation, and deviation are ultimately applied in the interpretation of the developmental history of the 5 streams of development in combination with direct observations from the developmental evaluation (Table 10.3). Gross motor delay with a developmental quotient of 50 or less is consistent with a diagnosis of cerebral palsy, regardless of the developmental quotients in other streams. Delay (DQ<70) in both streams of language and visual-motor (nonverbal) skills is diagnostic of intellectual disability and is generally accompanied by delays in adaptive skills, and perhaps social skills as well. Delay in the language stream in the presence of normal visual-motor skills exemplifies dissociation between the cognitive streams of development and indicates a communication disorder. Communication disorders may be accompanied by deficits in social skills as well and should signal the need for a historical review of autism symptoms and behavioral rating scales for autism symptoms (see Chapter 11, Making Developmental-Behavioral Diagnoses).

Table 10.3. Diagnostic Interpretation of Delay and Dissociation				
	Cerebral Palsy	**Intellectual Disability**	**Communication Disorder**	**Autism**
Gross Motor	DQ<50	Normal or delayed	Normal or delayed	Normal or delayed
Language	Normal or delayed	DQ<70	Delayed	Delayed
Visual Motor or Nonverbal	Normal or delayed	DQ<70	Normal	Normal or delayed
Adaptive	Normal or delayed	Delayed	Normal	Normal or delayed
Social	Normal or delayed	Normal or delayed	Normal or delayed	Delayed

A diagnostic summary clarifies the findings of the child being evaluated and also opens the evaluation to consideration of associated deficits and potential future risks. A child with motor delay and physical findings consistent with a hemiplegic pattern of cerebral palsy should be evaluated for common associated findings, such as homonymous hemianopsia and seizures, while the child whose motor delay yields a pattern of spastic diplegia is at greater risk of co-occurring intellectual disability. Similarly, the child with language delay and associated low muscle tone may have co-occurring attentional deficits but should also be considered as having an established risk of language-based learning disabilities and should be monitored for academic underachievement as he or she advances in the school environment. Knowledge of patterns of associated comorbidities of developmental diagnoses and estimation of future risk of subsequent developmental hurdles provides parents with appropriate expectations and anticipatory guidance that is specific to their child with atypical development.

The diagnostic conclusions of the neurodevelopmental evaluation may be enhanced or supported by further assessment by local early intervention teams, which also assist in securing, directing, and organizing services. Finally, once the descriptive developmental-behavioral diagnoses are made (see Chapter 11, Making Developmental-Behavioral Diagnoses), the primary pediatric health care professional is also responsible for further medical workup in an attempt to establish an etiological diagnosis to account for the child's neurodevelopmental/neurobehavioral impairments (see Chapter 4, Biological Influences on Child Development and Behavior and Medical Evaluation of Children With Developmental-Behavioral Disorders).

Conclusion

The developmental evaluation of children suspected of developmental delay based on failed surveillance and/or screening involves a structured, comprehensive evaluation of all streams of development. The basic components of the developmental evaluation include (1) a thorough history to assess historical and established risk for developmental disabilities and to establish a historical pattern of developmental delays; (2) complete general physical, neurological, and dysmorphology examinations; (3) direct neurodevelopmental evaluation of the 5 streams of development using standardized evaluation measures, including behavioral measures when indicated; and (4) consideration of an etiological evaluation to determine cause, prognosis, and recurrence risk of disabilities. The conclusion of the evaluation should generate a summary of diagnoses, a hypothesis as to the etiology of the developmental-behavioral diagnoses, and a strategy for providing appropriate interventions and community resources to optimize outcome and school readiness.[44]

References

1. American Academy of Pediatrics Council on Children With Disabilities; Section on Developmental Behavioral Pediatrics; Bright Futures Steering Committee; Medical Home Initiatives for Children with Special Needs Project Advisory Committee. Identifying infants and young children with developmental disorders in the medical home: an algorithm for developmental surveillance and screening. *Pediatrics*. 2006;118(1):405–420

2. Boyle CA, Boulet S, Schieve LA, Cohen RA, Blumberg SJ, Yeargin-Allsopp M, Visser S, Kogan MD. Trends in prevalence of developmental disabilities in US children, 1997–2008. *Pediatrics*. 2011;127(6):1034–1042

3. American Board of Pediatrics. *Workforce Data 2015–2016*. http://www.abp.org/sites/abp/files/pdf/workforcebook. pdf. Accessed November 22, 2017

4. Voigt RG, Accardo PJ. Formal speech-language screening not shown to help children. *Pediatrics*. 2015;136(2):e494–e495

5. Accardo PJ, Accardo JA, Capute AJ. A neurodevelopmental perspective on the continuum of developmental disabilities. In: Accardo P, ed. *Capute & Accardo's Neurodevelopmental Disabilities in Infancy and Childhood*. 3rd ed. Baltimore, MD: Paul H. Brookes Publishing Co.; 2008:3–26

6. Gesell A, Amatruda CS. *Developmental Diagnosis: Normal and Abnormal Development*. New York, NY: Paul B. Hoeber;1947

7. Capute AJ, Shapiro BK. The motor quotient: a method for the early detection of motor delay. *Am J Dis Child*. 1985;139(9):940–942

8. Capute AJ. Early neuromotor reflexes in infancy. *Pediatr Ann*. 1986;15(3):217–226

9. Capute AJ, CAT/CLAMS Pearls of Wisdom. In: *The Capute Scales: CAT/CLAMS Instruction manual*. Baltimore, MD: Kennedy Fellows Association; 1996

10. Cattell P. *The measurement of intelligence of infants and young children*. New York, NY: Harcourt Assessment; 1940

11. Sheridan MD. Development of auditory attention and the use of language symbols in young children. In: Renfrew C, Murphy K, eds. *The Child Who Does Not Talk*. Clinics in Developmental Medicine. Vol 13. London, UK: Spastics International Medical Publications; 1964:1–10

12. Lock TM, Shapiro BK, Ross A, Capute AJ. Age of presentation in developmental disability. *J Dev Behav Pediatr*. 1986;7(6):340–345

13. Osterman MJK, Kockanek KD, MacDorman MF, Strobino DM, Guyer B. Annual report on vital statistics: 2012–2013. *Pediatrics*. 2015;135(6):1115–1125

14. Abrahams BS, Geschwind DH. Advances in autism genetics: on the threshold of a new neurobiology. *Nat Rev Genet*. 2008;9(5):341–355

15. Murphy K. Development of normal vocalization and speech. In: Renfrew C, Murphy K, eds. *The Child Who Does Not Talk*. Clinics in Developmental Medicine. Vol 13. London, UK: Spastics International Medical Publications; 1964:11–16

16. Levy SE, Kruger H, Hyman SL. Treatments for children with autism spectrum disorders. In: Accardo P, ed. *Capute & Accardo's Neurodevelopmental Disabilities in Infancy and Childhood*. 3rd ed. Baltimore, MD: Paul H. Brookes Publishing; 2008:523–543

17. Montgomery TR. Neurodevelopmental assessment of school-age children. In: Accardo P, ed. *Capute & Accardo's Neurodevelopmental Disabilities in Infancy and Childhood*. 3rd ed. Baltimore, MD. Paul H. Brookes Publishing Co.; 2008:405–417

18. Accardo PJ, Capute AJ, eds. *The Capute Scales: Cognitive Adaptive Test and Clinical Linguistic and Auditory Milestone Scale (CAT/CLAMS)*. Baltimore, MD: Paul H. Brookes Publishing Co.; 2005

19. Newborg J. *Battelle Developmental Inventory*. 2nd ed. Rolling Meadows, IL: Riverside Publishing; 2005

20. Mullen EM. *Mullen Scales of Early Learning: AGS Edition*. Circle Pines, MN: Pearson Assessments; 1995

21. Brigance AH, French BF. *Brigance Inventory of Early Development III*. North Billerica, MA: Curriculum Associates; 2013

22. Glascoe FP, Robertshaw NS. *PEDS: Developmental Milestones*. Nashville, TN: Ellsworth & Vandermeer Press; 2007

23. Gesell Institute of Child Development. *Gesell Developmental Observation–Revised*. New Haven, CT: Gesell Institute of Child Development; 2012

24. Fluharty NB. *Fluharty Preschool Speech and Language Screening Test—2*. Austin, TX: Pro-Ed Inc.; 2001

25. Wiig EH, Secord WA, Semel E. *Clinical Evaluation of Language Fundamentals—Preschool (CELF-P 2)*. 2nd ed. San Antonio, TX: Psychological Corporation; 2004

26. Dunn LM, Dunn DM, *Peabody Picture Vocabulary Test*. 4th ed. Bloomington, MN: NCS Pearson Inc.; 2007

27. Brownell R. *Expressive One-Word Picture Vocabulary Test*. Novato, CA: Academic Therapy Publications; 2000

28. Illingsworth RS. *The Development of the Infant and Young Child: Normal and Abnormal*. 3rd ed. Baltimore, MD: The Williams and Wilkins Company; 1966

29. Harris DB. *Goodenough-Harris Drawing Test*. New York, NY: Harcourt Brace & World, Inc.; 1963

30. Roid GH, Miller CH, Pomplun M, Koch C. *Leiter International Performance Scale*, 3rd ed. Torrance, CA: Western Psychological Services; 2013

31. Raven CJ. *Raven's Coloured Progressive Matrices.* San Antonio, TX: Pearson; 1989

32. Brown L, Sherbenou RJ, Johnsen SK. *Test of Nonverbal Intelligence,* 4th ed. Torrance, CA: Western Psychological Services; 2010

33. Wilkinson GS, Robertson GJ. *Wide Range Achievement Test.* 4th ed. Lutz, FL: Psychological Assessment Resources, Inc.; 2006

34. Brigance AH. *Comprehensive Inventory of Basic Skills—Revised.* North Billerica, MA: Curriculum Associates; 1999

35. Hammill DD, Larson SC. *Test of Written Language.* 3rd ed. Austin, TX: Pro-ed Inc.; 1996

36. American Academy of Pediatrics Subcommittee on Attention Deficit/Hyperactivity Disorder; Steering Committee on Quality Improvement and Management, Wolraich M, et al. ADHD: clinical practice guideline for the diagnosis, evaluation and treatment of attention-deficit/hyperactivity disorder in children and adolescents. *Pediatrics.* 2011;128(5):1007–1022

37. American Academy of Pediatrics. *National Institute on Children's Health Quality Vanderbilt Assessment Scale.* 2nd ed. Elk Grove, IL; 2011

38. Conners CK. *Conners Comprehensive Behavior Rating Scale.* Torrance, CA: Western Psychological Services; 2008

39. Schopler E, Van Bougordien ME. *Childhood Autism Rating Scale,* 2nd ed. Torrance, CA: Western Psychological Services; 2010

40. Johnson CP, Myers SM, American Academy of Pediatrics Council on Children with Disabilities. Identification and evaluation of children with autism spectrum disorder. *Pediatrics.* 2007:120(5):1183–1215

41. Gilliam JE. *Gilliam Autism Rating Scale,* 3rd ed. Austin TX: Pro-Ed; 2014

42. Rutter M, Bailey A, Lord C. *Social Communication Questionnaire.* Torrance, CA: Western Psychological Services; 2003

43. Birmaher B, Brent D A, Chiappetta L, Bridge J, Monga S, Baugher M. (1999). Psychometric properties of the Screen for Child Anxiety Related Emotional Disorders (SCARED): A replication study. *J Am Acad Child Adolesc Psychiatry.* 1999;38(10):1230–1236

44. American Academy of Pediatrics Council on Early Childhood, Council on School Health. The pediatrician's role in optimizing school readiness. *Pediatrics.* 2016;138(3): pii: e21062293

CHAPTER 11

Making Developmental-Behavioral Diagnoses

Robert G. Voigt, MD, FAAP

Introduction

Developmental and behavioral disorders are the most prevalent chronic medical diagnoses encountered by primary pediatric health care professionals.[1] Given their frequent, longitudinal contact with children and their families, primary pediatric health care professionals are ideally positioned to identify children with possible developmental delays and behavioral problems within the medical home through the processes of developmental surveillance and screening (see Chapter 9, Developmental and Behavioral Surveillance and Screening). Once a failed screen provides a chief complaint of a developmental or behavioral concern, a medical approach to making developmental-behavioral diagnoses begins with obtaining comprehensive medical, social, family, and developmental histories, performing physical and neurological examinations, and completing direct developmental evaluations[2] (see Chapter 10, Developmental Evaluation). Once this process has been completed, primary pediatric health care professionals need to make specific developmental-behavioral diagnoses, such as intellectual disability (ID), autism spectrum disorder (ASD), cerebral palsy (CP), learning disabilities (LD), attention-deficit/hyperactivity disorder (ADHD), and developmental coordination disorder (DCD), and to attempt to determine a specific medical etiology to account for the developmental-behavioral diagnoses made. However, to fully understand any single specific diagnosis, given overlap in symptomatology and frequent comorbidities, one first needs to appreciate the entire spectrum and continuum of developmental-behavioral diagnoses.

Developmental Versus Etiological Diagnosis

The process of making comprehensive developmental-behavioral diagnoses is twofold—each child requires a descriptive developmental-behavioral diagnosis (eg, CP, ID, LD, ADHD, ASD), but it is also imperative to pursue an appropriate laboratory workup (eg, chromosome microarray analysis, DNA testing for fragile X syndrome, metabolic studies, head imaging, whole-exome sequencing) in an attempt to establish an etiological diagnosis to account for each child's descriptive developmental-behavioral diagnoses (see Chapter 4, Biological Influences on Child Development and Behavior and Medical Evaluation of Children With Developmental-Behavioral Disorders). For example, a child who exhibits a static pattern of severe global developmental delays may receive a descriptive developmental diagnosis of ID; however, laboratory workup may reveal the child to have a chromosomal deletion syndrome. The specific chromosomal deletion is the etiology to account for the child's ID. Similarly, a child described as evidencing the developmental-behavioral patterns that meet criteria for a descriptive developmental diagnosis of CP may be found at brain magnetic resonance imaging (MRI) to have periventricular leukomalacia. The hypoxic-ischemic event that produced the periventricular leukomalacia is the etiology of the child's CP.

The distinction between descriptive and etiological diagnoses for children with developmental-behavioral disorders is illustrated in Figure 11.1. Etiological diagnoses for all neurodevelopmental/neurobehavioral disorders result from an interaction between neurobiological factors (genetic/epigenetic, metabolic, toxic, infectious, etc) and environmental experiences (developmental stimulation received in home or child care environments, exposure to toxic stress, etc.; see Chapter 2, Nature, Nurture and Interactions in Child on Development and Behavior; Chapter 3, Environmental Influences on Child Development and Behavior; and Chapter 4, Biological Influences on Child Development and Behavior and Medical Evaluation of Children With Developmental-Behavioral Disorders). This interaction can result in what has been described as "developmental brain dysfunction,"[3,4] which produces a pattern of neurocognitive, neurobehavioral, and/or neuromotor impairments represented by Caput's triangle (which will be described herein).[5,6] Once this pattern of impairments has been established, descriptive developmental-behavioral diagnoses (eg, ID, ASD, CP, LD, ADHD) can be made along the spectrum and continuum of developmental-behavioral disorders.

The descriptive nature of developmental-behavioral diagnoses is illustrated by the fact that the same developmental-behavioral diagnosis can be caused by multiple different genetic etiologies (eg, ID is caused by multiple different genetic etiologies), and the same genetic etiology can cause multiple different developmental-behavioral diagnoses (eg, ID, autism, or schizophrenia can all be caused by the same copy number variant).[7,8] Further, descriptive developmental-behavioral diagnoses may change over time in the same individual. For example, Nelson and Ellenberg reported that just over half of children who were diagnosed with CP at 1 year of age no longer had this diagnosis at 7 years of age.[9] However, despite this loss of one descriptive developmental-behavioral diagnosis, children who "outgrew" CP were more likely at age 7 years to have other neurodevelopmental diagnoses, such as ID, speech articulation disorders, and seizures.[9] Similarly, Helt et al reported that up to 25% of children diagnosed to have ASD will lose that descriptive developmental-behavioral diagnosis over time.[10] However, children who "outgrow" autism appear to be at higher risk for residual vulnerabilities affecting higher-order communication and attention, tics, depression, and phobias.[10] Finally, Barbaresi et al reported that among children diagnosed with ADHD, only about 30% continued to have a descriptive developmental-behavioral diagnosis of ADHD as adults.[11] However, adults who "outgrew" the diagnosis of ADHD were at increased risk of multiple neurobehavioral disorders, including substance use disorders, antisocial personality disorder, anxiety, hypomania, and depression.[11] In each of these cases, the descriptive developmental-behavioral diagnoses changed over time in the same individuals, but the "developmental brain dysfunction" caused by the interaction of each individual's neurobiology and environmental experiences remains the etiological diagnosis for the range of descriptive developmental-behavioral diagnoses encountered over time.

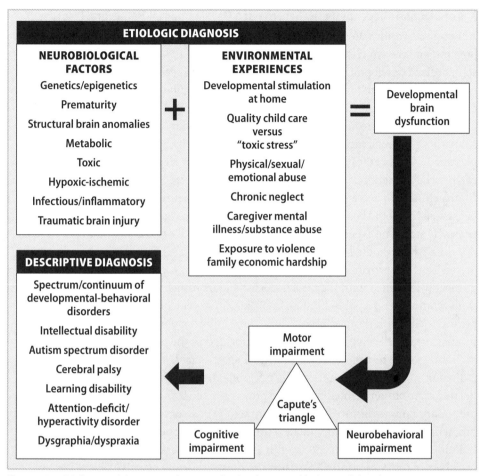

Figure 11.1. Etiologic and descriptive diagnoses for developmental-behavioral disorders.

The more severe the developmental-behavioral disorder, the more likely a specific etiological diagnosis will be identified. However, across the spectrum of developmental-behavioral disorders, mild disorders predominate over severe disorders; thus, while all children with developmental-behavioral disorders will receive a descriptive diagnosis, the specific etiological diagnosis remains unknown for a majority of children. With rapid advances in genetic testing and neuroimaging techniques, however, more and more children with developmental-behavioral diagnoses will receive etiological diagnoses in the future. While it is only each child's longitudinal pattern of specific developmental strengths and weaknesses that should guide predictions about prognosis and recommendations for educational and therapeutic interventions, a specific etiological diagnosis allows for genetic counseling for families and may lead to detection of associated anomalies or medical problems and prevent medical complications; it rarely (as in the case of treatable metabolic disorders) provides treatment options but often provides parents peace of mind in knowing specifically why their child has a developmental-behavioral disorder.

Age at Diagnosis Depends on the Severity of a Developmental-Behavioral Disorder

Although it is critical to make developmental-behavioral diagnoses at as early an age as possible, and the American Academy of Pediatrics (AAP) has recommended the use of standardized developmental screening instruments at specified ages to identify delays early,[12] it is important to note that mild disabilities are much more common than severe disabilities. Further, the more subtle the developmental-behavioral disorder, the older a child must be before his or her development or behavior is appreciably different from similarly aged peers, such that the developmental or behavioral disorder can be reliably identified.[13] Alternatively, the more severe the disability, the younger the age at which it can be reliably identified. For example, a child with severe ID is likely indistinguishable from a child with average intelligence on a newborn neurodevelopmental assessment, but severe ID should be suspected by one year of age—at one year of age, children with severe ID would be expected to show developmental skills at the level of a 6-month old or below, which should be clearly distinguishable at 1 year of age. However, of all children with ID, approximately 85% will have mild ID[14]; many of these children may not be reliably identified until they reach at least 3 years of age, when their developmental skills would be expected to be at an approximate 2-year-old level or below, clearly behind their similarly aged peers. Thus, some children with mild ID may well not be identified by developmental screens performed in the first 3 years of life, when such screens are recommended at specified ages. In fact, it appears likely that many individuals with mild ID are actually never identified. While statistically, based on a normal distribution of intelligence, the prevalence of ID should be between 2% and 3%, prevalence rates determined by ascertainment are closer to 1% due to methodological problems in identifying individuals with mild ID—it appears that as adults, many individuals with mild ID blend in with and become indistinguishable from other members of the community.[14] Further, the most subtle of cognitive disabilities, the specific learning disabilities (LD), such as dyslexia, certainly cannot be diagnosed in the first 3 years of life and are typically not diagnosed until a child begins to have difficulty keeping up with peers at school. Similarly, while intensive early intervention strategies have been shown to benefit children with ASD,[15] not all children with ASD can be identified by screening in the birth-to-3-year population.[16] The behavior of children with milder cases of high-functioning ASD might not be recognized to be significantly different from that of peers until older ages, when there are increasingly complex demands for peer social interaction and communication. Thus, while early recognition and intervention should always be the primary goal, it remains difficult to identify the much more common milder disabilities in the birth-to-3-year age range with the use of standardized developmental screening techniques.

Primary Developmental-Behavioral Diagnosis and Associated Deficits (Comorbidities)

As opposed to adult neurology, where acquired focal neurological deficits derivative of etiologies such as cerebrovascular accidents are common, the neuropathology in developmental-behavioral disorders of childhood tends to be more diffuse. While each child with a developmental-behavioral disorder will typically receive a primary developmental-behavioral diagnosis (eg, CP, ID, LD, ASD, or ADHD), associated deficits or comorbidities are the rule, rather than the exception, in children with these disorders. For example, approximately 13% of children with ID also have CP,[17] and 30% of children with ID have ADHD.[18] Approximately 50% of children with CP also have ID.[17] Further, about 40% of children with ASD also have ID.[19] In addition, about 60% of children with ADHD have LD,[20] and 50% have motor coordination disorders.[21]

Such diffuse neurological dysfunction should not be unexpected given the etiological entities that typically cause developmental-behavioral disorders. For example, a child with a chromosomal abnormality, such as a trisomy or chromosome deletion, would evidence the chromosomal abnormality in every neuron of the brain. Thus, diffuse neurodevelopmental dysfunction should be expected to result from such diffuse brain involvement. Similarly, other hypoxic-ischemic, metabolic, infectious, or toxic causes of brain dysfunction or the effects of environmental neglect or understimulation on a developing brain would also be expected to cause more diffuse rather than focal neurodevelopmental impairments. Therefore, while in this chapter a spectrum of developmental-behavioral disorders from mild to severe will be described within each of 3 primary streams of development (motor, cognitive, and neurobehavioral streams), one must remember that there is also a continuum of developmental-behavioral disorders across developmental streams: Children with primary motor disorders are likely to have associated cognitive, learning, or behavioral difficulties; children with primary cognitive disorders are likely to have associated neurobehavioral and motor issues; and children with primary neurobehavioral disorders are likely to have associated learning, cognitive, and/or motor impairments.

Delay, Dissociation, and Deviation

Developmental-behavioral disorders occur along a spectrum and continuum from high-prevalence, lower-morbidity conditions (eg, DCD, LD, and ADHD) to low-prevalence, higher-morbidity conditions (eg, CP, ID, and ASD). Capute and Accardo have described a model for enhancing developmental-behavioral diagnosis through understanding this spectrum and continuum via analysis of 3 fundamental neurodevelopmental processes: delay, dissociation, and deviation.[22, 23] *Developmental delay* refers to a significant lag in the attainment of developmental milestones; as reviewed previously, given that the etiological entities that result in developmental-behavioral disorders tend to produce diffuse neurological dysfunction, developmental delay is most commonly represented by a more global delay across all streams (cognitive, neurobehavioral, motor) of development.

Developmental dissociation describes a significant difference between the developmental rates of two streams of development, with one stream significantly more delayed. Developmental dissociation thus describes significant scatter or unevenness across different streams of development. Given that developmental delays are typically more global in nature, dissociations between developmental streams are less commonly encountered and should be recognized as atypical, even in a setting where dissociation exists without corresponding significant developmental delay. For example, specific LD represents an example of developmental dissociation. Specific LD has traditionally been defined by a significant discrepancy, or dissociation, between intelligence and academic achievement. Learning disabilities may also be defined by a significant dissociation between verbal and nonverbal cognitive abilities. In language-based LD (LLD), a significant dissociation exists between relatively stronger nonverbal and relatively weaker verbal cognitive abilities, while in nonverbal LD (NVLD), there exists a significant dissociation between relatively weaker nonverbal versus relatively stronger verbal cognitive abilities. Similarly, ADHD can be defined as a dissociation between neurobehavioral and cognitive streams of development, as children with ADHD have levels of inattention, poor impulse control, and excessive motor activity that are discrepant from their levels of cognitive development (ie, these behaviors are developmentally inappropriate compared to their cognitive abilities).

Developmental deviation represents nonsequential unevenness in the achievement of developmental milestones (ie, achieving higher-age-level developmental milestones in a typical developmental sequence prior to achieving lower-age-level developmental milestones); such deviated acquisition of developmental milestones is considered to be atypical at any age.[22] While developmental dissociation refers to significant scatter or unevenness of developmental abilities across different developmental streams, developmental deviation is defined by significant scatter or unevenness of abilities within a single developmental stream. Developmental deviation in motor development is most often observed in children with CP. For example, a child with CP may be observed to exhibit higher-level motor milestones, like being able to stand next to a table (which is expected at around 8 months of age), before exhibiting lower-level developmental milestones, such as rolling over (expected at around 4 to 5 months) or sitting independently (expected at 6 to 7 months), with the ability to stand being secondary to lower extremity spasticity or to a persistent positive support primitive reflex. Children with ASD most often exhibit developmental deviation in cognitive and neurobehavioral development. For example, deviation in the language component of cognitive development may be observed in a child with ASD who has a 50-word vocabulary (expected at 24 months) prior to using a specific "mama" and "dada" to refer to his or her parents (expected at 10 months). Many children with ASD persist in using echolalia and confusing pronouns (atypical after 30 months) despite having higher-age-level, single-word vocabularies. Deviation in social and neurobehavioral development observed in children with ASD can be defined as behavior that is atypical at any age. Thus, deviation in social development is exemplified by the impairment in reciprocal social interaction and lack of interest in peers observed in ASD, while an example of deviation in neurobehavioral development is the atypical attention observed in children with ASD, who exhibit fleeting attention to maintaining eye contact, but who are overly focused or perseverative on restricted areas of interest.

While every individual exhibits a unique pattern of developmental strengths and weaknesses, the terms *dissociation* and *deviation* are applied to describe more significant scatter or unevenness of developmental abilities, both across (dissociation) and within (deviation) developmental streams, than is typically encountered. This model postulates that developmental delay, dissociation, and deviation reflect underlying central nervous system (CNS) dysfunction. Consequently, the amount of delay, dissociation, and/or deviation encountered increases as one moves from the mild to severe end of the spectrum and continuum of developmental-behavioral disorders. Increasing levels of developmental delay, dissociation, and deviation reflect increasingly atypical development, and increasingly atypical development is usually accompanied by increasingly atypical behavior. As will be discussed herein, this model predicts that the most atypical pattern of neurobehavioral development, as observed in children with ASD, is most commonly accompanied by the most delayed, dissociated, and deviated patterns of cognitive development.

Capute's Triangle: Spectrum and Continuum

The AAP annually presents the Dr Arnold J. Capute Award to recognize a physician who has made notable contributions to the health and well-being of children with developmental disabilities through service and/or advocacy. Dr Capute described a model for making developmental-behavioral diagnoses that distills the highly complex functions of the brain into a triangle of 3 primary streams of development: motor, cognitive, and neurobehavioral (see Figure 11.2).[5,6] The motor stream of development includes gross motor, fine motor, and oral motor development. The cognitive stream of development includes the language and visual-motor problem solving developmental streams, which come together to form the social (which is primarily communicative [eg, social smile, gestured language, pragmatic language]) and adaptive (which primarily depends on visual-motor abilities [spoon feeding, tying of shoes, etc]) streams.[22] The neurobehavioral stream of development could be considered to contain all of neuropsychiatry, but this chapter will focus on the neurobehavioral streams of attention and activity level.

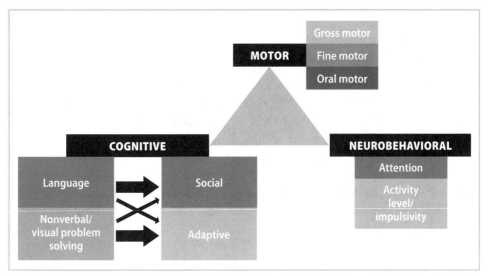

Figure 11.2. Capute's triangle. Adapted from Capute AJ. The expanded Strauss syndrome: MBD revisited. In: Accardo PJ, Blondis TA, Whitman BY, editors. *Attention Deficit Disorders and Hyperactivity*. 1991; New York: Marcel Dekker, Inc. p 28.

Developmental-behavioral disorders exist across a spectrum of severity, from mild to severe, *within* each of the 3 primary developmental streams, with mild disabilities predominating over severe disabilities. There is also a continuum of developmental-behavioral disorders *across* these 3 developmental streams, as primary developmental-behavioral diagnoses in one stream are usually accompanied by associated deficits or comorbidities in one or both of the other developmental streams.

While the extreme ends of the spectrum and continuum of developmental-behavioral disorders are easily differentiated, the concept of a spectrum and continuum of disorders implies a lack of exact cutoff points and a blending of diagnoses across the spectrum and continuum, with typically indistinct borders between specific developmental-behavioral diagnoses. For example, in the spectrum of motor disorders, it is easy to differentiate a mild DCD from severe CP, but it may be difficult to decide whether an individual with motor difficulties more in the middle of this spectrum is best described as evidencing a severe motor coordination disorder or mild CP. Similarly, in the continuum of cognitive and neurobehavioral streams of development, it is easy to separate a child with dyslexia and associated ADHD from one with severe deficits in social interaction/social communication and repetitive and stereotypic behavior characteristic of ASD, but it may be difficult to distinguish whether an individual in a more intermediate position in this continuum has a severe language disorder or LLD with associated social and behavioral concerns versus a mild ASD.

After a child has failed a developmental screen, the primary pediatric health care professional will then ascertain the child's degree of developmental delay, dissociation, and deviation within and across the motor, cognitive, and neurobehavioral streams of development via a comprehensive developmental history and direct developmental evaluation (see Chapter 10, Developmental Evaluation). An analysis of the degree of developmental delay, dissociation, and deviation that a child evidences within and across the motor, cognitive, and neurobehavioral streams of development directs the clinician in choosing the most appropriate developmental-behavioral diagnoses to apply along the spectrum and continuum of developmental-behavioral disorders.

The following will describe a framework for conceptualizing the relationship among the various developmental-behavioral diagnoses. It is hoped that this model will provide a structure for primary pediatric health care professionals to more confidently make developmental-behavioral diagnoses within the medical home. Of course, this model should not substitute for using currently accepted diagnostic criteria when a specific developmental-behavioral disorder (eg, ASD, ADHD, LD) is suspected. Chapters to follow will specifically review current diagnostic criteria for each developmental-behavioral diagnosis; this model serves to introduce the relationship among these overlapping descriptive entities.

The Spectrum of Global Developmental Delay

As reviewed previously, the etiologies for developmental-behavioral disorders, such as chromosomal anomalies, tend to affect the brain diffusely, and thus, the most common pattern of developmental delay is global delay across all developmental streams. For example, a 4-year-old child with the cognitive abilities of a 2-year-old most often exhibits behaviors that are characteristic of a 2-year-old (not of a 4-year-old) and motor skills that are generally commensurate with this cognitive level. While some children with delays in cognitive development will show age-appropriate acquisition of early motor milestones, as motor milestones increase in complexity and begin to involve more motor planning over time (eg, hopping on one foot, skipping, riding a bicycle), levels of motor development most typically become generally commensurate with levels of cognitive development.

The cognitive stream of development is composed of 4 primary domains of central processing: language, social, adaptive, and visual-motor problem solving. In the spectrum of global developmental delay, delays in verbal, nonverbal, social, and adaptive development are generally equivalent (without any significant dissociation or deviation) and increase in severity as one moves from the mild to severe end of the spectrum of global developmental delay. This spectrum provides the most distinct diagnostic entities, as diagnoses in this spectrum are defined by specific IQ and adaptive behavior scores in a normal distribution (see Figure 11.3).

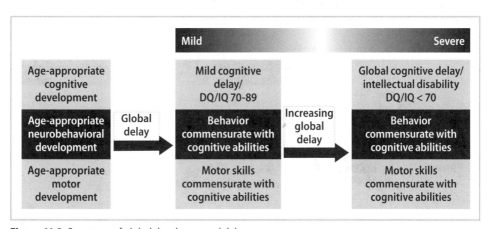

Figure 11.3. Spectrum of global developmental delay.

At the mild end of this spectrum, the Wechsler Intelligence Scale for Children—Revised previously classified IQ scores between 80 and 89 as the "dull" range of intelligence.[24] Currently, while children who function in this range of intelligence are classified as "low average" by the Wechsler Intelligence Scale for Children, Fifth Edition,[25] they might more descriptively be referred to as "slower learners," as they typically experience significant difficulties keeping up in regular classroom settings.[26] As the global developmental delay becomes more severe across this spectrum, children with IQ scores between 70 and 79 are described as evidencing borderline intelligence, and those with IQ and adaptive behavior standard scores below 70 are defined as having ID (see Chapter 15, Cognitive Development and Disorders). As with disorders across all developmental streams, mild global developmental delays predominate over severe global developmental delays, as 23% of the population evidences slower learning or borderline intelligence, while statistically only between 2% and 3% of the population would be expected to evidence ID (although only 1% of the population is actually identified as evidencing ID due to methodological problems in identifying individuals with mild ID).[14]

Global developmental delay is the most typical developmental-behavioral presentation, while developmental dissociation and deviation are less common and more atypical developmental presentations. However, within each of the primary streams of development—motor, cognitive, and neurobehavioral—there exists a spectrum of dissociated and deviated developmental-behavioral diagnoses, which will be reviewed herein.

The Spectrum of Motor Dissociation and Deviation

The motor stream of development includes the development of gross motor, fine motor, and oral motor (speech, chewing/swallowing) skills. There is a spectrum of motor disorders within each of these motor areas, with mild motor disorders occurring more frequently than more severe disorders (see Figure 11.4). As one moves across the spectrum of dissociated motor disorders from mild to severe, increasing deviation occurs, as motor deviation is commonly observed in children with CP.

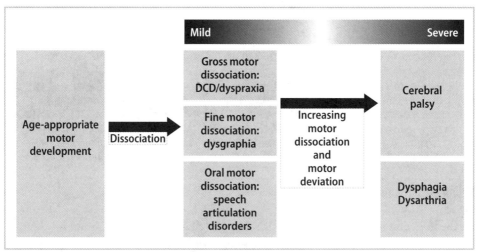

Figure 11.4. Spectrum of motor dissociation and deviation. Abbreviation: DCD, developmental coordination disorder.

The mild end of the spectrum of motor dissociation and deviation has in the past been described as the "clumsy child syndrome" or "developmental dyspraxia,"[27] but it is described in the *Diagnostic and Statistical Manual of Mental Disorders,* Fifth Edition (*DSM-5*), as "developmental coordination disorder" or DCD.[28] At this mild end of the motor spectrum, children evidence mild gross motor delays and difficulties with motor planning, and many evidence "soft" neurological signs (eg, synkinesias, choreiform movements, dysdiadochokinesis, and posturing of the upper extremities with stressed gaits).[29] As motor delay increases in severity within this spectrum, and is accompanied by "hard" neurological signs (persistent primitive reflexes, brisk deep tendon reflexes, spasticity, dyskinesia, ataxia, hypotonia), a diagnosis of CP becomes more appropriate. Minor fine motor deficits produce difficulties with handwriting (dysgraphia) and delays in accomplishing activities of daily living, such as buttoning and tying shoes, while more severe fine motor delays are also seen in quadriparetic and hemiparetic forms of CP. From an oral motor standpoint, the mild end of this spectrum includes mild speech articulation difficulties and milder feeding issues, while the severe end includes the dysphagia and dysarthria that frequently accompany more severe forms of CP. Consistent with disorders within all streams of development, mild motor disorders predominate over severe motor disorders. There are many more children with gross motor clumsiness, handwriting difficulties, and speech articulation disorders (with an estimated prevalence of DCD of 10%)[27] than there are with CP (which has a prevalence of 2.9 per 1,000 or only 0.29%)[30] (see Chapter 14, Motor Development and Disorders).

The Spectrum of Cognitive Dissociation and Deviation

The cognitive stream of development consists of the language and visual-motor problem-solving streams that come together to form the primarily communicative social and primarily visual-motor–dependent adaptive streams.[22] Within the spectrum of global developmental delay described previously, there is no significant discrepancy or dissociation among these cognitive streams of development. However, such discrepancies between cognitive streams and deviations within these cognitive streams can and do occur, and they exist across a spectrum from mild to severe.

The Spectrum of Language Dissociation and Deviation

When children evidence discrepant and disproportionate delays in their language development relative to their nonverbal visual-motor problem-solving development, their developmental diagnoses will lie within the spectrum of language dissociation and deviation (see top portion of Figure 11.5). Of course, when a child presents with discrepant delays in speech or language development, primary pediatric health care professionals first need to formally confirm the child's hearing status prior to making a diagnosis within this spectrum. As one moves from the mild to severe end of this spectrum, in addition to evidencing dissociated delays in more diffuse aspects of language relative to nonverbal problem solving, increasing amounts of developmental deviation in language milestone acquisition and social communication are observed.

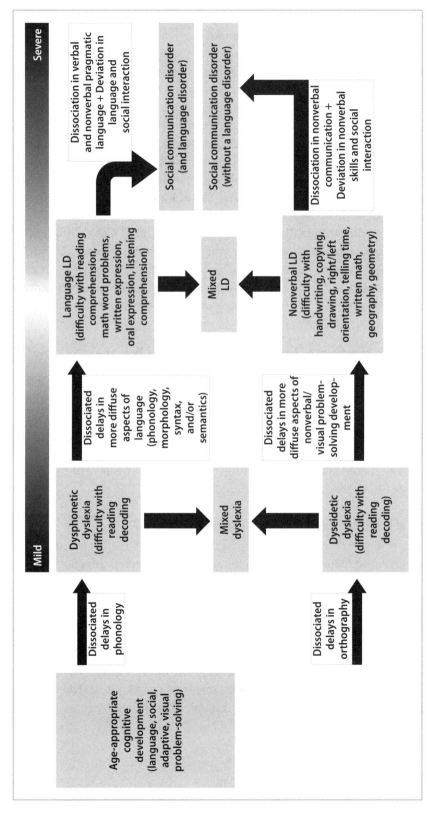

Figure 11.5. Spectrum of cognitive dissociation and deviation. Abbreviation: LD, learning disability.

Language consists of 5 components: phonology, morphology, syntax, semantics, and pragmatics, with phonology, morphology, and syntax comprising the "form of language," semantics comprising the "content of language," and pragmatics comprising the "use of language" (see Chapter 16, Speech and Language Development and Disorders). The mild end of the spectrum of language dissociation and deviation thus involves a dissociation in only one of these domains: phonology. Such a relatively focal deficit in phonological processing is the primary neuropsychological deficit observed in children with dyslexia,[31] and children with phonological processing deficits can be described as having dysphonetic dyslexia (see Figure 11.5). Children with phonological processing deficits have difficulty rhyming words and associating sounds with written symbols. They have difficulty with reading decoding (given their difficulty in sounding out words that they do not know), although they may be able to visually memorize lists of sight words (given their preserved nonverbal orthographic processing abilities). They can also understand material that is read to them, given that the components of language development other than phonology (morphology, syntax, semantics, and pragmatics) are preserved. Most children with reading disabilities evidence underlying difficulties with phonological processing, and they have traditionally been identified by schools based on a dissociation between their IQ scores and their discrepantly low achievement scores in reading. When comparing the cognitive component at the mild end of the spectrum of global developmental delay (slower learning) with the mild end of the spectrum of language dissociation and deviation (dysphonetic dyslexia), it is again confirmed that more diffuse or global cognitive dysfunction predominates over more focal or dissociated cognitive dysfunction, as more global slower learning affects 23% of the population, while discrepancy-based reading disabilities affect only 8%.[32]

As more diffuse components of receptive and expressive language become discrepantly delayed (or dissociated) compared to nonverbal visual-motor problem-solving, an individual can be described as evidencing a language disorder, which can also be described as developmental dysphasia or a specific language impairment. As more diffuse aspects of the form and content of receptive and expressive language (phonology, morphology, syntax, and/or semantics) become discrepantly delayed, verbal reasoning is negatively impacted, and a point is reached where verbal reasoning is found to be significantly below nonverbal reasoning on IQ testing. Such a significant discrepancy or dissociation between verbal and nonverbal IQ is often classified as LLD. Rather than evidencing a relatively isolated difficulty in reading decoding as seen in dyslexia, individuals with LLD evidence more diffuse academic difficulties in listening comprehension, oral expression, reading comprehension, written expression, and math word problems.

As one moves toward the most severe end of the spectrum of language dissociation and deviation, dissociated delays in the pragmatic component of language occur, and pragmatic language use or social communication is discrepantly delayed (dissociated) compared to the level of language form (morphology/word structure and syntax/grammar). These discrepant delays in pragmatic language include both verbal (difficulties with greeting, requesting, commenting, etc) and nonverbal (difficulties with eye contact, understanding and using facial expressions and gestures, etc) aspects of social communication. As one moves toward the severe end of this spectrum, increasing developmental deviation also tends to occur. This includes deviated acquisition of language milestones (eg, having a 50-word vocabulary but not yet using gestured language or a specific "Mama" or "Dada"; persistent use of echolalia or pronoun confusion despite upward deviation in more rote aspects of language [such as rote auditory memory, including memorizing song lyrics or having a large vocabulary based on the memorization of labels]) and deviated or atypical social interaction (eg, impairments in reciprocal social interaction, lack of interest in peers). Thus, individuals at the severe end of this spectrum have both language disorders and impairments in the pragmatic/social use of language that are described as social communication disorders. Both language disorders and social communication disorders have specific diagnostic criteria in the *DSM-5*[28] (see Chapter 16, Speech and Language Development and Disorders, and Chapter 19, Autism Spectrum Disorder).

The language and social communication deficits observed at the severe end of the spectrum of language dissociation and deviation represent the most developmentally dissociated and deviated end of the language and social domains of cognitive development, and thus represent the most atypical presentation of language/communication development. As reviewed previously, the more atypical the cognitive development, the more atypical the behavior is expected to be. As will be reviewed herein, in the continuum of developmental-behavioral disorders, this most dissociated and deviated pattern of language/social communication development is often accompanied by the most atypical neurobehavioral manifestations of what was defined in the *Diagnostic and Statistical Manual of Mental Disorders,* Fourth Edition (*DSM-IV*) as "autistic disorder"[33] and is currently defined in *DSM-5* as "autism spectrum disorder with a language disorder."[28]

The Spectrum of Nonverbal Dissociation and Deviation

When children evidence discrepant and disproportionate delays in their nonverbal visual-motor problem-solving development relative to their language development, their developmental diagnoses lie within the spectrum of nonverbal dissociation and deviation (see bottom portion of Figure 11.5). Of course, when a child presents with discrepant delays in visual-motor problem-solving development, primary pediatric health care professionals first need to formally confirm the child's vision status prior to making a diagnosis within this spectrum. As one moves from the mild to the severe end of this spectrum, in addition to evidencing dissociated delays in more diffuse aspects of nonverbal visual-motor problem-solving abilities, increasing amounts of developmental deviation in the nonverbal domain are observed.

Visual-motor problem-solving development consists of multiple components, including visual-spatial perception, visual-motor integration, visual sequencing, visual memory, visual closure, and nonverbal communication. At the mild end of this spectrum, the dissociation in nonverbal visual problem-solving development involves a relatively focal deficit in orthographic processing, which involves the visual processing of letter identity and letter position within words.[34] Children with orthographic processing deficits have difficulty with visual-spatial feature analysis, which initially results in difficulty in remembering the shapes of letters and how to use the correct sequence of strokes to form letters, and goes on to result in letter reversals ("b" and "d") and reversals of whole words ("saw" for "was") in reading and writing.[35,36] Children with orthographic processing disorders have difficulty with memorizing sight words, resulting in dyseidetic dyslexia, but they are able to sound out words, and they can spell phonetically, given their preserved language skills, including their preserved phonological processing.

While this chapter has described both dysphonetic and dyseidetic dyslexia as specific entities, and it will describe LLD and NVLD as specific entities, it is important to note that children may have mixed deficits in aspects of both phonological and orthographic processing, resulting in mixed dyslexia, or mixed deficits in aspects of both language-based and nonverbal-based learning, as in a mixed LD (see Figure 11.5 and Chapter 17, Learning Disabilities).

As more diffuse aspects of nonverbal visual problem solving become discrepantly delayed, nonverbal reasoning is negatively impacted, and a point is reached where nonverbal reasoning is found to be significantly below verbal reasoning on IQ testing. Such a significant discrepancy between nonverbal and verbal IQ is often classified as NVLD. Rather than evidencing a relatively isolated difficulty in the orthographic processing of letters and words, individuals with NVLD evidence more diffuse difficulties in visual-spatial, visual-perceptual, and visual-motor processing. Children with NVLD have deficits in the discrimination and recognition of visual detail and in visual-spatial orientation, including difficulties with right-left orientation, telling time on a clock, and reading maps. These children also have difficulty understanding spatial relations, including getting lost in familiar places and lacking appreciation of appropriate boundaries of interpersonal space. From an academic standpoint, children with NVLD have difficulties with the visual-spatial and conceptual aspects of mathematics (eg, aligning columns for multidigit calculations and geometry), and their visual-motor deficits negatively impact their writing.[36]

As one moves toward the most severe end of the spectrum of nonverbal dissociation and deviation, increasing developmental deviation in the visual problem-solving domain tends to occur, and the dissociated delays in nonverbal abilities include discrepant delays in nonverbal pragmatic communication. Thus, despite their significant relative strengths in verbal ability and verbal reasoning compared to nonverbal reasoning, individuals at the severe end of this spectrum have deficits in the pragmatic/social use of nonverbal communication (difficulties with eye contact, maintaining a topic of conversation, taking turns during conversations, understanding figurative language, etc) that can be described as a social communication disorder without a language disorder. The nonverbal and social communication deficits at the severe end of this spectrum represent the most developmentally dissociated and deviated end of the nonverbal domain of cognitive development and thus represent the most atypical presentation of a nonverbal disorder. As reviewed previously, the more atypical the cognitive development, the more atypical the behavior is expected to be. As will be reviewed herein, in the continuum of developmental-behavioral disorders, this most dissociated and deviated pattern of nonverbal development is often accompanied by the most atypical neurobehavioral manifestations of what previously was defined in the *DSM-IV*[33] as "Asperger disorder," and what is currently defined in the *DSM-5* as "autism spectrum disorder without a language disorder."[28]

The Spectrum of Neurobehavioral Dissociation and Deviation

It is essential to appreciate the wide behavioral variation of typically developing children and the importance of always interpreting behavior within the context of a child's underlying developmental level and family, social, and cultural environments. However, neurobehavioral disorders are defined as disorders of behavior, thought, or emotion that are associated with dysfunction in the CNS. While this stream of development includes all of neuropsychiatry, the focus of this chapter will be the neurobehavioral domains of attention and activity level. As reviewed previously, within the spectrum and continuum of developmental-behavioral disorders, the processes of developmental dissociation and deviation are markers of increasing CNS dysfunction; behavior that is dissociated from cognitive expectations sits at the mild end of this spectrum of neurobehavioral disorders, while behavior that is deviated, or atypical at any age, sits at the severe end of this spectrum (see Figure 11.6).

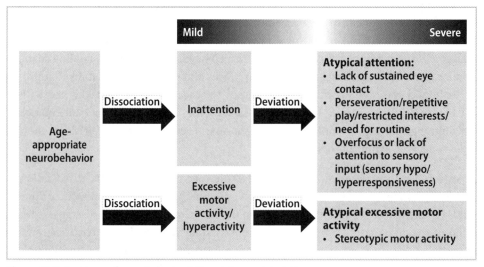

Figure 11.6. Spectrum of neurobehavioral dissociation and deviation.

At the mild end of the spectrum of neurobehavioral dissociation and deviation are children whose levels of attention and activity are discrepantly delayed from what is expected based on their cognitive abilities, and these neurobehavioral difficulties impair the child's functioning across settings. Children who exhibit this dissociation between attention span and/or activity level and cognitive expectations are at risk of a *DSM-5* diagnosis of ADHD[28] (see Chapter 18, Attention-Deficit/Hyperactivity Disorder).

As one moves to the more severe manifestations of this neurobehavioral spectrum, in place of the dissociated difficulties with inattention and easy distractibility observed in children with ADHD, a pattern of more developmentally deviated atypical attention is observed. Such deviated attention may be manifested by a short attention span that is present to such a severe degree that eye contact is difficult to maintain, while at the same time, the child becomes highly overfocused, and either visually or verbally perseverative, on repetitive behaviors or restricted interests.[6] This significantly atypical attention may also be manifested by underfocus or overfocus on sensory stimuli, such as evidencing a high pain threshold or intolerance to certain noises, tightly fitting clothes, or food textures. Rather than evidencing the dissociated increased activity level and fidgetiness seen in ADHD, a child at the severe end of this spectrum may evidence more atypical and developmentally deviated stereotypic motor activity, such as hand flapping, body rocking, and spinning (see Figure 11.6).

As will be reviewed in the section on the continuum of developmental-behavioral disorders, it is important to note that these more atypical behavioral manifestations at the severe end of the spectrum of neurobehavioral dissociation and deviation are characteristically associated with the more atypical manifestations of the spectrum of cognitive dissociation and deviation. Given that increasing developmental delay, dissociation, and deviation within the cognitive stream of development signal increasingly atypical information processing, it should be expected that the more atypically an individual processes information, the more likely that the individual's behavior will be similarly atypical. Thus, the repetitive and stereotyped behavior observed at the severe end of the spectrum of neurobehavioral dissociation and deviation is characteristically observed in continuum with either profound ID (significant global cognitive delay) or social communication disorders (significant dissociation and deviation in either language or nonverbal development).

The Continuum of Developmental-Behavioral Disorders

As reviewed previously, it is clear that diffuse developmental-behavioral dysfunction is more common than focal dysfunction among children with developmental-behavioral disorders: Associated deficits or comorbidities are the rule rather than the exception. In addition to a spectrum of disorders from mild to severe within each stream of development, there also exists a continuum of disorders from mild to severe across developmental streams. The primary developmental-behavioral diagnosis applied to each child's unique pattern of developmental delays, dissociation, and/or deviation is rarely unaccompanied by secondary diagnoses.

Continuum Across Motor and Cognitive Streams

The continuum of developmental-behavioral disorders may be most easily conceptualized by the continuum across motor and cognitive streams of development at the severe end of each of these spectra. There is a significant continuum or overlap of disability across motor and cognitive streams, as approximately 50% of individuals with CP also have ID, and about 13% of individuals with ID also have CP.[17] In addition, those individuals with CP who do not have ID are at higher risk than those without CP for other cognitive and neurobehavioral difficulties, including slower learning, LD, ADHD, and ASD.[17,37]

Continuum Across Cognitive and Neurobehavioral Streams

There is also a continuum of developmental-behavioral disorders across cognitive and neurobehavioral streams of development at the mild end of each of these spectra (see Figure 11.7). Although an outdated term that has been generally discredited, the mild end of the cognitive and neurobehavioral continuum was previously described as representing *minimal brain dysfunction*.[38] This term implies mild but diffuse developmental-behavioral dysfunction across developmental streams.[39] Epidemiological research has supported this concept of mild but diffuse dysfunction across cognitive, neurobehavioral, and motor streams of development, as, for example, children with ADHD are much more likely than children without ADHD to have associated LD, gross motor clumsiness, handwriting difficulties, and speech articulation disorders.[40] Certainly, not every individual with ADHD evidences all of these comorbidities, but it is rare to identify an individual with ADHD who does not evidence some comorbid developmental or behavioral diagnoses (see Figure 11.7 and Chapter 18, Attention-Deficit/Hyperactivity Disorder).

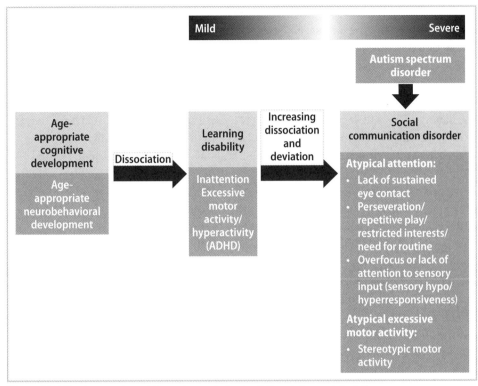

Figure 11.7. Continuum of cognitive and neurobehavioral dissociation and deviation.

At the severe end of the cognitive and neurobehavioral continuum lies what the *DSM-IV* termed the *pervasive developmental disorders.*[33] While these disorders shared a pervasive primary deficit in reciprocal social interaction, this term was somewhat misleading, as the cognitive component of these disorders typically involved scattered, uneven, discrepant, dissociated, and deviated cognitive profiles, rather than pervasive cognitive delays across cognitive domains.[41,42] The pervasive developmental disorders, as defined in the *DSM-IV*,[33] included the diagnoses of autistic disorder, Asperger disorder, and pervasive developmental disorder not otherwise specified, but this classification was not retained in the *DSM-5*.[28] In the *DSM-5*, there is a single classification of ASD: What was "autistic disorder" in *DSM-IV* is now "autism spectrum disorder with a language disorder" in *DSM-5*, and what was "Asperger disorder" in *DSM-IV* is now "autism spectrum disorder without a language disorder" in *DSM-5*.[28,33]

Within the spectrum and continuum of developmental-behavioral disorders, ASD consists of a continuum between the most developmentally dissociated and deviated cognitive profile observed in social communication disorders combined with the most developmentally deviated restricted, repetitive, and stereotypic behaviors observed at the severe end of the spectrum of neurobehavioral dissociation and deviation (see Figure 11.7). Children with ASD and a language disorder have social communication disorders at the severe end of the spectrum of language dissociation and deviation. In addition to their relative strengths in visual-motor problem solving and dissociated deficits in receptive and expressive language, these children also exhibit deviated reciprocal social interaction (impairment in reciprocal social interactions, lack of interest in peers, etc), dissociated delays in their verbal and nonverbal pragmatic/social communication (including difficulties with eye contact, response to name, greeting, requesting, and gestured communication), and deviation in their acquisition of language milestones (eg, having a 50-word vocabulary but not yet using a specific "Mama" or "Dada" to refer to their parents or continuing to use echolalia and to confuse pronouns when other [more rote and memorized] aspects of their language development extend beyond a 30-month level). Given their dissociated strengths in nonverbal visual problem-solving development, the repetitive behaviors and restricted interests of children with ASD and a language disorder typically include visually perseverative behaviors, such as lining up and sorting objects and visual perseveration on spinning objects, flashing lights, water flowing, or opening and closing doors repetitively. Their strengths in aspects of nonverbal visual problem solving might also be expressed through abilities in art, direction sense (ie, noticing changes in usual car routes), and visual memory. Consistent with this model of a spectrum and continuum of developmental-behavioral disorders, studies have confirmed that individuals with ASD with a language disorder (what used to be termed *autistic disorder*) tend to evidence dissociated delays in early language relative to visual problem solving development[42-44] and often evidence language-based learning disabled cognitive profiles as they get older, with discrepancies between higher nonverbal IQs relative to lower verbal IQs.[45-48]

Children with ASD without a language disorder have social communication disorders at the severe end of the spectrum of nonverbal dissociation and deviation. In addition to their dissociated nonverbal deficits, these children also exhibit deviated reciprocal social interaction and dissociated delays in their nonverbal pragmatic/social communication (including difficulties with eye contact, understanding and use of facial expressions and gestured communication, and visually "reading" social situations). Despite their relative verbal strengths, children with ASD without a language disorder (what used to be termed *Asperger disorder*) experience difficulty with speech prosody, taking turns during conversation, maintaining the topic of conversation, and understanding figurative language, including humor, sarcasm, and idioms. Given their dissociated strengths in language, the repetitive behaviors and restricted interests of children with ASD without a language disorder typically include verbally perseverative behaviors, such as engaging in pedantic, one-sided conversations that tend to list factual information about restricted interests, such as dinosaurs, train schedules, baseball statistics, or the weather. Consistent with this model of a spectrum and continuum of developmental-behavioral disorders, studies have confirmed that most individuals with ASD without a language disorder (what used to be called Asperger syndrome) evidence nonverbal learning-disabled cognitive profiles with discrepancies between higher verbal IQs relative to lower nonverbal IQs.[49, 50]

When reviewing the continuum of developmental-behavioral disorders, it is important to remember that diagnoses at the mild end of the continuum occur more commonly than those at the more severe end. For example, while LD and ADHD occur in approximately 7% to 8% of the population, ASD occurs in only 1.5% of the population.[19,32,51] It is also important to note that developmental dissociation and deviation occur more commonly in the setting of developmental delay. For example, while most children with ID exhibit behavior consistent with their mental ages, they are at higher risk for both the dissociated neurobehavioral pattern of ADHD (30% of children with ID have ADHD versus 7.4% of children without ID).[18,51] and the dissociated and deviated social communication disorder cognitive profile and deviated neurobehavioral pattern of ASD (28% of children with ID have ASD versus a 1.5% prevalence in the general population).[17] Figure 11.8 illustrates the entire spectrum and continuum of developmental-behavioral disorders described in this chapter.

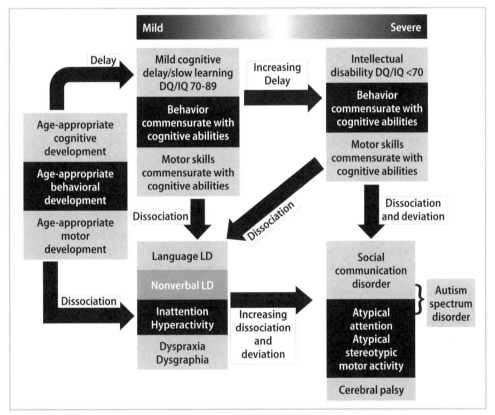

Figure 11.8. Spectrum and continuum of developmental-behavioral diagnoses. Abbreviations: DQ, developmental quotient; IQ, intelligence quotient; LD, learning disability.

Conclusion

Developmental-behavioral disorders are the most prevalent chronic medical conditions encountered by primary pediatric health care professionals within the medical home; however, there is a dearth of pediatric subspecialists in the fields of neurodevelopmental disabilities and developmental-behavioral pediatrics to whom primary care professionals can refer their patients, and long waiting lists at tertiary care developmental evaluation centers. Thus, the vast majority of children with developmental-behavioral disorders need to be identified, diagnosed, and managed by their primary pediatric health care professionals within the medical home in collaboration with local early intervention and special education professionals. The AAP recommends the use of standardized developmental screening tests at specified ages,[12] but it is important for primary pediatric health care professionals to know that while low-prevalence, higher-morbidity developmental-behavioral problems should be identified by early screening, much more prevalent mild developmental-behavioral problems may not be identifiable by screening at younger ages.[13] In addition, while standardized screening and evaluation instruments certainly facilitate making accurate developmental and behavioral diagnoses, expert panels have endorsed that the clinical judgment of an experienced clinician is the gold standard for making developmental-behavioral diagnoses.[16] Given the prevalence of these conditions in primary care practice, primary pediatric health care professionals need to be such experienced clinicians in this field. Certainly, in clinical practice, not every child with a developmental-behavioral concern always fits neatly into the diagnostic framework described in this chapter, and currently accepted diagnostic criteria need to be used when a specific developmental-behavioral disorder (eg, ASD, ADHD, LD, ID) is suspected. However, a thorough understanding of the key neurodevelopmental principles underlying the spectrum and continuum of developmental-behavioral disorders (as outlined in Box 11.1) may enhance clinical judgment and improve the confidence and diagnostic acumen of primary pediatric health care professionals in identifying children with developmental or behavioral disorders at the earliest possible age.

Box 11.1. Key Neurodevelopmental Principles

- 3 primary streams of development
  - Motor
  - Cognitive (including language, social, adaptive, and visual problem solving)
  - Neurobehavior
- The more severe the developmental-behavioral disorder, the younger the age that it can be reliably identified
- There is a spectrum of disorders within each developmental stream
  - Mild disorders predominate over severe disorders within each stream
- There is a continuum of developmental-behavioral disorders across streams
  - More diffuse/global developmental-behavioral dysfunction predominates over more isolated/focal dysfunction (comorbidities are the rule rather than the exception)
- Developmental delay, dissociation, and deviation reflect underlying CNS dysfunction
- The more delayed, dissociated, and deviated the development, the more atypical the behavior should be expected to be

Abbreviation: CNS, central nervous system.

Making Developmental-Behavioral Diagnoses: Cases

The following cases will illustrate the key points of this chapter.

At his well-child health maintenance visit, a 24-month-old boy fails a standardized developmental screen; his mother is concerned that he is exhibiting a delay in his speech and language development. A comprehensive medical (including birth history, past medical history, and a complete review of systems), family, and social history do not indicate any increased risk for a developmental-behavioral disorder. His physical and neurological examinations and his hearing and vision are all normal.

DEVELOPMENTAL HISTORY FOR CASE 1

MOTOR STREAM

This boy's mother reports that he sat at 1 year of age (expected at around 6 months of age), and he just started taking independent steps last week (expected at around 12 months). Thus, this developmental history indicates a static pattern of delayed acquisition of gross motor milestones, with gross motor skill acquisition at approximately 50% of the expected rate.

COGNITIVE STREAM

Visual-Motor Problem Solving/Adaptive: This boy's mother reports that he began reaching for objects at 1 year of age (expected at around 5 months) and finger feeding himself at 18 months of age (expected at around 9 months). She reports that he just began to uncover hidden toys (expected at around 10 months of age), and to release objects intentionally (expected at around 12 months of age). She reports that he does not yet feed himself with a spoon (expected at around 14 months). Thus, this developmental history indicates a static pattern of delayed acquisition of visual-motor problem solving/adaptive milestones, with visual-motor problem solving/adaptive skill acquisition at approximately 50% the expected rate.

CASE 1

Language/Social Communication: This boy's mother reports that he began babbling at 1 year of age (expected at around 6 months), he began waving bye-bye at 18 months of age (expected at around 9 months), and he just started using a specific "Mama" and "Dada" about a month ago (expected at around 10 months). He now has a 2-word vocabulary (expected at around 12 months), and he just began following single-step gestured commands (expected at 12 months) and pointing with his index finger to indicate needs (protoimperative pointing) this week (expected at around 12 months). However, he does not yet point to share interest (protodeclarative pointing; expected at around 14 months) or engage in immature jargon (expected at 14 months). She reports that he shows good eye contact (visually focusing on a face, expected by 1 month), follows a point (expected at around 9 months), responds preferentially when his name is called (expected at around 10 months), and has recently begun sharing objects of interest with others (expected at around 12 months). Thus, this developmental history indicates a static pattern of delayed acquisition of language/social communication milestones, with language/social communication skill acquisition at approximately 50% the expected rate.

NEUROBEHAVIORAL STREAM

This boy's mother reports that he is not able to sit and attend in circle time as long as his classmates, and his overall behavior seems "immature" compared to his classmates at his Mother's Morning Out program. However, he does not have any atypical or restricted interests or need for routine, he does not engage in any stereotypic motor mannerisms, he is not a picky eater, and he is not bothered by noises.

Developmental Evaluation for CASE 1: On direct developmental observation using a standardized developmental evaluation instrument, this boy receives the following age equivalent scores:

- Gross Motor = 12 months
- Fine Motor = 12 months
- Adaptive = 12 months
- Visual-Motor Problem Solving = 12 months
- Receptive Language = 12 months
- Expressive Language = 12 months
- Social = 12 months

CASE 1

Thus, formal developmental evaluation confirms the developmental history provided by this boy's mother. He presents with a developmental history of a static pattern of globally delayed developmental milestone acquisition, with a historical rate of developmental milestone acquisition of approximately 50% of the expected rate across all developmental streams. On formal developmental evaluation, his globally delayed developmental milestones are confirmed, with his current developmental age equivalents scoring at 50% of his chronological age of 24 months across all developmental streams.

Developmental-Behavioral Diagnosis for CASE 1: This boy is exhibiting *global developmental delays* (and is at risk for a future diagnosis of ID). Although his mother's presenting concern based on standardized developmental screening was his delay in speech and language development, this chief complaint represented only the tip of an iceberg of more global underlying developmental difficulties. In the model for making developmental-behavioral diagnoses presented in this chapter, it is stated that the causes of developmental delays in children (eg, chromosomal deletions) tend to affect the brain diffusely, and therefore, more globally delayed developmental milestones are more frequently encountered than focal delays in a single developmental stream relative to the other streams (dissociation) or nonsequential unevenness of milestone acquisition within a stream of development (deviation). Thus, it should not be surprising to this boy's primary pediatric health care professional that despite the chief complaint of speech and language delay, this boy actually exhibits a global developmental delay across all streams of development. Also, it should not be unexpected that other than behaving in an "immature" fashion (which is consistent with what would be expected of his behavior given his global developmental delays), this boy does not exhibit any atypical behaviors, as he does not exhibit the atypical developmental patterns of dissociation and/or deviation. Hence, this boy's behavior and his motor skills are commensurate with his cognitive abilities, consistent with a global developmental delay.

CASE 2

At his well-child health maintenance visit, a 24-month-old boy fails a standardized developmental screen; his mother is concerned that he is exhibiting a delay in his speech and language development. A comprehensive medical (including birth history, past medical history, and a complete review of systems), family, and social history do not indicate any increased risk for a developmental-behavioral disorder. His physical and neurological examinations and his hearing and vision are all normal.

DEVELOPMENTAL HISTORY FOR CASE 2

MOTOR STREAM

This boy's mother reports that he walked at 12 months of age (expected at around 12 months), he can walk up and down stairs with both feet to each step (expected at around 21 months), and he recently began jumping up, getting both of his feet off the floor (expected at 24 months). She reports that he does not yet pedal a tricycle (expected at 30 to 36 months). Thus, this developmental history indicates age-appropriate acquisition of gross motor milestones, with gross motor skill acquisition at 100% the expected rate.

COGNITIVE STREAM

Visual-Motor Problem Solving/Adaptive: This boy's mother reports that he began releasing objects intentionally at 1 year of age (expected at around 12 months), he has been able to scribble spontaneously since 18 months of age (expected at around 18 months), and he has recently started to imitate horizontal and vertical strokes with a crayon (expected at 24 months). She reports that he is able to unzip and to feed himself with a fork (expected at around 21 months), and she has observed him aligning 4 blocks horizontally to build a train of blocks (expected at around 24 months). She reports that he does not yet draw a circle (expected at around 36 months) or even attempt to draw a circle as a circular motion (expected at around 30 months), and he does not yet recognize colors (expected at around 36 months). Thus, this developmental history indicates age-appropriate acquisition of visual-motor problem-solving/adaptive milestones, with visual-motor problem-solving/adaptive skill acquisition at 100% of the expected rate.

CASE 2

Language/Social Communication: This boy's mother reports that he began babbling at 1 year of age (expected at around 6 months), and he just started using a specific "Mama" and "Dada" about a month ago (expected at around 10 months). She reports that he now has 2 other specific words in his vocabulary (expected at around 12 months), and he just began following single-step gestured commands (expected at 12 months), but he does not yet engage in immature jargon (expected at 14 months). She reports that despite his delays in speech, he attempts to compensate for his delayed verbal development by attempting to communicate nonverbally. She reports that he waves bye-bye (expected at around 9 months) and points with his index finger to what he wants (protoimperative pointing; expected at around 12 months) and to share interest (protodeclarative pointing; expected at around 14 months). She has never had concerns about his ability to understand or use facial expressions. She reports that he has always shown good eye contact (visually focusing on a face expected by 1 month), he responds preferentially when his name is called (expected at around 10 months) and shares objects of interest with others (expected at around 12 months, and he imitates household tasks (expected at 18 months). Thus, this developmental history indicates a static pattern of delayed acquisition of language milestones with language milestone skill acquisition at approximately 50% the expected rate.

NEUROBEHAVIORAL STREAM

This boy's mother reports that he sometimes gets frustrated with communication breakdowns, but he otherwise enjoys interacting with adults and other children. He does not like to play alone, he is not a picky eater, he is not bothered by noises, he does not have any need for routine or atypical or restricted interests, and he does not engage in any stereotypic motor mannerisms.

Developmental Evaluation for CASE 2: On direct developmental observation using a formal standardized developmental evaluation instrument, this boy receives the following age equivalent scores:

- Gross Motor = 24 months
- Fine Motor = 24 months
- Adaptive = 24 months
- Visual-Motor Problem Solving = 24 months
- Receptive Language = 12 months
- Expressive Language = 12 months
- Social = 18 months

CASE 2

Thus, formal developmental evaluation confirms the developmental history provided by this boy's mother: He presents with a developmental history of discrepant delays (dissociation) in his speech/language development, with a historical rate of language milestone acquisition of approximately 50% of the expected rate, and on formal developmental evaluation, his dissociated delays in speech/language development were confirmed, with his current speech/language age equivalent at 50% of his chronological age.

Developmental-Behavioral Diagnosis for CASE 2: This boy is exhibiting age-appropriate motor and visual-motor/adaptive development, but he is exhibiting dissociated delays in his language development, consistent with a **language disorder** (and placing him at risk for a future LLD). Despite his delayed speech/language milestones, he attempts to compensate for his verbal delays through using nonverbal communication, and he does not exhibit dissociated or deviated pragmatic/social communication when compared to his level of language development or any concerns about atypical behavior. It is important to note that despite his delayed acquisition of language developmental milestones, this boy is acquiring language milestones in the typical sequence; thus, he is not exhibiting any developmental deviation in his language milestone acquisition.

CASE 3

At his well-child health maintenance visit, a 24-month-old boy fails a standardized developmental screen; his mother is concerned that he is exhibiting a delay in his speech and language development. A comprehensive medical (including birth history, past medical history, and a complete review of systems), family, and social history do not indicate any increased risk for a developmental-behavioral disorder. His physical and neurological examinations and his hearing and vision are all normal.

DEVELOPMENTAL HISTORY FOR CASE 3

MOTOR STREAM

This boy's mother reports that he walked at 12 months of age (expected at around 12 months). He can walk up and down stairs with both feet to each step (expected at around 21 months), and he just recently began jumping up, getting both of his feet off the floor (expected at 24 months). She reports that he does not yet pedal a tricycle (expected at around 30 to 36 months of age). Thus, this developmental history indicates age-appropriate acquisition of gross motor milestones, with gross motor skill acquisition at 100% the expected rate.

COGNITIVE STREAM

Visual-Motor Problem-Solving/Adaptive: This boy's mother reports that he began releasing objects intentionally at 1 year of age (expected at around 12 months), he has been able to scribble spontaneously since 18 months of age (expected at around 18 months), and he can copy horizontal and vertical lines in the appropriate orientation (expected at 30 months), but he does not yet draw a circle (expected at 36 months). She reports that he is able to unzip (expected at around 21 months), but he will not attempt to feed himself with a fork (expected at around 21 months), as he prefers to feed himself with his hands. She reports that he does not yet unbutton (expected at around 36 months). However, she reports that she has observed him building very complex structures with blocks, he can complete puzzles designed for 5-year-olds, he seems very good at remembering where his family's car is parked when they go to the supermarket, and he seems to notice when the usual route is not taken when their family drives to a familiar location. She reports that he has been recognizing colors (expected at 36 months) and all letters of the alphabet (a kindergarten-level skill) since he was 18 months of age, and he can also recognize complex shapes, such as an octagon and dodecagon. Thus, this developmental history indicates at least age-appropriate acquisition of visual-motor problem-solving milestones (at least 100% of the expected rate), with upward deviation in his ability to recognize colors, shapes, and letters of the alphabet and to complete puzzles to at least a 5-year-old level.

CASE 3

Language/Social Communication: This boy's mother reports that he began babbling at 1 year of age (expected at around 6 months), and he said his first word ("circle") at around 2 years of age. She reports that he now has about a 10-word (expected at around 18 months) vocabulary (other than for names of colors, shapes, and letters), and while she has heard him use a nonspecific "mama" and "dada" (expected at around 8 months), he does not yet use a specific "Mama" or "Dada" to refer to his parents (expected at around 10 months). These 10 other words in his vocabulary are just used to label objects and not to spontaneously communicate. She reports that he does not yet wave bye-bye (expected at around 9 months) or point (expected at around 12 months), he rarely attempts to communicate with others, and when he does, he will only do so by leading someone else by the hand and placing their hand on his desired item. She reports that he just started following a point (expected at around 9 months) and following single-step gestured commands (expected at around 12 months), but he does not follow single-step commands without a gesture (expected at around 16 months). She reports that he does not make eye contact with others (visually focusing on a face; expected at around 1 month), his face tends to be devoid of expression, and he does not seem to understand the facial expressions of others. She reports that he does not respond preferentially when his name is called (expected at around 10 months), or make any attempts to share objects of interest with others (expected at around 12 months). She reports that he tends to ignore other children, he only approaches his parents when he needs something opened or turned on, and he prefers to be alone. Thus, this developmental history indicates a static pattern of delayed acquisition of language milestones, but it also indicates nonsequential unevenness or deviated acquisition of language milestones, with difficulties beginning at a 9-month level (lack of waving bye-bye) but with upward deviation in his vocabulary to an 18-month level; however, while he reportedly has a 10-word vocabulary (as expected at 18 months), he is not using a specific "Mama" or "Dada" (as expected at 10 months), and despite this vocabulary, his mother reported that he rarely makes attempts at communicating. In association with these delayed and deviated language milestones, he also presents with delayed and deviated (both nonsequential social milestone acquisition [ie, lack of eye contact as expected by 1 month, but he is able to follow a point as expected at 9 months] and social behavior that is atypical at any age [ie, ignores other people; prefers to be alone, etc]) social communication.

CASE 3

NEUROBEHAVIORAL STREAM

This boy's mother reports that he engages in repetitive play, such as lining up objects, watching the same part of a video over and over, and repetitively turning lights on and off, opening and closing doors, and watching the toilet flush. She reported that he is very attracted to objects with spinning parts or flashing lights, he loves to watch flowing water, and he likes to hold plastic letters of the alphabet in his hands at all times. She reported that he has a strong need for routine and becomes upset with changes or transitions. She reported that he is a very picky eater, he is bothered by noises, he refuses to wear socks, and he seems to have a high pain threshold, as he does not cry after he falls. She reported that he flaps his hands when he is excited, and he tends to walk on his toes.

Developmental Evaluation for CASE 3: On direct developmental observation using a formal standardized developmental evaluation instrument, this boy receives the following age equivalent scores:

- ▶ Gross Motor = 24 months
- ▶ Fine Motor = 24 months
- ▶ Adaptive = 18 months
- ▶ Visual-Motor Problem Solving = 33 months
- ▶ Receptive Language = 12 months
- ▶ Expressive Language = 16 months
- ▶ Social = 6 months

Thus, formal developmental evaluation confirms the developmental history provided by this boy's mother—he presents with a developmental history of discrepant delays (dissociation) in his language/social communication development, and his direct developmental evaluation confirms this history. In addition, he also presents with a history of significant developmental deviation in his language/social communication development.

CASE 3

Developmental-Behavioral Diagnosis for CASE 3: This boy is exhibiting age-appropriate motor milestones, and while his visual-motor problem solving skills exceed his chronological age of 24 months on formal developmental evaluation, he exhibits atypical developmental deviation in his acquisition of visual-motor problem-solving skills (as he is not yet able to draw a circle [as expected at 36 months], but he precociously recognized all the letters of the alphabet at 18 months of age, he recognizes complex shapes, he completes puzzles designed for older children, and he seems to have an exceptional visual memory). He also exhibits discrepant delays (dissociation) in his language and social communication development relative to his visual-motor problem solving development, with significant deviation in his acquisition of language and social milestones. Thus, this boy is exhibiting a language disorder and social communication disorder. However, as reviewed in this chapter:

▶ Developmental delay, dissociation, and deviation represent underlying CNS dysfunction.

▶ Dissociation and deviation are atypical compared to more global developmental delays.

▶ The more delayed, dissociated, and deviated the cognitive development, the more atypical the behavior is expected to be.

This boy is exhibiting **delayed** language/social communication development, his language and social communication are **dissociated** from his nonverbal/visual-motor problem-solving development, and he is exhibiting significant **deviation** in his acquisition of both language/social communication and nonverbal/visual-motor problem-solving developmental milestones. Given that this extent of developmental delay, dissociation, and deviation is atypical, it should be expected that this boy's neurobehavior would be similarly atypical. Given his significant weaknesses in language/social communication and significant strengths in nonverbal/visual-motor problem solving, it is not surprising that this boy exhibits atypical attention, lacking the attention to make eye contact in language confrontational social situations while overly focusing or perseverating on restricted, repetitive, visually stimulating behaviors (lining up objects, watching objects spin, etc) and either over- or under-focusing on various sensory stimuli (high pain threshold, upset with noises, picky eating, etc). It should also not be surprising that such atypical dissociated and deviated cognitive development would be accompanied by atypical motor activity, such as hand flapping and toe walking. This combination of a social communication disorder (with a language disorder) and associated atypical neurobehavior represents ASD (with an associated language disorder).

Summary of Cases

In each of these 3 cases, concerns were elicited from a mother through standardized developmental screening about her 24-month-old boy's speech and language development. Through recognition of the different patterns of developmental delay, dissociation, and deviation for each of these cases, combined with an understanding of the spectrum and continuum of developmental-behavioral disorders, the primary pediatric health care professional is able to make the correct developmental-behavioral diagnoses (global developmental delay, language disorder, and ASD with a language disorder) for each of these cases.

References

1. Lipkin PH. Epidemiology of the developmental disabilities. In: Capute AJ, Accardo PJ, eds. *Developmental Disabilities in Infancy and Childhood: Second Edition*. Baltimore, MD: Paul H. Brookes;1996:137–158
2. Voigt RG, Accardo PJ. Formal speech and language screening not shown to help children. *Pediatrics*. 2015;136(2):e494–e495
3. Moreno-De-Luca A, Myers SM, Challman TD, Moreno-DeLuca D, Evans DW, Ledbetter DH. Developmental brain dysfunction: revival and expansion of old concepts based on new genetic evidence. *Lancet Neurol*. 2013;12(4):406–14
4. Myers SM. Diagnosing developmental disabilities. In: Batshaw ML, Roizen NJ, Lotrecchiano GR, eds. *Children with Disabilities*. 7th ed. Baltimore, MD: Brookes Publishing; 2013:243–266
5. Accardo PJ. The father of developmental pediatrics: Arnold J. Capute, MD, MPH (1923–2003). *J Child Neurol*. 2004;19:978–981
6. Capute AJ. The expanded Strauss syndrome: MBD revisited. In: Accardo PJ, Blondis TA, Whitman BY, eds. *Attention Deficit Disorders and Hyperactivity*. New York, NY: Marcel Dekker, Inc.; 1991:27–36
7. Coe BP, Girirajan S, Eichler EE. The genetic variability and commonality of neurodevelopmental disease. *Am J Med Genet C Semin Med Genet*. 2012;160C(2):118–129
8. Rosenfeld JA, Patel A. Chromosomal microarrays: understanding genetics of neurodevelopmental disorders and congenital anomalies. *J Pediatr Genet*. 2017;6(1):42–50
9. Nelson KB, Ellenberg JH. Children who "outgrew" cerebral palsy. *Pediatrics*. 1982;69(5):529–536
10. Helt M, Kelley E, Kinsbourne M, Pandey J, Boorstein H, Herbert M, Fein D. Can children with autism recover? If so, how? *Neuropsychol Rev*. 2008;18(4):339–366
11. Barbaresi WJ, Colligan RC, Weaver AL, Voigt RG, Killian JM, Katusic SK. Mortality, ADHD, and psychosocial adversity in adults with childhood ADHD: a prospective study. *Pediatrics*. 2013;131(4):637–644
12. American Academy of Pediatrics Council on Children with Disabilities, Section on Developmental and Behavioral Pediatrics, Bright Futures Steering Committee, and Medical Home Initiatives for Children with Special Needs Project Advisory Committee. Identifying infants and young children with developmental disorders in the medical home: an algorithm for developmental surveillance and screening. *Pediatrics*. 2006;118(1):405–420
13. Voigt RG, Accardo PJ. Mission impossible? Blaming primary care providers for not identifying the unidentifiable. *Pediatrics*. 2016;138(2):pii:e20160432
14. Walker WO, Johnson CP. Mental retardation: overview and diagnosis. *Pediatr Rev*. 2006;27(6):204–211
15. Myers SM, Johnson CP. American Academy of Pediatrics Council on Children With Disabilities. Management of children with autism spectrum disorders. *Pediatrics*. 2007;120(5):1162–1182
16. Filipek PA, Accardo PJ, Ashwal S, et al. Practice parameter: screening and diagnosis of autism: report of the Quality Standards Subcommittee of the American Academy of Neurology and the Child Neurology Society. *Neurology*. 2000;55(4):468–479
17. Van Naarden Braun K, Christensen D, Doernberg N, et al. Trends in the prevalence of autism spectrum disorder, cerebral palsy, hearing loss, intellectual disability, and vision impairment, metropolitan Atlanta, 1991–2010. *PLoS One*. 2015;10(4):e0124120
18. Voigt RG, Barbaresi WJ, Colligan RC, Weaver AL, Katusic, SK. Developmental dissociation, deviance, and delay: occurrence of attention-deficit/hyperactivity disorder among individuals with and without borderline-to-mild intellectual disability in a population-based birth cohort. *Dev Med Child Neurol*. 2006;48(10):831–835
19. Christensen DL, Baio J, Van Naarden Braun K, et al. Prevalence and characteristics of autism spectrum disorder among children age 8 years—autism and developmental disabilities monitoring network, 11 sites, United States, 2012. *MMWR Surveill Summ*. 2016;65(3):1–23

20. Barbaresi WJ, Katusis SK, Colligan RC, Weaver AL, Jacobsen SJ. Modifiers of long-term school outcomes for children with attention-deficit/hyperactivity disorder: does treatment with stimulant medication make a difference? Results from a population-based study. *J Dev Behav Pediatr.* 2007;28(4):274–287

21. Pitcher TM, Piek JP, Hay DA. Fine and gross motor ability in males with ADHD. *Dev Med Child Neurol.* 2003;45(8):525–535

22. Accardo PJ, Accardo JA, Capute AJ. A neurodevelopmental perspective on the continuum of developmental disabilities. In: Accardo PJ, ed. *Capute & Accardo's Neurodevelopmental Disabilities in Infancy and Childhood.* 3rd ed. Baltimore, MD: Paul H. Brookes; 2008:3–26

23. Capute AJ, Accardo PJ, The infant neurodevelopmental assessment: a clinical interpretive manual for CAT-CLAMS in the first two years of life, part 1. *Curr Probl Pediatr.* 1996;26(7):238–257

24. Wechsler D. *Manual for the Wechsler Intelligence Scale for Children—Revised.* San Antonio, TX: The Psychological Corporation; 1974

25. Wechsler D. *Wechsler Intelligence Scale for Children—Fifth Edition. Administration and Scoring Manual.* San Antonio, TX: The Psychological Corporation; 2014

26. Belmont I. Belmont L. Is the slow learner in the classroom learning disabled? *J Learn Disabil.* 1980;13(9):496–499

27. Gibbs J, Appleton J, Appleton R. Dyspraxia or developmental coordination disorder? Unraveling the enigma. *Arch Dis Child.* 2007;92(6):534–539

28. American Psychiatric Association. *Diagnostic and Statistical Manual of Mental Disorders.* 5th ed. Arlington, VA: American Psychiatric Publishing; 2013

29. Accardo PJ, Blondis TA, Roizen NJ, Whitman BY. The physical examination of the child with attention deficit hyperactivity disorder. In: Accardo PJ, Blondis TA, Whitman BY, eds. *Attention Deficit Disorders and Hyperactivity.* New York, NY: Marcel Dekker, Inc.; 1991:121–139

30. Durkin MS, Benedict RE, Christensen D, et al. Prevalence of cerebral palsy among 8-year-old children in 2010 and preliminary evidence of trends in its relationship to low birthweight. *Paediatr Perinat Epidemiol.* 2016;30(5):496–510

31. Shaywitz SE, Shaywitz BA. Dyslexia (specific reading disability). *Pediatr Rev.* 2003;24(5):147–153

32. Katusic SK. Colligan RC. Barbaresi WJ. Schaid DJ. Jacobsen SJ. Incidence of reading disability in a population-based birth cohort, 1976–1982, Rochester, Minn. *Mayo Clin Proc.* 2001;76(11):1081–1092

33. American Psychiatric Association. *Diagnostic and Statistical Manual of Mental Disorders.* 4th ed. Washington, DC: American Psychiatric Association; 1994

34. Mariol M, Jacques C, Schelstraete MA, Rossion B. The speed of orthographic processing during lexical decision: electrophysiological evidence for independent coding of letter identity and letter position in visual word recognition. *J Cogn Neurosci.* 2008;20(7):1283–1299

35. Kelly DP. Aylward GP. Identifying school performance problems in the pediatric office. *Pediatr Ann.* 2005;34(4):288–298

36. Thompson S. Nonverbal learning disorders. http://www.ldonline.org/article/6114. 1996. Accessed January 10, 2018

37. Odding E. Roebroeck ME. Stam HJ. The epidemiology of cerebral palsy: incidence, impairments and risk factors. *Disabil Rehabil.* 2006;28(4):183–191

38. Rutter M. Syndromes attributed to "minimal brain dysfunction" in childhood. *Am J Psychiatry.* 1982;139(1):21–33

39. Brown FRIII, Voigt RG, Elksnin N. Attention-deficit/hyperactivity disorder: neurodevelopmental perspectives. *Contemp Pediatr.* 1996;13(6):25–44

40. Rappley MD. Clinical practice. Attention deficit–hyperactivity disorder. *N Engl J Med.* 2005;352(2):165–173

41. Johnson CP. Myers SM. American Academy of Pediatrics Council on Children With Disabilities. Identification and evaluation of children with autism spectrum disorders. *Pediatrics.* 2007;120(5):1183–1215

42. Voigt RG, Childers DO, Dickerson CL, et al. Early pediatric neurodevelopmental profile of children with autistic spectrum disorders. *Clin Pediatr (Phila).* 2000;39(11):663–668

43. Rapin I. Dunn M. Language disorders in children with autism. *Semin Pediatr Neurol.* 1997;4(2):86–92

44. Morgan B, Mayberry M, Durkin K. Weak central coherence, poor joint attention, and low verbal ability: independent deficits in early autism. *Dev Psychol.* 2003;39(4):646–656

45. Shah A, Frith U. Why do autistic individuals show superior performance on the block design task? *J Child Psychol Psychiatry.* 1993;34(8):1351–1364

46. Caron MJ, Mottron L, Rainville C, Chouinard S. Do high functioning persons with autism present superior spatial abilities? *Neuropsychologia.* 2004;42(4):467–481

47. Nowell KP, Schanding GT, Kanne SM, Goin-Kochel RP. Cognitive profiles in youth with autism spectrum disorder: an investigation of base rate discrepancies using the Differential Ability Scales—Second Edition. *J Autism Dev Disord.* 2015;45(7):1978–1988

48. Joseph RM, Tager-Flusberg H, Lord C. Cognitive profiles and social-communicative functioning in children with autism spectrum disorder. *J Child Psychol Psychiatry.* 2002;43(6):807–821

49. Klin A, Volkmar FR, Sparrow SS, Cicchchetti DV, Rourke BP. Validity and neuropsychological characterization of Asperger syndrome: convergence with nonverbal learning disabilities. *J Child Psychol Psychiatry.* 1995;36(7):1127–1140

50. Rourke BP, Ahmad SA, Collins DW, Hayman-Abello SE, Warriner EM. Child clinical/pediatric neuropsychology: some recent advances. *Annu Rev Psychol.* 2002;53:309–339

51. Barbaresi WJ, Katusic SK, Colligan RC, et al. How common is attention-deficit/hyperactivity disorder? Incidence in a population-based birth cohort in Rochester, Minn. *Arch Pediatr Adolesc Med.* 2002;156(3):217–224

CHAPTER 12

Social and Emotional Development

John C. Duby, MD, FAAP, CPE

Healthy social and emotional development sets the foundation for promoting all other domains of children's development. After all, children learn to think, reason, communicate, run, jump, climb, care for themselves, and play in the course of social interactions with caregivers and peers. Children's development progresses in the context of the dynamic transactions between their biological and genetic tendencies and their life experiences. Life experiences are rooted in social and emotional relationships. Children who grow up in supportive, predictable, and nurturing environments are better prepared for a healthy, productive, adulthood and healthy, lifelong relationships.

During the first 18 months of life, the social and emotional areas of the brain grow and develop more rapidly than the language and cognitive areas.[1] These right brain nonverbal systems build from social-, relational-, and attachment-based experiences and create the emotional regulation and stress regulatory systems of the body that may last a lifetime. Therefore, the quality of the child's early social and emotional experiences may have lasting implications. The young child who is raised in a nurturing, predictable, and safe environment is likely to be more resilient when faced with stressful experiences later in life. Conversely, the young child who is faced with stressful, chaotic, or traumatic early experiences may suffer lifelong consequences.

As children grow and develop through early childhood, middle childhood, and adolescence, the quality of their interactions with caregivers, extended family, peers, teachers and coaches, and other community members has an ongoing impact on their social and emotional development. The monitoring of social and emotional development and family relationship patterns from infancy through adolescence is a vital component of health supervision.

America's Promise Alliance has identified 5 key resources or "promises" that correlate with success in youth and adulthood.[2] Children who grow up in homes with caring adults, in safe places where they have opportunities for constructive use of time, with a healthy start and healthy development, with effective education for marketable skills and lifelong learning, and with opportunities to make a difference through helping others have a much greater chance of experiencing success.[2] Teens who receive 4 of these 5 promises are nearly two-thirds more likely than those who have only 0 or 1 promise to be generous, respectful, and empathetic, and to resolve conflicts calmly. Younger children with 4 or more promises are twice as likely as their peers to be socially competent than their peers with 0 or 1 promise. Unfortunately, research performed by America's Promise Alliance indicates that more than two-thirds of children from 6 to 17 years of age are not receiving sufficient resources to place them on a path for success.

Felitti[3] and Shonkoff and Garner[14] have documented that adverse childhood experiences, especially inadequacies in early parental care, are associated with higher rates of both acute and chronic psychosocial disorders in adulthood. Most long-term sequelae seem to depend on a series of short-term links, some related to continued elevated risks of environmental adversity, others related to psychological vulnerabilities and resiliencies and problems in intimate social relationships. Primary pediatric health care professionals are well positioned to work with families to promote social competence at individual, practice, and community levels and potentially reduce the risk for long-term concerns in social and emotional health.

Key Points

- ▶ Social and emotional development progresses through predictable stages.
- ▶ Consider the developmental and environmental context when assessing any social-emotional concerns.
- ▶ Clearly identify and address the family's concerns.
- ▶ Perform surveillance using open-ended trigger questions.
- ▶ Attend to your observations of parent-child interaction and the child's interaction with you.
- ▶ Use standardized screening tools that match the level of risk in the population you serve.
- ▶ Explore options for offering evidence-based interventions in the medical home.
- ▶ Use evidence-based strategies for behavior management as part of your anticipatory guidance.
- ▶ Promote community-based linkages and resources to support families to promote resilience and to address social-emotional concerns.

Social and Emotional Milestones

Social and emotional development progresses through predictable stages in healthy children. Monitoring the milestones of social and emotional development is an important component of health supervision from infancy to young adulthood. Multiple observations will provide opportunities to identify variation from the expected path of development early, facilitating early identification and treatment. Failure to achieve expected milestones at any age should trigger further investigation and consideration of referral.

During the infant and toddler period, the major tasks of social and emotional development are to experience and regulate emotions, develop secure relationships, and begin to explore and learn. Even in the first few months of life, the infant's temperamental characteristics will emerge. Chess and Thomas[5] have described 3 functional constellations of temperament. The "easy" group includes 40% of children. These children demonstrate regularity, positive approach responses to new situations, high adaptability to change, and a mild-to-moderate, predominantly positive mood. About 10% of children have a "difficult" temperament. These children have irregularity in biological functions, negative withdrawal responses to new situations, poor or slow adaptation to change, and intense, often negative moods. The "slow to warm up" temperament is seen in 15% of children. This group combines mild, negative responses to new situations with slow adaptability after repeated exposure. With additional opportunities with new experiences, these children will eventually show quiet and positive interest. Not all children fit into 1 of these 3 groups. Others will have a mix of temperamental characteristics. It is vital that the child's temperament be considered when assessing social and emotional development and parent-child interaction. The most important factor may be the "goodness of fit" between the child's temperament and the temperaments of his caregivers.

Information on the stages of social and emotional development outlined below is adapted from Bright Futures.[6]

The newborn is most responsive during short periods in a quiet, alert state. She recognizes the unique smell of her mother, can hear and prefers her parents' voices, responds favorably to gentle touch while withdrawing from unpleasant touches, and can imitate simple facial expressions from a distance of 7 to 8 inches.

Throughout the first 2 months, the infant becomes increasingly capable of consoling and comforting himself while becoming increasingly alert, smiling responsively, and responding to calming actions when upset. By 4 months, he smiles spontaneously, initiates, sustains, and reciprocates during social interactions, and shows an even greater capacity to comfort himself. He has discovered that he can control the movements of his hands and may use them to console and comfort.

By 6 months, she recognizes and responds specifically to familiar faces and is beginning to notice strangers. She has sustained interactions and jointly attends to actions and objects of interest with her parents and regular caregivers. At 9 months, she is apprehensive of strangers and actively seeks out her parents for play, comfort, and assistance. By 12 months, she has a strong attachment with her parents and significant caregivers and shows distress on separation from her parents. The 12-month-old plays interactive games like peek-a-boo and pat-a-cake and uses gestures to wave bye-bye and to indicate interests and needs. She will hand a toy or book to her parent when she wants to play or hear a story.

By 15 months, he is very interested in imitating whatever he sees. He may start to help with simple household tasks and will listen actively to stories. His interactions with his parent or caregiver should be robust, complex, continuous, and goal-directed. By 18 months, his temperament will be more and more evident in his approach to participating in new or familiar group settings. Temper tantrums frequently emerge. He may be interactive or withdrawn, friendly or aggressive. He will show increasing willingness to separate and explore on his own, testing boundaries and limits but will want his parent in close proximity for periodic, reassuring check-ins or encouragement. He is spontaneous with affection and laughs in response to others.

The 2-year-old is becoming increasingly independent. She refers to herself as "I" or "me." She may have a special attachment to a book, a toy, or a blanket to help her make the transition to independence more smoothly. She will show an eagerness to share, show, and engage with the parent, to the parent's delight. She plays alongside other children and is showing more pretend play. At 2.5 years, imaginative play is clearly evident, and she shows evidence of symbolic play, making an object into something new or different. Her play now includes other children. As she struggles with her newly found independence, she may be fearful of unexpected changes in daily life.

By 3 years of age, he will show much more elaborate imaginative play with themes and story lines. He enjoys interactive play and is delighted to show his parents his capacity for independence with feeding, dressing, and toileting. The 4-year-old is working to establish a comfortable place in an expanding world. Depending on his temperament and the history of his relationship patterns, he may be predominantly cooperative, friendly, and responsive or withdrawn, aggressive, or defiant. Extremes of behavior may be seen at times of stress. He is also able to see himself as an individual yet equally enjoys demonstrating his relational capacity as a communicator and entertainer. He knows his gender and age and can describe his interests and what he does well. He has favorite toys and favorite stories. He spends more time in fantasy play.

The 5- to 6-year-old is successful at listening, attending, and following simple rules and directions. However, she is also likely to test those rules. She is becoming comfortable with spending more time with a peer group. As she approaches 7 to 8 years of age, she more fully understands rules, relationships, and mores. She will consistently show cooperation and attention and is capable of taking on family responsibilities and chores. As her moral development progresses, her coping skills emerge. Her beliefs may be tested by her peers, as she turns more to them and other adults for new ideas and activities. She may have a best friend and will usually identify most with children of the same gender that have similar interests and abilities. By 9 to 10 years, her peer group takes on greater importance. Her growing need for independence from her family will often be a valuable incentive for her to make contributions at home in order to earn privileges with her friends. She will demonstrate increasingly responsible and independent decision-making. At times, she may disparage and dismiss the knowledge of adults. Her feelings of self-confidence can be bolstered by descriptive praise, affection, and quality time in a nurturing relationship with her family.

The Association of Maternal and Child Health Programs and the National Network of State Adolescent Health Coordinators have identified critical developmental tasks that indicate healthy progression through adolescence from 10 to 24 years of age.[7]

In the context of caring, supportive relationships with family, other adults, and peers, a child will have increasing opportunities to engage in positive activities in his community that will promote a sense of self-confidence, hopefulness, and well-being. As the 11- to 14-year-old approaches adolescence, there is a greater drive for independence and a growing commitment to the peer group. Concurrently, the young adolescent develops a capacity for abstract and symbolic thinking that enables deeper and more creative cognitive analysis along with the tendency to challenge his own thinking and that of the adult authority figures in his life. As a result, he may engage in risky behavior to impress his peers. He will respond well to authoritative parenting that is firm, accepting, and democratic. Social networks will form, break down, and then form again. He will usually cope well with these stressful experiences and should be encouraged and supported while making more and more independent decisions. As the adolescent approaches young adulthood, school and work and its activities are the central focus of his life. It becomes increasingly important to monitor for emotional problems and risk-taking behaviors.

By understanding the expected path of social and emotional development from infancy through adolescence, the primary pediatric health care professional will be well positioned to anticipate areas for timely guidance and to identify variations in development that warrant intervention (Table 12.1).

The fourth edition of *Bright Futures: Guidelines for Health Supervision of Infants, Children, and Adolescents* outlines the components of health supervision and places special emphasis on promoting child development, mental/behavioral health, and life-long health for families and communities, along with resources for key themes to be addressed in the well-child visits.[6] Bright Futures recommends that each preventive health visit include establishing a context for the visit, setting priorities for the visit, a review of the interval history, observation of parent-child interaction, surveillance of development, a physical examination, screening, immunizations, other practice-based interventions, inquiry into relevant social contexts and family transitions or stressors, including screening for maternal depression, and offering anticipatory guidance. The American Academy of Pediatrics (AAP) has published recommendations for developmental surveillance and screening of young children.[8] The components of surveillance include eliciting and attending to the parents' concerns, identifying risks and protective factors, maintaining a developmental history, making accurate observations of the child, and documenting the process and findings. These components can be reviewed in the context of the Bright Futures framework. All of these elements can contribute significantly to the understanding of a child's social and emotional development and assist in identifying opportunities to build on strengths within the child, family, and community, as well as identifying concerns that may require additional support and intervention.

Table 12.1. Social-Emotional Milestones[6,7]	
Age	**Milestones**
Newborn	Is most responsive in a quiet, alert state. Recognizes the unique smell of her mother. Prefers her parents' voices. Responds favorably to gentle touch and withdraws from unpleasant touches. Imitates simple facial expressions from a distance of 7–8 inches.
2 months	Consoles and comforts self. Is increasingly alert. Smiles responsively. Responds to calming actions when upset.
4 months	Smiles spontaneously. Initiates social interactions. Shows greater capacity to comfort self. Controls the movements of his hands and may use them to console and comfort.
6 months	Recognizes familiar faces and is beginning to notice strangers. Sustains interactions. Jointly attends to actions and objects of interest to her caregivers.
9 months	Has clear apprehension with strangers. Seeks out her parents for play, comfort, and assistance. Plays interactive games like peek-a-boo and pat-a-cake. Waves bye-bye. Looks preferentially when name is called.
12 months	Uses protoimperative pointing; uses gestures to indicate needs. Hands a toy or book to her parent when she wants to play or hear a story.
15 months	Uses protodeclarative pointing to indicate interests. Imitates whatever he sees. Helps with simple household tasks. Listens actively to stories.
18 months	Temperament will be more and more evident in new or group settings. Is willing to separate and explore on his own but will want his parent close by. Is spontaneous with affection. Laughs in response to others.
2 years	Is more independent. Refers to herself as "I" or "me." May have a special object to assist with transition to independence. Plays alongside other children. Shows more pretend play.

Table 12.1. Social-Emotional Milestones[6,7] *(continued)*	
Age	**Milestones**
2.5 years	Shows imaginative play. Shows symbolic play, making an object into something new or different. Play includes other children. May be fearful of unexpected changes in daily life.
3 years	Shows much more elaborate imaginative play with themes and story lines. Enjoys interactive play. Is independent with feeding, dressing, and toileting.
4 years	Extremes of behavior may be seen at times of stress. Sees himself as an individual. Knows gender and age. Describes interests and strengths. Has favorite toys and favorite stories. Spends more time in fantasy play.
5–6 years	Listens, attends, and follows simple rules and directions. Tests rules. Spends more time with a peer group.
7–8 years	More fully understands rules, relationships, and mores. Shows cooperation and attention. Takes on family responsibilities and chores. May have a best friend. Identifies most with children of the same gender with similar interests and abilities.
9–10 years	Peer group takes on greater importance. Demonstrates increasingly responsible and independent decision-making.
11–14 years	Has a greater drive for independence and a growing commitment to the peer group. May engage in risky behavior to impress her peers. Forms and breaks down social networks. Copes well with stressful experiences. Makes more and more independent decisions.
15–24 years	School, extracurricular activities, and work become central focus. Forms caring, supportive relationships with family, other adults, and peers. Participates in the community. Demonstrates resilience with everyday life stressors. Increases independence in decision-making. Shows self-confidence and hopefulness.

Context

When assessing a child's social and emotional development, it is important to consider a number of contexts. At any health care encounter, it is vital to consider the child's age, developmental level, and psychosocial, socioeconomic, and cultural circumstances in order to accurately interpret any concerns regarding social and emotional development.

Squires et al recommend considering the following variables: setting/time, development, health, and family/cultural considerations.[9] First, where and when a behavior occurs may lead to different interpretations of the behavior. A child who is hitting or biting his younger sibling may have that behavior accidentally rewarded when it draws attention from his mother. However, the same behavior may quickly disappear in a child care setting where the child is redirected and given descriptive praise for gentle touching and has models for appropriate play with peers. Timing makes a difference as well. A child who experiences a major traumatic event early in life may experience lasting effects, while the same experience for an adolescent with strong coping skills may lead to only a temporary setback.

Second, it is vital that demands and expectations placed on the child be matched to the child's overall level of development, including cognition, language, academic, and motor skills. Children with isolated or global delays in development may develop secondary behavioral or emotional symptoms due to frustration or a tendency to avoid tasks that may be too difficult for them. There may be wide variation in achieving various milestones. Opportunities for serial observations allow the primary pediatric health care professional to establish whether the child is progressing as expected over time. However, the health care professional should not dismiss problems based on the assumption that they are simply due to normal variation.

Third, health variables may also affect children's social and emotional functioning. The child with obstructive sleep apnea may be irritable and inattentive at school. A child with atopic dermatitis may be so uncomfortable with pruritus that she may be noncompliant. Children with special health care needs may develop a pattern of learned helplessness because of their chronic illness and its accompanying challenges.

Finally, the patterns of interactions and communication within family relationships in the context of family values and culture have a significant role in determining children's social and emotional responses. Some cultures allow their emotions to flow freely and openly, while others expect children to hold their emotions inside. Various cultures have different expectations regarding when children should sleep on their own, be weaned, master toileting, and dress themselves.[10] Children who grow up in families affected by parental mental illness,[11] marital discord and domestic violence,[12] high levels of stress,[4] or poverty[13,14] may show changes in their social and emotional functioning in an attempt to cope with these challenges.

Priorities

The needs, concerns and resources of the family should be given first priority during each visit. Because as many as 25% of children have social or behavioral problems,[15] it is likely that concerns about social and emotional development will be raised during many preventive health visits. It may be necessary to give up one's professional priorities for the visit in order to address the family's and child's concerns. The American Academy of Pediatrics recommends routine screening for behavioral and emotional problems.[16] In addition, Bright Futures recommends that maternal and family functioning be a priority for all health supervision visits,[6] including screening for maternal depression in early infancy.[17] A focus on social and emotional functioning and parent-child interactive patterns should be emphasized during early infancy, between 18 and 30 months, and at the transitions to kindergarten, middle school, and high school. These times coincide with anticipated challenges to social and emotional competence.

Social-Emotional Surveillance and Interval History

When social and emotional development is identified as a priority for the visit, several open-ended questions can set the stage for a productive, targeted discussion. Asking parents to share emerging abilities, behavior and personality can be a good starting point. Following this by asking whether there are any concerns about the child's development, behavior, or learning can be very productive. Parents' concerns about their child's development, behavior, and learning are substantiated at least 70% of the time.[18,19]

Additional trigger questions to assess social and emotional functioning include[20]

* How are things going for you as a parent?
* What changes have you seen in your child's development or behavior since the last visit?
* What does your child do really well? With you? At school? In the community?
* What kind of child is she? Tell me about your child's personality or temperament.
* What are your child's favorite play or recreational activities?
* What do you enjoy doing together?
* Have there been any significant changes or stressful events in the family since the last visit?
* Has anything bad, sad, or scary happened to you or your family since our last visit?
* What do you find most difficult about caring for your child now?
* How do you and your child solve problems?

The Classification of Child and Adolescent Mental Diagnoses in Primary Care: Diagnostic and Statistical Manual for Primary Care (DSM-PC)[21] provides a framework for assessing protective factors and environmental challenges. When faced with a child or family who appears at risk, this framework can provide a structured approach to identify opportunities to further support social competence and for remediation.

Once children reach the age of 3 or 4 years and through adolescence, these questions can be adapted and asked directly of the child. The primary pediatric health care professional may be reassured by the response or may feel a need to probe further.

Children have a full set of emotions by 3 years of age.[22] By 5 years of age, most children are skilled at describing their feelings. It is appropriate to ask school-aged children to describe examples of what leads them to feel various emotions.

- What makes you happy? Sad? Mad?
- What makes you afraid?
- What do you worry about? Do you have any worries about your body or about your health?
- Are there things you are afraid might happen to you or to people you care about?
- Have you ever thought about hurting yourself or running away? If so, have you made a plan? If you ever do think of hurting yourself, is there an adult you can talk to about your feelings?
- Do you have a best friend? What do you like to do with your friends? Are you being bullied?
- What would you like to change about yourself? What would you like to change about school? What would you like to change about your family?
- If you had 3 wishes, what would they be?

All of these questions can assist the primary pediatric health care professional in determining whether further history, evaluation, or referral may be indicated.

As children approach middle childhood and adolescence, it is often important to interview the child alone. This provides an opportunity to discuss risk-taking behaviors or to identify any perceived risk within the family system.

Observation of Parent-Child Interaction

Beginning in the newborn period, and on through adolescence, observation of parent-child interaction can offer insight into family relationships, parenting style, and the child's social and emotional well-being. Often much can be learned by observing what is happening when the health care professional opens the examination room door. Is the infant held in the mother's lap in a loving embrace with good eye contact and nice vocalizations? Or is the child tearing apart the office and climbing on the cupboards while the father is intent on reading a magazine? Neither of these observations should lead to a diagnostic conclusion, but one might offer the opportunity to provide descriptive praise, while the other might serve as an opportunity for incidental teaching. Yet, it is within the family relational and behavioral patterns that one sees, firsthand, the strengths and vulnerabilities of social-emotional developmental competency.

It is also important to attend to the quality of the interaction between the child and the health care professional. Are the child's responses developmentally appropriate? Does the child make good eye contact? Is the toddler showing joint attention skills and protoimperative and protodeclarative pointing? Is the child's mood and affect appropriate or flat or withdrawn? Is the child anxious about what is going to happen next? Is the parent or the child flushed or visibly nervous? These observations may add to the assessment of the child's social and emotional functioning.

Healthy children are better prepared to explore and learn. Parents who actively protect and promote their children's health, including maintaining the recommended immunization schedule, help to secure the foundation for healthy social and emotional development. In addition, observation of the child's behavior during the immunization process can provide additional insight into her coping skills and into the parent-child interaction. The administration of immunizations may provide an opportunity for the health care professional to model and teach coping and relaxation skills.

Physical Examination

The physical examination offers an additional opportunity to observe the child's adaptation to and compliance with the health care professional's requests and to observe the parent's response as well. Is the child cooperative or overly anxious or defiant? Is the parent encouraging and supportive or overly protective or coercive? The child's vital signs might be an indicator of stress if the child's blood pressure or heart rate is high for no other apparent reason. It is important to look for any subtle dysmorphic features that may indicate a genetic disorder that may present with developmental delays, including social or emotional concerns. The neurological and mental status examinations may contribute to an understanding of any social and emotional concerns. It is also important to look for any signs of accidental, intentional, or self-inflicted injuries.

Screening

Perrin and Stancin[23] and Weitzman and Wegner[16] have published comprehensive reviews of behavioral screening that include extensive lists of available instruments. Primary pediatric health care professionals can use their own interview or questionnaire, but there are advantages to using a published standardized questionnaire. These include the ability to compare responses with national norms, compare responses from several observers, and quantify and document change over time. A combination of an interval history, as outlined above, with a standardized questionnaire, if concerns are identified, may be most beneficial. At the same time, it may be beneficial to routinely administer a standardized tool to assess social and emotional functioning of children and their caregivers at key well-child visits (Table 12.2). Universal screening may provide an opportunity to introduce a difficult topic and reduce the tendency to rely on normal variation to explain concerns. For example, the AAP has recommended that all children have a standardized screen for autism, a primary disorder in social relatedness, at 18 and 24 months of age.[24]

Table 12.2. Screening and Assessment Tools				
Screening	**Instrument**	**Age Range**	**Time**	**Source**
Caregiver functioning	Edinburgh Postnatal Depression Screening	Adults	5 min	https://www.aap.org/en-us/advocacy-and-policy/aap-health-initiatives/practicing-safety/Documents/Postnatal%20Depression%20Scale.pdf
	Center for Epidemiologic Studies Depression Scale	Adults	5–10 min	https://www.brightfutures.org/mentalhealth/pdf/professionals/bridges/ces_dc.pdf
	Patient Health Questionnaire-2	Adults	1 min	https://brightfutures.aap.org/Bright%20Futures%20Documents/PHQ-2%20Instructions%20for%20Use.pdf
	Patient Health Questionnaire-9 & 9A	Adolescents and Adults	5 min	http://www.integration.samhsa.gov/images/res/PHQ%20-%20Questions.pdf http://www.uacap.org/uploads/3/2/5/0/3250432/phq-a.pdf
	Depression, Anxiety, and Stress Scale	17 y and up	10 min	http://www2.psy.unsw.edu.au/dass/
	Parenting Stress Index–Short Form	Parents of 1 mo to 12 y	10 min	https://www.parinc.com/Products/Pkey/333
	Adverse Childhood Experiences Score	Adults	5 min	www.acestudy.org
Temperament	Carey Temperament Scales	1 mo to 12 y	15 min	www.b-di.com
Infancy to early childhood	Ages & Stages Questionnaires: Social-Emotional, 2nd Edition	1–72 mo	10–15 min	http://www.brookespublishing.com/resource-center/screening-and-assessment/asq/asq-se-2/
	Communication and Symbolic Behavior Scales Developmental Profile Infant-Toddler Checklist	6–24 mo	5–10 min	http://products.brookespublishing.com/Communication-and-Symbolic-Behavior-Scales-Developmental-Profile-CSBS-DP-First-Normed-Edition-Toy-Kit-P30.aspx
	Brief Infant-Toddler Social Emotional Assessment	12–36 mo	7–10 min	http://www.pearsonclinical.com/childhood/products/100000150/brief-infant-toddler-social-emotional-assessment-bitsea.html
Early childhood to adolescence	Eyberg Child Behavior Inventory	2–16 y	5 min	https://www.parinc.com/Products/Pkey/97
	Pediatric Symptom Checklist	4–18 y	5 min	http://www.massgeneral.org/psychiatry/services/psc_forms.aspx
	Pictorial Pediatric Symptom Checklist	4–18 y	5 min	http://www.massgeneral.org/psychiatry/services/psc_forms.aspx

Table 12.2. Screening and Assessment Tools *(continued)*				
Screening	**Instrument**	**Age Range**	**Time**	**Source**
Assessment				
Multidimensional	Infant-Toddler Social Emotional Assessment	12–36 mo	25–30 min	http://www.pearsonclinical.com/childhood/products/100000652/infant-toddler-social-emotional-assessment-itsea.html
	NCAST Parent Child Interaction Feeding and Teaching Scales	12–36 mo	Feeding: length of meal Teaching: 1–6 min	http://ncast.org/index.cfm?category=2
	CHADIS	Birth to adolescence	10–20 min	http://www.chadis.com/site/
	Achenbach System of Empirically Based Assessments	1.5 y to adult	20–30 min	http://www.aseba.org/
	Behavioral Assessment Scale for Children, 3rd Edition	2–21 y	10–20 min	http://www.pearsonclinical.com/education/products/100001402/behavior-assessment-system-for-children-third-edition-basc-3.html
	Conners Comprehensive Behavior Rating Scales	6–18 y	10–20 min	http://www.pearsonclinical.com/psychology/products/100000523/conners-3rd-edition-conners-3.html?
	Child Symptom Inventories-5	5–18 y	20–30 min	http://www.checkmateplus.com/product/casi5.htm
	NICHQ Vanderbilt Parent and Teacher Assessment Scales, 2nd Edition	6–12 y	5–10 min	https://shop.aap.org/Caring-for-Children-with-ADHD-A-Resource-Toolkit-for-Clinicians/
Single dimension attention-deficit/hyperactivity disorder	Conners 3 Short Forms	6–18 y	5–20 min	http://www.pearsonclinical.com/psychology/products/100000523/conners-3rd-edition-conners-3.html?
	Attention Deficit Disorders Evaluation Scales, 4th Edition	4–18 y	12–15 min	http://www.hawthorne-ed.com/pages/adhd/ad1.html
	Brown Attention Deficit Disorder Scales	3 y to adult	10–20 min	http://www.drthomasebrown.com/assessment-tools/
Single dimension anxiety/depression	Beck Youth Inventories	7–18 y	5 min	http://www.pearsonclinical.com/psychology/products/100000153/beck-youth-inventories-second-edition-byi-ii.html
	Screen for Child Anxiety Related Emotional Disorders (SCARED)	8–18 y	10 min	http://www.pediatricbipolar.pitt.edu/resources/instruments

– Caregiver Functioning

There is growing attention to the importance of screening for maternal depression,[17] especially in the first 6 months when postpartum depression is prevalent, but also at any time there is a concern regarding a child's behavior. Observation without screening tools fails to identify most mothers with depressive symptoms. From 2004 to 2013, the rates of routine screening for maternal depression by pediatricians increased from 33–44%, leading to ongoing missed opportunities for identification and referral for treatment.[25]

Several tools are available to screen for maternal depression. The Edinburgh Postnatal Depression Screening is the most widely studied and uses a 10-item tool that includes anxiety symptoms as well as symptoms of depression. The Patient Health Questionnaire-9 includes a question regarding suicidality, but it also includes questions on somatic complaints that may reduce its reliability.[26] The Center for Epidemiologic Studies Depression Scale (CES-D) is a 20-item measure of psychological distress.[27] The Patient Health Questionnaire-2 (PHQ-2) has 2 questions that assess the presence and frequency of concerns about mood and anhedonia in the prior 2 weeks.[28] It has been validated in primary care and obstetric settings. Olson et al[29] evaluated the PHQ-2 in a pediatric setting and found that it added no more than 3 additional minutes to the length of the visit. Prolonged discussion was uncommon, requiring 5 to 10 minutes in 3% of well-child visits and more than 10 minutes in just 2% of well-child visits. Moreover, if these straightforward questions generate extended discussion, it can be assured that the issue was germane, so the time taken was needed and well served.

Recent studies have also documented the high prevalence of perinatal anxiety disorders.[30] Additional tools are available to assess broader dimensions of parental and caregiver functioning. For example, the Depression, Anxiety, and Stress Scale (DASS)[31] is a 42-item instrument designed to measure depression, anxiety, and tension/stress. It can be downloaded at no charge. The Parenting Stress Index[32] is available in 36-item and 120-item forms. The Parenting Stress Index is designed for the early identification of parenting and family characteristics that raise the risk for difficulties in social and emotional functioning and parent-child interaction. It can be used with parents of children as young as 1 month up to 12 years of age. The Adverse Childhood Experiences (ACE) score is used to assess the sources and cumulative total amount of stress during childhood and has demonstrated that as the number of ACE increase, the risk for physical and mental health problems increases in a strong and graded fashion.[33]

– Temperament

Parents will benefit from understanding their child's temperament and its influence on parent-child interaction as well as adaptation to new experiences. Medoff-Cooper and associates[34] have developed a number of questionnaires that can assist parents and health care professionals in understanding children's temperamental characteristics as early as 4 months of age. When combined with the interval history and observation of the parent-child interaction, a temperament questionnaire can be a useful tool for better understanding the caregiver and child's individuality and behavior. A series of questionnaires are available for various age groups.[35]

Infancy and Early Childhood

Provence[36] suggested that asking parents to describe a typical day from arousal to bedtime can be a useful tool to identify sources of harmony and potential areas of difficulty. A number of standardized tools are also now available to screen specifically for social and emotional development. The Ages & Stages Questionnaires: Social-Emotional, 2nd Edition (ASQ:SE-2) is a parent-completed child-monitoring system for social-emotional behaviors in children from 1 to 72 months of age.[9] The areas screened include self-regulation, compliance, social-communication, adaptive functioning, autonomy, affect, and interactions with people. Questionnaires can be photocopied and take 10 to 15 minutes for parents to complete and 1 to 3 minutes to score. The ASQ:SE-2 can be used routinely at key well-child visits, such as at 12 and 36 months, or as needed if surveillance indicates the need for standardized information. The Communication and Symbolic Behavior Scales Developmental Profile[37] identifies predictors of later language and communication problems by assessing social skills, including the use of gestures, emotions and eye gaze, communication, and object use. A 24-question checklist can be completed by the caregiver of a 6- to 24-month-old child in 5 to 10 minutes. Early concerns can identify those at risk for social and emotional or communication disorders. A more comprehensive questionnaire and a structured observation of behavior are available for further assessment when the initial checklist raises concerns.

The Brief Infant-Toddler Social-Emotional Assessment Scale (BITSEA)[38] is a first-stage screening of social and emotional development that is appropriate for all children from 12 to 36 months of age. Parents can complete the 42 items in 7 to 10 minutes. If concerns are evident, they can be further characterized by administering the more comprehensive Infant-Toddler Social Emotional Assessment (ITSEA).[39]

Early Childhood to Adolescence

The Eyberg Child Behavior Inventory[40] is designed to assess parental report of behavioral problems in children and adolescents from 2 to 16 years of age. It measures the number of difficult behavior problems and the frequency with which they occur. It takes 5 minutes to complete and 5 minutes to score.

The Pediatric Symptom Checklist (PSC)[41,42] is a first-stage screening appropriate for all children from 4 to 18 years of age. It focuses on broad concerns that reflect general psychological functioning. Parents can complete either a 17- or 35-item checklist in less than 5 minutes. Subscales identify internalizing, externalizing, and attention problems. Cut-off scores are established, and it is available free of charge. It is also available in a pictorial format. The PSC is not a diagnostic instrument but rather a tool that will indicate whether further assessment of social and emotional development is warranted. It may be worthwhile to administer a tool such as the Eyberg Child Behavior Inventory or the PSC at annual visits from preschool through adolescence.

– Multidimensional Tools

The Center for Promotion of Child Development through Primary Care has developed CHADIS,[43] a Web-based diagnostic, management, and tracking tool designed to assist health care professionals in addressing parents' concerns about their child's behavior and development. Parents complete online questionnaires from home that are based on the *DSM-PC*. CHADIS analyzes the responses and provides the health care professional with decision support, handouts, and community resources. Additional information is available at www.chadis.com.

Numerous, more extensive multidimensional scales are available to provide additional information when initial surveillance or screening tests raise concerns.[16] None of these tools should be considered a substitute for a thorough clinical assessment. Therefore, it may be appropriate to consider referral to a mental/behavioral health professional when screening assessments raise concerns. Examples of multidimensional scales include the Achenbach System of Empirically Based Assessments,[44] the Behavioral Assessment Scale for Children, second edition,[45] the Conners Comprehensive Behavior Rating Scales,[46] the Child Symptom Inventories-4,[47] and the National Institute for Children's Health Quality (NICHQ) Vanderbilt Parent and Teacher Assessment Scales.[48] The Vanderbilt Scales are in the public domain.

– Screening for Adolescent Depression

The US Preventive Services Task Force recommends screening for depression for 12- to 18-year-old adolescents in the primary care setting when systems are in place to provide further evaluation and treatment.[49] Richardson and colleagues have evaluated the Patient Health Questionnaire-9 and have established a higher cut point for adolescents compared to adults. They found that its ease of administration and scoring make it an excellent tool for adolescent depression screening in the primary care setting.[50]

Practice-based Interventions

A variety of practice-based interventions have been developed to assist primary pediatric health care professionals in promoting healthy social and emotional development and in addressing concerns. Options range from written materials for parents, Internet resources, and seminars, to innovative models for offering health supervision and collaborative interdisciplinary practice models for addressing social and emotional concerns.

The AAP publishes a variety of brochures, books, and other materials that focus on promoting healthy social and emotional development. American Academy of Pediatrics resources are available at the AAP Online Bookstore at https://shop.aap.org/. Zero to Three has a variety of resources to help parents support social-emotional development.[51] The Centers for Disease Control and Prevention (CDC) has developed a series of 2-page downloadable handouts entitled *Positive Parenting Tips for Healthy Child Development* that offer suggestions for parents to promote social and emotional development from infancy through adolescence.[52] The CDC also hosts a series of videos entitled *Essentials for Parenting Toddlers and Preschoolers*.[53] The ASQ:SE-2 Kit includes a series of activity sheets for parents that focus on promoting social and emotional development from infancy to 6 years of age.[9]

Parent Training Programs

Among a number of parent training programs that have been developed, Incredible Years and Triple P are two that have a strong body of evidence to support their implementation. Parent training programs can be offered in the health care setting or the primary pediatric health care professional can work with community partners to ensure that such services are available to the families they serve.

The Incredible Years series targets children from 2 to 10 years of age, their parents, and their teachers. The program is designed to promote emotional and social competence and to prevent, reduce, and treat children's behavioral and emotional problems.[54] Videotaped scenes are used to encourage group discussion, problem-solving, and sharing of ideas. The core program includes 12 to 14 two-hour weekly sessions. The program teaches parents how to play with children, help children to learn, give effective praise and incentives, use limit setting, and handle misbehavior. Supplemental sessions emphasize parents' interpersonal skills, including communication, anger management, problem-solving between adults, and enhancing parent support. The Incredible Years series also includes a child-training component, which seeks to improve peer relationships and reduce aggression. The teacher training program emphasizes classroom management skills.

The Triple P, Positive Parenting Program is a tiered system of behavioral family intervention that includes a public health component and may benefit from application at a population rather than practice level.[55,56] There are 5 levels of Triple P services. The first level involves raising public awareness of the challenges of parenting and supporting families who are concerned about their child's social and emotional functioning to seek help early. The second and third levels of Triple P may be offered in the primary care setting or throughout the community. Brief, problem-specific advice is offered either as anticipatory guidance or to manage a discrete, short-lived, mild problem in an otherwise well-functioning family. The fourth level of Triple P is a more in-depth, broad-based curriculum for parents of children who have more longstanding and challenging behavioral concerns. Parents learn and practice the principles of functional behavioral assessment. Parents learn to monitor their child's behavior, determine the cause of the problem behavior, use strategies to promote social competence and self-control, and manage misbehavior. The fifth level offers assistance to parents who may be struggling with lack of partner support, high levels of stress, lack of coping skills, or difficulty with anger management. Families can enter Triple P at any level so that sufficient services are offered to match the nature of the behavioral or emotional concern. Sanders, Baker, and Turner completed a randomized controlled trial of an intensive 8-module version of Triple P Online and found high levels of parental satisfaction with the program, reduced child behavioral problems, and improved parenting practices after intervention.[57]

Expanding the primary care pediatric practice to include parent training can set the foundation for the possibility of developing more broad-based interdisciplinary services within pediatric practice. For example, the Healthy Steps for Young Children Program[58] is a model for enhanced well-child care that includes child development and family health checkups, home visits at key developmental points, written materials that emphasize prevention, a Healthy Steps telephone information line, parent groups, and linkages to community resources. An early childhood specialist works with primary pediatric health care professionals to deliver this enhanced approach. Piotrowski, Talavera, and Mayer completed a systematic review of 13 studies that have evaluated Healthy Steps. They found that the Healthy Steps program is effective in preventing negative child and parent outcomes and enhancing positive outcomes, and they recommended that the Healthy Steps program be more widely disseminated to relevant stakeholders.[59]

Group well-child visits are another innovation that may facilitate the development of social competence in families. Osborn and Woolley[60] examined the use of group discussions of 45 minutes followed by brief, individualized examinations with 4 to 6 families. Mothers were more assertive, asked more questions, and initiated discussions of more topics. There was greater coverage of recommended content and a decrease in advice-seeking between visits. Coker et al found evidence that group well-child care visits can be as effective as 1:1 visits.[61]

In the Video Interaction Project, a child development specialist covers a curriculum focused on promoting supportive parent–child interaction and then facilitates interactions in play and shared reading by reviewing a video of the parent and child interacting. This offers an opportunity to discuss developmental, behavioral, and emotional issues. Fifteen 30- to 45-minute sessions are offered through the first 3 years of life.[62] Mendelsohn et al performed a randomized, controlled trial with poor Latino children whose mothers had not completed high school and found that there were significant benefits in cognitive and language development for the children whose mothers had completed 7th to 11th grade, but not for those who completed the 6th grade or below. Other findings have included less media exposure, enhanced provision of toys, more shared reading, more teaching, and more parental verbal responsivity at 6 months old for the Video Interaction Project group.[63,64] When children were 33 months old, parents who participated in the Video Interaction Project were less stressed, and their children were more likely to have normal cognitive development and less likely to have any delayed development.[65]

Colocation and/or collaborative practice models with mental/behavioral health professionals is another approach to offering interdisciplinary services to families to address social and emotional concerns.[66] An integrated model of health care may increase the likelihood that families will pursue mental/behavioral health services and provides opportunities for support and collaboration among pediatric and mental/behavioral health professionals.

Mental/behavioral health professionals can offer parent training programs, as well as individual, group, and family therapy services that will augment routine pediatric care. Services could include opportunities to address early concerns about temperament mismatch, attachment disorders, or family violence.

Mental/behavioral health professionals can also offer cognitive behavioral therapy to parents and children for depression and anxiety. The goals of cognitive behavioral therapy are to teach the adult or child to identify their stressors and experiment with new ways of thinking and doing. Examples of promising cognitive behavioral approaches include The Optimistic Child[67] and the Coping Cat program.[68] Similar manualized approaches are available to teach relaxation and stress reduction.[69]

Anticipatory Guidance to Promote Family Relationships

The content of anticipatory guidance will be determined by the context, priorities, surveillance of development, physical examination, and screening completed during health supervision. Bright Futures suggests that anticipatory guidance should be timely, appropriate to the child and family, and relevant.[6] When concerns about social and emotional development rise to the surface, it is likely that the information in this section will prove helpful.

Carey[70] has suggested that information on temperament be part of basic education for all parents on child-rearing. Temperament refers to a child's behavioral style, or the "how" of behavior. Individual differences in temperament are real and have a significant impact on the parent-child interaction, including the parents' feelings of competency in child-rearing. It may be especially helpful in the first months of life to provide guidance related to the role of temperament in influencing children's social and emotional development.

The principles of positive parenting outlined in Triple P[71-73] (a prevention-oriented, early intervention program that aims to promote positive, caring relationships between parents and their children and to help parents develop effective management strategies for dealing with a wide variety of childhood behavior problems and common developmental issues) can serve as a framework for providing additional anticipatory guidance regarding social and emotional development.

Teaching parents skills for promoting their children's development, social competence, and self-control with evidence-based strategies will enhance their self-sufficiency in managing children's behavior. Additional benefits should include a reduction in the parents' use of coercive and punitive disciplinary methods, improved communication between parents, and less parental stress related to raising their children. Parents can be encouraged to ensure a safe and developmentally stimulating environment, create a positive learning environment using assertive discipline, have realistic expectations, and take care of themselves as parents.

A number of strategies can encourage positive relationships between parent and child. These include spending quality time with children and adolescents. Frequent, brief amounts of time, even for a few minutes, engaged in a child-preferred activity can be highly beneficial. These brief interactions offer opportunities for children to self-disclose and practice conversational skills and for adolescents to enjoy parent contact and maintain a positive relationship. Talking to children and adolescents during brief conversations about an activity or interest of the child promotes vocabulary and conversational and social skills, and gives adolescents the chance to voice opinions and to discuss issues important to them. Showing physical affection (eg, hugging, touching, cuddling, tickling, patting) and being certain to avoid public embarrassment for adolescents provides opportunities to become comfortable with intimacy and physical affection in appropriate ways.

Examples of strategies for encouraging desirable behavior for all ages are summarized here. Using descriptive praise provides encouragement and approval by describing behavior that is appreciated. This might include behaviors such as speaking in a pleasant voice, playing cooperatively, sharing, drawing pictures, reading, and compliance with instructions. Providing positive nonverbal attention (eg, a smile, wink, pat on the back, watching) will also encourage appropriate behavior. Additional strategies include arranging the child's physical and social environment to provide interesting and engaging activities, materials, and age-appropriate toys; creating opportunities for adolescents to explore and try out new social and recreational activities; and encouraging independent play and interests while promoting appropriate behavior when in community settings.

Parents can also benefit from guidance in teaching new skills and behaviors. By setting a good example, parents can demonstrate desirable behavior. Through modeling, children learn how to behave appropriately, especially in relation to interpersonal interactions and moral issues. Incidental teaching is a technique in which a series of questions and prompts is used to respond to child-initiated interactions and promote learning. This approach promotes language, problem-solving, cognitive ability, and independent play in children older than 1 year. "Ask, Say, Do" is another strategy to gradually build the confidence and skills of children 3 years of age and older. In a stepwise approach, children are first given verbal, then gestural, and then manual prompts to teach new skills.

Behavior charts are effective tools for providing social attention and backup rewards contingent on the absence of a problem behavior or the presence of an appropriate behavior. They are useful for children 2 years and older.

Adolescents can benefit by being coached in problem-solving skills. This helps them to deal with a problem in a constructive and effective way and promotes independence. Adolescents can also benefit from behavior contracts. An agreement can be negotiated to deal with a dispute or a distressing issue. This promotes development of personal responsibility. Family meetings can also be a valuable tool with this age group. By organizing a set time for family members to work together to set goals for change, adolescents learn compromise, decision-making, and personal responsibility. Scheduling a review session to check on how the strategies worked and offering suggestions for the future can reinforce the strategies that emerge from family meetings. Parents of adolescents should be encouraged to establish networks with their friends' parents to assist with monitoring their children's behavior, identify opportunities to reinforce desirable behavior, and address problem behaviors.

Regular family meals have been linked to lower levels of adolescent risk-taking behavior. Adolescents who frequently eat meals with their family are less likely to engage in risk behaviors than those who never or rarely eat with their families.[74]

Parents frequently seek guidance regarding managing misbehavior. It is important to keep in mind that focusing attention on promoting positive relationships and encouraging desirable behavior will greatly reduce the need to manage misbehavior. At the same time, numerous simple techniques are effective in managing misbehavior. Distracting the young child by drawing her attention away from a problematic activity to an acceptable activity is often beneficial. Children older than 3 years of age will respond to fair, specific, and enforceable ground rules that have been negotiated in advance. This will clarify expectations and avoid casual conflict. The use of directed discussion for rule breaking permits children to identify and rehearse the correct behavior after rule breaking. This is especially helpful for minor rule breaking and initial violations following the application of a new rule. Planned ignoring is a useful strategy for minor behavior problems in 1- to 7-year-olds. The parent can be advised to withdraw attention while the problem behavior continues and ignore attention-seeking behavior.

One of the most important suggestions for parents is to become competent in giving clear, calm instructions. Children older than 2 years of age will respond well to receiving a specific instruction to start a new task or to stop a problem behavior and start a correct behavior. It is critical that the child be told what to do rather than what not to do. Instructions should be backed up with logical consequences. The consequence should involve the removal of an activity or privilege from the child or the child from an activity for a set time. This is effective for children older than 2 years of age when dealing with noncompliance and mild behavior problems that do not occur very often.

Quiet time for misbehavior can be a valuable tool for children 18 months to 10 years of age. The child can be removed from an activity in which a problem has occurred and be instructed to sit on the edge of the activity for a set time. This can be helpful for noncompliance and for children who repeat a behavior after a logical consequence. By staying at the edge of the activity, children have a chance to see what they are missing, increasing their incentive to demonstrate desirable behavior when they return to the activity.

Time-out should be reserved for serious misbehavior in 2- to 10-year-olds. The child should be removed to an area away from others for a set time. The family may need to identify a safe place where all attention can be withdrawn from the child. It is important to consider the function of the problem behavior before deciding to use time-out. Time-out will generally be effective for attention-seeking behavior rather than avoidant behavior. If a child is acting out in order to avoid a certain request or activity, time-out may actually be an accidental reward. Time-out is helpful for children who refuse to sit in quiet time and for those having temper outbursts and aggressive or destructive behavior.

Parents of adolescents may be challenged by their child's emotional behavior. Parents may need assistance in helping their adolescent manage unpleasant or intense emotional responses that interfere with effective problem-solving or lead to more conflict and distress. For example, parents should be encouraged to acknowledge their adolescent's distress, ask what he wants his parent to do, and then coach him to problem-solve. If this is not effective, he may need a cooling-off period while setting a later time to talk again. The parent should be encouraged to stay calm and use a cooling-off period for herself, if necessary. It is also important for parents to consider the possibility that emotional behavior is being used to avoid something the adolescent should do. If that is the case, the behavior should be ignored.

Particular challenges come with addressing risky behavior in adolescents. It is important for parents to anticipate events that may lead to risk-taking behavior and prevent unexpected demands from leading to conflict or decision-making under pressure. Parents can be sure their adolescent has accurate information about the potentially risky behavior. Primary pediatric health care professionals can offer this type of information during a visit or with appropriate resources. Parents can role-play with their adolescent to give them an opportunity to practice the words they will use when pressured into a possible risky behavior. Parents should be sure their adolescent knows they will be available to rescue them if they find themselves in an uncomfortable situation. Parents can work with their child in advance to negotiate a fair set of rules with preordained consequences. This approach will ensure that important decisions are not made on inaccurate assumptions and that the adolescent has the chance to participate in peer activities with a clearly established plan to support her in avoiding risky behavior.

Promoting Community Relationships and Resources

Primary pediatric health care professionals are in a unique position to foster the development of community relationships to address the social and emotional development of children. In the course of daily practice, it is likely that assets that are available in the community to support children and families will become evident (see Chapter 25, Social and Community Services for Children With Developmental Disabilities and/or Behavioral Disorders and Their Families). This information can be shared on the practice's Web site, in information kiosks in the office, on bulletin boards, and in the course of a visit. In addition, opportunities for the development of new programs and services will become apparent through repeated contacts with families and community leaders.

There are numerous evidence-based programs that have been developed as preventive and intervention models related to address the social and emotional development of children. When opportunities arise to promote development of community relationships and resources, it is important to consider whether existing, proven, or promising programs from across the country and across the world may be applicable in the primary pediatric health care professional's local community.

The primary pediatric health care professional has an important role in linking families with early intervention services.[75] Children who exhibit concerns in their social-emotional development may benefit from early intervention services through Part C of the Individuals with Disabilities Education Act (see Chapter 6, Early Intervention). Programs like Help Me Grow, which has over 20 affiliate partner states,[76] have trained health care professionals to perform effective developmental surveillance, created resource inventories of community-based services, and developed a referral and monitoring system to link young children and their families with early childhood services and support.

Several programs have included home visits as core components. The Nurse-Family Partnership is a prenatal and early infancy home visiting program that has demonstrated better infant emotional and language development and improved maternal independence.[77] The Infant Health and Development Program (IHDP)[78-80] was a multicenter, comprehensive early intervention program for low-birth-weight (≤2,500 g) and premature (≤37 weeks) infants that has proven to reduce the infants' health and developmental problems. The IHDP was designed as a randomized, clinical trial that combined early child development and family support services with pediatric follow-up for the first 3 years of life. The intervention services, provided free to participating families, consisted of 3 components: home visits, child attendance at a child development center, and parent group meetings. Infants participated in pediatric follow-up, which comprised medical, developmental, and social assessments, with referral for pediatric care and other services as indicated.

Early Head Start is a federally funded, community-based program for low-income pregnant women and families with infants and toddlers up to age 3 years. Its mission is to promote healthy prenatal outcomes for pregnant women, enhance the development of children from birth to 3 years of age, and support healthy family functioning. Services include child development services delivered in home visits, child care, comprehensive health and mental health services, parenting education, nutrition education, health care and referrals, and family support. Each community has the opportunity to select options for providing services that best meet the community's needs.[81,82]

Promoting First Relationships[83] is a curriculum designed to guide caregivers in building nurturing and responsive relationships with children from birth to 3 years of age. The program focuses on promoting the development of trust and security in infancy and promoting healthy development of self during toddlerhood, while assisting caregivers in understanding and intervening with children's challenging behaviors.

Big Brothers Big Sisters[84] is a program that matches unrelated mentors who serve as role models for children to promote positive development and social responsibility. This program has been shown to reduce rates of alcohol, tobacco, or illegal drug use and appears promising in reducing violent behavior and serious conduct problems and in performing at grade level.

A number of school-based programs are promising as well. For example, the Cognitive Relaxation Coping Skills program[85] is designed to increase sixth to eighth graders' ability to control their emotions. Students are taught relaxation methods and strategies to change attitudes. By learning how to control their anger, they avoid frustrating situations. The Reaching Educators, Children, and Parents program[86,87] is a semistructured, school-based skills training program designed for children experiencing internalizing and externalizing problems. The primary goal of the program is to reduce the level of children's psychological problems, as well as preventing the development of more serious problems among children who are not referred for formal mental health services. The Social Decision Making/Problem Solving program[88,89] can be provided to any student, rather than targeting those with special characteristics. The program seeks to develop children's self-esteem, self-control, and social awareness skills, including identifying, monitoring, and regulating stress and emotions; increasing healthy lifestyle choices; avoiding social problems, such as substance abuse, violence, and school failure; improving group cooperation skills; and enhancing the ability to develop positive peer relationships.

Additional information on the programs outlined here and on similar promising or proven programs is available at **www.promisingpractices.net.**

The Good Behavior Game is a classroom management strategy focused on improving attention and social skills that has demonstrated improved classroom behavior and long-term reductions in rates of antisocial personality disorder, tobacco, drug, and alcohol use, violence, and suicidal ideation in young adulthood.[90]

It is also important to consider that the media, including television and the Internet, may have broad applications for reaching large populations of people to promote healthy social and emotional development. In 2005 in the United Kingdom, a 5-episode television series, *Driving Mum and Dad Mad,* aired on prime-time television. In a project called The Great Parenting Experiment,[91] 500 families who viewed the series and had access to Web support and self-help materials reported improved confidence in managing their children's behavior. For some parents, television may be the only way they will access parenting information.

Text4Baby is a mobile information service designed to promote maternal and child health through text messaging. Pregnant women and new mothers who enroll receive 3 free text messages per week that are timed to their delivery date and continue through their child's first birthday. Preliminary evaluation findings indicate that Text4Baby is increasing the users' health knowledge, facilitating interaction with their health providers, improving their adherence to appointments and immunizations, and improving their access to health services.[92]

Boston Basics offers many resources, including booklets and videos to support families with young children in providing nurturing, supportive environments.[93]

There are many evidence-based prevention and intervention strategies available. As primary pediatric health care professionals identify needs in their community, it will be important to investigate and advocate for implementation of strategies that have been shown to be effective in other settings.

Conclusion

Healthy social and emotional development is rooted in the quality of relationships with parents, extended family, caregivers, peers, teachers, coaches, and other adults. It is vital for primary pediatric health care professionals to consider the dynamic interactions between the child's genetics, biology, and temperament with the environment in which he or she is expected to grow and develop. By following the Bright Futures recommendations for promoting child development and mental/behavioral health, while also promoting community relationships and resources, the primary pediatric health care professional will be well positioned to support children, adolescents, and their families in fostering healthy social and emotional development. Each preventive health visit provides an opportunity to establish a context for the visit and to set priorities for the visit. Should these identify social and emotional development as a priority, then an appropriate review of the interval history, observation of parent-child interaction, surveillance of development and behavior, a physical examination, and screening will provide a fund of information to guide anticipatory guidance, office-based interventions, and referral to community resources.

References

1. Cozolino L. *The Neuroscience of Human Relationships: Attachment and the Developing Social Brain.* New York, NY: W.W. Norton & Company; 2006
2. America's Promise Alliance. The five promises change lives. http://www.americaspromise.org/promises. Accessed November 22, 2017
3. Felitti VJ, Anda RF, Nordenberg D, et al. The relationship of adult health status to childhood abuse and household dysfunction. *Am J Prev Med.* 1998;14(4):245–258
4. Shonkoff JP, Garner AS; American Academy of Pediatrics Committee on Psychosocial Aspects of Child and Family Health; Committee on Early Childhood, Adoption, and Dependent Care; Section on Developmental and Behavioral Pediatrics. The lifelong effects of early childhood adversity and toxic stress. *Pediatrics.* 2012;129(1):e232–e246
5. Chess S, Thomas A. The development of behavioral individuality. In: Levine MD, Carey WB, Crocker AC, eds. *Developmental-Behavioral Pediatrics.* 3rd ed. Philadelphia, PA: W. B. Saunders Company; 1999:89–99
6. Hagan JF, Shaw JS, Duncan PM, eds. *Bright Futures: Guidelines for Health Supervision of Infants, Children, and Adolescents.* 4th ed. Elk Grove Village, IL: American Academy of Pediatrics; 2017
7. Fine A, Large R. *A Conceptual Framework for Adolescent Health: A Collaborative Project of the Association of Maternal and Child Health Programs and the National Network of State Adolescent Health Coordinators.* Baltimore, MD: The Annie E. Casey Foundation; 2005
8. American Academy of Pediatrics Council on Children With Disabilities; Section on Developmental and Behavioral Pediatrics; Bright Futures Steering Committee; Medical Home Initiatives for Children With Special Needs Project Advisory Committee. Identifying infants and young children with developmental disorders in the medical home: an algorithm for developmental surveillance and screening. *Pediatrics.* 2006;118(1):405–420
9. Squires J, Bricker D, Twombly, E. *The ASQ: SE-2 User's Guide for the Ages and Stages Questionnaires: Social-Emotional-2.* Baltimore, MD: Paul H. Brookes Publishing Co.; 2015
10. Carlson VJ, Harwood RL. What do we expect? Understanding and negotiating cultural differences concerning early developmental competence: the six raisin solution. *Zero to Three.* 1999;20:19–24
11. Singleton L. Parental mental illness: the effects on children and their needs. *Br J Nurs.* 2007;16(14):847–850
12. Fantuzzo JW, Mohr WK. Prevalence and effects of child exposure to domestic violence. *Future Child.* 1999;9(3):21–32
13. American Academy of Pediatrics Council on Community Pediatrics. Poverty and child health in the United States. *Pediatrics.* 2016;137(4):e20160339
14. Pascoe JM, Wood DL, Duffee JH, et al. mediators and adverse effects of child poverty in the United States. *Pediatrics.* 2016;137(4):e20160340

15. Costello EJ, Edelbrock C, Costello AJ, Dulcan MK, Burns BJ, Bren D. Psychopathology in pediatric primary care: the new hidden morbidity. *Pediatrics.* 1988;82(3 Pt 2):415–424

16. Weitzman C, Wegner L, American Academy of Pediatrics Section on Developmental and Behavioral Pediatrics, Committee on Psychosocial Aspects of Child and Family Health, Council on Early Childhood, and Society for Developmental and Behavioral Pediatrics. Promoting optimal development: screening for behavioral and emotional problems. *Pediatrics.* 2015;135(2):384–395

17. Earls MF. American Academy of Pediatrics Committee on Psychosocial Aspects of Child and Family Health. Incorporating recognition and management of perinatal and postpartum depression into pediatric practice. *Pediatrics.* 2010;126(5):1032–1039

18. Glascoe FP, Maclean WE, Stone WL. The importance of parents' concerns about their child's behavior. *Clin Pediatr (Phila).* 1991;30(1):8–11

19. Mulhern S, Dworkin PH, Bernstein B. Do parental concerns predict a diagnosis of attention deficit-hyperactivity disorder (ADHD). *Am J Dis Child.* 1993;147:419

20. Solomon R. Pediatricians and early intervention: everything you need to know but are too busy to ask. *Infants Young Child.* 1995;7(3):38–51

21. American Academy of Pediatrics Taskforce on Coding for Mental Health in Children. Wolraich, ML, Felice ME, Drotar D, eds. *The Classification of Child and Adolescent Mental Diagnoses in Primary Care: Diagnostic and Statistical Manual for Primary Care (DSM-PC) Child and Adolescent Version.* Elk Grove Village, IL: American Academy of Pediatrics; 1996

22. Anastasiow NJ. *Emotions, Affects, and Attachment, Development and Disability.* Baltimore, MD: Paul H. Brookes; 1986:95–110

23. Perrin E, Stancin T. A continuing dilemma: whether and how to screen for concerns about children's behavior. *Pediatr Rev.* 2002;23(8):264–276

24. Plauche-Johnson C, Meyers SM; American Academy of Pediatrics Council on Children With Disabilities. Identification and evaluation of children with autism spectrum disorders. *Pediatrics.* 2007;120(5):1183–1215

25. Kerker BD, Storfer-Isser A, Stein RE, Garner A, Szilagyi M, O'Connor KG, Hoagwood KE, Horwitz SM. Identifying maternal depression in pediatric primary care: changes over a decade. *J Dev Behav Pediatr.* 2016;37(2):113–120

26. Myers ER, Aubuchon-Endsley N, Bastian LA, et al. *Efficacy and Safety of Screening for Postpartum Depression.* Comparative Effectiveness Review 106. (Prepared by the Duke Evidence-based Practice Center under Contract No. 290–2007–10066-I.) AHRQ Publication No. 13-EHC064-EF. Rockville, MD: Agency for Healthcare Research and Quality; April 2013. www.effectivehealthcare.ahrq.gov/reports/final.cfm.

27. Radloff LS. The CES-D scale: a self-report depression scale for research in the general population. *Appl Psychol Meas.* 1977;1:385–401

28. Kroenke K, Spitzer RL, Williams JB. The Patient Health Questionnaire-2: validity of a two-item depression screener. *Med Care.* 2003;41(11):1284–1292

29. Olson AL, Dietrich AJ, Prazar G, Hurley J. Brief maternal depression screening at well-child visits. *Pediatrics.* 2006;118(1):207–216

30. Fairbrother N, Young AH, Zhang A, Janssen P, Antony MM. The prevalence and incidence of perinatal anxiety disorders among women experiencing a medically complicated pregnancy. *Arch Womens Ment Health.* 2017;20(2):311–319

31. Crawford JR, Henry JD. The Depression Anxiety Stress Scales (DASS): normative data and latent structure in a large non-clinical sample. *Br J Clin Psychol.* 2003;42(Pt 2):111–131

32. Abidin RR. *Parenting Stress Index.* 3rd ed. Lutz, FL: Psychological Assessment Resources; 1995

33. Felitti VJ, Anda RF, Nordenberg D, et al. The relationship of adult health status to childhood abuse and household dysfunction. *Am J Prev Med.* 1998;14(4):245–258

34. Medoff-Cooper B, Carey WB, McDevitt SC. The early infancy temperament questionnaire. *J Dev Behav Pediatr.* 1993;14(4):230–235

35. B-di.com. Understanding behavioral individuality. http://www.b-di.com/shoppingindex.html. Accessed November 22, 2017

36. Provence S. An interview for one day. In: Green M, Haggerty R, eds. *Ambulatory Pediatrics II.* Philadelphia, PA: W. B. Saunders Company; 1977:947–948

37. Wetherby AM, Prizant BM. *Communication and Symbolic Behavior Scales Developmental Profile.* Baltimore, MD: Paul H. Brookes Publishing; 2002

38. Briggs-Gowan MJ, Carter AS, et al. The Brief Infant-Toddler Social and Emotional Assessment: screening for social-emotional problems and delays in competence. *J Pediatr Psychol.* 2004;29(2):143–155

39. Carter AS, Briggs-Gowan MJ, Jones SM, Little TD. The Infant-Toddler Social Emotional Assessment (ITSEA): factor structure, reliability, and validity. *J Abnorm Child Psychol.* 2003;31(5):495–514

40. Eyberg S, Ross AW. *The Eyberg Child Behavior Inventory.* Lutz, FL: Psychological Assessment Resources; 1999

41. Jellinek MS, Murphy JM, Robinson J, Feins A, Lamb S, Fenton T. Pediatric Symptom Checklist: screening school-age children for psychosocial dysfunction. *J Pediatr.* 1988; 112(2):201–209

42. Murphy JM, Bergmann P, Chiang C, et al. The PSC-17: subscale scores, reliability, and factor structure in a new national sample. *Pediatrics.* 2016;138(3):pii:e20160038

43. Sturner R, Howard BJ, Morrel T, Rogers-Senuta K. *Validation of a Computerized Parent Questionnaire for Identifying Child Mental Health Disorders and Implementing DSM-PC.* Pediatric Academic Societies Meeting; 2003

44. Achenbach T. *Medical Practitioners' Guide for the ASEBA.* Burlington, VT: Research Center for Children, Youth, and Families, Inc; 2007

45. Reynolds CR, Kamphaus RW. *Behavior Assessment System for Children.* 2nd ed. Bloomington, MN: Pearson Assessments; 2004

46. Conners CK. *Conners Comprehensive Behavior Rating Scales.* Los Angeles, CA: Western Psychological Services; 2008

47. Gadow KD, Sprafkin J. *Child Symptom Inventory-4.* Los Angeles, CA: Western Psychological Services; 1998

48. Wolraich ML, Hannah JN, Pinnock TY, et al. Comparison of diagnostic criteria for attention-deficit hyperactivity disorder in a county wide sample. *J Am Acad Child Adolesc Psychiatry.* 1996;35(3):319–324

49. US Preventive Services Task Force. Screening and treatment for major depressive disorder in children and adolescents: US Preventive Services Task Force Recommendation Statement. *Pediatrics.* 2009;123(4):1223–1228

50. Richardson LP, McCauley E, Grossman DC, et al. Evaluation of the Patient Health Questionnaire (PHQ-9) for detecting major depression among adolescents. *Pediatrics.* 2010;126(6):1117–1123

51. Zero to Three. Social-emotional development. https://www.zerotothree.org/resources/series/developing-social-emotional-skills. Accessed November 22, 2017

52. Centers for Disease Control and Prevention. Positive parenting tips. https://www.cdc.gov/ncbddd/childdevelopment/positiveparenting/. Accessed November 22, 2017

53. Centers for Disease Control and Prevention. Essentials for parenting toddlers and preschoolers. https://www.cdc.gov/parents/essentials/index.html. Accessed November 22, 2017

54. Webster-Stratton C, Reid MJ, Hammond M. Treating children with early-onset conduct problems: intervention outcomes for parent, child, and teacher training. *J Clin Child Adolesc Psychol.* 2004;33(1):105–124

55. Sanders MR, Markie-Dadds C, Turner KMT. *Theoretical, Scientific, and Clinical Foundations of Triple P-Positive Parenting Program: A Population Approach to the Promotion of Parenting Competence. Parenting Research and Practice Monograph No. 1.* Queensland, Australia: Parenting and Family Support Centre, University of Queensland; 2003

56. Prinz RJ, Sanders MR. Adopting a population-level approach to parenting and family support interventions. *Clin Psychol Rev.* 2007;27(6):739–749

57. Sanders M R, Baker S, Turner KMT. A randomized controlled trial evaluating the efficacy of Triple P Online with parents of children with early onset conduct problems. *Behav Res Ther.* 2012;50(11):675–684

58. Minkovitz CS, Hughart N, Strobino D, et al. A practice-based intervention to enhance quality of care in the first 3 years of life: the Healthy Steps for Young Children Program. *JAMA.* 2003;290(23):3081–3091

59. Piotrowski CC, Talavera GA, Mayer JA. Healthy steps: a systematic review of a preventive practice-based model of pediatric care. *J Dev Behav Pediatr.* 2009;30(1):91–103

60. Osborn FM, Woolley FR. Use of groups in well child care. *Pediatrics.* 1981;67(5):701–706

61. Coker TR, Thomas T, Chung PJ. Does well-child care have a future in pediatrics? *Pediatrics.* 2013;131(suppl 2):S149–S159

62. Mendelsohn AL, Cates CB, Weisleder A, Berkule SB, Dreyer BP. Promotion of early school readiness utilizing pediatric primary care as an innovative platform. *Zero to Three.* 2013;34(1):29–40

63. Mendelsohn AL, Dreyer BP, Flynn V, et al. Use of videotaped interactions during pediatric well-child care to promote child development: a randomized, controlled trial. *J Dev Behav Pediatr.* 2005;26(1):34–41

64. Mendelsohn AL, Dreyer BP, Brockmeyer CA, et al. Randomized controlled trial of primary care pediatric parenting programs: effect on reduced media exposure in infants, mediated through enhanced parent-child interaction. *Arch Pediatr Adolesc Med.* 2011;165(1):42–48

65. Mendelsohn AL, Valdez PT, Flynn V, Foley GM, Berkule SB, Dreyer BP. Use of videotaped interactions during pediatric well-child care: impact at 33 months on parenting and on child development. *J Dev Behav Pediatr.* 2007;28(3):206–212

66. Stancin T, Perrin EC. Psychologists and pediatricians: opportunities for collaboration in primary care. *Am Psychol.* 2014;69(4):332–343

67. Seligman MEP. *The Optimistic Child: A Proven Program to Safeguard Children Against Depression and Build Lifelong Resilience.* New York, NY: Houghton Mifflin Company; 1995

68. Flannery-Schroeder EC, Kendall PC. Group and individual cognitive-behavioral treatments for youth with anxiety disorders: a randomized clinical trial. *Cognit Ther Res.* 2000;24(3):251–278

69. Davis M, Robbins-Eshelmann E, McKay M. *The Relaxation and Stress Reduction Workbook.* Oakland, CA: New Harbinger Publications; 2000

70. Carey WB. Teaching parents about infant temperament. *Pediatrics.* 1998;102:1311–1315

71. Turner KMT, Sanders MR, Markie-Dadds C. *Practitioner's Manual for Primary Care Triple P.* Milton, Queensland, Australia: Triple P International Pty. Ltd.; 1999

72. Sanders MR, Ralph A. *Practitioner's Manual for Primary Care Teen Triple P.* Milton, Queensland, Australia: Families International Publishing Pty. Ltd.; 2001

73. Sanders MR. *Every Parent: A Positive Approach to Children's Behaviour.* Camberwell, Victoria, Australia: Penguin; 2004

74. Skeer MR, Ballard EL. Are family meals as good for youth as we think they are? A review of the literature on family meals as they pertain to adolescent risk prevention. *J Youth Adolesc.* 2013;42(7):943–963

75. Adams, RC, Tapia C, American Academy of Pediatrics Council on Children With Disabilities. Early intervention, IDEA Part C services, and the medical home: collaboration for best practice and best outcomes. *Pediatrics.* 2013;132(4):e1073–e1088

76. Jones E. *Help Me Grow Promotes Optimal Child Development by Enhancing Protective Factors.* Hartford CT: Help Me Grow National Center; 2013

77. Olds DL. The nurse-family partnership: an evidence-based preventive intervention. *Infant Ment Health J.* 2006;27(1):5–25

78. Ramey CT, Bryant DM, Waski BH, Sparling JJ, Fendt KH, LaVange LM. Infant health and development program for low birth weight, premature infants: program elements, family participation, and child intelligence. *Pediatrics.* 1992;89(3):454–465

79. McCormick MC, McCarton C, Tonascia J, Brooks-Gunn J. Early educational intervention for very low birth weight infants: results from the infant health and development program. *J Pediatr.* 1993;123(4):527–533

80. McCarton CM, Brooks-Gunn J, Wallace IF, et al. Results at age 8 years of early intervention for low-birth-weight premature infants. *JAMA.* 1997;277(2):126–132

81. Love JM, Kisker EE, Ross CM, et al. *Making a Difference in the Lives of Infants and Toddlers and Their Families: The Impacts of Early Head Start, Vol I, Final Technical Report.* Princeton, NJ: Mathematica Policy Research, Inc., and New York, NY: Columbia University's Center for Children and Families at Teachers College; 2002

82. Roggman LA, Boyce LK, Cook GA, Hart AD. How much better than expected? Improving cognitive outcomes in Utah's Bear River Early Head Start. In: *The Early Head Start Research Consortium,* eds. *Making a Difference in the Lives of Infants and Toddlers and Their Families: The Impacts of Early Head Start, Vol III: Local Contributions to Understanding the Programs and Their Impacts.* Princeton, NJ: Mathematica Policy Research, Inc.; 2002:127–138

83. Kelly JF, Zuckerman T, Rosenblatt S. Promoting first relationships: a relationship-focused early intervention approach. *Infants Young Child.* 2008;21(4):285–289

84. Morrow KV, Styles MB. *Building Relationships With Youth in Program Settings: A Study of Big Brothers/ Big Sisters.* Philadelphia, PA: Public/Private Ventures; 1995

85. Deffenbacher JL, Lynch RS, Oetting ER, Kemper CC. Anger reduction in early adolescents. *J Couns Psychol.* 1996;43(2):149–157

86. Kataoka SH, Stein BD, Jaycox LH, et al. A school-based mental health program for traumatized Latino immigrant children. *J Am Acad Child Adolesc Psychiatry.* 2003;42(3):311–318

87. Stein BD, Jaycox LH, Kataoka SH, et al. A mental health intervention for schoolchildren exposed to violence: a randomized controlled trial. *JAMA.* 2003;290(3):603–611

88. Elias MJ. Improving coping skills of emotionally disturbed boys through television-based social problem-solving. *Am J Orthopsychiatry.* 1983;53(1):61–72

89. Elias MJ, Gara M, Ubriaco M, Rothbaum PA, Clabby JF, Schuyler T. Impact of a preventive social problem-solving intervention on children's coping with middle-school stressors. *Am J Community Psychol.* 1986;14(3):259–275

90. Poduska, JM and Kurki, A. Guided by theory, informed by practice: training and support for the good behavior game, a classroom-based behavior management strategy. *J Emot Behav Disord.* 2014;22(2):83–94

91. Sanders M, Calam R, Durand M, Liversidge T, Carmont SA. Does self-directed and web-based support for parents enhance the effects of viewing a reality television series based on the Triple P Positive Parenting Programme? *J Child Psychol Psychiatry.* 2008;49(9):924–932

92. Remick AP, Kendrick JS. Breaking new ground: the text4baby program. *Am J Health Promot.* 2013;27(3 suppl):S4–S6

93. Boston Basics. http://boston.thebasics.org/en/. Accessed November 22, 2017

CHAPTER 13

Sensory Impairments: Hearing and Vision

Desmond P. Kelly, MD, FAAP

Stuart W. Teplin, MD, FAAP

Introduction

The ability to accurately receive and interpret a variety of environmental and internal somatic signals comprises the domain of sensory neurological functioning. In addition to the 5 major sensory systems (vision, hearing, touch, taste, and smell), other internal sensory systems provide and integrate other types of information about the body's current status and safety. These include sensations of pain, hunger, and temperature, as well as integrated awareness of body position in, and movement through, space (kinesthesia), using vestibular and proprioceptive functions.

This chapter focuses on the conditions resulting from impairments or loss of **hearing** and/or **visual function**. Although these 2 major sensory systems and their respective dysfunctions differ considerably, the following descriptions also illustrate several common features: As infants and children progress through normal neuro-developmental stages, both visual and auditory information are integral components of *other* central nervous system (CNS) domains, eg, language and nonverbal concept development, motor skills, and social interactions. When these sensory signals are distorted or diminished, the child's CNS can learn to rely more on alternative sensory information in the child's quest for understanding, interacting with, and moving through his or her world. For primary pediatric health care professionals, similar broad diagnostic and intervention goals emerge for both vision- and hearing-impaired children and their families. These goals include the following: systematic screening/ early detection and accurate diagnosis; coordinated early intervention services and targeted special education; awareness of recent trends in technology for screening, diagnosis, and treatment; and the critical importance of advocacy for families and helping them find supports.

Hearing Impairment

Even mild degrees of hearing loss can impede language, social, and learning abilities. Universal newborn hearing screening has significantly lowered the average age of identification of hearing loss, but many eventually identified children, especially those with progressive or delayed onset of hearing loss or those with inadequate or inconsistent access to health care, are unfortunately still diagnosed only after crucial developmental opportunities have been missed.[1,2] Comprehensive treatment with early identification, amplification of hearing, and educational interventions to promote communication facilitate optimal outcomes. Primary pediatric health care professionals must therefore be knowledgeable regarding screening and diagnosis of hearing impairment and the interventions that enable optimal functional outcomes for children with hearing loss.[1,2]

Epidemiology and Etiology

The prevalence of hearing loss varies depending on the population studied, but the overall rate of congenital severe-to-profound bilateral sensorineural hearing loss (SNHL) has remained stable at about 1 to 2 per 1,000 live births.[3] A further 2 to 3 per 1,000 subsequently acquire severe loss. Many more children suffer milder degrees of hearing impairment or unilateral hearing loss. The broad categories of hearing impairment include *sensorineural* (dysfunction of the cochlea and/or its neural connections to the cortex) and *conductive* hearing loss (interruption along the conductive pathways, eg, the pinna, external auditory canal, tympanic membrane, and middle ear structures]), or a combination of SNHL and conductive hearing loss.

A genetic etiology is the most likely explanation in about 50% of cases, if other investigations have failed to identify a definite cause for a child's hearing loss. In children with an identified genetic cause, 30% have an identified syndrome. Table 13.1 lists a few of the more common syndromes that are associated with hearing loss. Of those children with nonsyndromic hearing loss, 80% have an autosomal recessive pattern of inheritance, frequently with no family history of hearing loss or external physical manifestations of the disorder.[4] X-linked and mitochondrial inheritance account for only 1% to 2% of nonsyndromic hearing loss.[5] More than 100 loci for genes associated with nonsyndromic hearing impairment have been identified.[4,5] Mutations in the gap junction proteins beta 2 and beta 6 (GJB2 and GJB6) are a common cause of hearing impairment, and a mutation of GJB2, which encodes the connexin protein 26 (critical for potassium homeostasis in the cochlea), is responsible for up to 50% of the hearing loss in certain populations.[5]

Prenatally acquired causes of hearing impairment include congenital infections (eg, toxoplasmosis, rubella, cytomegalovirus, herpes simplex, and Zika virus[6]), and prenatal exposure to toxins such as alcohol and mercury.[2,3] Extremely premature infants are at increased risk of hearing loss due to a variety of factors including hypoxia, acidosis, hypoglycemia, hyperbilirubinemia, high levels of ambient noise, and ototoxic drugs, such as aminoglycosides and diuretics. Immunization has decreased the incidence of bacterial meningitis, which is associated with SNHL in up to 10% of cases.[3] Audiological follow-up of these children is essential, as the hearing loss can be progressive.

Prolonged exposure to loud noise, either environmental or recreational (especially related to the use of audio headphones or ear pieces), is an increasingly common cause of high-frequency hearing loss (Table 13.2).

Table 13.1. Genetic Syndromes That Are Associated With Hearing Loss	
Syndrome	**Associated Clinical Features**
Autosomal Dominant	
Waardenburg	White forelock, heterochromia iridis, lateral displacement of inner canthus of eyes, and vestibular dysfunction
Alport	Progressive high-frequency SNHL and specific form of glomerulonephritis
Branchio-oto-renal	Preauricular pits and pinna abnormalities, renal anomalies (hypoplasia/dysplasia), mixed hearing loss; can have temporal bone abnormalities
Stickler	Cleft palate, flat facies, myopia, retinal detachment, high-frequency SNHL, spondyloepiphyseal dysplasia, and hypotonia
Treacher Collins	Bilateral symmetrical pinna abnormalities, malar hypoplasia, down-slanting palpebral fissures, and malformation of external ear (conductive hearing loss)
Autosomal Recessive	
Usher	Retinitis pigmentosa and vestibular dysfunction (3 types with varying degrees of hearing loss—progressive)
Pendred	Progressive high-frequency loss, enlarged vestibular aqueduct, incomplete partitioning of the cochlea, and thyroid dysfunction
Jervell and Lange-Nielsen	Absent vestibular function (motor incoordination) and cardiac conduction problems (prolonged QT interval)

Table 13.2. Degree and Effects of Hearing Loss[a]		
Degree of Hearing Loss	**Hearing Level (dB)**	**Effects (if not corrected)**
Normal	0–15	• Can detect all aspects of speech
Minimal	16–25	• May miss up to 10% of speech • May respond inappropriately • Peer social interaction affected
Mild	26–40	• May miss up to 50% of speech • May be labeled as "behavior problem" and "poor listener"
Moderate	41–55	• May miss 50% to 100% of speech • Speech quality likely to be poor • Vocabulary limited • Has compromised communication ability
Moderate/ Severe	56–70	• One hundred percent of normal volume speech lost • Can have delayed speech and poor intelligibility • Social isolation is likely
Severe	71–90	• Loud voices heard only within 12 inches of the ear • Has delayed speech and language if loss is prelingual • Has declining speech ability and atonal voice if loss is postlingual
Profound	90+	• Sound vibrations felt rather than heard • Is unable to communicate other than through visual or tactile cues

[a] Adapted with permission from Bachmann KR, Arvedson JC. Early identification and intervention for children who are hearing impaired. *Pediatr Rev.* 1998;19:155–165.

Identification

The key to an optimal outcome for the child with a hearing impairment is early identification and intervention. In 2007, the Joint Committee on Infant Hearing, which includes representatives from the American Academy of Pediatrics (AAP), issued an updated position statement reaffirming the recommendation for universal screening of newborns for hearing loss.[2] The US Preventive Services Task Force, in its 2008 update, affirmed that there is good evidence that newborn hearing screening is highly accurate with limited evidence about harms of screening.[7] It is also recommended that all infants who have risk indicators for delayed onset or progressive hearing loss should have regular assessment of hearing every 6 months until age 3 years.

The Centers for Disease Control and Prevention (CDC) Early Hearing Detection and Intervention Program has set "1–3–6" goals. These goals are hearing screening before 1 month of age, diagnostic audiological evaluation for children with hearing loss before 3 months of age, and early intervention for these children before 6 months of age.[1] Despite the success of the hearing screening initiative (more than 95% of newborns are screened for hearing loss), diagnosis is often delayed. Less than 60% of newborns who fail screening have a documented diagnosis, and 77% of those diagnosed with hearing loss receive intervention services by 6 months of age. The US Department of Health and Human Services held an invitational workshop in 2008, with recommendations subsequently published, to improve the quality of tracking following newborn hearing screening and to follow up for diagnosis and early intervention.[1] Recommendations included goals to (1) improve screening protocols and diagnostic testing before discharge from the NICU, (2) link infants who did not pass screening with a medical home provider, (3) increase timely access to effective early intervention services, (4) develop initiatives to improve access to loaner hearing aids, and (5) create a systematic process for monitoring developmental outcomes with the involvement of families and children. Primary pediatric health care professionals must also be alert to recognize signs of delayed or progressive hearing loss in children, especially those with risk factors as outlined in Box 13.1.

Primary pediatric health care professionals should not rely only on behavioral symptoms to identify hearing loss, although such symptoms might lead parents to raise concerns. The obvious manifestations of hearing loss include failure of an infant to startle to loud noises or to turn to localize a sound. Toddlers might not respond to environmental sounds or might appear to ignore requests or instructions or request a higher volume on electronic sound sources. Hearing loss might also manifest as social-emotional developmental delays, including behaviors that could be interpreted as features of autism spectrum disorder (ASD). A key clinical sign in children with severe to profound hearing loss is the failure to develop "canonical babbling" (use of discrete syllables such as "ba," "da," and "na") by 11 months. It should be noted that youngsters with even a profound hearing loss will begin to vocalize before 6 months of age, although further language development is impeded. If there is any suspicion of hearing loss or any delays in language development or social communication, there should be no delay in referring that child for formal audiological evaluation. Likewise, in children with otitis media with persistent middle ear effusion, the level of hearing loss should be documented and monitored closely.

Box 13.1. Risk Factors and Red Flags for Delayed Onset of Hearing Loss

- ▸ Caregiver concern regarding hearing, speech, language, or developmental delay
- ▸ Family history of permanent childhood hearing loss
- ▸ Neonatal intensive care of more than 5 days or any of the following regardless of length of stay:
  - – ECMO
  - – Assisted ventilation
  - – Exposure to ototoxic medications (gentamicin and tobramycin) or loop diuretics (furosemide)
  - – Hyperbilirubinemia requiring exchange transfusion
- ▸ In utero infections (eg, cytomegalovirus, rubella, syphilis, herpes, toxoplasmosis, or Zika virus)
- ▸ Craniofacial anomalies (involving the pinna, ear canal, ear tags, ear pits, and temporal bone anomalies)
- ▸ Syndromes associated with progressive hearing loss such as neurofibromatosis, osteopetrosis, Usher syndrome, and other more commonly identified syndromes (see Table 13.1)
- ▸ Neurodegenerative disorders such as Hunter syndrome
- ▸ Sensory motor neuropathies such as Friedreich ataxia and Charcot-Marie-Tooth syndrome
- ▸ Postnatal infections associated with SNHL including bacterial and viral (herpesvirus and varicella) meningitis
- ▸ Head trauma, especially basal skull/temporal bone fractures
- ▸ Chemotherapy

Abbreviation: ECMO, extracorporeal membrane oxygenation.

Adapted with permission from American Academy of Pediatrics, Joint Committee on Infant Hearing. Year 2007 position statement. Principles and guidelines for early hearing detection and intervention programs. *Pediatrics.* 2007;120(4):898–921.

Developmental Impact of Hearing Loss

Delayed development of speech is a universal symptom of hearing impairment, and even milder persistent degrees of hearing impairment can cause difficulties with language development, especially the processing and production of the softer, higher frequency sounds, such as some consonants (eg, "s" and "t"). Some degree of impairment of later *language development* and function is likely in children whose hearing loss is not corrected before 12 months of age. The degree of language delay is dependent on the severity and timing (prelingual or postlingual) of the hearing loss and the adequacy of intervention. Although expert opinions have varied over the years, it is now agreed that deafness per se does not impart limitations to *cognition*. However, some children who are deaf have less cognitive flexibility.

Most thought processes are mediated by language, and studies of children with deafness show that they place greater reliance than hearing children do on visual-spatial, short-term memory rather than on temporal-sequential coding.[8] Some studies indicate more efficient visual processing abilities. Children with associated vestibular dysfunction are at increased risk for difficulty with balance, equilibrium, and related *motor skills.* Children who are deaf or hard of hearing have been described as less socially mature. Language and communication is, of course, a central component of all social exchanges. A hearing evaluation should be the first step in the evaluation of any child suspected of having ASD. Although there has been a paucity of research regarding attention deficits in children who are deaf, it is clear that a youngster who is reliant on visual input for learning and communication would be at double jeopardy for learning problems if he or she also had attention weaknesses. Studies utilizing parent and teacher questionnaire ratings at a residential school for children who are deaf found that the overall prevalence of attention deficits in children who are deaf was not higher than for the general population. However, in that study, children with acquired deafness, eg, as a consequence of bacterial meningitis, manifested an increased prevalence of both attention deficits and learning disabilities.[9]

The most recent *Annual Survey of Hearing-Impaired Children and Youth* by Gallaudet University in 2010 reported that 39% of deaf children were classified as having educationally significant associated disabilities, with many of those being related to the same factor that caused the deafness.[10] Children with hearing impairment are at particularly increased risk for reading disabilities. In the Gallaudet University survey, 95% of students received some type of assistive services, with the most common being audiological follow-up and speech and language therapy, followed by 12% receiving occupational or physical therapy. Learning resource services were received by 12% and tutoring services by 8%.[10]

Unilateral hearing loss was previously considered to have little long-term effect on development. However, in a more recent study, children with hearing loss in one ear demonstrated lower oral language scores than their siblings with normal hearing, with an associated increased risk for subsequent learning problems.[11]

Assessment of Hearing

Screening of hearing in the clinical office setting using automated *otoacoustic emission* (OAE) measuring devices or audiometers can be a useful first step. If there is any question of hearing impairment, the child should be referred for formal audiological evaluation.[12]

Objective measures are most reliable in infants and younger children who cannot provide consistent behavioral responses. *Auditory evoked potentials* are electrophysiological responses that assess auditory function and neurological integrity. A click is introduced by an earphone or headphone at the external canal and the transmission of the low-energy evoked potential through the brainstem pathways to the auditory cortex is recorded by means of scalp electrodes. It is important to note that auditory brainstem response (ABR) testing does not measure how the sound is being interpreted and processed, and it should be used in conjunction with behavioral audiometry whenever possible. OAE testing measures the integrity and sensitivity of the cochlea as well as indirectly reflecting middle ear status. The OAE are a form of acoustic energy produced by active movements of the outer hair cells of the cochlea in response to sound.

Testing entails the introduction of a click via a probe in the ear canal with measurement of the emissions from the inner ear by a microphone. This test is relatively simple and highly sensitive, but it is less specific than ABR testing and can be affected by outer ear canal obstruction and middle ear effusion. Otoacoustic emissions testing can also be inaccurate in specific circumstances, including auditory neuropathy, in which the outer cochlear hair cells are normal but the inner hair cells and/or auditory nerve are dysfunctional.

Hearing tests that elicit *behavioral responses* allow for more frequency-specific testing and confirmation that sound is being perceived by the child. *Behavioral observation audiometry* can be used in very young infants (birth—6 months) to establish estimated levels of hearing. This technique entails controlled observation of an infant's behavioral response to sound stimulation under controlled conditions. These responses include the auro-palpebral reflex, startle and arousal responses, and rudimentary head turning. This type of testing is prone to relatively high false-negative and false-positive responses. *Visual reinforcement audiometry* can be used in children by 6 months of age, and it is particularly helpful in the 1- to 4-year-old age range. The child is conditioned to animated, lighted toys placed such that when the child turns in response to sound from the speaker, the toy at that speaker is lit to reinforce the response. After conditioning, the sound is presented before the toy lights up. *Play audiometry* can be used in children 2 years of age and older as attention spans increase. The child responds to sound by performing tasks such as dropping or stacking blocks or placing rings on pegs. *Pure tone and speech audiometry* provide more accurate measurement of responses to pure tones or speech where older children are asked to respond to signals generated by a calibrated audiometer. The use of speakers has the limitation of reflecting hearing only "in the better-hearing ear," and once children accept the use of headphones, more accurate assessments can be made for each ear. The results of hearing tests are represented graphically on an audiogram, which displays the auditory threshold in decibels as a function of frequency in hertz.

Medical Evaluation

When hearing loss has been identified, further medical assessment is necessary. A thorough history can establish risk factors and potential etiologies.[2] In children with SNHL, it is essential to rule out any associated conductive component. A detailed, general physical examination should include pneumatic otoscopy and tests of vestibular function. Comprehensive evaluation is important to look for associated disabilities. For example, unexplained fainting spells in a deaf child might signal a cardiac conduction defect (long QT interval) of Jervell and Lange-Nielsen syndrome. Ophthalmological evaluation is also essential to rule out conditions such as retinitis pigmentosa with progressive loss of vision, which occurs in children with Usher syndrome. Chorioretinitis accompanies some of the congenital infections, and this finding might help establish an etiological diagnosis. Routine evaluation for refractive errors is important to ensure optimal vision for these children, who are more reliant on visual input for communication and learning.

The extent of special investigations to be performed depends partly on clinical presentation. It is currently recommended that all children with SNHL should have a high-resolution computed tomography (CT) scan of the temporal bone to rule out conditions such as an enlarged vestibular aqueduct (associated with progressive hearing loss) or abnormalities of the cochlea and semicircular canals. Magnetic resonance imaging scans, especially 3-dimensional, can identify anatomical abnormalities (eg, cochlear anomalies that might preclude cochlear implantation) or neoplasms, and a CT brain scan might also reveal calcifications indicating congenital infection. Genetic testing is evolving rapidly and enabling specific diagnosis in many children previously classified as having hearing loss of undetermined etiology.[5] In addition to molecular testing for *GJB2,* the identification of other mutations, including *SLC26A4* (the second most common nonsyndromic form of SNHL, which may also cause Pendred syndrome) and *A1555G* (a mitochondrial gene mutation that causes deafness due to extreme sensitivity of the cochlea to aminoglycosides), could be considered. If more complex genetic testing is being considered, consultation with a geneticist is recommended both for interpretation of test results and counseling regarding associated risks. Next-generation sequencing and other advanced techniques will likely soon enable definitive diagnosis of all possible genetic causes of hearing loss.[5] Other special investigations could include tests of renal function or metabolic function, immunological testing, or an electrocardiogram depending on clinical findings. If congenital or acquired infection is suspected, consultation by a pediatric infectious disease specialist is helpful in ordering and interpreting immunological tests (cytomegalovirus, toxoplasmosis, rubella, herpes, syphilis, and Zika virus).

Developmental Evaluation

Although hearing loss is not associated with cognitive impairment (unless there has been associated neurological damage in those children with acquired hearing loss), careful assessment of language and learning abilities is essential to ensure appropriate planning for developmental and educational interventions.

Formal assessment of cognitive, language, and social abilities should be carried out by professionals who have experience in testing children with hearing impairment. Tests of cognition can include the performance subtests of the Wechsler Intelligence Scales[12] (WISC-V), the Leiter International Performance Scale–Revised,[13] and the Differential Ability Scales, Second Edition, Nonverbal Reasoning Index.[14] The latter two assessments have been shown to produce equivalent results when administered to children with hearing loss.[15]

Treatment

Comprehensive management should include attention to medical conditions, interventions to promote language development, educational interventions, use of assistive devices, and support and advocacy.[16,17] This is best accomplished by a team of professionals working in partnership with families, the primary pediatric health care professional, otolaryngologist, audiologist, speech-language pathologist, and an educator of children who are deaf or hard of hearing.

Primary pediatric health care professionals, working with parents and other health care professionals, provide the medical home to facilitate and coordinate many of these interventions. Audiologists confirm the existence and degree of hearing loss and provide recommendations for amplification and assistive technology. Otolaryngologists will be able to assess middle ear function and evaluate for any surgically correctable causes of hearing loss, such as cholesteatoma, ossicular abnormalities, or other anomalies of the conductive system. They can also provide consultation regarding candidacy for cochlear implantation.

When a significant hearing loss has been discovered, the child should be fitted with a hearing aid as soon as possible. Hearing aids can be fitted in infants based on estimates of hearing thresholds from ABR measurements. Once a child is old enough to participate in behavioral hearing tests, these results can be incorporated into more precise calibration of hearing aids. The goal of amplification is to make speech and other environmental sounds audible while avoiding high-intensity sound levels that are aversive or could damage residual hearing. A variety of forms of amplification are available, including behind-the-ear or ear-level hearing aids that fit behind the pinna with amplified sound transmitted to the ear canal via the custom-fit ear mold. Smaller, in-ear devices are not recommended for young children because of the risk of swallowing or aspiration. Amplification devices can also be used with telephones and with direct input from FM auditory systems, where the primary speaker (usually the classroom teacher) wears a microphone that transmits the speaker's voice directly to the hearing aid. Bone conduction devices are used for children with certain types of conductive hearing loss, such as atresia of the external auditory canal.[15]

While hearing aids are effective for children with moderate to severe hearing loss, cochlear implants have revolutionized the treatment of profound hearing loss.[17] Components of cochlear implants include a microphone, usually worn behind the ear, that transmits sounds to a speech processor that converts the sound into an electric code. An external coil then transmits the signal across the skin to the internal receiver system implanted within the temporal bone and connected to multichannel electrodes placed within the cochlea. The electrodes are located at different sites to use the tonotopic organization of the spiral ganglion cells within the cochlea. Cochlear implants provide significant improvement in appreciation of sound in everyday situations, speech recognition and understanding, and expressive language abilities. Recent studies have demonstrated lack of significant surgical complications and positive functional outcomes, even in children who receive their implants before 12 months of age.[18] Implantation before 2 years of age (preferably before 12 months of age) has been found to provide the greatest advantage with regard to speech perception and language development, with studies suggesting that most children with profound deafness who receive implants will enter school with near-normal language skills. Children who use any form of amplification device, and especially those who have cochlear implants, need comprehensive and coordinated follow-up with specialized speech and language therapy and auditory training to help them understand the meaning of the newly amplified sounds and to develop optimal language abilities.

A variety of assistive devices are available, including telecommunication devices for the deaf, closed captioning of television, and adapted warning devices such as vibrating devices or flickering lights that indicate a ringing alarm or telephone. Advances in information technology have, of course, enabled enormously increased opportunities for communication for individuals with hearing impairment. The Internet and e-mail, as well as smartphone text messaging and voice-to-text technology, have broken down barriers at many levels.

Early intervention to promote language development remains the most critical management challenge for children with hearing impairment.[19] The child with profound hearing loss and his or her parents and other caregivers should receive professional assistance to establish a functional system of communication as soon as possible. There are many differing opinions regarding the most appropriate communication and instructional techniques. Options include sign language (manual communication), lip reading and use of speech (oral communication), or a combination (total communication). Children with profound hearing loss who have not received cochlear implants usually experience great difficulty learning to read lips and speaking fluently; they are best served by early exposure to visual and manual forms of communication such as sign language. However, children with milder degrees of loss, and those who have received cochlear implants, are better able to communicate with those who have normal hearing by developing their oral language skills. Children will be best served by early intervention providers who have specialized knowledge and skills related to working with children who are deaf or hard of hearing and who have the professional qualifications to optimize the child's development and the child's and family's well-being.

The advent of universal, newborn hearing screening has provided a unique opportunity to study the effects of early intervention on child development, particularly as related to hearing impairment. Studies involving children in the Colorado Home Intervention Program[20] definitively established that early intervention services for families with infants with hearing loss identified in the first few months of life resulted in significantly better language, speech, and social-emotional development. Children who were diagnosed and received services before 6 months of age did significantly better than those diagnosed later, in whom intervention kept language delays from increasing but did not enable them to catch up with regard to delays that were already present at the time of diagnosis.[20]

For school-aged children, educational interventions should be tailored to the individual needs of each student. These services are mandated through the Individuals with Disabilities Education Act (IDEA). Options for those whose hearing loss has not been fully corrected range from use of interpreters in a regular school and classroom to special programs in a regular school or enrollment in a school for the deaf. Students with hearing impairment have the right to receive the range of amplification and technological interventions in the school setting, which were described earlier, as well as testing accommodations and regular reevaluations (usually every 3 years) to determine whether any additional learning difficulties have emerged. They must have the opportunity for full participation in both academic and social activities. The optimal school setting to achieve this goal depends on individual characteristics of the child and the educational system in that geographic region.

Parents of the child with newly diagnosed hearing loss are dealing with significant grief, while at the same time being faced with enormous amounts of information and the need to make decisions regarding treatment approaches.[19] Counseling can be helpful in assisting the parents to work through their feelings and adapt to their new roles. The primary pediatric health care professional can be a vital source of information and support for parents, who often receive conflicting advice regarding both medical and educational interventions deemed necessary for the child. Parents face numerous stressors, including adjustment to the diagnosis and the need to learn new forms of communication, and their primary pediatric health care professional is well-positioned to assist them in accessing the most appropriate therapies and interventions for their child.

The AAP program for Early Hearing Detection and Intervention (EHDI) provides extensive informational resources and toolkits to assist primary pediatric health care professionals in meeting the needs of children who are deaf or hard of hearing and their families.[21] (A listing of resources for professionals and parents regarding children with hearing impairment is located at the end of this chapter.)

Hearing Impairment: Conclusion

As the consistent provider of longitudinal care for children with hearing impairment, the primary pediatric health care professional has a crucial role in their lives from early identification of problems to coordination of the subsequent evaluation and management interventions. The health care professional's support and advocacy for the child and family as he or she progresses through the educational system can be a crucial factor in the child's ultimate success as an adult.

Vision Impairment

In humans, of the 5 primary senses and their respective CNS networks for processing information, vision is unique. Unlike touch, smell, and taste, vision enables reception of environmental information that is both near and distant. While it shares with hearing an important role in processing discontinuous, *sequential* bits of information (particularly critical for use in receptive language), vision also provides *simultaneous* and *continuous* reception of immense chunks of contextual information in a gestalt. Because of this power, vision assumes a unique role in enabling rapid synthesis of information pouring in from all of the senses and thereby automatically boosting the efficiency of the brain's associative and executive functions. For infants and toddlers, it also serves as a powerful motivator for further exploration, which in turn stimulates increasingly precise reaching, grasping, and moving through space. Vision therefore facilitates safe locomotion and bodily coordination. For young, typically developing children, most learning of new information and skills is not taught by others but rather through incidental acquisition of information and automatic feedback from experiences within their environments. It has been estimated that as much as 80% of this learning is visually mediated.

Visual impairment is a relatively low-incidence disability, often associated with neurological comorbidities, which can have a profound influence on how children learn, move, and experience the world. Some vision-impairing medical conditions, when detected early enough, can be treated and prevented from causing permanent and/or significant loss of visual functions. For other ophthalmological and vision-related CNS disorders for which there is no medical or surgical treatment available, early detection followed promptly by tailored educational interventions, environmental modifications (eg, enlarging print size, reducing glare, increasing contrast), use of low-vision devices to augment any residual visual function, and provision of support services for families can make a major difference in the child's ultimate learning, functional independence, and social-emotional adjustment.

Definitions of Blindness and Visual Impairment

The term *blindness* implies a best-corrected visual acuity of 20/400 or worse, including no light perception. *Legal blindness*, a term used only in the United States, refers to best-corrected distance visual acuity in the better eye of 20/200 or worse, a restriction of visual field in the better eye to 20 degrees or less, or both. An individual with visual acuity of 20/200 must be 20 feet or closer from the target in order to see visual detail that someone with normal vision could discriminate at a distance of 200 feet. Approximately 75% of legally blind children have some useful vision. Traditionally, corrected visual acuity between 20/70 and 20/200 in the better eye is considered *low vision (or visual impairment),* and in many states, is sufficient to establish a child's eligibility for special education services based on visual impairment. However, because visual function in children is determined by many factors in addition to distance visual acuity, planning medical and educational interventions for the child with any significant visual impairment should ideally be based on a thorough evaluation of visual function that includes such parameters as distance and near acuity, visual fields, sensitivity to contrast, depth perception, preferred head and eye positions, variability of visual function from day to day, responses to illumination and glare, color vision, eye motility, and responses to stationary versus moving visual targets.

Epidemiology and Etiology

The reported prevalence of visual impairment and blindness in children varies depending on definitions of severity, methods of ascertainment/surveillance, and populations' classification regarding economic wealth and poverty. For many regions of the world, epidemiological data are sparse, so regional prevalence rates should be viewed as rough estimates. Worldwide, as of 2015, an estimated 1.14 million children from birth to 16 years of age were blind or severely visually impaired (visual acuity <20/400),[22] and in 2010 roughly 17.5 million children had "low vision" (acuity between 20/60 and 20/400).[23]

Of those who are blind, roughly 10% live in developed countries.[24] In the United States and other industrialized countries, the prevalence of childhood blindness (variously including milder levels of visual impairment) ranges from approximately 10 to 22 per 10,000 children.[22] In contrast, the combined prevalence in some developing countries ranges from 30 to >65 per 10,000.[22,25] If visual impairment due to uncorrected major refractive errors is included, the prevalence in developing areas ranges from 0.6% to 2.6% of children.[24]

The epidemiology of childhood visual impairment also depends largely on the relative balance between genetic and environmental risk factors on the one hand and access to health services, ophthalmological care, and advanced medical technology on the other. In developed countries, the most common cause of unilateral, preventable, permanent visual impairment is amblyopia (functional reduction in visual acuity, usually unilateral, due to abnormal early visual development), affecting up to 5% of children and adults worldwide.[26] In developed countries, the most prevalent causes of childhood blindness/ severe visual impairment are related to underlying CNS conditions (ie, cerebral or cortical visual impairment [CVI]), sequelae of extreme prematurity, and genetic conditions. In contrast, most children with visual impairments in more impoverished developing countries have eye conditions caused by infections (eg, trachoma, toxoplasmosis, and onchocerciasis), nutritional deficiencies (eg, vitamin A deficiency), and inadequate access to ophthalmological treatments (eg, amblyopia due to lack or delay of treatment of infantile cataracts, corneal scarring, or strabismus).

Several classification systems are used to catalogue the causes of visual impairment in children, either by primary anatomical site (eg, cornea, retina, optic nerve, etc.), etiological process (eg, infectious, genetic, etc.), or timing of onset. In some settings, interactions of multiple etiologies may be causative. For example, a simple traumatic corneal abrasion of an infant's eye could become exacerbated by poor hygiene, infection, undernutrition, and lack of medical treatment, allowing eventual, permanent unilateral corneal scarring, resulting in amblyopia.

Prenatal causes of visual impairment include genetic conditions, fetal malformations, prenatal infections, and hypoxia. Congenital abnormalities of the brain and/or eye may be limited to one specific structure in the eye or brain (eg, isolated coloboma of the iris, diminished number of rod cells in the retina, etc.), might affect multiple parts of the visual system (eg, bilateral retinal dysfunction and anomalous routing of optic nerve fibers in oculocutaneous albinism), or could be part of a multisystem syndrome that is, for example, chromosomal (eg, Down syndrome), metabolic, or epigenetic in origin (eg, the CHARGE syndrome[27]). In the perinatal period, visual impairments may result from CNS hypoxia/ischemia, retinopathy of prematurity, and/or infection. Postnatal etiologies include amblyopia, tumors, nutritional deficiencies, trauma (including nonaccidental injury secondary to child abuse[28]), infection, increased intracranial pressure, and systemic conditions.

In industrialized countries, more than half of all children with visual impairment have additional disabilities,[29, 30] including intellectual disability, epilepsy, cerebral palsy,

ASD, and hearing impairment. In general, severity of visual impairment correlates with higher risk for comorbid disabilities. Hereditary conditions account for roughly half of all childhood blindness in developed regions.[31] However, in economically poor countries, infectious and nutritional diseases affecting the eyes continue to play a major role. Worldwide, a majority of conditions causing blindness in children can be either prevented or treated.[25]

Among preschoolers in the United States, the most common causes of severe visual impairment, in decreasing order of frequency, are CVI, retinopathy of prematurity (ROP), optic nerve hypoplasia (ONH), structural abnormalities of the eye, and albinism.[30] CVI is most commonly caused by perinatal hypoxia, prematurity, hydrocephalus, and congenital CNS anomalies.[25] See Table 13.3 for features of these common causes of childhood blindness and visual impairment. For a more complete listing, please refer to the table in Teplin et al.[32]

Identification

One of the most important responsibilities for primary pediatric health care professionals is early detection of significant visual impairment as well as conditions that, if not treated successfully, can create high risk for persisting vision loss. If vision is significantly impaired due to an ocular condition beginning early in infancy, parents and others are likely to notice persisting wandering nystagmus and poor visual regard and/or tracking by 3 to 6 months of age. Sometimes other worrisome signs emerge during the first 1 to 2 years, which should prompt medical attention (eg, persisting excessive tearing and redness of the eye, significant strabismus, and/or leukocoria [white pupil]). However, other common causes of visual impairment in children, eg, amblyopia, may be more insidious and therefore unsuspected until detected via systematic screening.

Routine vision screening by primary pediatric health care professionals has become increasingly efficient and effective; positive findings should prompt referral to an eye specialist for definitive diagnosis and treatment. Evidence shows that early detection and treatment of amblyopia does improve visual outcomes, and screening for and treating refractive problems boosts educational outcomes.[33] In 2016, an updated policy statement[34] and accompanying set of clinical guidelines[35] regarding vision screening was issued jointly by the American Academy of Pediatrics (AAP), the American Academy of Ophthalmology (AAO), and other eye care professional organizations. Recommendations include routinely screening for eye disorders and vision at birth to 6 months, 6 to 12 months, 1 to 3 years, 4 to 5 years, and then at each subsequent annual well-child visit. Indications for referral to an eye specialist include the following:

1. Persistent parental concerns, abnormal red reflex, history of prematurity (also see updated AAP guidelines regarding ophthalmological monitoring of premature infants[36])
2. Relevant metabolic/systemic conditions

3. Family history of childhood cataract
4. Retinoblastoma, retinal dysplasia, or glaucoma
5. Failure to fix and follow a visual target by 3 months of age
6. Abnormal eye alignment
7. Pupillary asymmetry of ≥1 mm
8. Asymmetry of corneal diameter
9. Ptosis or other obstruction of visual axis
10. Visual acuity discrepancy between the two eyes of ≥2 lines on a standardized acuity chart
11. Abnormal instrument-based vision screening results
12. Nystagmus
13. Abnormal visual acuity on age-based direct screening (abnormal fix/follow for newborn to 3-year-olds, acuity worse than 20/50 in one or both eyes for 1- to 3-year-olds, acuity worse than 20/40 for 4- to 6-year-olds, and acuity worse than 20/30 for ≥6-year-olds)

In addition to obtaining an appropriate history of visual behavior and family history, recommended primary care evaluation procedures include the following:

1. An examination of external eye structures
2. Red reflex testing
3. Pupil examination
4. Direct ophthalmoscopy in children who can cooperate with instructions (generally ≥ 3 to 4 years)
5. Assessment of ocular alignment and motility in preschool and early school-aged children (ie, early detection of strabismus and risk for amblyopia)
6. Evaluation of distance visual acuity for each eye. For **school-aged** children, Sloan or Snellen letter charts are recommended. For most **preschoolers and other pre-verbal children** who cannot comply with direct acuity testing, observation of visual fixation and tracking of an interesting object remains useful. In addition, instrument-based vision screening technology (ie, automated photoscreening and autorefraction) now has sufficient sensitivity and specificity in a primary care setting to detect risk for amblyopia in young children (12 months to approximately age 4 years) and in children with developmental disabilities.[34] By 3 to 4 years of age, visual acuity can be screened directly using validated optotypes (eg, LEA symbols or HOTV letter charts). If single optotypes (rather than the preferred visual target of several symbols aligned in a row) must be used to achieve child cooperation, it is important to surround the isolated figure or letter with "crowding bars" in order to accurately detect amblyopia. Use of picture card systems (eg, Allen cards) has not been adequately standardized and is therefore not recommended.

Table 13.3. Common Disorders Causing Childhood Blindness or Visual Impairment

Condition	Pathophysiology and Exam Findings	Commonly Associated Eye, Neurological, and Systemic Disorders	Common Developmental/Behavioral Features and Resources
Cortical/ Cerebral Visual Impairment	Injury to or maldevelopment of optic radiations and/or visual processing areas of the brain (all posterior to the optic chiasm). Typically normal ocular and optic nerve structure and function, but comorbid ocular disorders may complicate the clinical picture. Origin may be prenatal (eg, genetic/metabolic disorder), perinatal (eg, hypoxic-ischemic brain damage, periventricular leukomalacia, etc.), or postnatal (eg, nonaccidental brain trauma, meningitis, etc.). CVI is often a hidden comorbidity associated with cerebral palsy and treated hydrocephalus. Potentially affected CNS regions include primary optic radiations, occipital lobe, and visual association centers and their connecting pathways (eg, ventral and dorsal "streams" connecting occipital with temporal or parietal regions). Exam: normal eye exam and pupillary function, but often poor central visual fixation and tracking; usually without nystagmus (unless there is comorbid ocular disorder).	Extremely heterogeneous, depending on locations, extent, and timing of brain abnormalities. Clinical manifestations fall roughly into 3 broad categories: profound visual impairment (often associated with multiple disabilities), functionally useful vision associated with intellectual disabilities, functionally useful vision, and normal cognitive skills with subtle visual-perceptual difficulties.[a,b] Often associated with one or more neurological problems (eg, seizures, cerebral palsy, motor or verbal dyspraxia, intellectual disabilities, learning disabilities, hearing loss, and ASD). Due to dysfunction of "dorsal stream" (ie, connections between posterior parietal and occipital visual centers and these with motor and frontal cortical centers), difficulties with mapping environments, visually searching in a cluttered array, using visually mediated movement, or reaching for/grasping objects despite seemingly sufficient visual acuity, especially when fatigued. Clinically, this can be misinterpreted as "clumsiness or dyspraxia."[b] Dysfunctions of "ventral stream"[b] pathways (ie, connections between temporal and occipital visual processing centers) include functional difficulties in recognition of familiar objects or faces. Visual function may fluctuate from hour to hour and day to day. Visual function often improves over first 1–3 years. Experts in neurology, ophthalmology, neonatology, and education of children with visual impairment may still disagree regarding terminology, pathophysiology, and prognosis.[c]	Extremely heterogeneous clinical features, depending on multiple factors (eg, anatomical locations, severity, and developmental timing of brain injuries, presence and severity of co-occurring disabilities, child's temperament and motivations, history of environmental interactions, experiences, and interventions, etc.). Child may become lost despite being in a familiar environment; may have poor eye contact or look away from other person when communicating; may prefer reliance on color, tactile features, or voice to identify objects or people rather than recognition of shapes or faces. May be anxious about or avoid walking on uneven or sloping terrain; may frequently probe with foot to check level of ground. May show heightened anxiety in crowded, noisy environments. **Parent Resources** • **Books** – Lueck AH, Dutton GN. *Vision and the Brain: Understanding Cerebral Visual Impairment in Children.* New York, NY: AFB Press; 2015 – Roman-Lantzy C. *Cortical Visual Impairment: An Approach to Assessment and Intervention.* New York, NY: AFB Press; 2007 • **Web sites** – American Foundation for the Blind (www.familyconnect.org/info/after-the-diagnosis/1 browse-by-condition/cortical-visual-impairment/123) – CVI Scotland (cviscotland.org)

Table 13.3. Common Disorders Causing Childhood Blindness or Visual Impairment (*continued*)

Condition	Pathophysiology and Exam Findings	Commonly Associated Eye, Neurological, and Systemic Disorders	Common Developmental/Behavioral Features and Resources
Retinopathy of Prematurity (ROP)	Disorder of retinal neovascularization affecting immature retinal vessels in premature infants. Risk for ROP increases with lower birth weights (especially <1,000 g) and with earlier gestational ages (especially <28 weeks). Retinal oxygen levels regulate secretion of VEGF. In addition to other factors, ROP is believed to result from overproduction of VEGF and insufficient IGF-I. ROP occurs in most extremely low birth weight premature infants (BW <1,000 g), but in the United States, spontaneously resolves in 90%. However, even with regressed ROP, children remain at some risk for late ocular complications (eg, glaucoma, retinal detachment), necessitating regular ophthalmological monitoring throughout childhood.	Extremely premature infants also have a higher incidence of strabismus, nystagmus, and high myopia. High prevalence of multiple disabilities in children with advanced stages of ROP; higher risk of other disabilities associated with worsening visual function.[d] Timely cryo- or laser-ablative therapy of avascular retina for "threshold" ROP disease can prevent retinal detachment and increase chances of better functional vision. Laser treatment is currently the procedure of choice. Recent treatment trials of intravitreal bevacizumab (an anti-VEGF agent) for stage 3+ ROP showed better results than traditional laser therapy, but additional studies of long-term safety are still necessary.[e] In wealthier, developed countries, VI due to ROP primarily affects babies born at GA ≤31 weeks, with BW <1,250 g contributing 3%–8% of prevalence of childhood blindness. In middle income countries, premature babies with higher GAs and BWs are affected, accounting for about 40% of childhood blindness.[f]	Sometimes associated with greater than expected difficulties with spatial awareness and motor coordination. Increased risk of behavior problems.[g] **Parent Resources** • **Web sites** – Association for Retinopathy of Prematurity and Related Disorders (http://www.ropard.org)

Table 13.3. Common Disorders Causing Childhood Blindness or Visual Impairment (*continued*)

Condition	Pathophysiology and Exam Findings	Commonly Associated Eye, Neurological, and Systemic Disorders	Common Developmental/Behavioral Features and Resources
Optic Nerve Hypoplasia (ONH)	Abnormal fetal development of optic nerve (diminished number of nerve fibers). Etiology is unknown, but likely multifactorial, including environmental factors; can be associated with a variety of other conditions (eg, maternal diabetes, fetal alcohol exposure, chromosomal abnormalities, Goldenhar syndrome, osteogenesis imperfecta, Apert syndrome, etc.). May be unilateral or bilateral. Eye exam: small optic nerve head appearing gray or pale, often surrounded by yellow margin and darker ring ("double ring sign"). Retinal vessels are tortuous; nystagmus is usually present if there is significant visual impairment. Variable peripheral field cuts. Important to rule out constellation of ONH, absent septum pellucidum, and endocrinopathies due to various degrees of hypopituitarism. These comprise the elements of septo-optic dysplasia. Important to obtain brain MRI and endocrine consultation. May present in newborn with jaundice (hypothyroidism), temperature instability, and/or hypoglycemic seizures (adrenal insufficiency).	Visual acuity highly variable, ranging from normal to no light perception; visual acuity is usually stable over time. Often associated with variety of CNS anomalies, each of which may have its own neurological characteristics. Overweight or obesity is common. All children with ONH should undergo early endocrinological evaluation. It is important to monitor for emerging signs of hypothalamic-pituitary dysfunction (eg, short stature, hospitalizations for dehydration or hypoglycemia) and to periodically recheck serum hormone levels. Symptoms may develop even in children whose initial brain MRI shows apparently normal pituitary gland. There may be an increased risk of sudden death during febrile illness or anesthesia (inadequate adrenal response to stress).	Often associated with feeding problems, food refusals. Some children have sensory integration problems with hypersensitivity to certain textures or sounds. Cognitively, there is wide variability with many having learning problems; some fall into the range of ASD, especially in those with profound visual impairment.[h] Some are gifted in certain domains (eg, music). The presence of major brain malformations and/or hypoplastic corpus callosum on MRI correlates with higher risk for developmental delays.[i]

Table 13.3. Common Disorders Causing Childhood Blindness or Visual Impairment *(continued)*

Condition	Pathophysiology and Exam Findings	Commonly Associated Eye, Neurological, and Systemic Disorders	Common Developmental/ Behavioral Features and Resources
Albinism	Two main types: oculocutaneous (AR) and ocular (XR), each of which has several subtypes, according to a combination of 13 genes. Altered gene activity results in reduced or no melanin pigment production in eyes (retina, iris) and/or skin and hair. Visual acuity is reduced. Other eye findings include: nystagmus, refractive errors, iris translucency, macular hypoplasia, difficulty with depth perception, and abnormal routing of optic nerve fibers through chiasm.	Visual acuity may actually improve after the first 4–6 months, and nystagmus may spontaneously improve later in childhood. Strabismus and photophobia are common. Corrected visual acuity is variable but typically is in the range of low vision (ie, between 20/70 to 20/200). A significant subgroup may have vision in the legally blind range (worse than 20/200).	No other associated disabilities. May have behavioral difficulties because of others' misinterpretation or misunderstanding of child's apparent aloofness (eg, difficulty with recognizing people at a distance due to nystagmus or poor acuity). There may be transient fine motor delays due to problems with visual tracking and depth perception. May be some emotional difficulties secondary to stigma of "differentness" (eg, becoming targets of bullying), especially for children whose family members have dark skin. Affected children benefit from consistent support from family, peers, and teachers. Low-vision interventions may include avoidance of glare, magnification aids, high-contrast materials, sunglasses, and small telescopes for distance viewing. **Parent Resources** • **Web site** – National Organization for Albinism and Hypopigmentation (NOAH) (http://albinism.org) • **Books** – National Organization for Albinism and Hypopigmentation (NOAH). *Raising a Child with Albinism: A Guide to the Early Years.* East Hampstead, NH: NOAH; 2008 – National Organization for Albinism and Hypopigmentation (NOAH). *Raising a Child with Albinism: A Guide to the School Years.* East Hampstead, NH: NOAH – Ryan MA. *My Fair Child.* Bloomington, IN: Trafford Publishing; 2009

Abbreviations: AR, autosomal recessive; ASD, autism spectrum disorder; BW, birth weight; CNS, central nervous system; GA, gestational age; IGF-I, insulin-like growth factor-I; MRI, magnetic resonance imaging; PVL, periventricular leukomalacia; VEGF, vascular endothelial growth factor; VI, visual impairment; XR, X-linked recessive.

[a] Lueck AH, Dutton GN. *Vision and the Brain: Understanding Cerebral Visual Impairment in Children.* New York, NY: AFB Press; 2015

[b] Philip SS, Dutton GN. Identifying and characterising cerebral visual impairment in children: a review. *Clin Exp Optom.* 2014;97(3):196–208

[c] Roman-Lantzy C. *Cortical Visual Impairment: An Approach to Assessment and Intervention.* New York, NY: AFB Press; 2007

[d] Msall ME, Phelps DL, DiGaudio KM, et al. Severity of neonatal retinopathy of prematurity is predictive of neurodevelopmental functional outcome at age 5.5 years. Behalf of the Cryotherapy for Retinopathy of Prematurity Cooperative. *Pediatrics.* 2000;106(5):998–1005

[e] Mintz-Hittner HA, Kennedy KA, Chuang AZ; BEAT-ROP Cooperative Group. Efficacy of intravitreal bevacizumab for stage 3+ retinopathy of prematurity. *N Engl J Med.* 2011;364(7):603–615

[f] Fiedler AR, Quinn GE. Retinopathy of prematurity. In: Taylor D, Hoyt CS eds. *Pediatric Ophthalmology and Strabismus.* 3rd ed. Edinburgh, UK: Elsevier Saunders: 2005:516–517

[g] Termote J, Schalij-Delfos NE, Donders RT, Cats BP. The incidence of visually impaired children with retinopathy of prematurity and their concomitant disabilities. *J AAPOS.* 2003;7(2):131–136

[h] Parr JR, Dale NJ, Shaffer LM, Salt AT. Social communication difficulties and autism spectrum disorder in young children with optic nerve hypoplasia and/or septo-optic dysplasia. *Dev Med Child Neurol.* 2010;52(10):917–921

[i] Ryabets-Lienhard A, Stewart C, Borchert M, Geffner ME. The optic nerve hypoplasia spectrum—review of the literature and clinical guidelines. *Adv Pediatr.* 2016;63(1):127–146

Adapted with permission from Teplin SW, Greeley J, Anthony TL. Blindness and visual impairment. In: Carey WB, Crocker AC, Coleman WL, Elias ER, Feldman HM, eds. *Developmental-Behavioral Pediatrics.* 4th ed. Philadelphia, PA: Saunders Elsevier; 2009:700–709.

Primary pediatric health care professionals should also keep in mind that not all visual impairment is due to ocular abnormalities; in fact, the most frequent cause of visual impairment in young children living in developed countries is *CVI*. This occurs when visual signals received from the retinas and optic nerves are not accurately or consistently interpreted by the brain's posterior visual pathways, either temporarily (eg, in delayed visual maturation) or permanently. The dysfunctions associated with CVI vary greatly from child to child; they can range from mild to severe, may be accompanied by ocular conditions, and often, but not always, are comorbid with other neurodevelopmental dysfunctions. Diagnosis is often difficult because the classic signs and symptoms of eye disorders are absent (eg, normal pupillary responses, eye movements, and eye examination). In addition, visual symptoms associated with CVI are often subtle and/or confusing (eg, difficulty recognizing faces but not objects, difficulty seeing a stationary visual target but no difficulty seeing the same object when it is moving) or only inconsistently apparent (eg, only when the child is fatigued, only under specific lighting conditions, or only when the visual target is obscured within a visually cluttered background).[37] CVI should be suspected whenever there are apparent vision difficulties despite a normal eye exam or eye findings that are insufficient to explain the vision symptoms. Other neurological, behavioral, or historical clues may further support a diagnosis of CVI (Table 13.3). Ideally, a team of professionals experienced in assessments of children with visual impairments (including medical and developmental specialists, a teacher of the visually impaired [TVI], and an orientation and mobility specialist) can solicit key features in the history and carry out the necessary diagnostic observations and examinations. Despite diagnostic complexities, it is important to make the diagnosis so that appropriate interventions can be implemented.[38] Please refer to Table 13.3 for additional clinical features and resources for parents of children with CVI.

When a patient presents with obvious or previously diagnosed neurodevelopmental disabilities in nonvisual domains, the possibility of unsuspected vision impairment(s) further complicating the child's clinical picture should always be considered by clinicians.[39] Earlier detection of possible visual problems in children with known developmental disabilities provides an opportunity to refer them for a thorough ophthalmological evaluation. This in turn may identify treatments to ameliorate the visual problem and improve the long-term outcome.[40]

Although impaired vision can complicate general learning, studies continue to support the scientific consensus that language deficits (especially phonological processing difficulties) lie at the core of primary dyslexia. Furthermore, visual abnormalities of convergence, contrast sensitivity, and accommodation, or eye problems such as strabismus, refractive error, and amblyopia, are not associated with significant reading impairments.[41] Despite popular assertions that significant or subtle visual deficits can be a significant causative factor in children's reading disorders and claims that various types of vision therapies (eg, eye movement exercises, behavioral visual therapy, and colored filters) result in improved reading skills and comprehension, robust evidence to support these concepts and practices is lacking.[42] However, as we learn more about the complex interregional brain connections associated with CVI and some associated learning difficulties,[38] this controversy may persist.

Development

– Motor

Wide variability is noted in the acquisition of motor skills by young children with visual impairment. Important determinants include the severity and type of visual impairment, comorbid disabilities (particularly those involving the motor system), and the degrees to which early environments are enriched with opportunities and encouragement for movement. For children with visual impairment but without other disabilities, early motor milestones that involve only stationary balance (eg, sitting and standing unaided) often occur on roughly the same timetable as for infants with normal vision. However, movement through space is typically delayed (eg, walking may not occur until 18 to 24 months). To prevent a tendency to remain passive and relatively immobile, it is important for these children to have active engagement with their environments. Invaluable services are provided by *certified orientation and mobility specialists* (COMS), whose job is to help children with visual impairments learn about the spatial arrangement of their environments, develop their own mental maps, and use this knowledge to move about efficiently and safely.[43] Some children with severe visual impairment can be taught (or learn spontaneously from accumulated experience and exploration) to use echolocation skills similar to those used by bats and other nocturnal animals. Sounds bouncing off surrounding objects can provide accurate information about the size, distance, and consistency of those objects or obstacles, thereby facilitating safe and efficient movement.

– Cognitive

For sighted infants, vision serves as a powerful motivator for further exploration, which in turn stimulates increasingly precise reach/grasp and movement through space in order to get to a desired person, place, or object. As they move and observe objects and other people move, young children with normal vision discover and repeatedly verify basic cognitive concepts (eg, object permanence and cause and effect). For infants with congenital blindness or severe visual impairment, understanding of these principles often takes longer, requiring learning via alternative sequences. Most severely visually impaired children have additional disabilities; for these children, greater fragmentation of incoming information creates more formidable obstacles to learning these fundamental concepts, causing greater delays in their acquisition. It is crucial that the young child with severe visual impairment be actively introduced to a variety of experiences, objects, physical qualities, spatial relationships (eg, hot/cold, loud/soft, above/below, in/out, curved/straight), and people to allow the child to use all available sensory functions to take in, store, and eventually integrate these concepts. For example, instead of a parent or teacher verbally explaining to a young child who is blind what a tree is, it is much more effective to physically "introduce" the child to a variety of trees during the explanation. This active experience should include simultaneously feeling the tree's bark and leaves, smelling the blossoms, and both feeling and listening to the branches swaying in the wind. Parents of blind or severely visually impaired young children often need guidance and encouragement initially to take advantage of spontaneous opportunities for incidental learning during a child's daily activities. Such learning (ie, through serendipitous observation and experience rather than via intentional instruction) is a major source of knowledge for sighted children. For the child with impaired vision, such experiences are equally important but often depend upon another person (eg, parent, teacher, sibling, etc.) being assertive enough to intentionally make them happen by introducing relevant concepts, vocabulary, emotions, and related experiences to help fill in the conceptual gaps that might arise. For example, at breakfast time, a parent could propose a fun game for the young child to guess what he or she will soon be eating by paying attention and thoughtfully using his or her intact senses (including residual vision)—touching a bowl and listening to the sound of dry cereal being poured into it, hearing and smelling eggs or bacon cooking, etc. Parents also need support in resisting the temptation to anticipate the young child's every need or desire, thus inadvertently restricting the child's learning opportunities. For example, a caregiver can become mindful of his or her tendency to automatically retrieve objects the child has dropped or to carry the child around excessively because of concern about inevitable but harmless collisions with nearby furniture. Caregivers need to understand how important it is for the child to experience the environment *actively*. The child should be given many opportunities to use developing language skills to verbally express needs and desires, listening skills and fine motor coordination to search for dropped objects, and using his or her body to move through space, even when this might be temporarily frustrating for both the child and parent.[44]

Learning abilities, and therefore necessary instructional methods, may vary according to whether a child's visual loss was congenital versus adventitious because of the latter's advantage in having had some prior visual experience.[45] This is especially evident regarding spatial orientation and spatial behaviors as well as acquisition of motor skills.[46] However, studies have shown no correlation between age of vision loss and overall cognitive abilities.[46] Teaching strategies for children whose blindness occurred prior to the establishment of visual memory (approximately age 5 years[45]) must rely much more on their nonvisual senses.

– Language
As receptive and expressive vocabulary develop, language becomes an increasingly powerful tool for the child with blindness to learn about the environment. For many cognitively typical children with severe visual impairment or blindness, the pace of single-word acquisition is often comparable to that seen in children with normal vision. Some differences, however, are notable.[47] Compared with sighted children, those with severe visual impairments are slower to acquire adjectives and verbs, have more prolonged phases of echolalic speech, are more likely to choose more egocentric topics to discuss, and have longer periods of pronoun confusion and reversals (eg, saying "You want a cookie?" when what they mean is, "I want a cookie"). As the child grows older, there may be gaps in understanding words that have more visual referents (eg, *sky* or *red*) or that represent very large objects that would be difficult for the child to experience as a whole (eg, a building).

– Play

Compared with young children with normal vision, preschoolers who are severely visually impaired but otherwise developmentally intact tend to engage in more solitary play and play with adults more than with peers. Compared with sighted preschoolers, there is about a 2-year delay across all categories of play. The level of visual functioning directly correlates with the sophistication of play. Vision plays a critical role in the acquisition of higher levels of play behavior among sighted children. For young children with severe congenital visual impairments, most of their spontaneous play is exploratory and focuses on simple manipulation with much less functional play and even less pretend and symbolic play (eg, imaginative doll play). They are not likely to learn how to play without some guidance from others. When with peers, they have difficulty sustaining their social connection when there is a verbal communication breakdown. These delays are likely to be even more substantial for children with visual impairment plus additional disabilities. Such difficulties also correlate with deficiencies in social skills.[48]

Strategies that can promote more interactive and educational play include providing toys and activities that are interesting to the child (eg, through tactile and auditory sensations), choosing play partners who have similar interests, and facilitating the child's awareness of the environment by use of verbal descriptions. Sighted peers can be shown how to interact with the child who is blind, with gradual fading of adult reinforcement and support.[49]

– Social and Emotional

Infants with severe visual impairment often have facial expressions that are passive-appearing or somewhat "serious;" their social smiles are more subtle and fleeting, making it difficult for caregivers to detect and read the baby's social cues. The important early phase of prelingual, mutual social interaction may be jeopardized by possible misinterpretations by the caregiver. For example, the mother of an infant who is blind might notice the infant's lack of smiling on hearing her voice and mistakenly assume that he or she does not recognize her voice or does not want to be with her. A teacher for the visually impaired (TVI) who is especially experienced with young children could help this mother to understand that, to some extent, smiling is learned by seeing others smile, that the infant's sudden stillness may be the result of the infant trying to *listen* to the mother's voice, or that the infant's particular hand positioning may be a subtle cue that he or she is, in fact, responding to her. The child with severe visual impairment remains at risk for emotional and behavioral problems largely related to difficulties in adapting to change and not having the abilities of sighted peers to consistently interpret others' social cues or see their own impact on others. These potential difficulties in social expression, pretend play, and emotionally meaningful interactions with parents can often be prevented or at least ameliorated in infants, toddlers, and preschoolers when parents and other early caregivers have access to services from TVIs who can help them learn to read the child's cues, learn to be aware of their own and others' emotional reactions to events,[50] respond reciprocally, and provide explicit modeling to promote the child's pretend play.[47] Often such TVIs are itinerant and work closely with local early intervention (EI) teams.

Role of the Primary Pediatric Health Care Professional and Additional Interventions – Diagnostic and Medical Issues

In his or her role as medical home, the primary pediatric health care professional should routinely provide surveillance and screening for possible ocular and CNS disorders and identify visual problems as early as possible. In addition to appropriate referrals to an eye care specialist for definitive diagnostic assessment of suspected eye or vision problems, other pediatric subspecialty referrals may also be indicated (eg, a neurologist, geneticist, and/or developmental-behavioral or neurodevelopmental pediatrician). An interdisciplinary developmental assessment team that includes a TVI and COMS can provide comprehensive evaluation of the child's strengths as well as the nature of his or her limitations related to the visual impairment. Other medical problems that are more frequently seen in children with visual impairments include sleep difficulties,[51] feeding problems in young children, and other sensory processing difficulties. The clinician may need to devote additional time to exploring these issues with parents or refer them to a developmental consultant as needed.

Diagnostic concerns about possible comorbid ASD in children who are severely visually impaired can present major clinical challenges. Children with visual impairments are at higher risk than sighted peers to have ASD, particularly those with the most severe visual impairments[52] and those with additional cognitive and/or motor deficits.[53] Studies have been conflicting as to whether children with certain etiologies of blindness (eg, retinopathy of prematurity, Leber congenital amaurosis, and septo-optic dysplasia) are also at higher risk for ASD. Great caution must be exercised when attempting to draw diagnostic conclusions about the presence of possible ASD based on the behaviors of children with significant visual impairment. Several common behavioral features of blind children who are otherwise developmentally age appropriate could lead to erroneous diagnosis of a comorbid ASD. These features include difficulties in establishing typical social relationships with peers; stereotypical, self-stimulatory behaviors (eg, hand-flapping, rocking, eye-poking, or light-gazing) when excited or upset; prolonged phase of echolalic language during the toddler and preschool periods; and what seems to be over- or underreactivity to other sensory signals (eg, oversensitivity to ambient noise and inappropriate touching or sniffing of objects and people). These stereotyped behaviors often spontaneously regress by adolescence.[54] Until then, however, ruling in or out a co-occurring diagnosis of ASD can be quite difficult and is best addressed by an interdisciplinary team of developmental specialists, preferably including input from a TVI or other professional who has had extensive experience working with children with visual impairments. On the other hand, the mistaken exclusion of a diagnosis of comorbid ASD in a child who is severely visually impaired is also possible, again highlighting the importance of careful monitoring and then interdisciplinary evaluation when behaviors suggestive of ASD persist. As noted, the risk of ASD among children with severe visual impairment is significantly higher than in sighted children, occurring in 8% to >50% of blind children, particularly among children whose blindness is congenital.[55,56]

– Infants, Toddlers, and Preschoolers

The primary pediatric health care professional should inquire about and confirm that the young child who is visually impaired is being served by appropriate EI services, in collaboration with TVI and COMS professionals. The clinician can also help reinforce the parents' important role in actively introducing their child to his or her surroundings via intact sensory systems (touch, hearing, residual vision). The young child's parents are also likely to benefit from contact with local, regional, and national organizations that are dedicated to supporting parents of children with visual impairments that are often related to specific medical diagnoses (please refer to the listing of general parent resources at the end of this chapter and disorder-specific parent supports in Table 13.3).

– School-aged Children

Federal law (the Individuals with Disabilities Education Act [IDEA]) mandates that all students, including those with visual impairment, are entitled to educational instruction and services that are appropriate to their unique educational needs, as spelled out in the student's Individualized Educational Program (IEP). For students with visual impairment, being in a "least restrictive" setting may require much more than physical presence in a classroom of students without disabilities. Students with disabilities often need access to specialized instructors, services, books, other instructional media (including braille) and specialized technology sufficient to provide equal access to core and specialized curricula.

A team approach is usually necessary to provide these services and media, particularly for students who have multiple disabilities. Whenever possible, this team should include a TVI and a COMS. These students' curricular needs often encompass a broader range of concepts and skills than those of their sighted peers, including, for example, orientation and mobility, social-emotional skills, use of low-vision devices (eg, stand magnifiers, a closed circuit TV, etc.), visual efficiency skills, independent living skills, etc. These needs comprise the American Foundation for the Blind (AFB)[57] Expanded Core Curriculum, and must be systematically taught.[32] Instructional materials must be available in appropriate media formats (eg, braille, large print, audio, and/or digital) at the same time that their sighted peers are studying comparable content. Ongoing assessments over time by the TVI will help guide the decisions concerning which formats are best suited to a student, and these needs may change over time. National Instructional Materials Accessibility Standards (NIMAS)[58] mandate that textbook publishers make available an electronic version of any newly published printed text material they publish for students. This allows easy conversion to whichever media formats are appropriate to the student with visual impairment.[32]

In the United States, most students with blindness or low vision currently attend their own local public schools, receiving a range of special education services according to their individual needs. However, some school districts have specialized programs, TVIs who are on staff, and adaptive books and equipment; other districts must scramble to find and obtain limited resources when a new child with visual impairment enters the system. Advanced planning can help considerably. Primary pediatric health care professionals, often in collaboration with the local EI program, can help parents of a toddler with visual impairment to advocate for current and future services (eg, establishing an early relationship with the school system's coordinator of special education, giving the system plenty of time to prepare for the child's entry at age 3 years, etc.). Often the intensity and format of these services varies over time. For example, during the early elementary years, a child may spend more time in a specialized resource setting with a TVI where he or she can focus on learning necessary compensatory skills unique to his or her disability (ie, Expanded Core Curriculum). Depending on a student's abilities and unique educational needs, he or she can often be successfully included into regular education classes for at least part of the day, if appropriate support or consultation services from the TVI and COMS are available. Students with low vision are entitled to specialized assessments including evaluation of functional vision to determine under what conditions (eg, lighting, magnification, contrast, etc.) vision can be used most effectively and what modifications to the classroom environment will be necessary. Other educational issues addressed by specialized assessments might include determining braille (tactile) versus large print (visual) versus auditory reception as a primary reading mode, promoting listening skills, determining which technology or devices might be appropriate and which orientation and mobility skills need emphasis. Accommodations and modifications in learning environments and test settings (eg, extra time, minimal auditory distraction during testing, use of braille or large-print materials, use of tactile objects or experiences instead of reliance on pictures, speech-access computer software, etc.) often need to be established as part of the IEP. For some students, intense skill-building courses (for example, during the summer at a state's residential school for the blind) may provide unique opportunities, which may be unavailable in the local school, to learn about specialized adaptive technologies (eg, computer software and devices that can interconvert braille, written text, and synthetic speech) while also offering socialization opportunities for students from distant schools who have similar disabilities and interests.

In addition to coping with unique developmental and academic hurdles, students with visual impairments may also require specific help in learning appropriate social skills, many of which can rely on tuning in to verbal and other nonvisual cues. They also may need guidance in self-regulation of common self-stimulatory behaviors and promotion of conversational skills, such as staying on topic, taking turns, and determining when to interrupt. As noted, these skills are among the unique learning needs specified in the American Foundation for the Blind's Expanded Core Curriculum[57] as requiring explicit, systematic, and sequential instruction to students with visual impairments. Primary pediatric health care professionals can help parents advocate for the inclusion of these instructional goals within their child's IEP.

– Adolescents

Adolescents with significant visual impairment must cope with the same upheavals and issues as youth with normal vision. However, as with most youth with chronic illness or other developmental disabilities, they also struggle with more basic issues of independent identity. Their success in activities leading to greater independence (eg, dating, exploration of job opportunities, higher skill levels) hinge to some extent on whether they have already mastered more basic self-help skills, such as personal grooming, food preparation, money management, and travel. They are at risk for distorted concepts about sexuality due to having missed typical visual cues during childhood regarding appropriate and inappropriate sexual behavior. Sex education needs to begin early. Through use of anatomically correct dolls and ongoing factual discussions, they can acquire knowledge of fundamental facts and vocabulary. As with sighted youth, sex education is most effective when embedded within learning about the emotional context of sexual relationships.

Deaf-Blindness

Children who have significant impairments of both vision and hearing constitute a special group because the educational interventions and support services required are different from those typically needed for children with either single disability. Deaf-blindness encompasses a range of severity of each disability. Approximately 17% are totally blind or have light perception only, 24% are legally blind, and 21% have low vision. Approximately 39%, 13%, and 14% have severe to profound, moderate, and mild hearing loss, respectively.[59] The most common etiologies include a variety of hereditary conditions, complications of prematurity, hypoxic-ischemic encephalopathy, CHARGE syndrome, postinfectious complications, and Usher syndrome. Approximately 85% of children with this dual sensory impairment have additional disabilities, particularly intellectual disabilities, speech-language disorders, and orthopedic conditions.[46] The most important developmental issues include social interaction, mobility, communication,[60] and cognitive grasp of concepts.[48] For individuals who are deaf-blind, their hands must be carefully, patiently, and consistently trained to become their primary sensory organs, as well as the main means of communication with others.

Vision Impairment: Conclusion

During recent decades, research interest and our knowledge base about developmental implications of blindness and visual impairment in children and adolescents has expanded, both supporting and challenging clinicians and TVIs to meet the unique developmental, educational, and social needs of these children. However, compared with other disabling conditions, blindness or visual impairment still represents a relatively small percentage of all children with special needs. As a result, much of the expanding knowledge base fails to get transferred and integrated into medical and educational practice where it is most needed. Primary pediatric health care professionals can help close this gap by maintaining awareness of professionals and specialized agencies in their communities or regions that have expertise and experience in working with infants, preschoolers, school-aged students, and adolescents who are visually impaired and making prompt referrals when encountered as patients. Referral to a pediatric eye care specialist is mandatory, but that is only the beginning. It will usually be the primary pediatric health care professional's medical home, not the ophthalmologist's expertise, that will continue reinforcing the family's resilience, monitoring the child's developmental status and obstacles, and smoothing the path toward educational and behavioral consultation in order to optimize the child's progress. As devastating as it may seem initially for the family (and clinician) to confront the reality of a child's blindness or severe visual impairment, the health care provider's practical and positive attitude and commitment to helping parents advocate for necessary services and supports will prove extremely valuable.

Resources

Hearing
Maternal and Child Health Bureau (MCHB)
The MCHB is part of the Health Resources and Services Administration (HRSA). For more than 75 years, the federal Title V Maternal and Child Health program has provided a foundation for ensuring the health of the nation's mothers, women, children and youth, including children and youth with special health care needs, and their families.
https://mchb.hrsa.gov

Centers for Disease Control and Prevention (CDC) National Center on Birth Defects and Developmental Disabilities (NCBDDD)
The NCBDDD provides research, basic information, and statistics regarding hearing loss, screening, and diagnosis, as well as current articles and educational materials for clinicians and families.
https://www.cdc.gov/ncbddd

National Center for Hearing Assessment and Management (NCHAM)
The NCHAM serves as the national resource center for the implementation and improvement of comprehensive and effective Early Hearing Detection and Intervention (EHDI) systems.
http://www.infanthearing.org/

Joint Committee on Infant Hearing
The Committee works to address issues that are important to the early identification, intervention, and follow-up care of infants and young children with hearing loss.
http://www.jcih.org/

Hands and Voices

Hands and Voices provides parent-to-parent support for families of children with hearing loss, providing unbiased information and promoting interventions that best suit the child's and family's needs.

http://www.handsandvoices.org/

Babyhearing.org

This is a resource for parents of children with hearing loss and for primary care providers; it provides education resources, fact sheets, and other materials on hearing loss screening and intervention.

https://www.babyhearing.org/

National Institute on Deafness and Other Communication Disorders (NIDCD)

The NIDCD is part of the National Institutes of Health (NIH); the agency conducts and supports research into the normal and disordered processes of hearing, balance, smell, voice, speech, and language.

https://www.nidcd.nih.gov/

American Academy of Pediatrics (AAP) Program for Early Hearing Detection and Interventions (EHDI)

Toolkits and further helpful resources and information available through the AAP program for Early Hearing Detection and Intervention (EHDI) at

https://www.aap.org/en-us/advocacy-and-policy/aap-health-initiatives/ PEHDIC/Pages/Early-Hearing-Detection-and-Intervention.aspx

Hearing resources list adapted from American Academy of Pediatrics Early Hearing Detection and Intervention Web site.

Vision

See also Table 13.3 for additional parent resources regarding the most common medical conditions that cause visual impairment in children.

American Association for Pediatric Ophthalmology and Strabismus (AAPOS)

The Web site has information about the latest research efforts; it provides concise overviews of common conditions causing visual impairment in children and the treatment approaches.

http://www.aapos.org

American Foundation for the Blind (AFB)

The AFB provides resources, materials, educational devices, toys, and useful suggestions for parents and teachers. Their special Web site for parents of children with visual impairments (**www.familyconnect.org**) has a wealth of information and supportive resources.

www.afb.org

American Printing House for the Blind (APH)

APH is a source of publications and adapted educational equipment for children and youth who are visually impaired.

www.aph.org

Blind Babies Foundation (a program of the Junior Blind)

Under "Programs," click on the link for "Blind Babies Foundation." On the right side of that page, click on the link for "Fact Sheets."

These fact sheets provide practical tips and activities for families and teachers of infants and toddlers who are visually impaired. There is also a fact sheet for parents on how to cope with and optimize a visit to the child's doctor or hospital.

www.juniorblind.org

National Federation of the Blind (NFB)

The NFB is a membership organization of blind people in the United States. NFB has numerous publications for parents and professionals on blindness and visual impairment and includes a national parent organization.

www.nfb.org

Perkins School for the Blind (Watertown, MA)

This is a comprehensive Web site with many instructive articles on topics related to visual impairment in children, educational approaches, assistive technology, and parent support.

http://www.perkins.org

Suggested Reading

Chen D. *Essential Elements in Early Intervention: Visual Impairment and Multiple Disabilities.* **2nd ed. New York, NY: American Foundation for the Blind Press; 2014**

This book explores in depth early experiential learning for infants and toddlers who are visually impaired, including those with additional disabilities.

Holbrook MC. *Children with Visual Impairments: A Parent's Guide.* **Bethesda, MD: Woodbine House; 2006**

This book is authored by an expert team of parents and professionals. It offers jargon-free advice to parents of young children from birth to age 7 who have visual impairments.

Lueck AH, Dutton GN. *Vision and the Brain: Understanding Cerebral Visual Impairment in Children.* **New York, NY: AFB Press; 2015**

The book is a comprehensive overview of the pathophysiology of cerebral visual impairment with correlations to a range of visual, behavioral, and learning challenges commonly seen in CVI.

Lueck AH, Chen D, Kekelis L. *Developmental Guidelines for Infants with Visual Impairment: A Manual for Early Intervention.* **Louisville, KY: American Printing House for the Blind; 1997**

This manual was written for professionals working with children from birth through 2 years of age who have visual impairments. The manual includes narrative chapters and developmental charts in the domains of social-emotional, communicative, cognitive, and motor development.

Pogrund RL, Fazzi DL. *Early Focus: Working with Young Children Who Are Blind or Visually Impaired and Their Families.* **2nd ed. New York, NY: American Foundation for the Blind Press; 2002**

This book addresses the needs of young children with visual impairments, including those with additional disabilities and their families. It includes intervention recommendations in all developmental domains, including early literacy, daily living skills, and orientation and mobility.

Roman-Lantzy C. *Cortical Visual Impairment: An Approach to Assessment and Intervention.* **New York, NY: AFB Press; 2007**

This book was the first to present a structured clinical approach for educators and other professionals toward indexing and understanding visual behaviors that often comprise a confusing clinical picture of children with cerebral/cortical visual impairment (CVI). Principles for planning educational and home modifications and interventions are explained in detail.

References

1. Russ SA, Dougherty D, Jagadish P. Accelerating evidence into practice for the benefit of children with early hearing loss. *Pediatrics*. 2010;126:S7–S18

2. American Academy of Pediatrics, Joint Committee on Infant Hearing. Year 2007 Position Statement. Principles and guidelines for early hearing detection and intervention programs. *Pediatrics*. 2007;120(4):898–921

3. Petersen NK, Jorgensen AW, Ovesen T. Prevalence of various etiologies of hearing loss among cochlear implant recipients: systematic review and meta-analysis. *Int J Audiol*. 2015;54(12):924–932

4. Parker M, Bitner-Glindzicz M. Republished: genetic investigations in childhood deafness. *Postgrad Med J*. 2015;91(1077):395–402

5. Chang KW. Genetics of hearing loss—nonsyndromic. *Otolaryngol Clin North Am*. 2015;48(6):1063–1072

6. Moore CA, Staples JE, Dobyns WB, et al. Characterizing the pattern of anomalies in congenital Zika syndrome for pediatric clinicians. *JAMA Pediatr*. 2017;171(3):288–295

7. US Preventive Services Task Force. Universal Screening for hearing loss in newborns: US Preventive Services Task Force recommendation statement. *Pediatrics*. 2008;122(1):143–148

8. Marschark M. *Psychological Development of Deaf Children*. New York, NY: Oxford University Press; 1993

9. Kelly DP, Kelly BJ, Jones ML, Moulton NJ, et al. Attention deficits in children and adolescents with hearing loss: a survey. *Am J Dis Child*. 1993;147(7):737–741

10. Gallaudet Research Institute. *Regional and National Summary Report of Data from the 2009-2010 Annual Survey of Deaf and Hard of Hearing Children and Youth*. Washington, DC: GRI, Gallaudet University; 2011

11. Lieu JE, Tye-Murray N, Karzon RK, Piccirillo JF. Unilateral hearing loss is associated with worse speech-language scores in children. *Pediatrics*. 2010;125(6):e1348–e1355

12. Wechsler, D. *Wechsler Intelligence Scale for Children–Fifth Edition*. Bloomington, MN: Pearson; 2014

13. Roid GH, Miller LJ. *Leiter International Performance Scale–Revised*. Wood Dale, IL: Stoelting; 2011

14. Elliot CD. *Differential Abilities Scale–II*. Bloomington MN, Pearson; 2007

15. Phillips J, Wiley S, Barnard H, Meinzen-Derr J. Comparison of two nonverbal intelligence tests among children who are deaf or hard of hearing. *Res Dev Disabil*. 2014;35(2):463–471

16. Tharpe AM, Gustafson S. Management of children with mild, moderate and moderately severe sensorineural hearing loss. *Otolaryngol Clin North Am*. 2015;48(6)983–994

17. Iselli C, Buchman CA. Management of children with severe, severe-profound and profound sensorineural hearing loss. *Otolaryngol Clin North Am*. 2015;48(6):995–1010

18. Ruffin CV, Kronenberger WG, Colson BG, Henning SC, Pisoni DB. Long-term speech and language outcomes in prelingually deaf children, adolescents and young adults who received cochlear implants in childhood. *Audiol Neurootol*. 2013;18(5):289–96

19. Yoshinaga-Itano C. Principles and guidelines for early intervention after confirmation that a child is deaf or hard of hearing. *J Deaf Stud Deaf Educ*. 2014;19(2)143–175

20. Yoshinaga-Itano C. From screening to early identification and intervention: discovering predictors to successful outcomes for children with significant hearing loss. *J Deaf Stud Deaf Educ*. 2003;8(1):11–30

21. American Academy of Pediatrics Program for Early Hearing Detection and Intervention (EHDI) https://www.aap.org/en-us/advocacy-and-policy/aap-health-initiatives/PEHDIC/Pages/Early-Hearing-Detection-and-Intervention.aspx. Accessed February 6, 2018

22. Rahi JS, Gilbert CE. Epidemiology and worldwide impact of visual impairment in children. In: Lambert SR, Lyons CJ, eds. *Taylor and Hoyt's Pediatric Ophthalmology and Strabismus*. 5th ed. Edinburgh: Elsevier; 2017:7–16

23. Pascolini D, Mariotti SP. Global estimates of visual impairment: 2010. *Br J Ophthalmol*. 2012;96:614–618

24. Isenberg SJ, Apt L. International pediatric ophthalmology. In: Rudolph CD, Rudolph AM, Lister GE, First LR, Gershon AA, eds. *Rudolph's Pediatrics*. 22nd ed. New York, NY: McGraw Hill Medical; 2011:2282–2284

25. Walton DS. Visual impairment in childhood. In: Rudolph CD, Rudolph AM, Lister GE, First LR, Gershon AA, eds. *Rudolph's Pediatrics*. 22nd ed. New York, NY: McGraw Hill Medical; 2011:2289–2290

26. Wong AMF. New concepts concerning the neural mechanisms of amblyopia and their clinical implications. *Can J Ophthalmol*. 2012;47:399–409

27. Bergman JE, Janssen N, Hoefsloot LH, et al. CHD7 mutations and CHARGE syndrome: the clinical implications of an expanding phenotype. *J Med Genet*. 2011;48:334–342

28. Binenbaum G, Forbes BJ. The eye in child abuse: key points on retinal hemorrhages and abusive head trauma. *Pediatr Radiol*. 2014;44 (Supplement 4):S571–S577

29. Van Naarden Braun K, Christensen D, Doernberg N, et al. Trends in the prevalence of autism spectrum disorder, cerebral palsy, hearing loss, intellectual disability, and vision impairment, Metropolitan Atlanta, 1991–2010. *PLoS One*. 2015;10(4):e0124120

30. Hatton DD, Schwietz E, Boyer B, Rychwalski P. Babies Count: the national registry for children with visual impairments, birth to 3 years. *J AAPOS*. 2007;11(4):351–355

31. Rudanko SL, Laatikainen L. Visual impairment in children born at full term from 1972 through 1989 in Finland. *Ophthalmology.* 2004;111(12):2307–2312

32. Teplin SW, Greeley J, Anthony TL. Blindness and visual impairment. In: Carey WB, Crocker AC, Coleman WL, Elias ER, Feldman HM, eds. *Developmental-Behavioral Pediatrics.* 4th ed. Philadelphia, PA: Elsevier; 2009:698–716

33. Mathers M, Kees M, Wright M. A review of the evidence on the effectiveness of children's vision screening. *Child Care Health Dev.* 2010;36:756–780

34. American Academy of Pediatrics Committee on Practice and Ambulatory Medicine, Section on Ophthalmology; American Association of Certified Orthoptists; American Association for Pediatric Ophthalmology; American Academy of Ophthalmology. Visual system assessment in infants, children, and young adults by pediatricians. *Pediatrics.* 2016;137(1):e20153596

35. Donahue SP, Baker CN; Committee on Practice and Ambulatory Medicine, Section on Ophthalmology; American Association of Certified Orthoptists; American Association for Pediatric Ophthalmology and Strabismus; American Academy of Ophthalmology. Procedures for the evaluation of the visual system by pediatricians. *Pediatrics.* 2016; 137(1):e20153597

36. Fierson WM; American Academy of Pediatrics Section on Ophthalmology, American Academy of Ophthalmology, American Association for Pediatric Ophthalmology and Strabismus, American Association of Certified Orthoptists. Screening examination of premature infants for retinopathy of prematurity. *Pediatrics.* 2013;13:189–195

37. Dutton GN. Disorders of the brain and how they can affect vision. In: Lueck AH, Dutton GN, eds. *Vision and the Brain: Understanding Cerebral Visual Impairment in Children.* New York, NY: AFB Press; 2015

38. Roman-Lantzy C. *Cortical Visual Impairment: An Approach to Assessment and Intervention.* New York, NY: AFB Press; 2007

39. Das M, Spowart K, Crossley S, Dutton GN. Evidence that children with special needs all require visual assessment. *Arch Dis Child.* 2010;95:888–892

40. Fulton AB, Mayer L, Miller KB, Hansen RM. Eye and vision care. In: Rubin IL, Crocker AC, eds. *Medical Care for Children and Adults with Developmental Disabilities.* Baltimore, MD: Paul H. Brookes; 2006:343–352

41. Handler SM, Fierson WM; Section on Ophthalmology (AAP); Council on Children with Disabilities (AAP); American Academy of Ophthalmology; American Association for Pediatric Ophthalmology and Strabismus; American Association of Certified Orthoptists. Learning disabilities, dyslexia, and vision. *Pediatrics.* Pediatrics. 2011;127:e818–e856

42. Creavin AL, Lingam R, Steer C, Williams C. Ophthalmic abnormalities and reading impairment. *Pediatrics.* 2015;135:1057–1065

43. Jan JE. The visually impaired child and family. In: Taylor D, Hoyt CS, eds. *Pediatric Ophthalmology and Strabismus.* 3rd ed. Edinburgh, UK: Elsevier Saunders; 2005:127

44. Fazzi DL, Klein MD. Developing cognition, concepts, and language. In: Pogrund RI, Fazzi DL, eds. *Early Focus: Working with Young Children Who Are Blind or Visually Impaired and Their Families.* 2nd ed. New York, NY: AFB Press; 2002

45. Huebner KM. Visual impairment. In: Holbrook MC, Koenig AJ, eds. *Foundations of Education: History and Theory of Teaching Children and Youths With Visual Impairment.* 2nd ed. New York, NY: American Foundation for the Blind; 2000:58

46. Warren DH. *Blindness and Children: An Individual Differences Approach.* New York, NY: Cambridge University Press; 1994: 54–55, 106–107, 110–111, 117

47. Lueck AH, Chen D, Kekelis LS. *Developmental Guidelines for Visually Impaired Infants: A Manual for Infants Birth to Two.* Louisville, KY: American Printing House for the Blind; 1997

48. Bishop M, Hobson RP, Lee A. Symbolic play in congenitally blind children. *Dev Psychopathol.* 2005;17:447–465

49. Hughes M, Dote-Kwan J, Dolendo J. A close look at the cognitive play of preschoolers with visual impairments in the home. *Except Child.* 2008;64:451–462

50. American Foundation for the Blind. Teaching empathy to visually impaired children. http://www.familyconnect.org/info/browse-by-age/infants-and-toddlers/transition-to-independence-iandt/teaching-empathy/1235. Accessed November 23, 2017

51. Jan JE. Sleep disorders in children with poor vision. In: Taylor D, Hoyt CS, eds. *Pediatric Ophthalmology and Strabismus.* 3rd ed. Edinburgh, UK: Elsevier Saunders; 2005:1106–1107

52. Ryabets-Lienhard A, Stewart C, Borchert M, Geffner ME. The optic nerve hypoplasia spectrum: review of the literature and clinical guidelines. *Adv Pediatr.* 2016;63(1):127–146

53. Mukaddes NM, Kilincaslan A, Kucukyazici G, Sevketoglu T, Tuncer S. Autism in visually impaired individuals. *Psychiatry Clin Neurosci.* 2007:61(1):39–44

54. Freeman RD, Goetz E, Richards DP, Groenveld M. Defiers of negative prediction: a 14-year follow-up study of legally blind children. *J Vis Impair Blind.* 1991;85:365–370

55. Jure R, Pogonza R, Rapin I. Autism spectrum disorders (ASD) in blind children: very high prevalence, potentially better outlook. *J Autism Dev Disord.* 2016;46(3):749–759

56. Hobson RP, Lee A. Reversible autism among congenitally blind children? A controlled follow-up study. *J Child Psychol Psychiatry.* 2010;51(11):1235–1241

57. American Foundation for the Blind. The Expanded Core Curriculum for Students Who Are Blind or Visually Impaired Web site. http://www.familyconnect.org/info/education/expanded-core-curriculum/13 Accessed November 23, 2017

58. New Hampshire Department of Education. National Instructional Materials Accessibility Standard (NIMAS). https://www.education.nh.gov/instruction/special_ed/nimas.htm. Accessed November 23, 2017

59. The National Center on Deaf Blindness. *The 2015 National Child Count of Children and Youth Who Are Deaf-Blind.* The National Center on Deaf-Blindness, The Research Institute, Western Oregon University. October 2016. https://nationaldb.org/pages/show/2015-national-deaf-blind-child-count/2015-national-child-count-of-children-and-youth-who-are-deaf-blind-report. Accessed November 23, 2017

60. Nelson C, Bruce SM. Critical issues in the lives of children and youth who are deafblind. *Am Ann Deaf.* 2016;161(4):406–411

CHAPTER 14

Motor Development and Disorders

Catherine Morgan, PhD

Michael E. Msall, MD, FAAP

Typical Versus Atypical Development

Motor milestones are rapidly achieved in the first year of life with very few differences noted cross-culturally. This is helpful for primary pediatric health care professionals, as the typical sequential attainment of milestones in early childhood provides a window into neurodevelopment. Variations in both timing and sequence of milestone acquisition are often the first red flags alerting clinicians that all is not well developmentally. Differentiating between typical development that is simply slower than average and early signs of a more global delay or a defined neurodevelopmental disorder is not always straightforward. Developmental assessments are based on a neuromaturational model of development; however, current indications are that development is not linear but is a result of interaction between multiple subsystems.[1] It has been shown in typically developing children that progression on formal testing is not stable, and infants can move between percentile ranks.[2] Moreover, most children with disabilities continue to make some progress, and it is often not until a series of assessments are carried out that the rate of development is regarded as significantly slow enough to warrant further investigations or intervention. Unfortunately, this approach often delays access to intervention in the period of most rapid neural change.

The WHO Multicentre Growth Reference Study[3] provides helpful windows of achievement of gross motor skills. This longitudinal study, which followed 816 children from 5 different cultural groups (Ghana, India, Norway, Oman, and the United States) from 4 to 24 months of age, demonstrated the normal variation in gross motor milestone achievement in healthy children (see Table 14.1). This study found that the sequence of development chiefly varied with respect to the timing of crawling on the hands and knees. Most infants achieved this skill prior to walking with assistance; however, 8.5% did not crawl until later, and a further 4.3% never achieved crawling on the hands and knees. In this study, the narrowest window of achievement was for independent sitting. Ninety-nine percent of infants were sitting by 9 months, and the average age for sitting was 5.9 months. The age for independent walking ranged from 8 to 17 months with a mean age of 12 months; however, the mean age for walking with assistance was significantly earlier at 9 months.

Table 14.1. Motor Milestones				
Motor Milestones (n = 816)				
	10% (months)	**25% (months)**	**50% (months)**	**95% (months)**
Sitting without support	4.6	5.2	5.9	8
Crawling on hands and knees	6.6	7.4	8.3	11.3
Walking with assistance	7.4	8.2	9.0	11.8
Standing alone	8.8	9.7	10.8	14.4
Walking alone	10.0	11	12	15.3

Adapted with permission from WHO Multicentre Growth Reference Study Group. WHO Motor Development Study: windows of achievement for six gross motor development milestones. *Acta Paediatr.* 2006;95(S450):86–95.

Hand function emerges early in life with simple holding of toys beginning at 2 months and quickly developing into intentional grasping and mouthing of toys at around 3 to 4 months. By 6 months, infants can reach unilaterally and grasp a toy, transfer toys between hands, and can use both hands in coordinated action by 7 months. Coordinated sequential actions and more refined grasps are present by 9 to 10 months.

Primary pediatric health care professionals have at their disposal a number of screening instruments that can be utilized to identify early signs of developmental delay. The Ages & Stages Questionnaires (ASQ) with the following 3 extra questions are a good place to start when parents present concern about their infants' motor development[4]:

1. Is there anything your baby (or child) is doing with his or her arms, legs or body movements that concerns you?
2. Is there anything your baby (or child) is not doing with his or her arms, legs and body movements that concerns you?
3. Is there anything that you have tried to teach your infant (or child) to do involving his or her hands or whole body movement that has taken longer to learn than you think it should?

The American Academy of Pediatrics (AAP) provides a useful algorithm for evaluation of motor delay beginning at 9 months of age.[5] Signs of motor delay, however, are often evident prior to 4 months of age, including poor head control in prone and supported sitting, as well as incomplete visual tracking. Early asymmetries in hand function are not regarded as normal, and handedness is not apparent until between 2 and 4 years of age. Any asymmetry ought to be closely monitored or investigated more thoroughly, including brain magnetic resonance imaging (MRI) and evaluation by a physician, occupational therapist, or physical therapist. The primary pediatric health care professional might not be able to determine if these early delays are purely motor or more global at this time; however, referral for more thorough assessment and early intervention ought not to be delayed.

Motor delays that should prompt referral for early intervention include:
1. Poor head control at 4 months in prone or supported sitting
2. Asymmetry in upper limb function at any age
3. Not using hands purposefully by 4 months
4. Not sitting independently or taking weight through the feet by 9 months
5. Parental concern based on rate of development or unusual postures or movements

Spectrum of Motor Disorders

The spectrum of motor disorders in childhood is wide ranging from high prevalence, lower morbidity disorders such as developmental coordination disorder [DCD], to low prevalence, higher morbidity conditions such as cerebral palsy [CP]. Some authors have postulated that a continuum exists between these disorders because both are nonprogressive and occur in the developing brain.[6]

Developmental Coordination Disorder

The terms *developmental dyspraxia, minimal/minor neurological dysfunction,* and *clumsy child syndrome* have all been used to describe the same clinical presentation; however, the most generally accepted terminology is now *developmental coordination disorder* or DCD. *Diagnostic and Statistical Manual of Mental Disorders,* Fourth Edition[7] criteria required other general medical conditions (eg, intellectual disability, epilepsy, or autism spectrum disorder [ASD] to be excluded and required the motor impairment to be disproportionately impaired compared to verbal and nonverbal cognitive abilities. However, as motor coordination difficulties are a common marker for higher risk for a spectrum of comorbid communicative, cognitive, attention, and autism spectrum disorders, a broader perspective is in order. The *Diagnostic and Statistical Manual of Mental Disorders,* Fifth Edition (*DSM-5*)[8] and the European Academy of Childhood Disability[9] have emphasized the critical importance of a qualitative and quantitative approach to this disorder linked to evidence-based support.

Developmental coordination disorder affects approximately 5% to 6% of school-aged children, and children born preterm are 6 to 8 times more likely to be diagnosed with the condition.[10] Developmental coordination disorder is often not diagnosed until at least 5 years of age, although screening and the start of treatment can occur earlier. Children with this condition experience significant difficulties with activities of daily living and academic achievement due to poor performance of gross and fine motor skills.[10]

Although DCD is regarded as a mild motor disorder when compared to CP, the effects on the child's and family's quality of life can be significant.[11] In 2011, the European Academy of Childhood Disability produced comprehensive clinical guidelines for the diagnosis, assessment, and management of DCD.[12,13] Among these recommendations was evidence that task-oriented training approaches were more effective in improving motor function than sensory motor integration therapies. A subsequent systematic review and meta-analysis confirmed that interventions such as neuromotor task training and cognitive orientation to occupational performance have a larger effect on outcome than traditional approaches.[14]

Cerebral Palsy

Cerebral palsy is a heterogeneous condition and the most common physical disability of childhood. Current prevalence is estimated at 1 in 500 live births in developed countries.

Cerebral palsy is defined as "a group of disorders of the development of movement and posture, which are attributed to non-progressive lesions of the developing fetal or infant brain. The motor disorders of cerebral palsy are often accompanied by disturbances of sensation, perception, cognition, communication, and behaviour, by epilepsy, and by secondary musculoskeletal problems."[15]

The diagnostic label "cerebral palsy" does not imply anything about etiology or severity and is regarded as a clinical descriptive diagnosis.[16] To achieve a level of consistency in the use of the term *CP*, worldwide CP register groups have adopted a set of inclusion and exclusion criteria.[17] However, some discrepancies remain. For example, the Surveillance for Cerebral Palsy in Europe excludes central hypotonia as a subgroup of CP, while other registers include these children as hypotonic CP.[18] Both groups, however, emphasize that this hypotonia is of central nervous system origin and does not involve hypotonia with flaccid weakness. The latter is characteristic of processes involving spinal cord, muscle, or peripheral nerves. There is very rarely one specific cause of CP, and hence the phrase "causal pathways to cerebral palsy" is best used to describe etiology.[19] Much research has been done to identify individual risk factors for CP; however, little is understood about how risk factors diverse in timing act together to produce an eventual diagnosis of CP.[20]

– Type and Topography

There are 3 major classifications used to describe cases of CP: physiological motor type, topography, and function. The motor type and topography classifications are more traditional but notoriously unreliable.[20] Major advances have occurred in describing gross motor, manual ability, communicative, eating and drinking, and self-care functioning.

When classifying based on physiological motor type, the movement disorder is described based on

1. spasticity (velocity-dependent resistance to stretch),
2. dyskinesia (choreoathetosis [hyperkinesia with hypotonia] or dystonia [hypokinesia with hypertonic movements characterized by involuntary twisting postures or repetitive movements]; includes nearly 4% to 7% of children with CP),
3. ataxia (loss of coordination with abnormal movement force, rhythm, and accuracy; includes 4% to 6% of children with CP), and
4. hypotonia (pure, generalized decreased muscle tone without flaccid weakness; includes only 2% of children with CP).[20]

When classifying based on topography, the following categories are used: hemiplegia/unilateral (involvement of 1 side of the body; includes about 38% of children with CP), diplegia (both lower limbs affected more so than upper limbs; includes about 36% of children with CP), and quadriplegia (all 4 limbs affected with upper limbs at least as affected as lower limbs; includes about 26% of children with CP). There are also rare cases in which only 1 limb is affected (monoplegia) or 1 upper limb is spared (triplegia). In Europe, diplegia and quadriplegia are collapsed into one category, known as bilateral CP, in order to increase reliability of classification.[20]

Functional classifications are very helpful for clinicians both for describing severity of impairment and for prognosticating about future needs. Two motor classifications for both gross motor function (Gross Motor Function Classification Scale [GMFCS]) and manual ability (Manual Ability Classification Scale [MACS]) are now widely used, and recently, a communicative functioning classification scale (CFCS) and an eating and drinking ability classification scale (EADACS) have been added.

The Gross Motor Function Classification Scale (GMFCS), considered to be the "contemporary gold standard" of CP classification, is a 5-level ordered scale describing an individual's functional mobility.[20,21] GMFCS classification is based on the child's ability to sit, transfer, and mobilize (see Figure 14.1).[20]

The GMFCS was initially developed for children from 6 to 12 years of age, but an expanded and revised version was later developed for ages 2 to 18 years.[22] It is also important to be cautious in using the current GMFCS among children under 2 years of age, as 40% will change their level.[23]

Motor development curves for CP incorporating GMFCS levels are widely used to discuss prognosis with families and plan achievable rehabilitation goals.[24] Longitudinal assessment of these curves demonstrates that children with CP achieve 90% of their gross motor development potential by age 5 years across all GMFCS levels.[24] In addition, children at GMFCS level V reach this point before 3 years of age.[24] When counseling families, it is important to note that, based on GMFCS prevalence rates, mild CP is more common than severe CP.[20]

GMFCS E & R between 6th and 12th birthday: Descriptors and illustrations

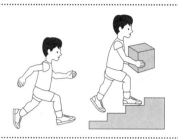

GMFCS Level I

Children walk at home, school, outdoors and in the community. They can climb stairs without the use of a railing. Children perform gross motor skills such as running and jumping, but speed, balance and coordination are limited.

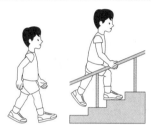

GMFCS Level II

Children walk in most settings and climb stairs holding onto a railing. They may experience difficulty walking long distances and balancing on uneven terrain, inclines, in crowded areas or confined spaces. Children may walk with physical assistance, a hand-held mobility device or used wheeled mobility over long distances. Children have only minimal ability to perform gross motor skills such as running and jumping.

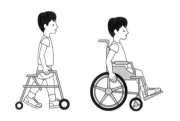

GMFCS Level III

Children walk using a hand-held mobility device in most indoor settings. They may climb stairs holding onto a railing with supervision or assistance. Children use wheeled mobility when traveling long distances and may self-propel for shorter distances.

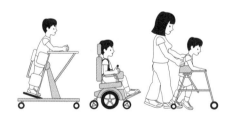

GMFCS Level IV

Children use methods of mobility that require physical assistance or powered mobility in most settings. They may walk for short distances at home with physical assistance or use powered mobility or a body support walker when positioned. At school, outdoors and in the community children are transported in a manual wheelchair or use powered mobility.

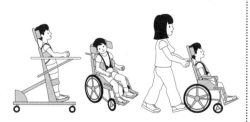

GMFCS Level V

Children are transported in a manual wheelchair in all settings. Children are limited in their ability to maintain antigravity head and trunk postures and control leg and arm movements.

GMFCS descriptors: Palisano et al. (1997) Dev Med Child Neurol 39:214-23
CanChild: www.canchild.ca

Illustrations Version 2 © Bill Reid, Kate Willoughby, Adrienne Harvey and Kerr Graham,
The Royal Children's Hospital Melbourne   ERC151050

Figure 14.1. Gross motor function classification scale (GMFCS).

Reproduced with permission. Copyright © Bill Reid, Kate Willoughby, Adrienne Harvey, and Kerr Graham, The Royal Children's Hospital; CanChild.

The Manual Ability Classification Scale (MACS) and mini-MACS (used prior to age 4 years) classify how children with CP use their hands in everyday activities.[25,26] These 5-level scales range from "handles objects easily and successfully" to "does not handle objects and has severely limited ability to perform even simple actions."[25, 26] Studies have shown there is not always a high correlation between MACS and GMFCS levels; however, the relationship is variable across subgroups of children with hemiplegia, diplegia, and quadriplegia.[27] It is recommended that both measures are used in clinical practice.

– Prevalence

Over 750,000 children and adults in the United States are affected by CP. The lifetime cost of CP was estimated to be $1 billion per individual and $1.2 billion in direct medical costs for all children born with CP in the year 2000.[28] However, because accurate population tracking similar to the Centers for Disease Control and Prevention (CDC) Autism Surveillance Network is not currently taking place in the United States, these aggregated costs should be viewed as a preliminary estimate.

– Diagnosing Cerebral Palsy
Risk Factors

Risk factors for CP are various, reflecting the heterogeneity of the condition. Approximately 40% of all children with CP were born preterm, yet less than 10% of all preterm infants go on to have CP.[29] Cerebral palsy has frequently been linked with both prematurity and low birth weight in the United States, Australia, Scandinavia, and Western Europe. In one European study, it was found that approximately 54% of children with CP were born at term gestation while 18% were born at 32 to 36 weeks' gestation, 16% were born at 28 to 31 weeks' gestation, and 11% were born at <28 weeks' gestation.[30]

There are 5 particularly important risk factors for CP in preterm cohorts. The first is the presence of parenchymal brain injury (intraventricular hemorrhage grade 3 or 4, ventriculomegaly, or cystic periventricular leukomalacia [PVL]). One study found that while cystic PVL was highly predictive of future CP, it was not predictive of outcome severity.[22] Furthermore, in this study, cystic PVL and a related lesion of periventricular hemorrhagic infarction (PVHI) could account for only 32% of CP cases and 13% of cognitive disability cases.[28] Therefore, it has been concluded that brain abnormalities other than PVHI and cystic PVL are likely responsible for a significant percentage of preterm CP cases.[28]

The second key risk factor for CP is multiple gestation. There is evidence that twin pregnancies have a higher rate of CP than singleton pregnancies (20 in 1,000 compared to 2 in 1,000) and that the rate continues to increase for pregnancies of triplets (100 in 1,000) and quadruplets (500 in 1,000).[28]

The other 3 key risk factors for CP are chronic lung disease (determined by the need for supplemental oxygen at 36 weeks' gestation), retinopathy of prematurity stage 4 or 5, and the presence of severe infection (eg, postnatal sepsis, necrotizing enterocolitis, meningitis).[28]

A key risk factor for CP in term infants is neonatal encephalopathy. These infants account for 25% of term children with CP. However, the majority of term CP infants have no identifiable risk factors around the time of birth.[31] A recent systematic review identified placental abnormalities, malformations, low birth weight, meconium aspiration, instrumental or emergency Caesarean delivery, birth asphyxia (unspecified timing/duration), neonatal seizures, respiratory distress syndrome, hypoglycemia, and neonatal infections as consistent risk factors for CP in term infants.[32] Other research has identified abnormal posturing, limited ability to lift head from floor in prone position, head lag, poor visual tracking, and poorly coordinated eye movements as developmental risk factors that may be useful in the early identification of CP.[20]

However, ultimately there are no biomarkers that can accurately predict which infants will have CP. Further, clinical risk factors can only partially identify subpopulations of infants who are at increased risk of CP.[20]

Diagnosis Timeline

Formal diagnosis of CP has traditionally occurred in the second year of life based on clinical examination and often after the exclusion of other conditions. About half of all children who are diagnosed with CP spend time in a neonatal intensive care unit or special care nursery as newborns. Theoretically, the risk for CP in these children ought to be established early, as they undergo multiple assessments and are monitored regularly in the first years of life. Register data indicates that infants with neonatal risk factors associated with more severe forms of CP, such as neonatal encephalopathy, are often diagnosed earlier. A recent population register study showed, however, that preterm infants were not more likely to be diagnosed earlier unless they had an abnormal cranial ultrasound (CUS).[33] Yet, some studies of preterms have shown that one-third of cases of CP are not detected when CUS alone is used as a neuroimaging modality.[34] In fact, earlier detection of CP does not routinely occur in these infants, often delaying access to intervention.[35]

For children with no apparent traditional risk factor, investigations typically begin when it becomes apparent that motor milestones are not being reached. However, as many standardized motor tests are not specifically predictive of CP, and as motor signs such as spasticity often do not appear until the second year, it can still be some time before an official CP diagnosis is given. Register data indicates that ambulant children with CP are not diagnosed until 17 months of age on average and that ambulant children with bilateral spastic CP have an even later median diagnostic age of 23.9 months.[31]

In recent years, a large body of evidence has accumulated that suggests CP can and should be diagnosed earlier. Many things should be taken into consideration when seeking to make an early diagnosis, including any history of CP risk factors, the presence of any brain structural abnormalities, abnormal general movement between 12 and 20 weeks' postterm equivalent age, abnormal neurological signs, poor feeding skills, eye tracking difficulty, the presence of opisthotonic postures in the supine position, and a lack of integration of strong primitive reflexes into voluntary motor patterns.[20] It is also important to determine a comprehensive quantitative and qualitative assessment framework for examining fine, gross, visual, and oral motor skills through the first 6 months of life. A systemic review has demonstrated that the absence of fidgety movements at 12 weeks post conception has a 98% sensitivity and 91% specificity for CP. This tool is superior to MRI (86%, 89-97%), neurological exam (88%, 87%), and cranial ultrasound (74%, 92%).[36]

Physical Examination

During the physical examination, the child should be in a relaxed state and nonintrusive observations should be the starting point. These observations include the infant's general state and his or her spontaneous demonstration of neurological skills, such as 360-degree visual tracking, strong sucking, symmetric facies, lifting the head and chest, and supporting weight on forearms or wrists in prone position. Other key observations occur with gentle handling and include head lag on pull to sit; flipping or early rolling in a nongraded fashion (which reflects abnormally persistent primitive reflexes); becoming unfisted and demonstrating midline and manipulative hand play; and batting at, obtaining, and transferring objects.[20]

An early diagnosis of CP can be established by considering motor delay in combination with indicators of abnormalities of tone, reflexes, and postural motor control.[20] Historically, Capute and Shapiro have emphasized the importance of the motor quotient involving observed postural skills.[37]

A recent consensus statement has emphasized the value of General Movement Assessment (98% sensitivity), term age brain MRI (86-89% sensitivity), and the Hammersmith Infant Neurological Evaluation (HINE) (90% sensitivity) before 5 months corrected age.[38]

After 5 months corrected age, the most predictive tools for detecting CP were a brain MRI (86-89% sensitivity), the HINE (90% sensitivity), and a standardized motor assessment with the Developmental Assessment of Young Children (89% predictive) or the Alberta Infant Motor Scale (86% predictive).[38]

Recently, Maitre and colleagues described standardization of the neurological exam using the HINE in high-risk infant follow-up programs.[39–41] Additionally, webinars and training workshops for general movements have been offered through the CP Research Foundation and the CP Alliance.

By definition, a CP diagnosis requires the presence of a movement and posture disorder that limits the child's ability to perform activities. These neurological impairments might include spastic weakness, unusual postures, and challenges during feeding. Of course, the younger the child is, the more difficult it is to observe these.[20]

Feeding Difficulty

Difficulty with oral feeding is one of the most frequently occurring and recognizable CP risk factors. Difficulty with oral feeding can also be recognized early, as it is an infant's first voluntary motor skill. Difficulty sucking and swallowing, extended feeding time for small volumes, and respiratory distress during feeding are all manifestations of poor oral feeding skills.[20] By 4 to 6 months of age, many children with CP exhibit feeding difficulty in addition to difficulty with head control and an abnormal neurological examination.[20]

Neuroimaging

Brain imaging is widely used to document the presence and extent of brain structural integrity in CP, and increasingly sophisticated tools are under development. A number of systematic reviews have demonstrated that certain defined patterns of injury in the grey and/or white matter nearly always lead to CP, indicating the importance of appropriately timed neuroimaging in the diagnostic process.[42,43] For example, MRI exams at 36 weeks postmenstrual age in former very low and extremely low birth weight preterm infants are incredibly valuable for the highest-risk cohort of preterm infants.[28] There is also considerable evidence that CP can be predicted with neuroimaging in the newborn period, provided the optimal sequences and timing are used.[44,45] Evidence-based recommendations for timing and use of preferred imaging modalities are available for preterm infants and those with neonatal encephalopathy;[46] however, recommendations for infants not considered high-risk are more complicated. The AAP suggests that the MRI be carried out in the case of increased tone,[5] and the American Academy of Neurology and the Child Neurology Society have produced an evaluation parameter, also recommending imaging be conducted during the diagnostic process.[47] However, clinical research also documents outcomes that do not seem to "match" imaging findings, and it is estimated that up to 15% of children with CP have normal neuroimaging. It should also be noted that although understanding of the etiology of CP is growing, methods of CP detection in high-risk populations still need much improvement, as there is currently no imaging strategy with 95% sensitivity and specificity and none that accurately predicts the severity of disability.[28] The combined use of neuroimaging, standard motor developmental assessment (General Movement Assessment, Test of Infant Motor Performance), and neurological examination provides the best information for early and accurate diagnosis of CP.[29] When a diagnosis of CP cannot be made with confidence due to nonspecific or conflicting clinical results, the designation "high risk of CP" should be given, and the infant should be referred for early intervention services.

Further Assessments

While all children diagnosed with CP will have a motor impairment, the motor impairment rarely exists in isolation. There are several impairments, diseases, and functional limitations that frequently co-occur with CP, all of which further impact a child's prognosis and independence and should be screened for during the diagnostic process.[48] In particular, epilepsy and intellectual disability combined with severe physical disability tend to impact prognosis and life expectancy the most.[20] There are many other comorbidities of CP. Chronic pain is one of the most common, affecting approximately 3 in 4 children with CP.[48] Others include cognitive impairment, which affects almost 50% of children with CP, and sleep disorders, which affect 20%.[49] Behavior disorders affect

25%, epilepsy 28%, scoliosis 7%, and hearing impairment 7%.[20,30] Some studies have shown that visual impairment affects 42% of children with CP, and that 10% are functionally blind.[30] Difficulties with feeding are also common, and 41% of children with CP experience functional walking limitations, 69% experience fine motor limitations, and 58% experience communication challenges.[30] In school-aged children, specific learning disorders often appear, including challenges with reading, mathematics, handwriting, attention deficit and executive function, anxiety, and ASD.

The natural history of CP usually involves secondary musculoskeletal impairment, and early hip surveillance is now considered the standard of care[50] due to the high prevalence of hip pathology, even in children as young as 2 to 3 years of age. Current recommendations are for the initial AP pelvic radiograph to be taken at 12 to 24 months of age or at the time of diagnosis if later.[51]

– Informing Families of Diagnosis

The primary goal when informing families of developmental diagnoses is to be supportive and link families to informed management resources that set achievable goals and allow them to feel empowered. The critical aim is to be proactive and give all children with evolving neurodevelopmental disability quality support while not being too pessimistic or overwhelming caregivers with either fear or a myriad of details.[20] Informing a parent of his or her child's diagnosis will be a difficult conversation, but it is important that it be done well. Many parents report being dissatisfied with the amount of information they receive at diagnosis and a lack of discussion about the likely impact of CP on their families. The parents' chief criticisms are unclear information and the clinician conveying a pessimistic future outlook in delivering the news.[20] When communicating news to families, primary pediatric health care professionals must recognize that parental acceptance of the CP diagnosis will be a shifting and ongoing process, and that continuous dialog will be needed.[20]

At the initial diagnosis, in their efforts to understand the news, parents of children with cerebral palsy will almost always ask whether the child will walk, talk, and be able to learn. Individual answers will depend on the severity of physical disability, the type of motor impairment, and the presence of comorbid conditions, most of which may be very difficult to determine during the neonatal period and in the first year of life.[20]

It is important for parents to understand that though CP currently has no cure, it does not mean that developmental progress does not occur. Primary pediatric health care professionals can comfort parents in the difficult task of coming to terms with an individual child's activity limitations by helping them to maintain hope. For example, knowing that mild CP is more common than severe CP can offer parents hope. In addition, there is currently substantial neuroprotection and neuroregenerative research under way that is investigating enhanced plasticity and potential cures.[52] Parents should be coached to be mindful of their child's function in the longer term rather than pursuing overly ambitious physical feats. Parents can also be reassured that severity of physical disability does not predetermine quality of life.[20]

The most important messages to convey to parents are highlighted in Box 14.1.

– Evidence-Based Interventions in Cerebral Palsy

Rehabilitative interventions are the standard of care for children with CP, and available interventions broadly fall into 3 categories based on their aims: (1) improving function, (2) preventing secondary impairments from occurring, and (3) adapting and enriching the child's environment.

High-quality evidence exists for some interventions that aim to improve motor function in children with CP; however, there are still many interventions with poor supporting evidence that are part of the standard care of children with CP. Traditional interventions based on facilitation and handling (including neurodevelopmental therapy) or passive stretching have been shown to be ineffective and should be abandoned now that alternative treatment options are available.[53]

A number of developmental and therapeutic interventions are offered in the neonatal period with the aim of optimizing the infant's comfort, parental attachment, and developmental outcome. None of these interventions are specific to CP, but it is possible that these interventions are helping to contribute to the reduced rate of CP following prematurity, which has been observed in recent years. These interventions are, therefore, an integral part of the standard care for infants with CP.[20]

– Early Intervention

The aim of early intervention is to harness neuroplasticity mechanisms at work in the infant brain. It is well accepted that intervention should start as soon as a permanent disability is suspected, as the corticospinal tract is still developing and targeted activity-based therapy can influence the development and connectivity of axon termi-nals.[54] The "wait-and-see" approaches does not optimize developmental outcomes.

Most early intervention research that has been done in preterm populations consistently demonstrates improvements in cognitive outcomes with little effect on motor skills.[55] Less is known about the effects of early intervention in infants with CP; however, emer-ging research suggests that interventions that are task specific, involve environmental enrichment, and are family centered can improve motor and cognitive outcomes.[56-58] Interventions should always be child focused and provided at a level that matches the child's ability yet is scaffolded to introduce increasing challenges as skills emerge. Active parental involvement in early intervention is vital, as sensitive and responsive parenting improves the child's cognitive and behavioral outcomes and allows for a more intense "dose" of therapeutic activity.

Infants with emerging hemiplegia may benefit from modified forms of constraint-induced movement therapy (CIMT), as cohort studies have demonstrated improved functional ability in children who had CIMT during infancy.[59] CIMT and training of bimanual hand function are equally effective in improving hand function when offered at the same dose.[60] These interventions ought to be offered to children with hemiplegic CP as a standard of care. Studies show that 60 hours of intervention are required to achieve long-term improvements. Finally, early treadmill training might bring forward the onset of independent walking and improve gait quality.[61]

– Goal-Directed and Functional Training

Goal-directed training (GDT) is an activity-based approach that involves intense and repeated practice of specific, everyday tasks that the child and family have chosen as the goals for therapy. These tasks could be in the areas of gross motor skills, self-care, communication, play, or school-based activities. This functional approach does not primarily try to "fix" the child by addressing muscle tone or strength but instead pro-vides opportunities in real-life environments for the child to achieve his or her goals. This might include adaptations to the environment. Best-practice home programs support functional training and improve outcomes.

– Splints and Orthoses

Ankle and foot orthoses are frequently used to help maintain range of movement and improve gait. Upper limb orthoses are frequently used to improve functional grasp or maintain range of motion.

– Assistive Technology

A vast array of equipment and assistive technology is now available for children to improve access to communication, the school environment, and to assist parents in caregiving. Early access to powered mobility for young children who are nonambulant is important for optimizing cognition and social inclusion.[62] Speech therapists, occupa-tional therapists, physical therapists, and assistive technology professionals are skilled at identifying appropriate equipment solutions for home and school to optimize the development of children with significant motor, speech, and language impairments.

– Medical Interventions

Spasticity management is an important component of the management of children with CP. Focal but temporary spasticity management can be achieved through the use of botulinum toxin-A (botox-A) injections. Botox-A injections should be related to specific functional goals and are most effective when combined with physical or occupational therapy postinjections.[63]

When spasticity affects many muscle groups, medications might be required. Baclofen, dantrolene, and diazepam are all used for spasticity management; however, side effects can limit their usefulness. Intrathecal baclofen is infrequently used when spasticity is difficult to manage with oral medications. There is some evidence that interventions of this sort have a positive effect in the short term.[64]

The effects of spasticity and reduced muscle activity result in contracture development over time, and many children with spasticity require surgery to maintain ambulation, reduce pain, or prevent further deterioration of joint integrity. To correct hip subluxation, soft tissue surgery may be all that is required if optimal surveillance is used and migration identified early. A systematic surveillance and prevention program conducted in Sweden has resulted in complete eradication of hip dislocation, indicating that its natural history can be interrupted through providing the right treatments at the right time.[65]

– Prognosis

Almost all children with CP live to adulthood. Children at the highest risk of early mortality are those with severe physical disability coupled with epilepsy and intellectual disability. About 5% to 10% of children with CP die during childhood, according to Norwegian and Swedish CP registers.[20]

Associated medical comorbidities of CP, including feeding and swallowing difficulties, seizures, visual and hearing impairments, and orthopedic deformities can develop over time. Many of these comorbidities can be managed, so the prognosis of a child with CP often depends on the type and severity of CP and the accompanying medical comorbidities.

The degree of community acceptance of a child with disability; the child's curiosity, determination, and problem-solving skills; and the accessibility of education and community supports also affect the outcomes of a child diagnosed with CP.[30] The main goal of any CP management program is to help optimize performance in mobility, functioning in daily activities, educational attainment, and social participation. Children with CP require ongoing care management for nutrition, sensory disorders, deformities, mobility skills, psychoeducational functioning, and adaptive equipment.[30]

– Quality of Life

Many challenges stem from overly focusing on motor impairments rather than promoting developmental, self-care, and communicative functioning. The caregivers' concerns might be more focused on their fears of an uncertain future rather than exploring current strategies that promote self-care, learning, and social competencies despite the child's motor impairments.

There are several crucial components for achieving independence: self-mobility, learning and problem-solving skills, educational achievement, family support, and community accessibility.[30] Among health professionals, it is important to have a life-cycle approach that continuously promotes the child's independence and has self-efficacy as a goal. The focus of caregivers should grow and change with the child. During early and middle childhood, caregivers of children with CP should be more concerned with their child's ability to perform self-care, communicate with peers, and learn in school. Throughout adolescence and young adulthood, educational achievement, friendships, relationships, and job attainment should be prioritized.[30]

Despite parental concerns regarding the mobility challenges of children with CP, on average, over half of children with CP learn to walk without aids, and an additional 20% learn to walk with assistive or mobility devices. It should be noted that individuals with hemiplegia have the highest rate of ambulatory function, and 100% learn to walk either independently or with aids. Furthermore, approximately 90% of individuals with diplegic CP learn to walk (GMFCS levels 1 to 3).[30]

Spina Bifida

In children with spina bifida, spinal level is typically classified as either thoracic, high lumbar (L1 or L2), midlumbar (L3), low lumbar (L4 or L5), or sacral, and the level is determined through a careful examination of motor function as well as sensation.[66] Some hip flexion and adduction, but no quadriceps strength, may be present in children with high lumbar myelomeningocele. Loss of sensation around the anus, perineum, and feet is common in children with low lumbar or sacral myelomeningocele, but it is possible to have lower sacral lesions with no loss of sensation.[66]

There is an extensive body of research reviewing functional mobility outcomes and the need for bracing in different levels of spina bifida.[66] Some children with thoracic or high lumbar lesions may be able to stand upright and walk, relying on considerable support of the hips, knees, and ankles.[66] Children with L3 paralysis typically rely on the use of forearm crutches and bracing above the knees, although most children with midlumbar spina bifida become increasingly reliant on wheelchairs as they age.[66] Children who have lesions in the sacral vertebrae can typically walk by age 2 or 3 years but may require some bracing at their ankles.[66]

Myelomeningocele affects motor and sensory nerves, as well as sacral parasympathetic nerves—which innervate the rectum, urethra, and walls of the bladder and are critical for sexual function—and lumbar sympathetic nerves that control the bladder outlet.[66]

Historically, prior to the fetal surgery era, most babies with myelomeningocele had a Chiari type II malformation of the brain. Chiari type II malformation involves displacement of the cerebellum, medulla, and fourth ventricle, elongation of the medulla and fourth ventricle, corpus callosum dysgenesis, the appearance of a small posterior fossa, and is often accompanied by associated hydrocephalus.[66] Chiari type II typically appears in the fifth week of gestation and is typically the result of abnormal neurulation. Often, the malformation is not accompanied by symptoms, although a variety of symptoms connected to compression of the brainstem and lower cranial nerve dysfunction may appear.[66] Symptoms of Chiari crisis include weak or absent crying, stridor, apnea and color change, feeding and swallowing disorders, arching of the neck, gastroesophageal reflux, and failure to thrive. Eighty percent (80%) of Chiari type II patients with sacral lesions receive a ventriculoperitoneal shunt, and the percentage increases to 90% for Chiari type II patients with higher-level lesions.[66] With fetal therapy in experienced centers, there have been decreased rates of hydrocephalus requiring shunting, decreased hindbrain herniation, and improved motor outcomes.[67]

Spina bifida has a significant and lasting impact on the functioning of affected individuals. There is evidence that children and adolescents with spina bifida tend to have a reduced health-related quality of life (HRQOL) when compared to individuals with other chronic health conditions, and that this difference tends to hold across sex, age, geographical location, and time.[66] Measures of the severity of spina bifida, including lesion level, continence status, and surgical procedure outcomes, are often not associated with HRQOL, but other factors, such as lack of mobility and the presence of shunted hydrocephalus, are significantly associated with HRQOL.[67] Pain levels, parental stress, social class, and other family factors can also be strong predictors of HRQOL effects.[68]

Individuals with spina bifida tend to experience lower levels of self-concept and high levels of depressive symptoms in late childhood when compared to unaffected individuals.[69] Children and adolescents with spina bifida also tend to experience social difficulties that can persist into young adulthood. These difficulties include being socially immature or passive, having fewer friends, being less likely to have social contacts outside of school, and dating less during adolescence.[68]

The mortality rate among individuals with spina bifida is approximately 1% per year between ages 5 and 30 years, and this rate is the highest among individuals with the highest level of lesions.[68] The quality of survivors' health typically declines from adolescence to young adulthood. This effect is likely caused by difficulties in transitioning to adult health care.[68] Adults with spina bifida are also at risk of depressive symptoms and anxiety, but they are less likely to engage in risky behaviors, possibly because of their lower rates of social integration.[68]

Individuals with spina bifida are less likely to go to college than typically developing young people (41% to 56% compared to 66%) and are employed full- or part-time at lower rates than typically developing young people and those with other chronic conditions.[68] Of those who are employed, over half work part-time positions and therefore earn annual salaries below the national average.[68] Approximately half of individuals with spina bifida are in a romantic relationship, which is a lower rate than that for typically developing young adults.[68] Between 43% and 77% of individuals with spina bifida live with their parents.[68] It has been found that levels of life satisfaction are the lowest in the areas of romantic relationships, employment, and financial independence for individuals with spina bifida.[68] Executive functioning deficits and specific learning disabilities, particularly nonverbal learning disabilities, are prevalent in adolescents with spina bifida and hydrocephalus and play a prominent role in the adolescent's ability to succeed at school, learn self-care, and master social skills.

Tic Disorders and Tourette Syndrome

Simple tics are very common in childhood, as 6% to 13% of all children will experience a transient tic at some time during childhood.[69] The childhood incidence of chronic tic disorder is around 1% to 2%, with an approximate 3:1 ratio of boys to girls.[69] Transient tic disorders can last between 4 weeks and 1 year, include single or multiple motor and/ or vocal tics, and most are simple rather than complex and do not usually cause great distress. However, a child with complex and distressing motor and vocal tics lasting a few months may be at risk for developing Tourette syndrome (TS).

Tourette syndrome is defined as the presence of multiple motor tics and at least 1 vocal tic (not necessarily concurrently), lasting over the course of at least 1 year, with tic-free periods lasting no longer than 3 months.[69] Onset must be before 18 years of age, and peak onset is around 5 to 8 years of age. The nature and severity of the tics may fluctuate, as these characteristics are associated with impaired function or distress.[69] Tic severity tends to peak at approximately 9 to 11 years of age, and tics often improve or even disappear during puberty.[69]

Tourette syndrome has a prevalence of about 0.3%, and it is more common in teenagers than in preteens and in white children than in black or Hispanic children.[69] Forty percent of children with TS also meet criteria for obsessive-compulsive disorder (OCD), and more than 20% of children with tic disorders have OCD.[69] Sixty-four percent of children with TS have been diagnosed with attention-deficit/hyperactivity disorder (ADHD), and half of all children with tic disorders have ADHD.[68] Clinical depression (impacting 36% of individuals with TS), anxiety (40%), developmental problems (28%), and learning difficulties (80%) are also common comorbidities of TS.[69]

There seem to be both genetic and nongenetic factors at play in the etiology of TS. Certain cortico-striato-thalamo-cortical circuits have been implicated because of their key roles in the initiation and inhibition of psychomotor activity and in the detection and avoidance of harm, and limbic, cognitive, and motor circuits work in tandem to suppress responses to both internal and external stimuli.[69]

Tics are fragments of normal behaviors that occur quickly and in isolation. Tics can be confused with normal behavior and are easy to mimic.[69] Tics are more repetitive and less variable than behaviors such as recurrent throat clearing and sniffing associated with allergies and habits like hair-twirling, nose-touching, and skin-picking. There is not a definitive test for the presence of tics, and so there are indistinct boundaries between simple tics and habits, as well as between complex tics and the compulsive symptoms of OCD.[69] When evaluating tic disorders, it is necessary to keep a few things in mind: (1) it is important to examine and consider the child's experience of the tics and any social or emotional impact; (2) it is important to rule out the presence of other movement disorders through physical and neurological examinations; (3) it can be useful to use neurodevelopmental examinations to look for processing problems, such as attention deficits; and (4) currently, no specific diagnostic tests for tics exist.[69]

The goals of management of tic disorders are to minimize stress, social isolation, and functional impairment. Education and demystification for the affected child, his or her family, and school personnel also help to promote support and tolerance. Treatments can include behavioral modification techniques, such as habit reversal and cognitive behavior therapy, as well as judicious pharmacotherapy. It should be noted that tics should be aggressively treated only if they are causing major functional impairment. The presence, scope, and severity of comorbid diagnoses (ADHD, OCD, and depression) should also be assessed in planning pharmacotherapy. Common psychopharmacological treatments for tics include alpha-2 norepinephrine agonists and antipsychotics/neuroleptics, and for comorbid diagnoses, stimulants for ADHD and tic disorders and selective serotonin reuptake inhibitors for OCD and tic disorders.

The child with recent onset of tics is a common patient presenting to primary pediatric health care professionals. If the child's first tic appeared less than a year in the past, the diagnosis is usually provisional tic disorder. Published reviews by experts[70-75] demonstrate a substantial consensus on prognosis in this situation: The tics will often disappear within a few months, having remained mild while they lasted.

– Pediatric Autoimmune Neuropsychiatric Disorders Associated with Streptococcal Infections (PANDAS)

Pediatric Autoimmune Neuropsychiatric Disorders Associated with Streptococcal Infections, or PANDAS, are closely related to Sydenham chorea of rheumatic fever. Circumstantial evidence suggests that PANDAS may result from antineuronal antibodies affecting basal ganglia function.[69] Some children appear susceptible to abrupt onset or sudden emergence of tics, compulsions, emotional lability, and anxiety during or following an acute episode of streptococcal pharyngitis. Recently, 2 pilot randomized controlled trials have explored the role of azithromycin and intravenous immunoglobulin (IVIG) in the acute management of those children with acute-onset PANDAS.[76,77]

Motor Stereotypies

Motor stereotypies, such as body rocking, head-banging, facial-grimacing, and hand-flapping, are rhythmic, patterned, repetitive, nonfunctional movements that can occur in both children with typical neurodevelopment as well as more frequently in children with intellectual disability, ASD, visual impairment, and sensorineural hearing loss. The age of onset of motor stereotypies is less than 2 years, and boys outnumber girls by 2:1.

Children with motor stereotypies are unaware of their occurrence, and unlike tics, motor stereotypies are not associated with an urge or compulsion. Repeated instructions to the child to stop are not effective. Unlike compulsive behaviors observed in OCD, motor stereotypies do not bother the child but can be distressing to parents. Children with motor stereotypies without intellectual disability, ASD, or sensory impairments are more likely to have ADHD, learning disabilities, or motor incoordination. Twenty-five percent of children with motor stereotypies have a positive family history of motor stereotypies, suggesting an underlying genetic abnormality.[78] Behavioral interventions are the primary treatment for motor stereotypies.

Neuromuscular Disorders of Childhood

Neuromuscular disorders present with hypotonia and weakness. In the neonatal period, these disorders may include congenital muscular dystrophy, Pompe disease, and congenital myotonic dystrophy. In early childhood, all children with motor delay, low muscle tone, and an uncoordinated gait should have a serum creatine kinase (CK) level (to rule out Duchenne muscular dystrophy [DMD] and related neuromuscular or inflammatory myopathies) and thyroid function testing performed. The most important diseases to manage and recognize are Duchenne muscular dystrophy, Pompe disease, and spinal muscle atrophy, as major advances are occurring in the diagnosis and treatment of neuromuscular disorders.[79,80]

Duchenne muscular dystrophy is one of the most common inherited genetic diseases and is caused by mutations to the DMD gene that encodes the dystrophin protein.[81] In addition to progressive muscular dystrophy, children with DMD are at increased risk of intellectual disability, learning disability, ADHD, and ASD. Over the course of the last century, the average life expectancy of patients with DMD has doubled, and it now stands at approximately 25 years.[82] This progress has been made possible through advances in the diagnosis, treatment, and long-term care of patients with DMD. Both basic science and clinical research, national and international scientific networks, and parent and patient support groups have all contributed to achieving this goal. The advent of molecular genetic therapies and personalized medicine has opened up new avenues and raised hopes that ameliorating the relentless course of this disease will be found. Recent advances in genome editing and gene therapy offer hope for the development of potential therapeutics. Truncated versions of the DMD gene can be delivered to the affected tissues with viral vectors and show promising results in a variety of animal models.

Myotonic dystrophy type 1 (DM1) is a multisystem disease arising from mutant cytosine-thymine-guanine (CTG) expansion in the nontranslating region of the dystrophia myotonica protein kinase gene.[83] While DM1 is the most common adult muscular dystrophy, with a worldwide prevalence of 1 in 8,000, age of onset varies from before birth to adulthood. There is a broad spectrum of clinical severity, ranging from mild to severe, which correlates with the number of DNA repeats. Importantly, the early clinical manifestations and management in congenital and childhood DM1 differ from classic adult DM1. In neonates and children, DM1 predominantly affects muscle strength, cognition, and the respiratory, central nervous, and gastrointestinal systems. Sleep disorders are often underrecognized, yet these represent a significant morbidity. Neuropsychological examinations in patients with myotonic dystrophy show a great variability of results from intellectual disability to more subtle cognitive impairments. It is unclear whether different clusters of neuropsychological deficits appear in different phenotypes of DM, or if there are patients with no cognitive deficit at all.[68] No effective disease-modifying treatment is currently available, and neonates and children with DM1 may experience severe physical and intellectual disability, which may be life limiting in the most severe forms. Novel therapies, which target the gene and the pathogenic mechanism of abnormal splicing, are emerging.

Spinal muscular atrophies (SMAs) are hereditary degenerative disorders of lower motor neurons associated with progressive muscle weakness and atrophy.[84] Proximal 5q SMA is caused by decreased levels of the survival motor neuron (SMN) protein and is the most common genetic cause of infant mortality. Its inheritance pattern is autosomal recessive, resulting from mutations involving the *SMN1* gene on chromosome 5q13. Unlike other autosomal recessive diseases, the *SMN1* gene has a unique structure (an inverted duplication) that presents potential therapeutic targets. Recently, pilot studies using gene therapy with an adeno-associated virus vector or intra-thecal nusinersen (an antisense oligonucleotide drug that increases production of survival motor neuron (SMN) protein) have resulted in improved survival, motor milestones, and independent respiration.[85,86] Advances in the multidisciplinary supportive care of children with SMA also offer hope for improved life expectancy and quality of life.

Conclusion

We are at a threshold of neuromodulation, neuroplasticity, and neurorestoration for children with cerebral palsy, spina bifida, muscular dystrophies, and spinal muscle atrophy. Even though the major disability may be motor, children with these complex disorders benefit from a whole child focus, surveillance for behavioral and learning problems, and advocacy to implement pathways to independence in self-care, communication, learning, and social skills. There have been major disparities in addressing the common developmental and behavioral disorders that often accompany these motor disorders and often result in missed opportunities for maximizing learning, behavior, and social competencies essential to well-being, community participation, and family life.

References

1. Thelen E, Smith L. Dynamic systems theories. In: Lerner WDR, ed. *Handbook of Child Psychology.* Vol 1. Hoboken, NJ: Wiley; 1998:563–634
2. Darrah J, Hodge M, Magill-Evans J, Kembhavi G. Stability of serial assessments of motor and communication abilities in typically developing infants—implications for screening. *Early Hum Dev.* 2003;72(2):97–110
3. WHO Multicentre Growth Reference Study Group. WHO motor development study: windows of achievement for six gross motor development milestones. *Acta Paediatr.* 2006;95(S450):86–95

4. Rosenbaum P, Missiuna C, Echeverria D, Knox S. Proposed motor development assessment protocol for epidemiological studies in children. *J Epidemiol Community Health.* 2009;63(Suppl 1):i27–i36

5. Noritz G, Murphy N, Hagan J, et al. Motor delays: early identification and evaluation. *Pediatrics.* 2013;131(6):e2016–e2027

6. Pearsall-Jones J, Piek J, Levy F. Developmental coordination disorder and cerebral palsy: categories or a continuum? *Hum Mov Sci.* 2010;29(5):787–798

7. American Psychiatric Association. *Diagnostic and Statistical Manual of Mental Disorders.* 4th ed. Text rev. Washington, DC: American Psychiatric Association; 2000

8. American Psychiatric Association. *Diagnostic and Statistical Manual of Mental Disorders.* 5th ed. Arlington, VA: American Psychiatric Association; 2013

9. Blank R. European Academy of Childhood Disability (EACD): recommendations on the definition, diagnosis, and intervention of developmental coordination disorder (pocket version) German-Swiss interdisciplinary clinical practice guideline S3-standard according to the Association of the Scientific Medical Societies in Germany. *Dev Med Child Neurol.* 2012;54(11):1–7

10. Zwicker J, Missiuna C, Harris S, Boyd L. Developmental coordination disorder: a review and update. *Eur J Paediatr Neurol.* 2012;16(6):573–581

11. Wuang YP, Wang CC, Huang MH. Health-related quality of life in chidlren with developmental coordination disorder and their parents. *OTJR (Thorofare N J).* 2012;32(4):142–150

12. Blank R, Smits-Engelsman B, Polatajko H, Wilson P. European Academy for Childhood Disability (EACD): recommendations on the definition, diagnosis, and intervention of developmental coordination disorder (long version). *Dev Med Child Neurol.* 2011;54(1):54–93

13. Blank R. Information for parents and teachers on the European Academy for Childhood Disability (EACD) recommendations on Developmental Coordination Disorder. *Dev Med Child Neurol.* 2012;54(11):54–93

14. Smits-Engelsman B, Blank R, van der Kaay A, et al. Efficacy of interventions to improve motor performance in children with developmental coordination disorder: acombined systematic review and meta-analysis. *Dev Med Child Neurol.* 2013;55(3):229–237

15. Rosenbaum P, Paneth N, Leviton A, et al. A report: the definition and classification of cerebral palsy April 2006. *Dev Med Child Neurol.* 2007;109:8–14

16. Badawi N, Watson L, Petterson B, et al. What constitutes cerebral palsy? *Dev Med Child Neurol.* 1998;40(8):520–527

17. Smithers-Sheedy H, Badawi N, Blair E, et al. What constitutes cerebral palsy in the twenty-first century? *Dev Med Child Neurol.* 2014;56(4):323–328

18. Australian Cerebral Palsy Register Group (ACPR Group), Badawi N, Balde I, et al. *Australian Cerebral Palsy Register Report 2016.* Sydney, Australia: Cerebral Palsy Alliance Research Institution CP Register;2016

19. Blair E, Stanley F. Aetiological pathways to spastic cerebral palsy. *Paediatr Perinat Epidemiol.* 1993;7(3):302–317

20. Novak I, Msall M. Cerebral Palsy. In: Malcolm W, ed. *Beyond the NICU: Comprehensive Care of the High Risk Infant.* New York, NY: McGraw Hill-Lange; 2015:376–410

21. Palisano R, Rosenbaum P, Walter S, et al. Development and reliability of a system to classify gross motor function in children with cerebral palsy. *Dev Med Child Neurol.* 1997;39(4):214–223

22. Rosenbaum P, Palisano R, Bartlett D, Galuppi B, Russell D. Development of the Gross Motor Function Classification System for cerebral palsy. *Dev Med Child Neurol.* 2008;50(4):249–253

23. Gorter J, Ketelaar M, Rosenbaum P, Helders P, Palisano R. Use of the GMFCS in infants with CP: the need for reclassification at age 2 years or older. *Dev Med Child Neurol.* 2009;51(1):46–52

24. Rosenbaum P, Walter S, Hanna S, et al. Prognosis for gross motor function in cerebral palsy: creation of motor development curves. *JAMA.* 2002;288(11):1357–1363

25. Eliasson A, Krumlinde-Sundholm L, Rosblad B, et al. The Manual Ability Classification System (MACS) for children with cerebral palsy: scale development and ecidence of validity and reliability. *Dev Med Child Neurol.* 2006;48(7):549–554

26. Eliasson A, Ullenhag A, Wahlstrom U, Krumlinde-Sundholm L. Mini-MACS: development of the Manual Ability Classification System for children younger than 4 years of age with signs of cerebral palsy. *Dev Med Child Neurol.* 2017;59(1):72–78

27. Carnahan K, Arner M, Hagglund G. Association between gross motor function (GMFCS) and manual ability (MACS) in chidlren with cerebral palsy: a population-based study of 359 children. *BMC Musculoskelet Disord.* 2007;8:50

28. Romantseva L, Msall M. Advances in understanding cerebral palsy syndromes after prematurity. *Neoreviews.* 2006;7:575–585

29. McIntyre S, Morgan C, Walker K, Novak I. Cerebral palsy—don't delay. *Dev Disabil Res Rev.* 2011;17(2):114–129

30. Msall M, Park J. Neurodevelopmental management strategies for children with cerebral palsy: optimizing function, promoting participation, and supporting families. *Clin Obstet Gynecol.* 2008;51(4):800–815

31. Smithers-Sheedy H, McIntyre S, Gibson C, et al. A special supplement: findings from the Australian Cerebral Palsy Register, birth years 1993 to 2006. *Dev Med Child Neurol.* 2016;58(Suppl 2):5–10

32. McIntyre S, Taitz D, Keogh J, Goldsmith S, Badawi N, Blair E. A systematic review of risk factors for cerebral palsy in children born at term in developed countries. *Dev Med Child Neurol.* 2013;55(6):499–508

33. Granild-Jensen J, Rackauskaite G, Flachs E, Uldall P. Predictors for early diagnosis of cerebral palsy from national registry data. *Dev Med Child Neurol.* 2015;57(10):931–935

34. Ancel P, Licinec F, Larroque B, Marret S, Arnaud C, Pierrat V. Cerebral palsy among very preterm children in relation to gestational age and neonatal ultrasound abnormalities: the EPIPAGE cohort study. *Pediatrics.* 2006;117(3):828–835

35. Hubermann L, Boychuck Z, Shevell M, Majnemer A. Age at referral of children for initial diagnosis of cerebral palsy and rehabilitation current practices. *J Child Neurol.* 2016;31(3):364–369

36. Bosanquet M, Copeland L, Ware R, Boyd R. A systematic review of tests to predict cerebral palsy in young children. *Dev Med Child Neurol.* 2013;55(5):418–426

37. Capute A, Shapiro B. The motor quotient. A method for the early detection of motor delay. *Am J Dis Child.* 1985;139(9):940–942

38. Novak I, Morgan C, Adde L, et al. Early accurate diagnosis and early intervention in cerebral palsy: advances in diagnosis and treatment. *JAMA Pediatr.* 2017;171:897–907

39. Maitre NL, Chorna O, Romeo DM, Guzzetta A. Implementation of the Hammersmith Infant Neurological Exam in a High-Risk Infant Follow-Up Program. *Pediatr Neurol.* 2016;65:31–38

40. Romeo DM, Ricci D, Brogna C, Mercuri E. Use of the Hammersmith Infant Neurological Examination in infants with cerebral palsy: a critical review of the literature. *Dev Med Child Neurol.* 2016;58(3): 240–245

41. Romeo, Domenico MM, et al. "Neurological assessment in infants discharged from a neonatal intensive care unit." *european journal of paediatric neurology* 17.2 (2013): 192–198

42. Arnfield A, Guzzetta A, Boyd R. Relationship between brain structure on magnetic resonance imaging and motor outcomes in children with cerebral palsy: a systematic review. *Res Dev Disabil.* 2013;34(7):2234–2250

43. Reid S, Dagia C, Ditchfield M, Carlin J, Reddihough D. Population based studies of brain imaging patterns in cerebral palsy. *Dev Med Child Neurol.* 2014;56(3):222–232

44. de Vries L, van Haastert I, Benders M, Groenendaal F. Myth: cerebral palsy cannot be predicted by neonatal brain imaging. *Semin Fetal Neonatal Med.* 2011;1(5):279–287

45. Massaro A, Evangelou I, Brown J, et al. Neonatal neurobehavior after therapeutic hypothermia for hypoxic ischemic encephalopathy. *Early Hum Dev.* 2015;91(10):593–599

46. Austin T, Boardman J, Harigopal S, et al. *Fetal and Neonatal Brain Magnetic Resonance Imaging: Clinical Indications, Acquisitions, and Reporting—A Framework for Practice.* British Association of Perinatal Medicine; 2016

47. Whelan MA. Practice parameter: diagnostic assessment of the child with cerebral palsy: report of the Quality Standards Subcommittee of the American Academy of Neurology and the Practice Committee of the Child Neurology Society. *Neurology.* 2004;63(10):1985–1986

48. Novak I. Evidence-based diagnosis, health care, and rehabilitation for children with cerebral palsy. *J Child Neurol.* 2014;29(8):1141–1156

49. Novak I, Hines M, Goldsmith S, Barclay R. Clinical prognostic messages from a systematic review on cerebral palsy. *Pediatrics.* 2012;130(5):e1285–e1312

50. Hagglund G, Lauge-Pedersen H, Wagner P. Characteristics of children with hip displacement in cerebral palsy. *BMC Musculoskelet Disord.* 2007;8(1):1

51. Wynter M, Gibson N, Kentish M, et al. Australian Hip Surveillance Guidelines for Children with Cerebral Palsy 2014. American Academy for Cerebral Palsy and Developmental Medicine Web site. https://www.aacpdm.org/UserFiles/file/IC292.pdf. Accessed February 2, 2018

52. Morgan C, Novak I, Badawi N. Enriched environments and motor outcomes in cerebral palsy: systematic review and meta-analysis. *Pediatrics.* 2013;132(3):735–746

53. Novak I, McIntyre S, Morgan C, Campbell L, Dark L, Morton N, et al. A systematic review of interventions for children with cerebral palsy: state of the evidence. *Dev Med Child Neurol.* 2013;55(10):885–910

54. Martin JH. The corticospinal system: from development to motor control. *Neuroscientist.* 2005;11(2):161–173

55. Spittle A, Orton J, Anderson P, Boyd R, Doyle L. Early developmental intervention programmes provided post hospital discharge to prevent motor and cognitive impairment in preterm infants. *Cochrane Database Syst Rev.* 2015;24(11):CD005495

56. Morgan C, Novak I, Badawi N. Enriched environments and motor outcomes in cerebral palsy: systematic review and meta-analysis. *Pediatrics.* 2013;132(3):e735–e746

57. Morgan C, Darrah J, Gordon A, et al. Effectiveness of motor interventions in infants with cerebral palsy: a systematic review. *Dev Med Child Neurol.* 2016;58(9):900–909

58. Morgan C, Novak I, Dale R, Guzzetta A, Badawi N. Single blind randomised controlled trial of GAME (Goals-Activity-Motor Enrichment) in infants at high risk of cerebral palsy. *Res Dev Disabil.* 2016;55:256–267

59. Nordstrand L, Holmefur M, Kits A, Eliasson A. Improvements in bimanual hand function after baby-CIMT in two-year-old children with unilateral cerebral palsy: a retrospective study. *Res Dev Disabil.* 2015;41–42:86–93

60. Gordon AM, Hung YC, Brandao M, et al. Bimanual training and constraint-induced movement therapy in children with hemiplegic cerebral palsy: a randomized trial. *Neurorehabil Neural Repair.* 2011;25(8):692–702

61. Mattern-Bazter K, McNeil S, Mansoor J. Effects of home-based locomotor treadmill training on gross motor function in young children with cerebral palsy: a quasi-randomized controlled trial. *Arch Phys Med Rehabil.* 2013;94(11):2061–2067

62. Logan SW, Feldner HA, Galloway JC, Huang HH. Modified ride-on car use by children with complex medical needs. *Pediatr Phys Ther.* 2016;28(1):100–107

63. Love S, Novak I, Kentish M, et al. Botulinum toxin assessment, intervention, and after-care for lower limb spasticity in children with cerebral palsy: international consensus statement. *Eur J Paediatr Neurol.* 2010;17(2):9–37

64. Hasnat MJ, Rice JE. Intrathecal baclofen for treating spasticity in children with cerebral palsy. *Cochrane Database Syst Rev.* 2015;11:CD004552

65. Hagglund G, Andersson S, Duppe H, Lauge-Pedersen H, Nordmark E, Westbom L. Prevention of dislocation of the hip in children with cerebral palsy. *Bone Joint J.* 2005;87(1):95–101

66. Sandler A. Children with spina bifida: key clinical issues. *Pediatr Clin North Am.* 2010;57(4):879–892

67. Heuer GG, Moldenhauer JS, Adzick NS. Prenatal surgery for myelomeningocele: review of the literature and future directions. *Childs Ner Syst.* 2017;33(1149–1155).

68. Copp A, Adzick N, Chitty L, Fletcher J, Holmbeck G, Shaw G. Spina bifida. *Nat Rev Dis Primers.* 2015;1:15007

69. Sandler A. Tic disorders and Tourette syndrome. In: Augustyn A, Zuckerman B, Caronna E, eds. *The Zuckerman Parker Handbook of Developmental and Dehavioral Pediatrics for Primary Care.* 3rd ed. Philadelphia, PA: Lippincott Williams & Wilkins; 2011:389–392

70. Dooley J. Tic disorders in childhood. *Semin Pediatr Neurol.* 2006;13(4):231–242

71. Kuperman S. Tics and Tourette syndrome in childhood. *Semin Pediatr Neurol.* 2003;10(1):35–40

72. Zinner S, Mink J. Movement disorders I: tics and stereotypies. *Pediatr Rev.* 2010;31(6):223–233

73. Jung H, Chung S, Hwang J. Tic disorders in children with frequent eye blinking. *J AAPOS.* 2004;8(2):171–174

74. Scahill L, Sukhodolsky D, Williams S, Leckman J. Public health significance of tic disorders in children and adolescents. *Adv Neurol.* 2005;96:240–248

75. Fourneret P, Desombre H, Broussolle E. From tic disorders to Tourette syndrome: current data, comorbidities, and therapeutic approach in children. *Arch Pediatr.* 2014;21(6):646–651

76. Murphy T, Brennan E, Johnco C, et al. A double-blind randomized placebo-controlled pilot study of azithromycin in youth with acute-onset obsessive-compulsive disorder. *J Child Adolesc Psychopharmacol.* 2017;27(7)640–651

77. Williams K, Swedo S, Farmer C, et al. Randomized, controlled trial of intravenous immunoglobulin for pediatric autoimmune neuropsychiatric disorders associated with streptococcal infections. *J Am Acad Child Adolesc Psychiatry.* 2016;55(10):860–867

78. Harris K, Mahone E, Singer H. Nonautistic motor stereotypies: clinical features and longitudinal follow-up. *Pediatr Neurol.* 2008;38(4):267–272

79. Shimizu-Motohashi Y, Miyatake S, Komaki H, Takeda S, Aoki Y. Recent advances in innovative therapeutic approaches for Duchenne muscular dystrophy: from discovery to clinical trials. *Am J Transl Res.* 2016;8(6):2471–2489

80. Ashizawa T, Sarkar P. Myotonic dystrophy types 1 and 2. *Handb Clin Neurol.* 2011;101:193–237

81. Robinson-Hamm J, Gersbach C. Gene therapies that restore dystrophin expression for the treatment of Duchenne muscular dystrophy. *Hum Genet.* 2016;135(9):1029–1040

82. Strehle E, Straube V. Recent advances in the management of Duchenne muscular dystrophy. *Arch Dis Child.* 2015;100(12):1173–1177

83. Ho G, Cardamone M, Farrar M. Congenital and childhood myotonic dystrophy: current aspects of disease and future directions. *World J Clin Pediatr.* 2015;4(4):66–80

84. Darras B. Spinal muscular atrophies. *Pediatr Clin North Am.* 2015;62(3):743–766

85. Finkel RS, Mercuri E, Darras BT, et al. Nusinersen versus Sham Control in Infantile-Onset Spina Bifida. *N Engl J Med.* 2017;377(18):1723–173

86. Mendell JR, Al-Zaidy S, Shell R, et al. Single-Dose Gene-Replacement Therapy for Spinal Muscular Atrophy. *N Engl J Med.* 2017;377(18):1713–172

CHAPTER 15

Cognitive Development and Disorders

Jill J. Fussell, MD, FAAP

Ann M. Reynolds, MD, FAAP

Cognitive Developmental Milestones

For the first 1 to 2 years of a child's life, when primary pediatric health care professionals are most often interfacing with young patients, cognitive development can be more difficult to appreciate than development in other domains, such as gross motor, fine motor, and language. This is because, in those early years, clues to a child's cognitive development are more indirectly expressed through the child's interactions with the environment. Developmental psychologist Jean Piaget described this phase of cognitive development as "sensorimotor intelligence." Attaining cognitive milestones during this stage is dependent on intact sensory systems (ie, vision and hearing), and children learn through sensory exploration. Children in this phase of development express mastery of cognitive milestones through physical manipulation of objects in their environment. Children with sensory impairments (blindness, deafness) or motor impairments, such as cerebral palsy, will therefore show lagging or notable variability in attainment of cognitive milestones during this early phase. This type of difference ultimately may not represent a true cognitive deficit but instead a function of the sensorimotor focus of cognitive development during this young age. Concerns about lack of interaction with the environment or delay in attainment of early cognitive milestones should prompt the primary pediatric health care professional to further assess vision and hearing and give more thought to the impact that overall motor development may be having on a child's ability to physically approach and access objects in the environment (gross motor) or his or her ability to manipulate objects (fine motor). Correctly identifying such impairments as early as possible in order to provide aid to a child and/or modifications in the environment can foster the progression of cognitive development.

Cognitive Development in Infancy

In the office, primary pediatric health care professionals should observe a child's physical manipulation of objects in the environment and expect to see much visual inspection, banging, mouthing, and throwing of objects between 4 and 10 months of age. During this time, infants begin to appreciate the association of "cause and effect," wherein they recognize how their actions lead to a response in the environment. By 9 months of age, most infants will show mastery of this concept, realizing that they cause lights or sounds to occur when they activate a push-button toy, for example. Understanding cause and effect is a powerful first step for infants to realize the impact they can have in interacting with and causing change in their environment.

A major milestone during this sensorimotor phase of cognitive development is that of object permanence (Table 15.1). The understanding that an object exists even if one cannot see it is typically mastered by 9 months of age. Out of sight is *not* out of mind once object permanence is achieved, so a child will look for a toy that has been completely covered from view. Once object permanence has developed, an infant can retain a mental picture of a parent when the parent has left the room, so separation anxiety also emerges at about the same age. Mastery of object permanence can be observed during a child's play or quickly elicited with a "peek-a-boo" game during a clinic visit.

Table 15.1. Cognitive Milestones		
Milestone	**Description**	**Approximate Age of Attainment**
Early object permanence	Follows an object falling out of sight; searches for a partially hidden object	4–8 months
Object permanence	Searches for an object completely hidden from view	9–12 months
Cause and effect	Realizes his/her action causes another action or is linked to a response	9 months
Functional use of objects	Realizes what objects are used for	12–15 months
Representational play	Pretends to use objects functionally on others and/or on dolls	18 months
Symbolic play	Uses an object to symbolize something else during pretend play	2–3 years
Preacademic skills	Knows colors, shapes, numbers, letters, and counts	3–5 years
Logical thinking	Understands conservation of matter, multistep problem-solving; realizes there can be differing perspectives	6–12 years
Abstract thinking	Able to hypothesize, think abstractly, draw conclusions	>13 years

One should be able to appreciate, either by observation or parent report, the development of a toddler's ability to understand the functional use of objects. Knowing what the objects they encounter in the environment are used for is a cognitive milestone typically mastered by 12 to 15 months of age. A child of that age might put a hairbrush on her head, she may hold a phone to her ear, or she may hold a key to a doorknob. A child whose thinking skills have progressed to a developmental level of 18 months or more will begin to demonstrate representational play. In this phase of development, a child may put a hair brush to a baby doll's head, pretending to brush its hair. Increased complexity comes at approximately the cognitive level of 2 to 3 years, wherein symbolic play emerges. Children are then capable of using objects to symbolize something else, so that they may place a stick to a baby doll's hair, pretending it is a hairbrush. At this level of functioning, play can become more imaginary and pretend, with symbolic play allowing children to think beyond the objects in their immediate vicinity in order to develop their play themes. Although the ages of acquisition are not at all absolute, a child's play can be a window into overall cognitive level, with the complexity providing some clues to a child's overall thinking abilities.

Cognitive Development in Preschoolers

In preschool-aged children (ages 3–5 years), cognitive development can be appreciated through their mastery of preacademic skills. Children in this age group begin to recognize colors, shapes, numbers, and letters. They begin to develop a concept of time and understand concepts such as big/little, up/down, before/after. They typically count objects up to 10 by the age of 5 years, and they respond correctly when asked their first and last name, gender, and age. Preschool children remain egocentric in their thinking and understand the world primarily by how it relates to them. Where expression of cognitive development was largely dependent on sensory and motor systems prior to this age, the domain of language becomes a primary factor in the appreciation of cognitive development in preschoolers. Preschoolers ask many questions (particularly "Why?" questions) and express their thinking and problem-solving skills largely through verbal communication. Therefore, one might make the mistake of assuming that a child with language impairment is cognitively delayed at this age. For children who seem to be lagging in attainment of preacademic milestones, primary pediatric health care professionals should pay specific attention to their acquisition of language milestones and obtain more formal assessment when necessary.

One must also be careful presuming cognitive level based on mastery of preacademic skills because children in environments lacking adequate developmental stimulation may have the cognitive potential to learn preacademics but lack exposure; therefore, assessing the environment is an important part of a clinician's conclusions regarding cognitive level. Primary pediatric health care professionals should encourage parents to provide the exposure to and opportunity to exercise preacademic skills at home or in a preschool setting.

Cognitive Development in School-aged Children and Adolescents

In the school-age years, thinking becomes less egocentric, and children can appreciate that other people have viewpoints different from their own. Typically developing school-aged children can think more logically, appreciate concepts such as conservation of matter, identify more subtle relationships, and consider multiple aspects of a problem they are attempting to solve. Children who are not progressing through this phase of cognitive development are likely to struggle in school, so a child with cognitive impairment may present to his or her primary pediatric health care professional because of school failure. Typically developing adolescents master more elaborate logical thinking, but they also develop the ability to think abstractly. Adolescents who are not progressing to that expected phase of abstract thought may struggle more with recognizing right and wrong in hypothetical scenarios and be less able to think and plan toward the future.

Intellectual Disability

Intellectual disability (ID) is defined by impaired general mental abilities and adaptive skills, with these deficits causing a person functional impairment. With the American Psychiatric Association's (APA) publication of the fifth edition of the *Diagnostic and Statistical Manual of Mental Disorders* (*DSM-5*) in May 2013, changes were made to the definition of ID.[1] One notable change is the name of the disorder itself. Previous wording in medical literature and prior editions of the *DSM* used the term *mental retardation;* currently, *intellectual disability* is the generally accepted and preferred terminology. A subtitle term included in *DSM-5* for this diagnosis is *intellectual developmental disorder (IDD),* to reference the fact that this is a diagnosis with symptoms presenting in the developmental period of life (not adulthood).

A second notable change with the *DSM-5* was the specific definition of ID or mental retardation, which had been, for several decades, defined as an intelligence quotient (IQ) score that was 2 standard deviations (SDs) below the mean (IQ <70) combined with adaptive function that is 2 SDs below the mean. The *DSM-5* definition puts relatively more emphasis on impairments in adaptive functioning instead of an IQ score in defining and diagnosing ID. An IQ score of 70 or below is still included in the supportive text for the ID definition in *DSM-5*, but it is no longer included as a primary diagnostic feature. Impairments in general mental abilities that begin during the developmental period are still symptoms of ID as described in *DSM-5*, but the diagnosis is based on the severity of the adaptive deficits.[1] Emphasis is placed not only on standardized assessment when making the diagnosis of ID, but also on clinical assessment. Interpretation of findings should be individualized within the context of a person's sociocultural environment and accounting for other conditions that might better explain a poor performance on an IQ measure, such as sensory impairment or language disorder.

Measurements of IQ and adaptive function compare an individual's performance or skill level to a same-aged sample from the general population. Population results therefore follow a "normal" or bell-shaped curve. Standard scores are based on a mean of 100 with a SD of 15. Most individuals (~95%) in a population will fall between a standard score of 70 and 130 (Figure 15.1). *Adaptive function* refers to how an individual functions in his or her environment and includes measures of socialization, communication motor skills, and activities of daily living, such as dressing and toileting. These adaptive functioning skills cluster into 3 main categories: conceptual, practical, and social. Skills included in the conceptual domain are those that tend to be more academic, such as reading, writing and math skills, but also include memory, language, problem-solving, and judgement in novel situations. The practical domain includes life skills, such as managing money, personal hygiene, occupational skills, and organizational skills. The social domain includes interpersonal communication skills, empathy, engagement in friendships, and social judgment. According to the APA, the level of severity of an ID diagnosis is defined by the level of impairment in adaptive functioning and the level of supports needed for day to day functioning.[1]

The definition of ID published by the American Association on Intellectual and Developmental Disabilities (AAIDD) is similar to the APA's. It is defined as a disability characterized by significant limitations in both intellectual functioning and in adaptive behavior as expressed in conceptual, social, and practical adaptive skills.[2] AAIDD agrees that culture, language, communication, sensory, motor, and behavioral factors must be considered in an ID diagnosis. AAIDD also makes the point, however, that it is important to recognize that limitations often occur with strengths. Limitations are described in order to determine needed supports, and a person with intellectual disability can gain functional skills over time with appropriate support systems in place.[2,3]

The diagnosis of ID is usually reserved for children 5 years of age or older due to the lack of good predictive validity for developmental and intelligence tests in younger children and the degree to which child development is changing in those early formative years. If a child younger than 5 years is failing to meet developmental milestones as expected, the APA defines this as global developmental delay (GDD).[1] This diagnostic category could also include children who are too young or older children who are otherwise unable to participate in standardized assessments of intellectual functioning. Repeated attempts at accurate standardized assessment over time is appropriate for children diagnosed with GDD to document improvements or ultimately to make a diagnosis of ID when appropriate.

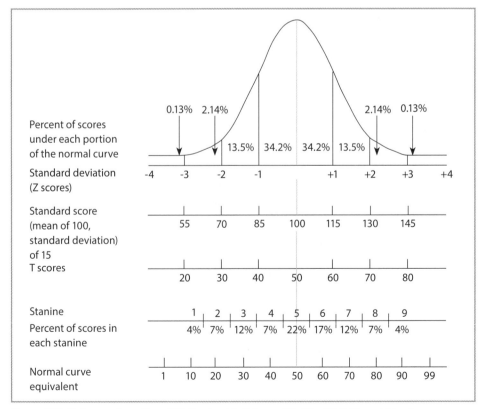

Figure 15.1. Bell curve. From Carey WB, Crocker AC, Coleman WL, Elias ER, Feldman HM, eds. *Developmental & Behavioral Pediatrics.* Philadelphia, PA: Elsevier; 2009:764, with permission from Elsevier.

The medical evaluation of children with ID and GDD should include a careful history, including a 3-generation family history and a thorough physical examination, including head circumference, a dysmorphology exam, a neurological exam, and a skin exam for neurocutaneous stigmata[4] (Table 15.2, Figure 15.2). A medical genetics evaluation should be offered to all families of an individual with ID or GDD. A specific diagnosis facilitates development of expectations for the future, access to family support organizations specific to the condition, education of primary pediatric health care professionals to monitor for potential associated medical and psychiatric comorbidities, education of families about potential research trials for targeted treatments, and genetic counseling in regard to risk of recurrence in future pregnancies. The diagnosis also often relieves parental anxiety about what they may have previously believed to have caused their child's cognitive disability.

Table 15.2. The Purposes of the Comprehensive Medical Genetics Evaluation of the Young Child With Global Developmental Delay or Intellectual Disability
1. Clarification of etiology
2. Provision of prognosis or expected clinical course
3. Discussion of genetic mechanism(s) and recurrence risks
4. Refined treatment options
5. Avoidance of unnecessary or redundant diagnostic tests
6. Information regarding treatment, symptom management, or surveillance for known complications
7. Provision of condition-specific family support
8. Access to research treatment protocols
9. Opportunity for co-management of appropriate patients in the context of a medical home to ensure the best health, social, and health care services satisfaction outcomes for the child and family

With permission from Moeschler JB, Shevell M; American Academy of Pediatrics Committee on Genetics. Comprehensive evaluation of the child with intellectual disability or global developmental delays. *Pediatrics.* 2014;134:e903–e918.

A parent or family's "need to know" may vary greatly. Decisions about etiological evaluation should include shared decision-making. While the specific genetic workup to consider in individuals with ID/GDD is rapidly evolving, current expert consensus suggests that the initial diagnostic work up should include fragile X molecular genetic testing and chromosomal microarray analysis (CMA), with consideration of a karyotype if there is a family history of multiple miscarriages, or fluorescence in situ hybridization (FISH) (testing if a specific etiology, such as Williams syndrome (WS), is suspected.[4,5] In the past, the ability to identify the etiology of ID in an individual increased when there were greater than 3 dysmorphic features or if the level of functioning was lower.[6] With the advent of new technology, such as whole-exome and whole-genome sequencing, the etiological yield in the future is likely to increase.

However, there are concerns regarding interpretation, cost, a potential to find a mutation with future clinical significance that is unrelated to ID or GDD, and the potential to miss epigenetic changes with these technologies. Currently, a CMA will be positive in about 6% of children with ID or GDD. This rate goes to 10% if the child has dysmorphic

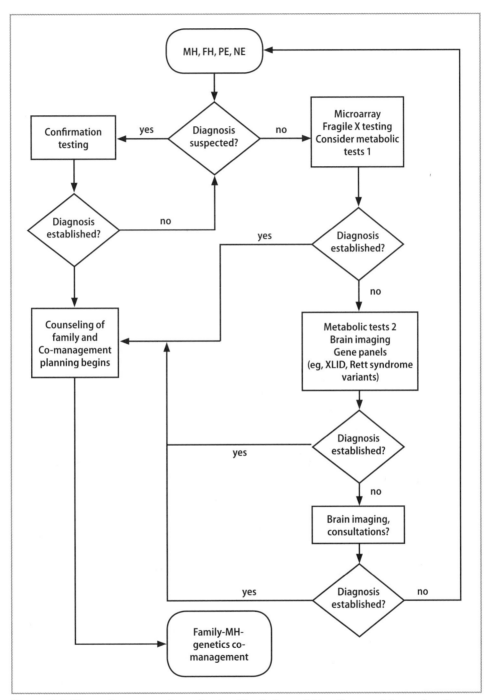

Figure 15.2. Diagnostic process and care planning. Metabolic test 1: blood homocysteine, acylcarnitine profile, amino acids; urine organic acids, glycosaminoglycans, oligosaccharides, purines, pyrimidines, GAA/creatine metabolites. Metabolic test 2 based on clinical signs and symptoms. Abbreviations: FH, family history; MH, medical history; NE, neurologic examination; PE, physical and dysmorphology examination.

Adapted with permission from Moeschler JB, Shevell M, American Academy of Pediatrics Committee on Genetics. Comprehensive evaluation of the child with intellectual disability or global developmental delays. *Pediatrics.* 2014; 134:e903–e918.

features. Fragile X DNA testing will be positive in about 2% to 3% of individuals with ID or GDD. A drawback to CMA is finding a copy number variation of unknown clinical relevance. A medical geneticist or certified genetic counselor should interpret abnormal values.[4] If the initial workup is negative, testing for nonsyndromic X-linked ID genes and high-density X-CMA in males and *MECP2* deletion, duplication, and sequencing in females should be considered. When microcephaly, macrocephaly, seizures, developmental regression, or neurological signs are present, magnetic resonance imaging (MRI) of the brain should be considered. A formal audiology evaluation is also indicated if the child has not had a hearing evaluation since birth. Ophthalmological examination and EEG should also be considered. Clinicians should also screen for medical conditions that frequently co-occur in children with ID, such as sleep problems, feeding problems, obesity, gastrointestinal disorders, and behavioral and psychiatric conditions.[4]

Metabolic testing for inborn errors of metabolism (IEM) is rarely positive in children with ID or GDD (0% to 5%), especially in the absence of "metabolic" symptoms, such as abnormal tone, ataxia, seizures, developmental regression or plateauing, failure to thrive, organomegaly, coarse facial features, abnormalities of skin or hair, or signs of hypothyroidism. Newborn screening typically identifies many children with treatable medical conditions; however, there are many treatable conditions that are not currently part of newborn screening, and the specific tests included in newborn screening vary from state to state. Controversy exists about the cost-benefit ratio of testing for rare metabolic disorders. A tiered approach to etiological workup is suggested.[4,7] Van Karnebeek et al, based on a review of the available literature in 2013 and expert consensus, proposed a 2-tiered approach to testing for IEM. They discuss 89 treatable types of IEM. This tiered approach is primarily based on "availability, affordability, yield, and invasiveness." Tier 1 tests, or nontargeted screening tests, include (1) blood tests for lactate, ammonia, plasma amino acids, total homocysteine, acylcarnitine profile, copper, and ceruloplasmin; and (2) urine tests for organic acids, purines and pyrimidines, creatine metabolism, oligosaccharides, and glycosaminoglycans (Figure 15.3). Other tests to consider are 7- and 8- dehydrocholesterol to screen for Smith-Lemli-Opitz syndrome and screening for congenital disorders of glycosylation. Some of these tests may be difficult to find outside of an academic center. Tests requiring cerebrospinal fluid (CSF) samples, or single tests per disease, are in the second tier, but these may be used in the first tier if clinically indicated.[4,7] First-tier tests recommended in the American Academy of Pediatrics (AAP) guidelines for the comprehensive evaluation of the child with ID or global developmental delays include (1) blood tests for plasma amino acids, total homocysteine, and acylcarnitine profile; and (2) urine tests for organic acids, purines and pyrimidines, creatine metabolism, oligosaccharides, and mucopolysaccharides.[4]

An app is available to help guide clinicians in the management of children with treatable causes of ID or GDD. The app is available at **www.treatable-id.org**. This app is free and accepted by members of the "rare disease community."[7] Potential treatments that may improve symptoms or slow progression of IEMs include appropriate management during illness or fasting, dietary interventions, cofactor supplements, vitamin supplements, substrate inhibition, stem cell transplants, and gene therapy.[7] The evidence to support these treatments is variable and often relies on expert opinion due to low numbers of subjects and the progressive nature of the disorders. Many treatable IEMs may present later or without developmental regression or plateauing in children with ID/GDD. Disorders such as ornithine carbamoyltransferase deficiency, which is X-linked, may also present with milder symptoms in females.[7] Finally, lead screening should be considered, especially in children with pica or who routinely mouth objects.

1st Tier: Nontargeted screening to identify 54 (60%) treatable IEMs

Blood
- Ammonia, lactate
- Plasma amino acids
- Total homocysteine
- Acylcarnitine profile
- Copper, ceruloplasmin

Urine
- Organic acids
- Purines & pyrimidines
- Creatine metabolites
- Oligosaccharides
- Glycosaminoglycans

2nd Tier: Targeted testing to identify 35 (40%) treatable IEMs requiring "specific testing"

- According to patient's symptomatology & clinician's expertise

- Utilization of textbooks & digital resources
  (WebApp: *www.treatable-ID.org*)

- Consider the following biochemical/molecular analyses:
  - Whole blood manganese
  - Plasma cholestanol
  - Plasma 7-dehydroxy-cholesterol:cholesterol ratio
  - Plasma pipecolic acid & urine AASA
  - Plasma very long chain fatty acids
  - Plasma vitamin B_{12} & folate
  - Serum & CSF lactate:pyruvate ratio
  - Enzyme activities (leukocytes): arylsulfatase A, biotinidase, glucocerebrosidase, fatty aldehyde dehydrogenase
  - Urine deoxypyridinoline
  - CSF amino deoxypyridinoline
  - CSF neurotransmitters
  - CSF: plasma glucose ratio
  - CoQ measurement fibroblasts
  - Molecular: *CA5A, NPC1, NPC2, SC4MOL, SLC18A2, SLC19A3, SLC30A10, SLC52A2, SLC52A3, PDHA1, DLAT, PDHX, SPR, TH*

Figure 15.3. Two-tiered algorithm for diagnosis of treatable inborn errors of metabolism in intellectual developmental disorder. The first tier testing comprises group metabolic tests in urine and blood that should be performed in every patient with IDD of unknown cause. Based on the differential diagnosis generated by the patient's signs and symptoms, the second tier test is ordered individually at a low threshold.

Adapted with permission from van Karnebeek CD, Shevell M, Zschocke J, Moeschler JB, Stockler S. The metabolic evaluation of the child with an intellectual developmental disorder: diagnostic algorithm for identification of treatable causes and new digital resource. *Mol Genet Metab.* 2014;111(4):428–438.

If no etiology is found after completing first- and second-tier genetic testing, metabolic screening, imaging, and neurophysiological testing (when indicated), additional testing such as *MECP2* mutations in males and Rett/Angelman phenotype panels in males and females may be considered on the recommendation of a geneticist. In addition, due to the considerable progress being made with technology, consideration of newer methodologies, such as whole exome sequencing and multiplex ligation assay, should also be considered. Routine follow-up is suggested due to changes in technology, possible emergence of phenotypic features as the child grows, and ongoing research into the development of targeted treatments for some genetic disorders.[4]

Specific Etiologies of Intellectual Disability

In the following sections, the medical, developmental, and behavioral features of the most common genetic (Down syndrome), inherited (fragile X syndrome), and preventable (fetal alcohol spectrum disorders [FASDs]) etiologies of ID will be described. Other genetic disorders with characteristic behavioral phenotypes will then be discussed. Many of these are detected by specific FISH probes or by CMA, which is capable of detecting small deletions or duplications of genetic material.

– Down Syndrome/Trisomy 21

Down syndrome/trisomy 21 is the most common genetic cause of ID, occurring in 1 in 600 births. The incidence increases with maternal age. It is caused by an extra copy of chromosome 21. The physical phenotype is well recognized and includes hypotonia, microbrachycephaly, epicanthal folds, up-slanting palpebral fissures, Brushfield spots in the iris, flat nasal bridge, small mouth, small ears, excess skin at the nape of the neck, single transverse palmar creases, short incurving fifth fingers (clinodactyly), and a widened "sandal gap" between the first and second toes (Figure 15.4). Medical conditions, such as congenital heart disease, hearing and vision problems, hypothyroidism, obstructive sleep apnea, celiac disease, and hematologic problems, are commonly associated with Down syndrome, and patients should be monitored for these potential medical comorbidities[8] (Table 15.3). Reactive airway disease may also be more frequent in children with Down syndrome[9], and overweight and obesity are common, with rates up to 70%.[10] Use of growth charts specific for children with Down syndrome are no longer recommended.[8]

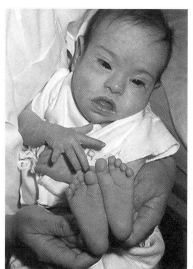

Figure 15.4. Down syndrome. A 6-month-old with Down syndrome with up-slanting palpebral fissures, epicanthal folds, and protrusion of the tongue.

From Marion RW. Facial dysmorphism. In: McInerny TK, Adam HM, Campbell DE, Kamat DM, Kelleher JS, eds. American Academy of Pediatrics Textbook of Pediatric Care. Elk Grove Village, IL: American Academy of Pediatrics; 2009.

Table 15.3 Medical Problems Common in Down Syndrome	
Condition	**%**
Hearing problems	75
Vision problems	60
Cataracts	15
Refractive errors	50
Obstructive sleep apnea	50–75
Otitis media	50–70
Congenital heart disease	40–50
Hypodontia and delayed dental eruption	23
Gastrointestinal atresias	12
Thyroid disease	4–18
Seizures	1–13
Anemia	3
Iron deficiency	10
Transient myeloproliferative disorder	10
Leukemia	1
Celiac disease	5
Atlantoaxial instability	1–2
Autism	10
Hirschsprung disease	<1

With permission from Bull MJ, American Academy of Pediatrics Committee on Genetics. Health supervision for children with Down syndrome. *Pediatrics*. 2011;128(2):393–406.

The AAP has published "Health Supervision for Children With Down Syndrome" (Table 15.4).[8] This policy statement provides essential information for management of individuals with Down syndrome. It is important for primary pediatric health care professionals and families to know that there is a broad range of cognitive and behavioral outcomes for children with Down syndrome, although a majority will have ID in a mild-to-moderate range. Children with Down syndrome classically tend to have fewer severe behavioral problems compared with other children with similar levels of ID, although approximately 10% will meet criteria for an autism spectrum disorder (ASD). Individuals with Down syndrome have an increased risk for depression and Alzheimer disease as they age.[11]

Table 15.4. Health Supervision for Children With Down Syndrome

	Prenatal	Birth–1 mo	1 mo–1 y	1–5 y	5–13 y	13–21 y
Counseling regarding prenatal screening test & imaging results	■					
Plan for delivery	■					
Referral to geneticist	■					
Parent-to-parent contact, support groups, current books and pamphlets	■	▓	■			
Physical exam for evidence of trisomy 21		▓		▓		
Chromosomal analysis to confirm the diagnosis		▓	▓	▓		
Discuss risk of recurrence of Down syndrome		■				
Echocardiogram		■	■			
Radiographic swallowing assessment if marked hypotonia, slow feeding, choking with feeds, recurrent or persistent respiratory symptoms, FTT		■				
Eye exam for cataracts		■				
Newborn hearing screen and follow-up		■				
History and PE assessment for duodenal or anorectal atresia		■				
Reassure parents delayed and irregular dental eruption, hypodontia are common			▓			
If constipation, evaluate for limited diet or fluids, hypotonia, hypothyroidism, GI malformation, Hirschsprung		Any visit				
CBC to R/O transient myeloproliferative disorder, polycythemia		■				
Hb annually; CRP & ferritin or CHr if possible risk iron deficiency or Hb <11g				Annually	Annually	
Hemoglobin						Annually
TSH (may be part of newborn screening)		■	6 and 12 mo	Annually	Annually	
Discuss risk of respiratory infection						

Legend: ■ Do once at this age ▓ Do if not done previously ▒ Repeat at indicated intervals

(continued on page 14)

Table 15.4. Health Supervision for Children With Down Syndrome *(continued)*

	Prenatal	Birth–1 mo	1 mo–1 y	1–5 y	5–13 y	13–21 y
If cardiac surgery or hypotonic: evaluate apnea, bradycardia, or oxygen desaturation in car seat before discharge		■				
Discuss complementary & alternative therapies			All health maintenance visits			
Discuss cervical spine positioning, especially for anesthesia or surgical or radiologic procedures			All health maintenance visits			
Review signs and symptoms of myopathy			All health maintenance visits			
If myopathic signs or symptoms: obtain neutral position spine films and, if normal, obtain flexion & extension films & refer to pediatric neurosurgeon or orthopedic surgeon with expertise in evaluating and treating atlantoaxial instability			Any visits			
Instruct to contact physician for change in gait, change in use of arms or hands, change in bowel or bladder function, neck pain, head tilt, torticollis, or new-onset weakness					Biennially	
Advise risk of some contact sports, trampolines				All health maintenance visits		
Audiology evaluation at 6 mo			▨	Every 6 mo		
If normal hearing established, behavioral audiogram and tympanometry until bilateral ear specific testing possible. Refer child with abnormal hearing to ENT				Every 6 mo		
If normal ear-specific hearing established, behavioral audiogram					Annually	
Assess for obstructive sleep apnea symptoms			All health maintenance visits			
Sleep study by age 4 years			■			
Ophthalmology referral to assess for strabismus, cataracts, and nystagmus			■			
Refer to pediatric ophthalmologist or ophthalmologist with experience with Down syndrome				Annually	Every 2 y	Every 3 y
If congenital heart disease, monitor for signs & symptoms of congestive heart failure			All visits			

■ Do once at this age ▓ Do if not done previously ▨ Repeat at indicated intervals

Table 15.4. Health Supervision for Children With Down Syndrome (*continued*)

	Prenatal	Birth–1 mo	1 mo–1 y	1–5 y	5–13 y	13–21 y
Assess the emotional status of parents and intrafamilial relationships	All health maintenance visits					
Check for symptoms of celiac disease; if symptoms present, obtain tissue transglutaminase IgA & quantitative IgA			All health maintenance visits			
Early intervention: physical, occupational, and speech therapies			Health maintenance visits			
At 30 months, discuss transition to preschool and development of IEP				■		
Discuss behavioral and social progress				Health maintenance visits		
Discuss self-help skills, ADHD, OCD, wandering off, transition to middle school					Health maintenance visits	
If chronic cardiac or pulmonary disease, 23-valent pneumococcal vaccine at age >2 y				Health maintenance visits		
Reassure regarding delayed and irregular dental eruption						
Establish optimal dietary and physical exercise patterns				Health maintenance visits		
Discuss dermatologic issue with parents					■	
Discuss physical and psychosocial changes through puberty, need for gynecologic care in the pubescent female						
Facilitate transition: guardianship, financial planning, behavioral problems, school placement, vocational training, independence with hygiene and self-care, group homes, work settings						Health maintenance visits
Discuss sexual development and behaviors, contraception, sexually transmitted diseases, recurrence risk for offspring						Health maintenance visits

■ Do once at this age   ▨ Do if not done previously   ▨ Repeat at indicated intervals

Abbreviations: ADHD, attention-deficit/hyperactivity disorder; CBC, complete blood cell count; CHr, reticulocyte hemoglobin; Hb, hemoglobin; GI, gastrointestinal; FTT, failure to thrive; IEP, Individualized Education Program; IgA, immunoglobulin A; OCD, obsessive compulsive disorder; PE, physical examination; R/O, rule out.

Reproduced with permission from Bull MJ, Committee on Genetics. Health supervision for children with Down syndrome. *Pediatrics.* 2011 Aug;128(2):393–406.

– Fragile X Syndrome

The most common inherited cause of ID is fragile X syndrome. Fragile X syndrome is caused by a trinucleotide repeat expansion (CGG) within the fragile X mental retardation 1 *(FMR1)* gene.[12] The *FMR1* gene typically includes about 30 repeats. If the repeat size expands to 200 or more repeats, the gene will become methylated and silenced. This will result in a deficiency of FMR1 protein and the classic fragile X syndrome phenotype.[13] The FMR1 protein is an RNA-binding protein that is found in most cells in the body.[14] One role of FMR1 is to regulate metabotropic glutamate receptor 5 (mGluR5). Individuals who carry the premutation have 54 to 200 repeats.[12] Previously, individuals with the premutation were thought to be unaffected; however, there is mounting evidence for a specific phenotype in these individuals. Women with the premutation have a higher incidence of premature ovarian failure.[15] Males with the premutation are at high risk for developing the fragile X–associated tremor/ataxia syndrome (FXTAS). FXTAS is a progressive neurodegenerative disorder that typically develops in male premutation carriers older than 50 years of age.[16] Individuals with the premutation have normal levels of FMR1 protein but increased levels of messenger RNA.[17,18] Approximately 1 in 250 women and 1 in 800 to 1,000 men within the general population are premutation carriers.[19,20] The repeat number usually expands when passed from a woman with the premutation to her offspring but not when a man with the permutation passes the premutation to his daughters.

The presentation of the full mutation (>200 repeats) varies between males and females because females have 2 copies of the X chromosome and experience random X inactivation. The portions of the X chromosome that are not present on the Y chromosome are randomly inactivated in each cell. The phenotype in females will thus depend at least in part on the pattern of X inactivation.[21,22] If the pattern of inactivation is skewed in one direction or the other, the female may be minimally affected or more significantly affected. In general, females are more likely to be more mildly affected than males.[22] Most males will present with ID in the mild-to-severe range.

The physical phenotype of fragile X syndrome in males is apparent prior to puberty but becomes more prominent after puberty. The phenotype includes macroorchidism, protuberant ears, a long, thin face, and a prominent jaw and forehead. Medical conditions frequently associated with fragile X syndrome include seizures, strabismus, otitis media, gastroesophageal reflux, mitral valve prolapse, and hip dislocation. The behavioral phenotype may include attention-deficit/hyperactivity disorder (ADHD), anxiety, sleep disturbance, perseverative language, hand flapping, gaze aversion, autism, and significant hypersensitivity to environmental stimuli.[23] Because the physical characteristics may not be present in young children, and because this is a relatively common disorder with a recurrence risk of 50%, specific DNA testing for fragile X syndrome is indicated in all children presenting with cognitive delays of unknown etiology.

Clinical guidelines have been established for health supervision in children with fragile X syndrome,[24] and treatment of children with fragile X syndrome has been reviewed.[25] Clinical trials are also being conducted to evaluate "targeted treatments" for fragile X syndrome, such as metabotropic glutamate receptor antagonists.[26] Genetic counseling is warranted in a family with a child with fragile X syndrome because of the 50% recurrence risk and implications for other family members. For example, a child with fragile X syndrome's mother and maternal grandfather may be at risk for issues associated with the premutation, such as FXTAS or premature ovarian failure. Families should also be informed about support groups.

– Fetal Alcohol Spectrum Disorders

FASDs are the most common preventable causes of ID and associated neurodevelopmental/neurobehavioral dysfunction in children. The FASDs include a broad range of outcomes that can be seen in individuals exposed to alcohol in utero. FASDs occur in about 1% to 5% of children.[27,28] There are several diagnostic schemas available. These include the updated clinical consensus guidelines for FASD developed by Hoyme et al and published in 2016.[29] The updated Hoyme guidelines clarify definitions for prenatal alcohol exposure and neurobehavioral dysfunction and update the definition of alcohol-related birth defects, the dysmorphology rating system, and the lip/philtrum guide for the North American white population. Despite the definition of prenatal alcohol exposure during pregnancy proposed by Hoyme et al, the AAP stipulates that no amount of alcohol during pregnancy is considered safe.[30] The Hoyme guidelines were intended to increase sensitivity to identify children with FASD by increasing head circumference, growth, and palpebral fissure percentile cutoffs from <3% to ≤10%.[29] The Hoyme guidelines also suggest that the diagnosis be made by a multidisciplinary team. Other diagnostic schemas for FASD include the Canadian guidelines for diagnosis,[31] National Task Force on Fetal Alcohol Syndrome and Fetal Alcohol Effects (2004),[32] and the FASD 4-digit diagnostic code.[33] The AAP also published a clinical report on FASD in 2015.[30]

Prior to diagnosing an FASD, other disorders with similar developmental and dysmorphic features that should be considered and/or ruled out include Cornelia de Lange, Williams, 22q11.2 deletion, 15q duplication, Noonan, and Dubowitz syndromes, as well as exposures to teratogens such as valproic acid and toluene. The dysmorphology rating system was designed to help determine the need to explore other diagnoses.[29]

Fetal Alcohol Syndrome

Fetal alcohol syndrome (FAS) refers to a full syndrome associated with prenatal alcohol exposure. The diagnosis can be made with or without confirmed maternal use of alcohol. The FAS diagnosis is made if all 4 of the following criteria are met: (1) at least 2 of 3 facial anomalies, including short palpebral fissures (≤10th percentile), thin upper lip, and smooth philtrum (the lip/philtrum guide is available for some races/ethnicities. [see Figures 15.5, 15.6]); (2) poor prenatal or postnatal growth (height or weight ≤10th percentile); (3) at least 1 structural or functional brain abnormality, such as poor brain growth (head circumference ≤10th percentile), morphogenesis, or neurophysiology (recurrent nonfebrile seizures with no other known etiology); and (4) neurobehavioral impairment.[29]

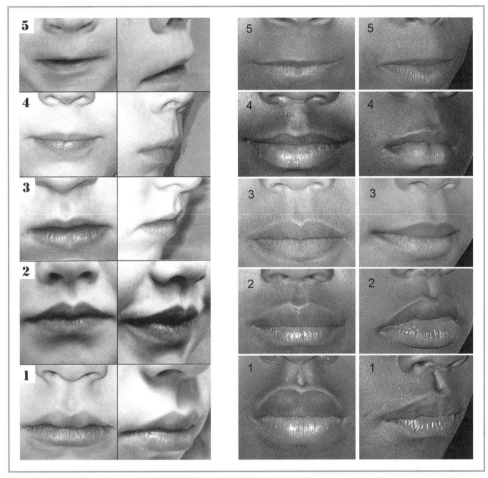

Figure 15.5. *(left)* With permission from Hoyme HE, Kalberg WO, Elliott AJ, et al. Updated clinical guidelines for diagnosing fetal alcohol spectrum disorders. *Pediatrics.* 2016;138(2):e20154256. *(right)* University of Washington Lip-Philtrum Guide 2 is used to rank upper lip thinness and philtrum smoothness for all other races with lips as full as African Americans. The philtrum is the vertical groove between the nose and upper lip. Guide 2 reflects the full range of lip thickness and philtrum depth with Rank 3 representing the population mean for African Americans. Ranks 4 and 5 reflect the thin lip and smooth philtrum that characterize the FAS facial phenotype. A separate Guide (Guide 1) is used for Caucasians and all other races with lips like Caucasians. Free digital images of these guides for use on smartphones and tablets can be obtained from astley@uw.edu. Copyright 2017, Susan Astley, PhD, University of Washington. Legend *(for right figure)* provided by Susan Astley, PhD.

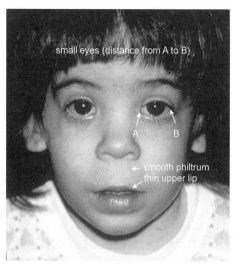

Figure 15.6. Child presenting with the 3 diagnostic facial features of FAS: (1) short palpebral fissure lengths (distance from A to B), (2) smooth philtrum; and (3) thin upper lip. Copyright 2017, Susan Astley, PhD, University of Washington. Legend provided by Susan Astley, PhD.

Partial Fetal Alcohol Syndrome

A diagnosis of partial FAS (pFAS) can also be made with or without a confirmed history of maternal alcohol use. If there is adequate documentation of prenatal alcohol exposure, then the child must have at least 2 facial anomalies as described earlier for FAS and neurobehavioral impairment. If there is not adequate documentation of prenatal alcohol exposure, the child must have at least 2 characteristic facial anomalies, a growth deficiency or brain abnormality, and neurobehavioral impairment.[29]

Alcohol-Related Neurodevelopmental Disorder

A diagnosis of alcohol-related neurodevelopmental disorder (ARND) requires confirmation of prenatal alcohol exposure and neurobehavioral impairment. This diagnosis cannot be made until after 3 years of age.[29]

Neurobehavioral Disorder with Prenatal Alcohol Exposure

A diagnosis of neurobehavioral disorder with prenatal alcohol exposure (ND-PAE) requires confirmation of prenatal alcohol exposure and neurobehavioral impairment in neurocognition, self-regulation, and adaptive functioning. This is a newly proposed mental health diagnosis intended to capture the behavioral and mental health effects of in utero exposure to alcohol in those with and without physical dysmorphia. Because of its relatively recent creation, the *DSM-5* added ND-PAE as a diagnosis with the caveat that more study was needed.[1]

Alcohol-Related Birth Defects

The diagnosis of alcohol-related birth defects requires confirmation of prenatal alcohol exposure and at least one major congenital malformation that has been associated with prenatal alcohol exposure in humans or animal models, such as malformations or dysplasias in cardiac, skeletal, renal, ocular, or auditory areas (eg, sensorineural hearing loss).[29]

Individuals with an FASD may have significant difficulty with complex cognitive tasks and executive function (planning, conceptual set shifting, affective set shifting, response inhibition, and fluency). Some individuals with an FASD process information slowly and have difficulty with attention and short-term memory. Some individuals with FASDs do well with simple tasks but are challenged by more complex ones. Individuals with FASDs are also at risk for social difficulties and mood disorders.[34] People with an FASD are more vulnerable to being involved with the criminal justice system.[35]

For children with an FASD, functional classroom assessments can be a very helpful supplement to psychoeducational evaluations. Methods that have been found to be helpful for individuals with FASD are visual structure (color code each content area), environmental structure (keep work area uncluttered, avoid decorations), and task structure (clear beginning, middle, and end). Cognitive control therapy is an intervention that has shown promising results for children with FASD.[36] A review of current evidence for interventions was published in 2017.[37] Primary pediatric health care professionals have a critical role in the prevention of FASD through education of families and adolescents.[38]

– Prader-Willi Syndrome

Prader-Willi syndrome is caused by a microdeletion on chromosome 15q11.2-q13 in an area that is imprinted. *Imprinting* refers to a gene being turned on or off depending on the parent of origin. The Prader-Willi/Angelman critical region was the first region of the human genome described to be affected by imprinting. A deletion in the same area gives a completely different phenotype (either Prader-Willi or Angelman syndrome) depending on the parent of origin. In 75% of children with Prader-Willi syndrome, the symptoms are caused by a deletion on the paternal chromosome; in 20% there are 2 copies of the maternal chromosome and no copy of the paternal chromosome 15 (uniparental disomy). In 5% there is a translocation or other structural anomaly of chromosome 15, and in 1% there is a problem with the imprinting center.[39] As with Angelman syndrome, there is some variation in the phenotype with different mechanisms.

Infants with Prader-Willi syndrome initially have failure to thrive and hypotonia. By age 2 years, the children begin to develop obesity and significant hyperphagia. They have hypogonadism and short stature. Consultation with an endocrinologist is indicated to consider the use of growth hormone, which has been found to have a positive impact on growth, muscle, bone mass, cognitive development, and metabolic parameters.[40] Sex hormone replacement is also sometimes recommended. Physical characteristics of children with Prader-Willi syndrome include almond-shaped eyes, a thin upper lip, and some may have hypopigmented skin, hair, and eyes (Figure 15.7).[39,41] Mean IQ scores of individuals with Prader-Willi have been reported in the mild range of ID (average IQ = 65), but cognitive abilities may extend from a low average range to the range of moderate ID.[41,42] They often have

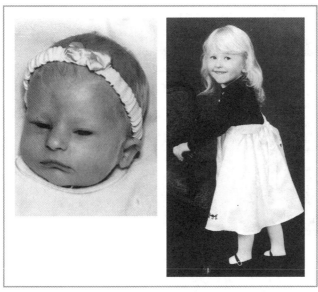

Figure 15.7. Prader-Willi syndrome. A 3-month-old female who has Prader-Willi syndrome (left). Note the almond-shaped eyes and down-turned mouth. The same patient at approximately 3 years of age (right).

Reproduced with permission from Jonas JM, Demmer LA. Genetic syndromes determined by alterations in genomic imprinting pathways. *NeoReviews*. 2007;8(3);e120–e126.

executive functioning deficits and impaired social cognition. They struggle specifically with Theory of Mind, which includes difficulty understanding the behavior and mental states of others and taking other's perspective. Over 25% meet diagnostic criteria for ASD.[42,43] Individuals with Prader-Willi syndrome often have obsessive-compulsive behaviors, including hyperphagia and skin picking. They can also have psychosis, a high pain tolerance, and disordered sleep.[39,41]

– Angelman Syndrome

Angelman syndrome is also associated with the imprinted 15q11.2-q13 region on chromosome 15. There are 4 known mechanisms that lead to the Angelman syndrome phenotype: (1) a deletion at 15q11.2-q13 on the maternal chromosome; (2) paternal uniparental disomy, which means that the individual has 2 copies of the paternal chromosome 15 instead of one from each parent; (3) imprinting defects; and (4) mutations in the ubiquitin-protein ligase E3A gene *(UBE3A)*.[44] The phenotype can vary depending on the genotype, and individuals with the deletion tend to have the most severe phenotype. Angelman syndrome is characterized by 4 routinely present features: (1) severe cognitive impairment, (2) expressive language more impaired than receptive language, (3) movement and gait disorders, and (4) a happy demeanor/frequent laughter (Figure 15.8, Box 15.1). Features that are present in greater than 80% of individuals with Angelman syndrome are small head, seizures, and characteristic electroencephalogram (EEG) abnormalities[45] (Figure 15.8, Box 15.1).

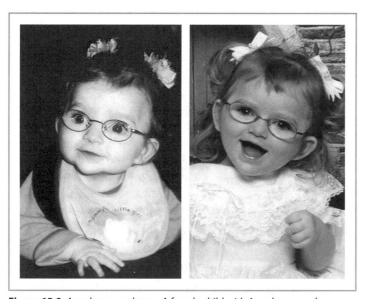

Figure 15.8. Angelman syndrome. A female child with Angelman syndrome.

Reproduced with permission from Jonas JM, Demmer LA. Genetic syndromes determined by alterations in genomic imprinting pathways. *NeoReviews.* 2007;8(3):e120–e126.

Box 15.1. Clinical Features of Angelman Syndrome[a]

A. Consistent (100%)

- Developmental delay, functionally severe.
- Movement or balance disorder, usually ataxia of gait, and/or tremulous movement of limbs. Movement disorder can be mild. May not appear as frank ataxia but can be forward lurching; unsteadiness; clumsiness; or quick, jerky motions.
- Behavioral uniqueness: any combination of frequent laughter/smiling; apparent happy demeanor; easily excitable personality, often with uplifted hand-flapping, or waving movements; hypermotoric behavior.
- Speech impairment, none or minimal use of words; receptive and nonverbal communication skills higher than verbal ones.

B. Frequent (more than 80%)

- Delayed, disproportionate growth in head circumference, usually resulting in microcephaly (2 SD of normal OFC) by age 2 years.
- Microcephaly is more pronounced in those with 15q11.2-q13 deletions.
- Seizures, onset usually <3 years of age. Seizure severity usually decreases with age but the seizure disorder lasts throughout adulthood.
- Abnormal EEG, with a characteristic pattern. The EEG abnormalities can occur in the first 2 years of life, and can precede clinical features, and are often not correlated to clinical seizure events.

C. Associated (20%–80%)

- Flat occiput
- Occipital groove
- Protruding tongue
- Tongue thrusting; suck/swallowing disorders
- Feeding problems and/or truncal hypotonia during infancy
- Prognathia
- Wide mouth, wide-spaced teeth
- Frequent drooling
- Excessive chewing/mouthing behaviors
- Strabismus
- Hypopigmented skin, light hair, and eye color (compared to family), seen only in deletion cases
- Hyperactive lower extremity deep tendon reflexes
- Uplifted, flexed arm position especially during ambulation
- Wide-based gait with pronated or valgus-positioned ankles
- Increased sensitivity to heat
- Abnormal sleep-wake cycles and diminished need for sleep
- Attraction to/fascination with water; fascination with crinkly items such as certain papers and plastics
- Abnormal food-related behaviors
- Obesity (in the older child)
- Scoliosis
- Constipation

Abbreviations: EEG, electroencephalogram; OFC, occipitofrontal circumference; SD, standard deviation.

[a] Reproduced with permission from Williams CA, Beaudet AL, Clayton-Smith J, et al. Angelman syndrome 2005: updated consensus for diagnostic criteria. *Am J Med Genet A*. 2006;140:413–418.

– Williams Syndrome

WS, also known as *Williams-Beuren syndrome*, is often recognized by characteristic facial features (periorbital fullness, short nose with bulbous nasal tip, long philtrum, wide mouth, full lips, and mild micrognathia) and a characteristic cognitive and behavioral phenotype. WS is caused by a microdeletion on chromosome 7 at 7q11 and is found in about 1 in 7,500 to 10,000 children. This chromosomal area is particularly vulnerable to rearrangements due to nonallelic homologous recombination (NAHR). A reciprocal duplication in the same region has been described and is distinct from WS.[46] WS is a contiguous gene deletion syndrome with a variable phenotype; however, there is a critical region. The WS critical region on chromosome 7 includes the elastin gene, which is expressed in connective tissue and leads to the characteristic facial features, cardiovascular defects, bladder and bowel diverticula, hoarse voice, and orthopedic issues observed in individuals with this syndrome.[46] The facial features (Figures 15.9, 15.10, and 15.11) become less classic with age. The most recent AAP health supervision guidelines for children with WS were published in 2001. Dr Barbara Pober updated medical comorbidities of children with WS in 2010.[47] High-frequency sensorineural hearing loss is common and often goes unrecognized.[47] About 75 to 80% of children with WS have congenital heart disease (usually supravalvular aortic stenosis [SVAS]), and 15% have idiopathic hypercalcemia. Table 15.5 lists the associated medical issues.

Individuals with WS have developmental delays, and 75% have ID. The most frequently reported cognitive pattern includes weak visuospatial skills with stronger language skills. While language is a strength, especially for concrete vocabulary and grammatical structure, pragmatic/social use of language may be weaker.[48] Children with WS also tend to be overly friendly ("cocktail personality"), anxious, empathetic, and have difficulty with sensory modulation.[46,49,50]

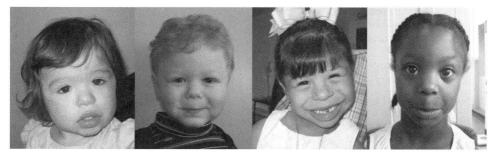

Figure 15.9. Young children with Williams syndrome (left to right): Asian female, age 19 months; Caucasian male, age 2 years; Hispanic female, age 3 years; African-American female, age 5 years.

Reproduced with permission from Morris CA. Introduction: Williams syndrome. *Am J Med Genet C Semin Med Genet.* 2010; 154C(2): 203–208.

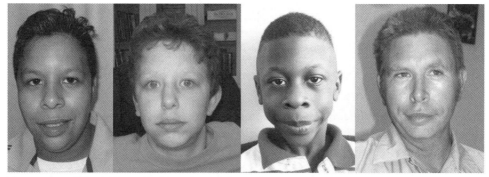

Figure 15.10. Older children and adult with WS (left to right): Hispanic male, age 9; Caucasian male, age 13; African American male, age 7; Caucasian male, age 30.

Reproduced with permission from Morris CA. Introduction: Williams syndrome. *Am J Med Genet C Semin Med Genet.* 2010; 154C(2): 203–208.

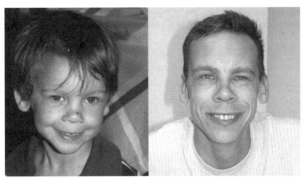

Figure 15.11. Changing facial phenotype over time in a male with WS: left, age 3.5; right, age 21.

Reproduced with permission from Morris CA. Introduction: Williams syndrome. *Am J Med Genet C Semin Med Genet.* 2010; 154C(2): 203–208.

Table 15.5. Common Features of Williams-Beuren Syndrome

Feature*	Comments†
Auditory and ear, nose, and throat	
Hyperacusis	Noise sensitivity can negatively affect quality of life
Mild-to-moderate high-tone sensorineural hearing loss	Clinically detected in adolescents and adults
Recurrent otitis media	
Cardiovascular	
Vascular stenosis (eg, SVAS, PPS)	Change in stenosis most likely to occur during childhood; surgery often indicated for greater-than-moderate SVAS
Hypertension	Renovascular cause occasionally found
Valve abnormality (eg, MVP)	
Intracardiac lesion (eg, VSD)	
Stroke	Very rare; can be secondary to intracranial stenosis
Sudden death	Very rare; risk factors are use of anesthesia, biventricular outflow obstruction, biventricular hypertrophy, coronary artery obstruction
Development and cognition	
Global cognitive impairment (mean IQ, about 55)	IQ ranges from 40 to 100; a few patients have IQs within the normal range
Characteristic pattern of cognitive strengths and weaknesses (known as the Williams-Beuren syndrome cognitive profile)	Strengths are in selected language skills and weaknesses in visuospatial skills
Dental	
Small or unusually shaped primary teeth	
Malocclusions	
Hypodontia	

Table 15.5. Common Features of Williams-Beuren Syndrome (continued)	
Feature*	**Comments†**
Endocrine	
Early onset of puberty	Menarche occurs about 2 years early
Glucose intolerance or diabetes mellitus	Reported in 75% of adults
Osteopenia or osteoporosis	Vitamin D or calcium supplementation should be used with caution
Hypothyroidism (subclinical)	Can be associated with mild thyroid hypoplasia; drug therapy required in minority
Hypercalcemia	Documented in a minority of patients; not restricted to infancy
Gastrointestinal and weight-related	
Colic, difficulty feeding, textured-food intolerance	
Abnormal weight gain	Many infants gain weight poorly; as adults, two thirds have a body mass index >25‡
Constipation	
Gastroesophageal reflux	
Abdominal pain of unclear cause	
Diverticular disease	Possibly occurs in up to one-third of patients; diverticulitis can occur in young adults
Rectal prolapse	
Celiac disease	
Genitourinary	
Delayed toilet training	
Voiding frequency, urgency, enuresis	
Structural renal anomalies	
Bladder diverticula	
Recurrent urinary tract infections	
Nephrocalcinosis	
Miscellaneous	
Short stature	Common but not obligatory; cause is probably multifactorial
Sleep dysregulation, possibly including restless legs syndrome	Prevalence is currently unknown
Musculoskeletal	
Joint laxity	
Joint contractures	Worsening lower-extremity contractures with increasing age
Lordosis	
Scoliosis	

Table 15.5. Common Features of Williams-Beuren Syndrome (*continued*)	
Feature*	**Comments†**
Neurologic	
Hypotonia	
Hyperreflexia	More prevalent in adolescents and adults than in younger patients, especially in lower extremities
Cerebellar findings	Poor balance and coordination
Type I Chiari malformation	
Ophthalmologic	
Strabismus	
Altered visual acuity	
Reduced stereopsis	
Narrowing of lacrimal duct	
Personality, behavior, and emotional well-being	
Friendly personality	Endearing, friendly personality that can confer vulnerability to inappropriate advances
Impulsivity and short attention span (ADHD)	Lifelong ADHD, declining hyperactivity after childhood
Anxiety and phobias, obsessive-compulsive traits	Anxiety and other traits develop over time and are present in a majority of adolescents and adults
Dysthymia	
Skin and integument	
Soft skin with mild premature aging	
Premature graying of hair	Can start in young adulthood
Inguinal (and other) hernias	

Abbreviations: ADHD, attention deficit–hyperactivity disorder; MVP, mitral-valve prolapse; PPS, peripheral pulmonary stenosis; SVAS, supravalvular aortic stenosis; VSD, ventricular septal defect. Reproduced with permission from Pober BR. Williams-Beuren syndrome. *N Engl J Med.* 2010 Jan 21;362(3):239–252.

* Common features are listed in descending order of prevalence.

† Comments are listed for the features for which the trajectory is particularly distinctive in Williams-Beuren syndrome.

‡ The body mass index is the weight in kilograms divided by the square of the height in meters.

— Smith-Magenis Syndrome/Potocki-Lupski Syndrome

Rearrangements on the short arm of chromosome 17, involving band 17 p11.2, lead to 2 distinct syndromes related to gene dosage. Smith-Magenis syndrome (SMS) is caused by a 3.6 Mb deletion at 17p11.2, and Potocki-Lupski syndrome (PTLS) is caused by a duplication in the same area. While both syndromes are contiguous gene syndromes and can typically be diagnosed with CMA, the retinoic acid inducible 1 gene (*RAI1*) has been found to be a major contributor to both phenotypes. Therefore, sequencing of the *RAI1* gene is recommended if an individual's phenotype is highly suggestive of SMS or PTLS and CMA does not find a copy number variation. Both syndromes have a prevalence of about 1 in 25,000.[51]

SMS is typically associated with ID, hypotonia, multiple congenital anomalies, hyperactivity, aggressive and self-injurious behaviors, and significant sleep disturbances. Individuals with SMS often engage in skin-picking, pulling out nails, hand-clasping, and self-hugs. Most individuals with SMS have moderate ID. Adaptive function is often more impaired than cognitive function due to maladaptive behaviors. Features of ASD are also frequently seen in individuals with SMS.[51,52] Cognitive and adaptive function have been found to vary with the size of the deletion.[53] Physical features of SMS are brachycephaly, broad face, midface hypoplasia, prognathism, everted upper lip, short stature, short hands, scoliosis, strabismus, myopia, and cardiac and renal anomalies. Hearing impairment is found in about 70%, EEG abnormalities in 50%, and seizures in 20%.[53] Hypotonia and facial dysmorphism can be mild and easily missed. Sleep and maladaptive behaviors are present in most individuals with SMS and have a significant impact on the quality of life for the child and family. Abnormal patterns of melatonin secretion have been found in individuals with the deletion and the point mutation on *RAI1*. Treatment of sleep problems is difficult and evidence is sparse. Melatonin at bedtime, with or without a beta-blocker during the day to suppress daytime melatonin secretion, may be helpful. Routine screening for comorbidities is recommended.[51]

PTLS has a much broader phenotype that includes hypotonia and failure to thrive in infancy, ID, ASD, apraxia of speech, behavioral problems (including poor attention, hyperactivity, and anxiety), cardiac anomalies (including aortic root dilation and rhythm disturbances), and unrecognized central and obstructive sleep apnea. Due to the variability in phenotype, parental studies are recommended. Routine screening for comorbidities is recommended.[51]

— Sex Chromosome Aneuploidies

Sex chromosome aneuploidies are the most common chromosomal abnormalities and occur in approximately 1 in 500 children. The most common conditions include XXY (Klinefelter syndrome) and XYY in males, and XXX (triple X) and 45,X (Turner syndrome) in females. Cognitive impairment in the intellectual disability range is rare in the trisomy conditions and in Turner syndrome; however, these groups have a high rate of learning disabilities. Interestingly, in XXY, XYY, and triple X syndromes, language-based learning disabilities are present in approximately 70% of patients with strengths in visual-perceptual skills, while in Turner syndrome, nonverbal learning disabilities occur in approximately 70% of patients with strengths in verbal skills.[54,55] ADHD is common across all of these conditions. Physical features of XXY, XYY, and triple X include tall stature, low muscle tone, mild hypertelorism, epicanthal folds, and clinodactyly. Males with XXY/Klinefelter syndrome also develop hypogonadism during puberty with findings of microorchidism, gynecomastia (in 50%), and azoospermia.[55] Treatment with testosterone is indicated.[56] Assistive reproductive technology and testicular sperm extraction have increased fertility in males with XXY.[57] Pubertal development and fertility are not typically affected in XYY and triple X. Girls with Turner syndrome present with short stature and can also have congenital heart abnormalities (40%), renal abnormalities (30%–40%), and ovarian dysgenesis/gonadal failure (90%).[54] The AAP has published health supervision guidelines for Turner syndrome.[58] Haploinsufficiency of the *SHOX* gene has been shown to be associated with the short stature in Turner syndrome, and thus overexpression of *SHOX* is postulated to be related to tall stature in the supernumerary conditions. Genes on the sex chromosomes related to the cognitive phenotypes have not yet been identified; however, in Turner syndrome, those with a small ring X chromosome are at increased risk for ID.[54] Other rarer variations, such as XXYY, XXXY, XYYY, XXXXY, tetrasomy X, and pentasomy X, can also occur, and the degree of physical and cognitive problems increases as additional X and Y chromosomes are added.

Educational Programming for Children With Cognitive Impairments

All children are entitled to a free and appropriate education, regardless of the presence of medical, emotional, or developmental disabilities. Federal law requires that education be provided in the learning environment that is most appropriate for that particular child. Schools are charged with accommodating or modifying for any disabling conditions that might interfere with a child's learning in the school setting, but also not to excessively limit learning potential, so that education is provided in the *least restrictive environment* (LRE).[59] Per the Individuals with Disabilities Education Act (IDEA; formerly the Education for All Handicapped Children Act), children with identified disabilities are deemed eligible for special education and related services. Related services include, but are not limited to, speech/language, occupational, and physical therapies, counseling, and transportation services. ID, LD, ASD, physical/motor impairments, emotional/behavioral disorders, and hearing and vision impairments are examples of conditions that qualify children for special educational services under this legislation. In addition, a variety of medical conditions that have the potential to interfere with learning (eg, epilepsy, ADHD) can be designated as "other health impairments" and therefore qualify for services under IDEA. Section 504 of the Rehabilitation Act is another legal avenue through which some children with disabilities may receive related services and/or modifications within the "regular" classroom setting, if they are not deemed to qualify for special education services under IDEA.

Specific to cognitive impairments, children who meet diagnostic criteria for intellectual disability qualify for special education and related services and, per IDEA, will have a written Individualized Education Program (IEP) developed for them by a multidisciplinary team. This team is composed of teachers, special education personnel, therapists, and other professionals and also includes the child's parents. Based on assessments of the child that document his or her profile of learning strengths and weaknesses and potential interferences for learning, the team develops an educational plan specific to that child. Primary pediatric health care professionals are encouraged to be a part of this team, and the AAP has described ways in which they can be involved in the IEP process.[60,61] Although schedules rarely allow for primary care providers to be able to physically attend IEP team meetings, they can still be active in the process through early developmental screening and identification, making referrals for additional assessments and IEP development, and reviewing IEPs to counsel families on plans that are developed (Box 15.2).

Primary pediatric health care professionals should remain aware of federal legislation regarding special education and amendments as they occur. The most recent amendments to IDEA were enacted in December 2004 (PL 108–446, IDEA Improvement Act of 2004, HR 1350) and reauthorized most recently in 2015. Some changes to the law within the most recent amendment include clarification that the transition process for a student with a disability should begin by age 16 years, a requirement that an IEP in place in one school be implemented in a new school when a child transfers there until a new IEP can be developed, and an option for multiyear IEPs in some states.[60] Primary pediatric health care professionals should be aware that special education can last through 21 years of age, and there are vocational rehabilitation programs to support job training, specifically for individuals with ID.

When developing an IEP, the educational conditions that provide the least restrictive environment remain a priority in decision-making, as a stipulation within IDEA. The intent of least restrictive environment is to provide children with disabilities the opportunity to be among their typically developing peers as much as possible during the school day. The *least restrictive environment* indicates that, whenever possible, children with disabilities will receive their education in the regular classroom environment, and "pull-out" services (eg, spending part of the school day in a specialized educational classroom or all day in a self-contained classroom) are to be provided only when receiving their education in the regular classroom is impossible. Children may receive accommodations (how a child accesses information or demonstrates mastery of a learning objective is adapted) or modifications (the learning material provided is modified for the child) within the regular classroom setting. There are several models for combining children with and without disabilities in educational environments, and theoretical arguments and controversy[62–66] exist around classroom designs and terms such as mainstreaming, inclusion, and full inclusion; however, that debate is beyond the scope of this discussion.

Box 15.2. Recommendations for Primary Care Involvement in Supporting Children in Need of IDEA Services in Schools[a]

▷ Perform developmental surveillance and screening to identify children who might benefit from services under IDEA.

 – For children age 3 years and under, specific guidance advises administering developmental screening at ages 9, 18, and 24 months.

▷ Refer for additional evaluations and consideration for IEP team development (or Individual Family Service Plan, IFSP, for children age 3 years and under) and share relevant information.

▷ Participate in the IEP team meetings and creation of the IEP, if time allows.

▷ Inform families of the interpretation of the IEP and their rights under IDEA.

▷ Provide a medical home, including the coordination of medically related services described within the IEP.

▷ Provide a liaison between family and school when necessary, remaining objective in the balance between realistic expectations and the family's hopes for the outcome.

▷ Advocate regarding educational services for children with disabilities, including involvement in local and state advisory and interagency committees.

▷ Work in school-based clinics and/or get involved administratively to improve school functioning for children with disabilities.

▷ Advocate for children with disabilities to receive appropriate services, particularly supporting families through times of transition (between schools, and/or from childhood to adolescence to adulthood).

▷ Remain current regarding knowledge of medical and educational needs of children with disabilities and their legal rights.

Abbreviations: IDEA, Individuals with Disabilities Act; IEP, Individualized Education Program.

[a] Derived from Lipkin PH, Okamoto J; American Academy of Pediatrics Council on Children With Disabilities and Council on School Health. The Individuals with Disabilities Education ACT (IDEA) for Children with Special Educational Needs. *Pediatrics*. 2015;136(6):e1650–e1662; American Academy of Pediatrics Council on Children With Disabilities; Cartwright JD. Provision of educationally related services for children and adolescents with chronic diseases and disabling conditions. *Pediatrics*. 2007;119:1218–1223; and American Academy of Pediatrics Council on Children With Disabilities, Section on Developmental and Behavioral Pediatrics; Bright Futures Steering Committee; Medical Home Initiatives for Children With Special Needs Project Advisory Committee. Identifying infants and young children with developmental disorders in the medical home: an algorithm for developmental surveillance and screening. *Pediatrics*. 2006;118(1):405–420. Reaffirmed August 2014.

Bullying is a chronic problem in the school setting for a proportion of all children, but children with disabilities appear to be at particular risk.[67] The degree of risk has been found to be somewhat influenced by the type of disability and/or classroom setting (restrictive versus inclusive setting).[68] Specific to students with ID, there is some suggestion that they are victims of direct (eg, physical) bullying in more restrictive settings (eg, self-contained specialized educational classrooms), but they are more often victims of relational bullying (eg, social isolation) in inclusive (regular education) settings.[69] Bullying prevention programs within schools should therefore include specific awareness regarding children with disabilities. Another concern about inclusion is the potential that the education of either group of children might be compromised by the presence of the other group because of different learning abilities.[70] This concern must be weighed against the potential benefits for both groups of children. Inclusion allows some "normalization" in the lives of children with disabilities. It has been shown to improve the academic performance of children with disabilities and to have a positive effect on their self-esteem and social skills.[62] Being among children with disabilities in the educational environment has also been linked to improved tolerance and awareness among the students without disabilities.[71,72]

Borderline Intelligence and Slow Learning

ID and specific learning disability are diagnoses included within IDEA legislation. The child who will not qualify for special education under IDEA but who has difficulty keeping up with average-performing peers in regular classroom environments is the one with borderline or low-average IQ scores (70–89). These individuals with borderline intellectual functioning (IQ 70–79) and slow learners (IQ 80–89) represent ~23% of the normally distributed population. Not all persons with borderline intellectual functioning or slower learning will have associated, significant impairments in adaptive functioning, but IQ scores in the 70 to 89 range do predict some risk for academic struggles and poorer adult outcomes.[73,74] Slow learners are a population at particular risk because their impairments may not be deemed significant enough to qualify for an IEP or special education services, but they are not learning at the same rate as peers with average IQ scores. Children with borderline intelligence may not be found to qualify for services in most jurisdictions and are at extremely high risk for school failure and dropping out. These children are often taught in the regular classroom setting, wherein the teacher is typically teaching at the pace of average learners, who have IQ scores in the average range of 90 to 110. An analogy that primary pediatric health care professionals can use with families is the "miles per hour" metaphor, wherein the typical learner with an average IQ is learning at a pace of 100 mph, but the child with a borderline IQ is learning at a pace of 75 mph. The child with the IQ of 75 is learning, but not as "fast," so that it will take the child longer to get to the destination, or to master the learning objective. In addition, there will be a limit to the complexity of academic material that children with slower learning can ultimately master. It has been estimated, for example, that individuals with slower learning will master only academic material in the range of mid-seventh to mid-ninth-grade level by the time of graduation from high school.[75]

Children with IQ scores in the borderline to low-average range require more time and practice to master academic material, and they need encouragement and emotional support to prevent them from losing motivation to succeed at school and to prevent school dropout. Primary pediatric health care professionals need to be aware that slow learners represent the largest group of children with learning problems in regular classroom settings and are at risk of being left behind in regular classrooms that do not provide accommodations and modifications to support their progress. Classroom accommodations that have had some success include scaffolding of information and reviewing the material in a more specific, systematic way for the slower learner (Table 15.6). Rather than grade retention, nongraded classrooms, learning in cooperative groups, basic and direct instruction of material, and direct instruction on study skills are more effective ways to support the learning of the child with borderline or low average intelligence.[76]

Table 15.6. Learning Difficulties Common for Slow Learners[a]		
Learning Difficulty	**Descriptions of Learning Difficulties**	**Teaching Strategies That Might Be Effective**
"Concrete" thinkers	Struggle to understand abstract concepts; understand only one dimension of a concept; cannot define, distinguish, analyze	Provide direct, systematic steps when teaching. Provide concrete, hands-on learning experiences.
Poorer auditory learning skills	Struggle to master information when provided initially (auditorily) in the typical classroom	Reinforce. Reteach. Use multimodality teaching techniques (visual, tactile, kinesthetic).
Do not learn well "incidentally"	Do not generally "pick up" on learning unless explicitly taught	Carefully target purpose of learning activity. Teach studying skills directly.
Difficulty transferring information	Have trouble applying what is learned in one academic subject or within one learning concept to another subject or another situation	Point out connections within learning and within academic subjects. Assist in making associations in learning.
Difficulty "shifting mental gears"	Take longer to mentally "get going," to engage in the learning process, and to maintain attention to task	Allow frequent breaks. Review information. Develop subtle prompts in the classroom to assist with remaining on task.
Work more slowly	Have trouble organizing thoughts; tend to be slow readers (which is the way children's knowledge is most often assessed); mental effort takes longer	Modify tests. Shorten homework assignments. Modify grading process.
Difficulty following directions	Struggle to follow through on 2- and 3-step instruction	Prompt for active listening skills. Give 1-step instructions.
Difficulty recognizing the most pertinent information for study	Struggle to determine what to study; overwhelmed by textbook learning; waste time trying to filter through the material	Supplement the textbook learning. Provide study guides. Highlight important information.

[a] Adapted from Johns K, Marshall C; Texas Education Agency. *The Slow Learner: An Advocate's View.* Austin, TX: Texas Education Agency; 1989.

Children with slower rates of learning are at increased risk for secondary social, emotional, and behavioral problems derivative of frustration caused by demands and expectations for their performance in regular classroom settings that exceed their abilities. Thus, when school-aged children present to their primary pediatric health care professionals due to behavioral concerns, it is critically important for the clinician to acquire information about a child's underlying cognitive abilities and to analyze whether the demands and expectations placed on the child at school are commensurate with the child's underlying abilities. Primary pediatric health care professionals should be aware of the interventions students with borderline IQ might be able to take advantage of and participate in, such as Response to Intervention (RTI), and advise parents about that. RTI (as defined in IDEA 2004) is a tiered system of intervention allowing identification of, and incremental support and intervention for, students struggling academically.

Research regarding borderline intellectual functioning has generally been quite limited, but one comprehensive 2014 literature review found consistent evidence that persons with borderline intellectual functioning struggle across the life course, not just during the school years.[74] They experience more neuropsychological, mental health, and social problems. Employment rates as adults were comparable to peers with average IQ scores, but wage earnings were notably lower among persons with borderline intellectual functioning.[74]

Gifted Children

Parents are often concerned when they interpret their child's developmental status as different from peers, and they will typically bring up those concerns for discussion with their primary pediatric health care professional. The concern can be that they see their child as lagging behind their peers, but it can also be that they believe their child has skills that surpass their peers or is gifted in one or more areas of development or learning. Of course, when counseling the parent whose child is gifted, primary pediatric health care professionals can and should be more optimistic and reassuring than when counseling the parent whose child is at the other end of the cognitive spectrum, with significant delay or impairment; however, gifted children have the potential for their own set of challenges and complications that a primary pediatric health care professional should be aware of in order to provide the best support to the family of a gifted child.

Gifted is a broad term that is poorly defined. Historically, it has indicated intellectual superiority, as demonstrated by results in the superior range on intelligence testing (IQ >120).[77,78] It has been a term used to describe children with particularly high ability in domains of intelligence that are most related to learning in an academic environment (linguistic and logical-mathematic abilities), but may also include children with other talents in areas outside of academics, such as music, arts, or athletics.[79,80] Early on, gifted children are often advanced in language and verbal abilities and demonstrate intuition and creativity that is precocious for their age.[78,79,81] Their advanced conversational ability, interests, sense of humor, and intellect can make them appear older than their actual age, but it also can make their age-appropriate social and emotional development appear to be more immature in contrast. The asynchronous nature of their development is one of several notable characteristics often seen in gifted children (Box 15.3) and, along with a tendency toward sensitivity and perfectionism, can lead gifted children to experience emotional problems, such as self-criticism, depression, and other internalizing behavioral symptoms.[78,82,83] Gifted children may underachieve academically related to this or intentionally do so, in order to fit in better with peers.

Box 15.3. Characteristics of Gifted Children[a]

- ▶ Asynchronous development across domains
- ▶ Advanced language and reasoning skills
- ▶ Conversation and interests like older children
- ▶ Insatiable curiosity and perceptive questions
- ▶ Rapid and intuitive understanding of concepts
- ▶ Impressive long-term memory
- ▶ Ability to hold problems in mind that are not yet figured out
- ▶ Ability to make connections between concepts
- ▶ Interest in patterns and relationships
- ▶ Advanced sense of humor for age
- ▶ Courage in trying new pathways of thinking
- ▶ Pleasure in solving and posing new problems
- ▶ Capacity for independent, self-directed activities
- ▶ Talent in a specific area (drawing, music, math, reading, etc)
- ▶ Sensitivity and perfectionism
- ▶ Intensity in feeling and emotion

[a] Adapted from Robinson NM, Olszewski-Kubilius PM. Gifted and talented children: issues for pediatricians. *Pediatr Rev.* 1996;17(12):427–434.

By making them aware of these characteristics, primary pediatric health care professionals can help parents to better understand their gifted child and be prepared to anticipate the support and enrichment their gifted child will need. With understanding and support from family and peers, gifted children can be happy and well adjusted, with a positive self-image and good social relationships.[84]

Although the US Department of Education states that gifted children "require services or activities not ordinarily provided in the schools,"[85] there is no federal requirement for distinct education of gifted and talented students.[83] Most states provide educational programs for gifted and talented students, but what is provided varies significantly among states and within communities. Some gifted programs include only certain age ranges, some schools provide in-class enrichment services, while others "pull out" gifted children for specialized education and activities. Parents will often consult primary pediatric health care professionals for advice on educational programming and on parenting specific to their gifted child. The fact that gifted children are such a heterogenous group makes such guidance a challenge to provide, but some general information that can be discussed with families is included in Box 15.4.

Box 15.4. Guidance That Primary Pediatric Health Care Professionals Can Provide Parents of Gifted Children

▶ **Provide enrichment specific to a child's talents, but do not push young children too hard to excel.** All children, regardless of any particular talent, should be provided choices and allowed to be creative and variable in their activities.[a]

▶ **Treat gifted children as "typical."** The same household rules of discipline apply, regardless of giftedness, and gifted children should not be excused from chores or other expectations. Gifted children can also have the same problems as nongifted peers, such as learning disabilities and attention-deficit/hyperactivity disorder.[b,c,d]

▶ **Advocate to make the gifted child's education as individualized as possible.** The best approach will not be the same for every gifted child. Some may be emotionally and socially mature enough for acceleration, such as skipping a grade or attending a higher-grade classroom for certain academic subjects. Alternatively, enrichment is a way to add depth to learning for a subset within the same age group and may include pull-out gifted programs, honors classes, or special interest clubs.[e,f]

▶ **Make connections with parents of other gifted children.** Such partnerships among families can bring some organization to advocating for gifted educational opportunities; allow for children with similar interests to find one another; and also allow shared learning regarding access to resources, effective parenting techniques, etc.

▶ **Be aware of the personality traits your gifted child may be prone to have, but do not worry excessively about them.** The odds are that a gifted child will grow up to be successful and well adjusted. Being aware that a gifted child tends to be a perfectionist, for example, just might make a parent more likely to praise a child when they try something new, even if the outcome is imperfect. Reminding the child it is acceptable and actually interesting to be "different" will help build a positive self-image.

▶ **Maintain awareness of legal and educational developments regarding gifted programming via Web sites and community advocacy chapters.** Reliable organizations include the National Research Center on the Gifted and Talented and the National Association for Gifted Children.

[a] Schechter NL, Reis SM, Colson ER. The gifted child. In: Levine MD, Carey WB, Crocker AC, eds. *Developmental-Behavioral Pediatrics*. 3rd ed. Philadelphia, PA: Elsevier Health Services; 1999:653–661.
[b] Nielsen ME. Gifted students with learning disabilities: recommendations for identification and programming. *Exceptionality*. 2002;10:93–111.
[c] Brody LE, Mills CJ. Gifted children with learning disabilities: a review of the issues. *J Learn Disabil*. 1997;30:282–296.
[d] Lovett BJ, Lewandowski LJ. Gifted students with learning disabilities: who are they? *J Learn Disabil*. 2006;39:515–527.
[e] Robinson NM, Olszewski-Kubilius PM. Gifted and talented children: issues for primary pediatric health care providers. *Pediatr Rev*. 1996;17:427–434.
[f] Jaffe AC. The gifted child. *Pediatr Rev*. 2000;21:240–242.

Suggested Resources

The Arc is a nonprofit organization dedicated to supporting families and individuals with developmental disabilities: **http://www.TheArc.org.**

The Center for Parent Information & Resources provides information for families of children with disabilities: **http://www.parentcenterhub.org/groups/cpir-group/forum/topic/resources-for-parent-centers/.**

Family Voices is a support network for those involved with children who have special health needs: **www.familyvoices.org.**

Educational materials and parent support information may be obtained at **www.fragileX.org** or **www.fraxa.org.**

Reliable Web sites about gifted and talented children include the *Renzulli Center for Creativity, Gifted Education, and Talent Development* (**www.gifted.uconn.edu**) and the *National Association for Gifted Children* (**www.nagc.org**).

References

1. American Psychiatric Association. *Diagnostic and Statistical Manual of Mental Disorders.* 5th ed. Washington, DC: American Psychiatric Association; 2013:xliv, 947

2. American Association on Intellectual and Developmental Disabilities. *Intellectual Disability: Definition, Classification, and Systems of Supports.* 11th ed. Washington, DC: American Association on Intellectual and Developmental Disabilities; 2010:6

3. American Association on Intellectual and Developmental Disabilities. *User's Guide: Intellectual Disability Definition, Classification, and Systems of* Support. 11th ed. Washington, DC: American Association on Intellectual and Developmental Disabilities; 2012:1

4. Moeschler JB, Shevell M, Committee on Genetics. Comprehensive evaluation of the child with intellectual disability or global developmental delays. *Pediatrics.* 2014 Sep;134(3):e903–e918

5. Miller DT, Adam MP, Aradhya S, et al. Consensus statement: chromosomal microarray is a first-tier clinical diagnostic test for individuals with developmental disabilities or congenital anomalies. *Am J Hum Genet.* 2010 May 14;86(5):749–764

6. Gillberg C. Practitioner review: physical investigations in mental retardation. *J Child Psychol Psychiatry.* 1997;38(8):889–897

7. Van Karnebeek CD, Shevell M, Zschocke J, Moeschler JB, Stockler S. The metabolic evaluation of the child with an intellectual developmental disorder: diagnostic algorithm for identification of treatable causes and new digital resource. *Mol Genet Metab.* 2014: 111(4):428–438.

8. Bull MJ, American Acdemy of Pediatrics Committee on Genetics. Health supervision for children with Down syndrome. *Pediatrics.* 2011;128(2):393–406

9. Roizen NJ, Magyar CI, Kuschner ES, et al. A community cross-sectional survey of medical problems in 440 children with Down syndrome in New York State. *J Pediatr.* 2014;164(4):871–875

10. Bertapelli F, Pitetti K, Agiovlasitis S, Guerra-Junior G. Overweight and obesity in children and adolescents with Down syndrome-prevalence, determinants, consequences, and interventions: A literature review. *Res Dev Disabil.* 2016;57:181–192

11. Dykens EM. Psychiatric and behavioral disorders in persons with Down syndrome. *Ment Retard Dev Disabil Res Rev.* 2007;13(3):272–278

12. Verkerk AJ, Pieretti M, Sutcliffe JS, et al. Identification of a gene (FMR-1) containing a CGG repeat coincident with a breakpoint cluster region exhibiting length variation in fragile X syndrome. *Cell.* 1991;65(5):905–914

13. Pieretti M, Zhang FP, Fu YH, et al. Absence of expression of the FMR-1 gene in fragile X syndrome. *Cell.* 1991;66(4):817–822

14. Loesch DZ, Huggins RM, Hagerman RJ. Phenotypic variation and FMRP levels in fragile X. *Ment Retard Dev Disabil Res Rev.* 2004;10(1):31–41

15. Sullivan AK, Marcus M, Epstein MP, et al. Association of FMR1 repeat size with ovarian dysfunction. *Hum Reprod.* 2005;20(2):402–412

16. Berry-Kravis E, Abrams L, Coffey SM, et al. Fragile X-associated tremor/ataxia syndrome: clinical features, genetics, and testing guidelines. *Mov Disord.* 2007;22(14):2018–2030, quiz 140

17. Hessl D, Tassone F, Loesch DZ, et al. Abnormal elevation of FMR1 mRNA is associated with psychological symptoms in individuals with the fragile X premutation. *Am J Med Genet B Neuropsychiatr Genet.* 2005;139(1):115–121

18. Primerano B, Tassone F, Hagerman RJ, Hagerman P, Amaldi F, Bagni C. Reduced FMR1 mRNA translation efficiency in fragile X patients with premutations. *RNA.* 2002;8(12):1482–1488

19. Crawford DC, Acuña JM, Sherman SL. FMR1 and the fragile X syndrome: human genome epidemiology review. *Genet Med.* 2001;3(5):359–371

20. Dombrowski D, Lévesque S, Morel ML, Rouillard P, Morgan K, Rousseau F. Premutation and intermediate-size FMR1 alleles in 10572 males from the general population: loss of an AGG interruption is a late event in the generation of fragile X syndrome alleles. *Hum Mol Genet.* 2002;11(4):371–378

21. Abrams MT, Reiss AL, Freund LS, Baumgardner TL, Chase GA, Denckla MB. Molecular-neurobehavioral associations in females with the fragile X full mutation. *Am J Med Genet.* 1994;51(4):317–327

22. de Vries BB, Wiegers AM, Smits AP, et al. Mental status of females with an FMR1 gene full mutation. *Am J Hum Genet.* 1996;58(5):1025–1032

23. Hagerman R. The physical and behavioral phenotype. In: Hagerman R, Hagerman P, ed. *Fragile X Syndrome: Diagnosis, Treatment, and Research.* 3rd ed. Baltimore, MD: John Hopkins University Press; 2002:3–109

24. Hersh JH, Saul RA, Committee on Genetics. Health supervision for children with fragile X syndrome. *Pediatrics.* 2011;127(5):994–1006

25. Lozano R, Azarang A, Wilaisakditipakorn T, Hagerman RJ. Fragile X syndrome: a review of clinical management. *Intractable Rare Dis Res.* 2016;5(3):145–157

26. van Karnebeek CD, Bowden K, Berry-Kravis E. Treatment of Neurogenetic Developmental Conditions: From 2016 into the Future. *Pediatr Neurol.* 2016;65:1–13

27. May PA, Baete A, Russo J, et al. Prevalence and characteristics of fetal alcohol spectrum disorders. *Pediatrics.* 2014;134(5):855–866

28. May PA, Keaster C, Bozeman R, et al. Prevalence and characteristics of fetal alcohol syndrome and partial fetal alcohol syndrome in a Rocky Mountain Region City. *Drug Alcohol Depend.* 2015;155:118–127

29. Hoyme HE, Kalberg WO, Elliott AJ, et al. Updated clinical guidelines for diagnosing fetal alcohol spectrum disorders. *Pediatrics.* 2016;138(2):pii:e20154256

30. Williams JF, Smith VC, American Academy of Pediatrics Committee on Substance Abuse. Fetal alcohol spectrum disorders. *Pediatrics.* 2015;136(5):e1395–e1406

31. Cook JL, Green CR, Lilley CM, et al. Fetal alcohol spectrum disorder: a guideline for diagnosis across the lifespan. *CMAJ.* 2016;188(3):191–197

32. Centers for Disease Control and Prevention, National Center on Birth Defects and Developmental Disabilities, National Task Force on Fetal Alcohol Syndrome and Fetal Alcohol Effects. Fetal alcohol syndrome: guidelines for referral and diagnosis. www.cdc.gov/ncbddd/fas/documents/FAS_guidelines_accessible.pdf. Accessed November 24, 2017

33. Astley SJ, Clarren SK. Diagnosing the full spectrum of fetal alcohol-exposed individuals: introducing the 4-digit diagnostic code. *Alcohol Alcohol.* 2000;35(4):400–410

34. Kodituwakku PW. Defining the behavioral phenotype in children with fetal alcohol spectrum disorders: a review. *Neurosci Biobehav Rev.* 2007;31(2):192–201

35. Popova S, Lange S, Bekmuradov D, Mihic A, Rehm J. Fetal alcohol spectrum disorder prevalence estimates in correctional systems: a systematic literature review. *Can J Public Health.* 2011;102(5):336–340

36. Kalberg WO, Buckley D. FASD: what types of intervention and rehabilitation are useful? *Neurosci Biobehav Rev.* 2007;31(2):278–285

37. Petrenko CL, Alto ME. Interventions in fetal alcohol spectrum disorders: an international perspective. *Eur J Med Genet.* 2017;60(1):79–91

38. Gahagan S, Sharpe TT, Brimacombe M, et al. Pediatricians' knowledge, training, and experience in the care of children with fetal alcohol syndrome. *Pediatrics.* 2006;118(3):e657–e668

39. Chen C, Visootsak J, Dills S, Graham JM Jr. Prader-Willi syndrome: an update and review for the primary pediatrician. *Clin Pediatr (Phila).* 2007;46(7):580–591

40. Grugni G, Marzullo P. Diagnosis and treatment of GH deficiency in Prader-Willi syndrome. *Best Pract Res Clin Endocrinol Metab.* 2016;30(6):785–794

41. Butler MG, Manzardo AM, Forster JL. Prader-Willi Syndrome: clinical genetics and diagnostic aspects with treatment approaches. *Curr Pediatr Rev.* 2016;12(2):136–166

42. Whittington J, Holland A. Cognition in people with Prader-Willi syndrome: insights into genetic influences on cognitive and social development. *Neurosci Biobehav Rev.* 2017;72:153–167

43. Bennett JA, Germani T, Haqq AM, Zwaigenbaum L. Autism spectrum disorder in Prader-Willi syndrome: a systematic review. *Am J Med Genet A.* 2015;167A(12):2936–2944

44. Buiting K, Williams C, Horsthemke B. Angelman syndrome—insights into a rare neurogenetic disorder. *Nat Rev Neurol*. 2016;12(10):584–593

45. Williams CA, Beaudet AL, Clayton-Smith J, et al. Angelman syndrome 2005: updated consensus for diagnostic criteria. *Am J Med Genet A*. 2006 Mar 1;140(5):413–418

46. Morris CA. Introduction: Williams syndrome. *Am J Med Genet C Semin Med Genet*. 2010;154C(2):203–208

47. Pober BR. Williams-Beuren syndrome. *N Engl J Med*. 2010;362(3):239–252

48. Mervis CB, Becerra AM. Language and communicative development in Williams syndrome. *Ment Retard Dev Disabil Res Rev*. 2007;13(1):3–15

49. Dykens EM. Anxiety, fears, and phobias in persons with Williams syndrome. *Dev Neuropsychol*. 2003;23(1–2):291–316

50. Klein-Tasman BP, Mervis CB. Distinctive personality characteristics of 8-, 9-, and 10-year-olds with Williams syndrome. *Dev Neuropsychol*. 2003;23(1–2):269–290

51. Neira-Fresneda J, Potocki L. Neurodevelopmental disorders associated with abnormal gene dosage: Smith-Magenis and Potocki-Lupski syndromes. *J Pediatr Genet*. 2015;4(3):159–167

52. Dykens EM, Smith AC. Distinctiveness and correlates of maladaptive behaviour in children and adolescents with Smith-Magenis syndrome. *J Intellect Disabil Res*. 1998;42(Pt 6):481–489

53. Madduri N, Peters SU, Voigt RG, Llorente AM, Lupski JR, Potocki L. Cognitive and adaptive behavior profiles in Smith-Magenis syndrome. *J Dev Behav Pediatr*. 2006;27(3):188–192

54. Bondy CA; Turner Syndrome Study Group. Care of girls and women with Turner syndrome: a guideline of the Turner Syndrome Study Group. *J Clin Endocrinol Metab*. 2007;92(1):10–25

55. Visootsak J, Graham JM, Jr. Klinefelter syndrome and other sex chromosomal aneuploidies. *Orphanet J Rare Dis*. 2006;1:42

56. Davis S, Howell S, Wilson R, et al. Advances in the interdisciplinary care of children with Klinefelter syndrome. *Adv Pediatr*. 2016 Aug;63(1):15–46

57. Aksglaede L, Juul A. Testicular function and fertility in men with Klinefelter syndrome: a review. *Eur J Endocrinol*. 2013;168(4):R67–R76

58. Frías JL, Davenport ML; American Academy of Pediatrics Committee on Genetics and Section on Endocrinology. Health supervision for children with Turner syndrome. *Pediatrics*. 2003;111(3):692–702

59. The Individuals with Disabilities Education Act. 20USC §1400 2004

60. American Academy of Pediatrics Council on Children With Disabilities; Cartwright JD. Provision of educationally related services for children and adolescents with chronic diseases and disabling conditions. *Pediatrics*. 2007;119(6):1218–1223

61. Lipkin PH, Okamoto J; American Academy of Pediatrics Council on Children With Disabilities; Council on School Health. The Individuals With Disabilities Education Act (IDEA) for children with special educational needs. *Pediatrics*. 2015;136(6):e1650–e1662

62. Cooney G, Jahoda A, Gumley A, Knott F. Young people with intellectual disabilities attending mainstream and segregated schooling: perceived stigma, social comparison and future aspirations. *J Intellect Disabil Res*. 2006;50(6):432–444

63. Delgado CE, Vagi SJ, Scott KG. Tracking preschool children with developmental delay: third grade outcomes. *Am J Ment Retard*. 2006;111(4):299–306

64. Kauffman JM, Hung LY. Special education for intellectual disability: current trends and perspectives. *Curr Opin Psychiatry*. 2009;22(5):452–456

65. Pilling N, McGill P, Cooper V. Characteristics and experiences of children and young people with severe intellectual disabilities and challenging behaviour attending 52-weeks residential special schools. *J Intellect Disabil Res*. 2007;51(3):184–196

66. Schenker R, Coster W, Parush S. Participation and activity performance of students with cerebral palsy within the school environment. *Disabil Rehabil*. 2005;27(10):539–552

67. Reiter S, Lapidot-Lefler N. Bullying among special education students with intellectual disabilities: differences in social adjustment and social skills. *Intellect Dev Disabil*. 2007;45(3):174–181

68. Rose CA M-A, Espelage DL. Bullying perpetration and victimization in special education: a review of the literature. *Remedial Spec Educ*. 2011;32(2):114–130

69. Rose CA, Stormont M, Wang Z, et al. Bullying and students with disabilities: examination of disability status and educational placement. *School Psych Rev*. 2015;44(4):425–444

70. Smith P. Have we made any progress? Including students with intellectual disabilities in regular education classrooms. *Intellect Dev Disabil*. 2007;45(5):297–309

71. Piercy M, Wilton K, Townsend M. Promoting the social acceptance of young children with moderate-severe intellectual disabilities using cooperative-learning techniques. *Am J Ment Retard*. 2002;107(5):352–360

72. Rillotta F, Nettlebeck T. Effects of an awareness program on attitudes of students without an intellectual disability towards persons with an intellectual disability. *J Intellect Dev Disabil*. 2007;32(1):19–27

73. Johns K, Marshall C, Texas Education Agency. *The Slow Learner: An Advocate's View*. Austin, TX: Texas Education Agency; 1989

74. Peltopuro M, Ahonen T, Kaartinen J, Seppälä H, Närhi V. Borderline intellectual functioning: a systematic literature review. *Intellectual Dev Disabil*. 2014;52(6):419–443

75. Dunalp HB. Minimum competency testing and the slow learner. *Educ Leadership*. 1979;36(5):327–329

76. Carnine D. Introduction to the mini-series: diverse learners and prevailing, emerging, and research-based educational approaches and their tools. *School Psych Rev*. 1994;23(3):341–350

77. Callahan CM. Intelligence and giftedness. In: Sternberg RJ, ed. *Handbook of Intelligence*. New York, NY: Cambridge University Press; 2000:159–175

78. Winner E. The origins and ends of giftedness. *Am Psychol*. 2000 Jan;55(1):159–169

79. Robinson NM, Olszewski-Kubilius PM. Gifted and talented children: issues for pediatricians. *Pediatr Rev*. 1996;17(12):427–434

80. Winner E. *Gifted Children: Myths and Realities*. New York, NY: Basic Books; 1996

81. Nielsen ME. Gifted students with learning disabilities: recommendations for identification and programming. *Exceptionality*. 2002;10(2):93–111

82. Eklund K, Tanner N, Stoll K, Anway L. Identifying emotional and behavioral risk among gifted and nongifted children: a multi-gate, multi-informant approach. *Sch Psychol Q*. 2015 Jun;30(2):197–211

83. Liu YH, Lien J, Kafka T, Stein MT. Discovering gifted children in pediatric practice. *J Dev Behav Pediatr*. 2005;26(5):366–367

84. Field T, Harding J, Yando R, et al. Feelings and attitudes of gifted students. *Adolescence*. 1998;33(10):331–342

85. Ross PO. National excellence: a case for developing America's talent. Office of Educational Research and Improvement. Washington, DC: 1993; Contract No.: ED359743

CHAPTER 16

Speech and Language Development and Disorders

Michelle M. Macias, MD, FAAP

Angela C. LaRosa, MD, MSCR, FAAP

Shruti Mittal, MD, FAAP

Language acquisition is one of the most important components of a child's development. Language represents objects or actions in symbolic form and communicates ideas, intentions, and emotions. Effective communication is necessary for social-emotional development and interactions, learning, and effective functioning in society. Speech and language disorders are one of the most common developmentally disabling disorders of childhood, and 30% of parents voice concerns about language development during primary care visits.[1] Functions of the pediatric primary care medical home include promoting language development, alleviating concerns about language development, and/or detecting language development problems. Early recognition of language delays and intervention are necessary to provide children with speech and/or language disorders with the best possible outcome.

Communication skill development begins at birth. Infants communicate nonverbally through facial expressions and gestures and verbally through sounds and primitive words, and they soon learn that speech is a more efficient means of communication. Language development occurs in an orderly and predictable manner for most children; however, variations can occur. Virtually any disruption in brain function can affect language acquisition; therefore, a variety of conditions affecting the brain are associated with language problems. Delays in comprehension and/or expression not associated with other developmental or neurological problems are found in 5% to 16% of children aged 2 to 5 years, with a significantly higher proportion of boys being affected.[2]

Primary pediatric health care professionals should be careful not to attribute cultural or gender differences as reasons for delayed language development. Children who learn 2 languages simultaneously follow the same pattern of speech and language development as monolingual language learners. The child may have a period when he or she mixes the 2 languages, but this should gradually disappear as language skills develop.[3] Studies have shown that girls are more talkative (have more total words) than boys at all ages, with significant gender differences found between 1 to 2.5 years of age.[4] Although some boys may develop expressive language more slowly than girls, it is generally only by a few months and still within the accepted time frame. Language development is almost never delayed because the child "doesn't need to speak" (eg, "her big sister always talks for her"). There is a tremendous motivation to improve communication, as the use of verbal labels allows the child to meet needs more efficiently than pointing.

The term *language delay* implies the delay will resolve, and the child will catch up at some point. This varies depending on the type of language delay. Natural history studies reveal a 40% persistence rate for children with expressive language delay alone but a 70% persistence rate for those with mixed receptive-expressive language delays.[2,5] More than 40% of children with early delayed language that normalizes demonstrate later reading or cognitive difficulties.[6] Preschoolers with language disorders are at higher risk for language-based learning disorders and social and behavioral problems.[7,8] Speech and/or language concerns should not be dismissed with reassurance that the child will "catch up," given the possibility of future difficulties and better outcomes with earlier detection of these problems.

Dimensions of Speech and Language

Speech produces complex acoustic signals that communicate meaning and is the result of interactions between the respiratory, laryngeal, and oral structures. This acoustic signal varies with regard to vocal pitch, intonation, and voice quality. The signals need to conform to the language code so that they can be decoded as meaningful communication.

Language involves both expressive and receptive components. Expressive language involves the communication of ideas, intentions, and emotions. Receptive language involves understanding what is said by someone else. Receptive language includes auditory comprehension (listening), literate decoding (reading), and mastery of visual signing.

Language has several components, as outlined in Table 16.1. The simplest "units" of language are *phonemes*, or individual sounds. Phonemes are combined to produce *morphemes*, which are the meaningful units of sound combined to produce a word.

Table 16.1. Components of Speech and Language	
Term	**Definition**
Speech	
Intelligibility	Ability of speech to be understood by others
Fluency	Flow of speech
Voice and resonance	Sound of speech, incorporating passage of air through larynx, mouth, and nose
Language	
Receptive language	Ability to understand language
Expressive language	Ability to produce language
Phoneme	Smallest units of sound that change the meaning of a word (eg, "map" and "mop")
Morpheme	Smallest unit of meaning in language (eg, adding "s" to the end of a word to make it plural)
Syntax	Set of rules for combining morphemes and words into sentences (grammar)
Semantics	The meaning of words and sentences
Pragmatics	The social use of language, including conversational skills, discourse, volume of speech, and body language

The *lexicon* (vocabulary) is the collection of all of the meaningful words in a language. *Syntax* (grammar) is the order of words in phrases and sentences. *Semantics* are the individual word and sentence meanings. The literal interpretation of words can be modified by *prosody* or vocal intonation. The social use of language is known as *pragmatics*.

Typical Speech and Language Development

The concept of "critical periods" is generally accepted for speech/language development in infancy and early childhood.[9] Table 16.2 shows the typical ages for attaining language milestones, although variability exists. Some skills may be demonstrated by the child during the office visit, while others may rely on parent report.

Table 16.2. Speech and Language Milestones		
Age	**Receptive Language**	**Expressive Language**
0–3 months	Alerts to voice	Cries, social smile Coos
4–6 months	Turns to voice, name	Laughs out loud Blows raspberries, clicks tongue Uses single consonant sounds, then begins babbling
7–9 months	Turns head toward sound	Says "Mama" and "Dada" indiscriminately
10–12 months	Enjoys "peek a boo" Understands the word "no" Follows 1-step command with gesture	Says "Mama" and "Dada" specifically Waves "bye-bye" Begins to gesture Shakes head "no" First word other than "Mama" or "Dada"
13–15 months	Follows 1-step command without gesture Points to 1 body part Points to ask for something or to get help	Nonspecific jargoning Uses 3 words (other than names)
16–18 months	Points to 1 picture Points to 2 body parts Points to object of interest to draw attention to it	Mature jargoning with true words Up to 10 words (other than names) Uses giant words: "all gone," "thank-you"
19–24 months	Begins to understand pronouns Follows 2-step commands Points to 5–10 pictures	Up to 50 words Two-word phrases, then sentences
25–30 months	Understands "just one" Points to parts of pictures	Uses pronouns correctly Speech is 50% intelligible to strangers
3 years	Knows opposites Understand simple prepositions (eg, on, under)	250+ words 3-word sentences Answers "what" and "where" questions Speech is 75% intelligible to strangers
4 years	Follows 3-step commands Points to 4 colors	Uses 4-word sentences Answers "when" questions Knows full name, gender, age Tells stories Speech is 100% intelligible
5 years	Begins to understand left and right Understands adjectives	Answers "why" questions Defines simple words

Pre-Speech Period

Children's communication development begins shortly after birth through social interactions with adults, which are necessary for bonding and having the infant's needs met. Infants are able to distinguish their mother's voice and show preference for familiar adults from early on in the first few months of life.[10] By a few months of age, the infant realizes that some sounds are important and specifically reacts to them. By 6 months of age, an infant recognizes the basic sounds of her native language and has clear self-driven imitation of other's speech, with a rich interplay between the infant and the older individuals in her life.

Vocal development begins with phonation in the first few months (guttural or throaty sounds), then progresses to primitive articulation or cooing between 2 to 4 months of age. This expands to full vowel sounds by 4 to 5 months of age, single consonant sounds by about 5 months (eg, "ah-guh"), and well-formed babbling (repeated consonant-vowel pattern, eg, "bababa") at around 6 months of age. Receptive language skills and social routines also develop in the first year of life. Six-month-old children may pause momentarily when they hear their name called, and by 10 months pause at the word "no." At approximately 10 months of age children begin to gesture, holding their arms up to be picked up, waving bye-bye, and engaging in social games such as peek-a-boo.

Naming Period

Around their first birthday, children respond appropriately to requests for identification of familiar people or objects. Pointing is also used in a variety of contexts and is an important expression of nonverbal communication. A child uses *protoimperative pointing* to a desired object in order to get an adult to obtain the object for him; the child "imperiously" implies, "I need that!" by pointing to the object. *Protodeclarative pointing* is used when a child attempts to get an adult's attention to look at something of interest to the child and is a key component of *joint attention*. A child may also point to an object and vocalize in a questioning tone in an attempt to have an adult name that object for him.

Formal vocabulary development usually begins with the first word by an infant's first birthday and may include immature words such as "ba" for bottle or "cu" for cup. Vocabulary steadily expands, and by 2 years, a child may add 1 new word a day to include approximately 200 words by 2.5 years of age and more than 10,000 words by the time a child enters first grade. A child's receptive vocabulary is much larger than the number of words he or she uses expressively.

At 13 to 15 months of age, a child begins to *jargon,* or mimic mature conversation, by varying intonation and pitch but initially does not use true words with this immature speech. Parents may report their child sounds like he is "talking in a foreign language." As new words are learned, they are incorporated into the child's speech patterns *(mature* jargoning). First words are usually nouns used to label objects. Between 12 and 18 months of age, a child uses single words to communicate desires (eg, "more"), emotions (eg, "no"), and specific objects (eg, "baby").[11]

Word Combination Period

At around 18 months of age, when a child has a 20-word vocabulary, she begins to combine words into phrases. Initially, word combinations tend to be "giant words" (ie, words the child often hears used together, such as "thank you" and "let's go"). Next, the child combines words into novel phrases (eg, "big truck"), and then into 2-word sentences (noun + verb, verb + object [eg, "want ___"]).[11]

Sentences

A rough rule of thumb is that 90% of children use 2-word sentences at 2 years of age, 3-word sentences by 3 years of age, and 4-word sentences by 4 years of age.[12] Sentences become increasingly complex as the child's understanding of grammar and language develop. By 3 to 4 years of age, children are able to understand and use prepositions (eg, "under" and "on"), adjectives, and adverbs. They begin to ask and answer questions. Semantics (word and sentence meaning) and syntax (grammar) improve over time, and by 5 years of age, children have complete mastery of grammatical tense marking. The child's pragmatic language skills also develop as the child learns the rules of social communication.

Promotion of Language Development

As with all areas of development and behavior, promotion of language development is a function of the primary care medical home and is a component of the strength-based approach to primary pediatric care. Optimal language development occurs when children experience stimulating environments with predictable and developmentally appropriate responses from adults. Some families may need guidance in strategies to encourage language development. Parents should be encouraged to "make their house a language house," essentially, talking throughout daily activities with their children, no matter how mundane the activity. Reading aloud to young children has known positive effects on language and later reading decoding skills, as evidenced by research on Reach Out and Read, a primary care–based literacy promotion program. Studies have shown that parents use more complex language and more book-to-life comparisons when they read to young children using picture books rather than when they read books with text.[13] This helps to promote oral language usage and conversational speech. The American Speech-Language-Hearing Association (ASHA) has handouts on language stimulation activities for young children that can be downloaded, reviewed, and provided to families (**http://www.asha.org/public/speech/development/Parent-Stim-Activities.htm**). Parents should be reminded that television is not a substitute for language and should be avoided in the first years of life. Babies and young children do not get the same language stimulation from television as they do from personal, verbal interactions.

Variations in Development

Children's speech and language development is generally an orderly process, but like most aspects of development, language emergence is characterized by variation. When a parent raises a concern about language, the child will ultimately fall somewhere on the continuum of language developmental *variation,* language *problem,* or language *disorder.* Administering a standardized general developmental screen or language-specific screen will help the clinician determine where the child lies on this continuum. If the child passes the screen or has a borderline score, then watchful waiting is an appropriate next step to the discussion of language stimulation activities, with close follow-up and repeat screening in the medical home. If the child fails the screen, then referral to early intervention or early childhood programs (Head Start, preschool) and referral to a speech and language pathologist is recommended.

A speech-language or communication disorder is defined as an impairment in the ability to receive, send, process, and/or comprehend verbal, nonverbal, or graphic symbol systems.[14] The most common variation in language development is language *delay.* The word *delay* inherently implies that catch-up will occur. Of children with early language delays, approximately 60% will catch up by 4 years of age with no persistent problems.[5] Another variation is language *dissociation.* This can occur either within the language domain, as seen when developmental rates differ between expressive and receptive language, or between different domains (eg, language and motor skills). *Deviation* in language development occurs when language development deviates from the norm, for example when children learn more advanced language-based concepts before they have mastered early language milestones. An example of this is a child who is able to recite the alphabet or TV jingles but is not yet able to communicate needs using words and phrases. Deviated language development can often be a sign of autism spectrum disorder (ASD).[15]

Young children with late language emergence, or "late talkers," can be especially perplexing to primary pediatric health care professionals. Which children are just slower to develop expressive language but will catch up, and which children will continue to experience language delay? Generally, late talkers are those children aged 18–23 months of age with expressive vocabularies fewer than 10 words and/or those children 24–34 months of age whose expressive vocabulary consists of 50 words or less and/or are not using 2-word combinations.[16] Factors associated with decreased risk of continued language problems include age-appropriate receptive language, a greater number of gestures used to compensate, a younger age at diagnosis, and continued progress with language development.

Some late talkers resolve or appear to resolve their expressive language delays. However, resolved late talkers (RLT), from childhood through adolescence, often score lower on language tests than children with typical language development. Language-related problems can emerge in the later school years when more advanced language-related skills are needed.[16]

Speech Disorders

Speech disorders reflect problems with creating the appropriate sounds representing the language symbols (the words). These problems include phonological *(articulation)* disorders, dysarthria, apraxia of speech, voice disorders, and speech fluency disorders. Speech disorders may or may not also include impairments in expressive language.[14]

Phonological or Articulation Disorder

A phonological or articulation disorder is characterized by the substitution, omission, addition, or distortion of phonemes and represents most speech therapy referrals. Children master sounds at different ages depending on the difficulty in producing the sound. In the first 2 years, children master simple sounds, including all vowels and the consonants /b/, /c/, /d/, /p/, and /m/. More difficult sounds, such as the consonants /j/, /r/, /l/, and /v/ and blends (ie, sh, ch, th, st), may not be mastered until 5 or 6 years of age.

Dysarthria

Dysarthrias are motor speech disorders that involve problems of articulation, respiration, phonation, or prosody as a result of paralysis, muscle weakness, or poor coordination.[17] Dysarthric speech is characterized by weakness in specific speech sound production and is frequently associated with cerebral palsy. Dysarthric speech may also encompass problems in coordinated breath control and head posture.

Apraxia of Speech or Dyspraxia

Apraxia of speech, or *dyspraxia,* is a speech disorder that arises from difficulties in complex motor planning and movement and involves problems in articulation, phonation, respiration, and resonance. This results in a child having difficulty correctly saying what he or she wants to say. The child has problems putting syllables together to form words and has more difficulty with longer words rather than shorter, simpler words. It is not due to weakness of the oromotor musculature as seen with dysarthria. Therefore, apraxia/dyspraxia can usually be differentiated from dysarthria by the lack of association with other oral-motor skills, such as chewing, swallowing, or spitting. Other neurological "soft signs," such as generalized hypotonia, may be present on examination and can result in fine motor or gross motor difficulties.[18] Apraxia can be categorized as acquired or developmental. Acquired apraxia/dyspraxia commonly results from head injury, tumor, stroke, or other problems affecting the parts of the brain involved with speaking and involves loss of previously acquired speech. It may co-occur with dysarthria or aphasia, a communication disorder impacting understanding or use of words caused by damage to the language centers of the brain. Developmental apraxia of speech, also referred to as *childhood apraxia of speech* (CAS), is present from birth. A hallmark feature of CAS that distinguishes CAS from phonological disorders (where speech errors are consistent) is the inconsistent error pattern on consonants and vowels in repeated productions of syllables or words observed in CAS. For example, a child with CAS might be able to say the /t/ in the word "top." However, when he or she says the /t/ in the word "water" the /t/ might sound like an /n/ or a /d/, resulting in "waner" or "wader." Individuals with apraxia or aphasia might have difficulty with verbal expression; however, apraxia on its own does not present a problem with language comprehension. Apraxia of speech is differentiated from an expressive language delay in that children with expressive language delay typically follow a normal language trajectory but at a slower pace. It can be difficult to differentiate between expressive language delay and apraxia before the age of 2 years. Development of receptive language is often unaffected in apraxia. Because individuals with apraxia of speech demonstrate similar language concerns as individuals with expressive language disorders and dysarthria, it is necessary for examiners to administer an oral-motor examination to help differentiate the 2 conditions. Some helpful aspects of the oral-motor exam might include pursing of the lips, blowing, using a straw, licking the lips, and elevating the tongue. Children with apraxia will generally have difficulty imitating oral-motor movements but will not demonstrate weakness. Children with dysarthria will exhibit decreased strength and coordination of speech musculature, and speech errors are usually distortions. Standardized tests for praxis can be completed by speech-language pathologists. In regard to treatment options, 2 motor treatments (Dynamic Temporal and Tactile Cueing for Speech Motor Learning [DTTC] and Rapid Syllable Transition [ReST]), and one linguistic treatment (Integrated Phonological Awareness Intervention) have the most evidence supporting their use.[19]

Voice Disorders

Variations in pitch, volume, resonance, and voice quality can be seen in isolation or in combination with a language delay. Impaired modulation of pitch and volume can be seen in children with ASD, nonverbal learning disorders, and some genetic syndromes. Hyper- or hyponasal voice quality suggests anatomical differences or sometimes neurological dysfunction, with hypernasal speech occurring secondary to velopharyngeal palatal incompetence and hyponasal speech arising from air impeded by large adenoids.[20] Velopharyngeal palatine incompetence (insufficiency) can be a marker of 22q11.2 microdeletion syndrome.

Fluency Disorders

A fluency disorder involves the interruption in the flow of speaking. Examples of dysfluent speech include pauses, hesitations, interjections, prolongations, and interruptions. This is common in early childhood (age 2.5 to 4 years), and at that time is categorized as *normal dysfluency of childhood*. Persistent or progressive dysfluency is more likely *stuttering*, which arises in the preschool years for most affected children. Red flags indicative of pathological dysfluency requiring speech therapy include repetitions associated with sound prolongations (eg, "ca-caaaaa-caaaaat"), multiple part-word repetitions (eg, "ca-ca-ca-cat"), hurried and jerky repetitions with associated self-awareness and frustration, associated articulation problems, or a home environment with a low tolerance for stuttering or high pressure for verbal communication.[21]

Normal dysfluency usually improves over time, and parents should be instructed to avoid bringing attention to the dysfluent speech by correcting the child or reminding him to slow down. Parents also should speak more slowly and spend time with the child individually, so that he can express himself in a noncompetitive environment. Encouraging families to take turns and not interrupt conversations during family activities is also beneficial. However, referral to a speech-language therapist is indicated if parents continue to be concerned.

Language Disorders

A language disorder, or specific language impairment (SLI), is an impairment in the ability to understand and/or use words in context, both verbally and nonverbally. The disorder may involve the *form* of language (phonology, morphology, and syntax), the *content* of language (semantics), and/or the *function* of language (pragmatics).[14] Language disorders are also classified as *receptive disorders* (trouble understanding others), *expressive* disorders (trouble sharing thoughts, ideas, and feelings), or *mixed receptive and expressive disorders.*

Receptive Language Disorder

Deficits in receptive language almost always occur in conjunction with expressive delays. There are situations in which a child may appear to have an isolated receptive delay, but on careful evaluation, deficits in both areas are present. For example, a child with ASD may appear to have normal or advanced expressive language skills due to extensive use of echolalia, but his or her functional communication delays are similar to the child's impaired receptive skills. Children with hydrocephalus (congenital or acquired) may have superficially appropriate or advanced expressive language skills but exhibit poor content of expression, known as "cocktail party syndrome."[22] In this case, receptive language lags behind expressive language and is felt to be secondary to hydrocephalus and related effects on the language centers of the brain.

Auditory Processing Disorder

Auditory processing disorder (APD), also known as Central Auditory Processing Disorder (CAPD), is a set of purported functional deficits in the processing of verbal information despite normal auditory thresholds. APD is not universally accepted as a disorder and does not appear in the *Diagnostic and Statistical Manual of Mental Disorders,* Fifth Edition (*DSM-5*).[23] However, it is well described as a disorder by the ASHA. Auditory processing involves recognition and interpretation of verbal information and sounds in the brain. The "disorder" part of APD reflects the situation when something is adversely affecting the brain's processing or interpretation of the information heard. There is some controversy in diagnosing APD, as some theories suggest APD is likely more due to deficits in working memory and/or a short attention span.[24] Children with APD concerns often do not recognize subtle differences between sounds in words, even though the sounds themselves are clear, and they may have difficulty comprehending verbal messages, especially in noisy environments, when others are talking, or when listening to complex information. Auditory processing entails many different processes at all levels of the nervous system, and poor-quality acoustic environments, peripheral ear functioning, behavioral factors involved in listening, and problems with the cochlea, nerve, brainstem, and cortex can all be involved. Empirical research is scarce regarding the validity of modality-specific auditory-perceptual dysfunction. The diagnosis is made using behavioral tests supplemented by electroacoustic measures. Audiological assessment is recommended, and the audiologist will give a testing battery to determine how well the child recognizes sounds in words. A comprehensive assessment with a speech-language pathologist, audiologist, psychologist, and physician is often necessary to diagnose this disorder, as it is often associated with and must also be differentiated from other language, learning, and attention problems. Attention-deficit/hyperactivity disorder (ADHD) and APD especially present overlapping symptomatology, specifically inattention and distractibility. Patients have long-term difficulty with understanding sounds in a noisy environment. Clearly these entities have an overlapping clinical profile, and controversy still exists as to whether they are clinically distinct entities.

Expressive Language Disorder

Expressive language disorders represent a broad spectrum of delays, including developmentally inappropriate short length of utterances, word-finding weaknesses, semantic substitutions, and difficulty mastering grammatical morphemes that contribute to plurals or tense. Signs of weakness in expressive language include circumlocutions (using many words to explain a word instead of using the specific term), excessive use of place holders ("um," "uh"), nonspecific words ("stuff" or "like"), using gestures excessively, or difficulty generating an ordered narrative.

Mixed Receptive-Expressive Language Disorder

Unless formal language testing using standardized instruments supports the presence solely of an isolated articulation disorder or specific receptive or expressive weakness, a child with a history of "language delays" should be presumed to have had some combination of language understanding and expression weaknesses. A variety of receptive-expressive subgroups have been described, including (1) *verbal auditory agnosia* (impairment in interpreting the phonology of aural information and resultant limited comprehension of spoken language), (2) *phonological-syntactic deficit* (extreme difficulty producing language with variable levels of comprehension), (3) *semantic-pragmatic deficit* (expressively fluent with sophisticated use of words but poor comprehension and superficial use of conversational speech), and (4) *lexical-syntactic deficit* (word-finding weakness and higher-order expressive skills weakness).[25] Table 16.3 outlines the various linguistic features seen with these subtypes of mixed receptive-expressive language disorders.

Table 16.3. Subtypes of Developmental Language Disorders								
	Receptive			Expressive				
	Phonology	Syntax	Semantics	Phonology	Syntax	Semantics	Pragmatics	Fluency
Verbal auditory agnosia	↓↓	↓↓	↓↓	↓↓	↓↓	↓↓	↓↓	↓↓
Phonological-syntactic deficit	↓	↓	↓	↓	↓	↓	↓	↓
Semantic-pragmatic deficit	NL	NL	↓↓	NL	NL	↓↓	↓↓	NL or ↓
Lexical-syntactic deficit	NL	↓	↓↓	NL	NL or ↓	↓↓	↓	NL or ↓
Verbal dyspraxia	NL	NL	NL	↓↓	↓↓	↓	NL	↓↓
Phonological production deficit (articulation)	NL	NL	NL	↓	↓	NL or ↓	NL	NL or ↓

Abbreviations: NL, normal; ↓, below average; ↓↓, significantly below average.

Impairment in both the receptive and expressive language domains raises the possibility of a more serious pathological process, including intellectual disability, ASD and other communication disorders, and deafness. Milder impairment often correlates with less severe forms of these disorders. An audiological evaluation can uncover hearing impairment or auditory processing disorder. Evaluation of a child's nonverbal problem-solving and adaptive skills can determine whether the child may have an underlying cognitive impairment. If there are concerns related to a child's social relatedness and social interactions, ASD should be suspected. There is considerable overlap among these underlying causes, especially considering the wide spectrum of severity in each area (Table 16.4).

Table 16.4. Developmental Delays in Intellectual Disability, Autism Spectrum Disorder, Deafness, and Auditory Processing Disorder				
	Intellectual Disability	ASD	Deafness	APD
Expressive language	↓	↓↓ to ↑↑	↓↓	↓↓
Receptive language	↓	↓↓	↓↓	↓↓
Nonverbal IQ	↓	↓ to ↑	NL	NL
Adaptive (self-help) skills	↓	↓ to ↑	NL	NL
Social relatedness	NL for DQ	↓↓	NL	NL
Audiology assessment	NL	NL	ABNL	NL

Abbreviations: APD, auditory processing disorder; ASD, autism spectrum disorder; NL, normal; ABNL, abnormal; DQ, developmental quotient; ↓, below average; ↓↓, significantly below average; ↑, above average; ↑↑, significantly above average.

Disorders of Pragmatic Language

Deficits in pragmatic skills involve the inability to use verbal and nonverbal language appropriately for social communication. Successful communication requires one to interpret words that are said in the context of one's knowledge and experience (linguistic context) as well as the use of words and gestures in the context of interpersonal communication. This involves interpreting the contextual meanings conveyed by words and conversation; one must be able to decipher a speaker's meaning along with having the linguistic competence to understand what has been said.[26] Children with pragmatic language problems may be unable to regulate social interactions or reciprocal body language or appropriately modulate their voice. They may stand too close or too far away from people or have improper voice pitch or volume. They commonly have difficulty initiating, maintaining, or terminating a conversation, modifying a topic for an audience, or including others in conversation.

Pragmatic language disorders are found in diverse clinical populations, including ASD, nonverbal learning disorder, and spina bifida with hydrocephalus.[27] Youth with ADHD can also have pragmatic language difficulties consistent with deficits in executive function; deficits are seen in appropriate listener-speaker roles and in using well-organized expressive language.[28] *Social (pragmatic) communication disorder* (SPCD) was introduced in *DSM-5*, and confusion exists around how this disorder relates to ASD and previous descriptions of pragmatic language impairment. Successful social communication abilities extend beyond pragmatics into the social cognition domain. Criteria include impairments in using communication for social exchange, adaptingcommunication style to the context/needs of the listener, following rules of conversation (eg, taking turns), and understanding implicit or ambiguous language. Diagnosing SPCD is problematic due to inconsistencies in terminology and lack of well-validated, reliable assessment measures. Social communication skills are also subject to significant cultural variation (eg, discourse rules such as taking turns, eye contact, and use of humor), and fewer normative data exist for these behaviors.[27]

Relationship Between Early Language Delays and Dyslexia

Developmental continuities exist between oral (including speech) and written (reading and written expression) language disorders. Specific language impairments affect fewer children than dyslexia does. By age 5 years, roughly 7.5% of children have oral language skills below age expectations,[2] and 25% of these children meet criteria for dyslexia in second, fourth, and eighth grades. Learning to read involves the association between the sounds (phonemes) of spoken language and the symbols (letters [or *graphemes])* of printed words. Oral language skills, including phonology, semantics, grammar, and pragmatics, are the foundation for reading. Dyslexia is therefore characterized by reading decoding problems with the core problem based in phonological (speech) processing problems. However, broader language skills, including vocabulary and comprehension processes, are involved and can modify the impact of phonological difficulties. Children with more diffuse language problems typically are at higher risk for reading comprehension deficits. Children with persistent SLI at 8.5 years of age have been shown to have pervasive problems with spelling, word-level reading, and reading comprehension at 15 years of age.[29]

Evaluation of Children Suspected of Having a Speech or Language Delay

It is important to take parental concerns about speech or language development seriously, as these concerns are valid up to 75% of the time.[1] The evaluation of a child suspected of having a speech or language delay should involve a thorough history and physical examination to determine the nature and extent of the problem but also to uncover the etiology whenever possible.

History

It is important to determine whether the delay involves expression alone or both expressive and receptive language abilities. Isolated delays in receptive language are extremely rare. Sometimes a child may appear to have normal or advanced expressive skills due to complex echolalia of entire sentences, but their spontaneous (or functional) language is delayed at least to the *same* degree as their receptive language (for example, with autism). Parental concerns are often focused on a child's inability to express himself or herself, and they may not be aware of associated delays in comprehension. Asking parents about any articulation or intelligibility difficulties is important. Inquiry about prenatal and delivery history, results of the newborn hearing screen, hearing loss, multiple ear infections, excessive drooling or difficulty feeding, and delays in other developmental domains will further elucidate an underlying cause. A detailed social history may uncover environmental causes of mild speech delay, including regression after a stressful event (eg, divorce or birth of a sibling), lack of stimulation, or the older siblings and parents overly anticipating the child's needs. As biological factors contribute to language development, a detailed family history inquiring about speech and language or learning difficulties is important. Twin and family aggregation studies have demonstrated high heritability of language disorders.[30]

Physical Examination

A simple conversation with the child may be all that is needed to determine the extent of his or her comprehension, expression, and deficits in speech delivery. This includes all attempts to communicate, whether it is verbal (eg, babbling, jargoning, words) or nonverbal (eg, facial expressions, gesturing or pointing, presence of joint attention, eye contact, and body posture). A neurological examination focused on oromotor skills should be completed, especially if there are also feeding difficulties or suspected speech apraxia. The oromotor examination should include imitation of tongue movements in all directions, observance of palatal elevation on phonation, and evaluation of the structural integrity of the oral cavity. Oromotor tone can be assessed by looking at mouth position (ie, open mouth suggesting hypotonia), drooling, trouble drinking from a straw, or difficulty blowing bubbles. Slurred, slow, or hypernasal speech are associated with dysarthria (versus dyspraxia). Inconsistent sound errors and slow pauses between sounds are seen in apraxia/dyspraxia.

Surveillance and Screening

Along with other developmental domains, surveillance of speech and language milestones should be performed at every well-child visit. This includes eliciting and attending to parental concerns, updating attainment of speech and language developmental milestones, determining risk and protective factors, and making accurate observations of the child.[31] A 25% delay in milestone attainment is cause for concern and indicates the need for more detailed screening and/or evaluation of speech and language skills. Red flags for delayed speech and language skills are outlined in Table 16.5.

Screening all children for delays in any of the developmental domains should be conducted at periodic intervals and whenever parents voice concerns about their child's development. The American Academy of Pediatrics has established guidelines for developmental screening and recommends screening for all children at ages 9, 18, and 24 to 30 months,[31] or at any time concerns are raised by a caregiver or primary pediatric health care professional, with additional screening for ASD at the 18- and 24-month visits.[15]

Table 16.5. Red Flags for Delayed Speech and Language Development	
Age	**Milestone**
6 months	No cooing responsively
10 months	No babbling
12 months	No basic gesturing (waving bye-bye, holding arms out to be picked up)
18 months	No words other than "Mama," "Dada" No understanding of simple commands No pointing to what he wants
24 months	<50 words No 2-word phrases <50% intelligibility
36 months	No 3-word sentences <75% intelligibility
4–5 years	Not able to tell a simple story

Several screening measures are available for quick evaluation in the pediatric office setting (Table 16.6). Parent-completed questionnaires, such as the Parents' Evaluation of Developmental Status (PEDS),[32] the Parents' Evaluation of Developmental Status: Developmental Milestones (PEDS:DM),[33] and the Ages and Stages Questionnaire-3 (ASQ),[34] are good "broadband" screens designed to assess multiple developmental domains. All 3 specifically screen language, and the PEDS:DM offers an assessment-level version that produces age-equivalent scores in expressive and receptive language. Parent questionnaires specifically designed to evaluate language that can be administered in a busy primary care practice include the Receptive-Expressive Emergent Language Test (REEL),[35] the MacArthur-Bates Communicative Development Inventories (CDI),[36] the Language Development Survey (LDS),[37] and the Communication and Symbolic Behavior Scales Developmental Profile Infant-Toddler Checklist (CSBS DP ITC).[38] If there are concerns about language and a possible ASD, the CSBS DP ITC screens for social, speech, and symbolic communication in children 6–24 months of age and helps to delineate between communication concerns in those realms. Direct, interactive evaluation measures include the Clinical Linguistic and Auditory Milestone Scale (CLAMS)[39] and the Early Language Milestones Scale (ELMS)[40] for children from birth to 36 months of age.

Table 16.6. Screening Measures for Speech and Language Delays		
Parent Questionnaires	**Developmental Age Range**	**Web Address**
General Screens		
Ages & Stages Questionnaires	0–5 years	www.agesandstages.com
Parents' Evaluation of Developmental Status (PEDS)	0–8 years	www.pedstest.com
Language-Specific Screens		
MacArthur-Bates Communicative Development Inventories (CDI)	0–3 years	www.brookespublishing.com
Language Development Survey (LDS)	18–35 months	www.aseba.org
Receptive-Expressive Emergent Language (REEL)	0–3 years	www.linguisystems.com
Communication and Symbolic Behavior Scales Developmental Profile Infant-Toddler Checklist (CSBS DP ITC)	6–24 months	www.brookespublishing.com
Directly Administered Evaluations		
Clinical Linguistic Auditory Milestone Scale (CLAMS)	Up to 36 months	www.brookespublishing.com
Early Language Milestones Scale (ELMS)	Up to 36 months	www.proedinc.com
Parents' Evaluation of Developmental Status: Developmental Milestones (PEDS DM)	0–8 years	www.pedstest.com

Evaluation of articulation disorders begins with good surveillance. A formula for the expected conversational intelligibility levels of preschoolers talking to unfamiliar listeners is: AGE IN YEARS / 4 x 100 = % understood by strangers:

Child aged 1.0 = 1/4 or 25% intelligible to strangers
Child aged 2.0 = 2/4 or 50% intelligible to strangers
Child aged 3.0 = 3/4 or 75% intelligible to strangers
Child aged 4.0 = 4/4 or 100% intelligible to strangers[12]

Any child older than 4 years with a speech intelligibility score of less than 66% (ie, less than two-thirds of utterances understood by unfamiliar listeners) should be considered a candidate for intervention.[41]

It may not be practical to formally assess specific language-based learning problems in a school-aged child in the pediatric office setting. However, a few surveillance questions may help identify the presence of difficulties in language-based learning (see Box 16.1).

Box 16.1. Surveillance Questions for Language-based Learning Problems

1. Does the child have trouble expressing her or his thoughts?
2. Is it difficult for the child to understand or follow directions?
3. Does the child express herself or himself through gestures rather than verbally?
4. Does the child have trouble finding the correct word (word retrieval)?
5. Does the child confuse words that sound alike (eg, "tornado" for "volcano"; auditory discrimination)
6. Does it seem to take a long time for the child to understand directions or answer questions (processing speed)?
7. Does the child seem to have to repeat things (out loud or to self) in order to understand them (processing speed)?
8. Can the child tell you the letter that comes after "s" without going through the alphabet (sequential processing)? Note: The days of the week, months, etc., could also be used.

Other Evaluations

If a speech or language delay is suspected, the child should be referred for a formal audiological examination, as a child may not have apparent hearing deficits by history. Even mild hearing loss can cause language delays and may not be picked up by a newborn hearing screening. If there are concerns for ASD, an autism-specific screening tool should be used in conjunction with general developmental or language-specific screening.

Referral to a developmental-behavioral or neurodevelopmental pediatrician or to a pediatric neurologist is recommended if there is a history of language regression or if there are delays in other areas. Specific disorders in the differential diagnosis of language regression include ASD, Rett syndrome, or Landau-Kleffner syndrome (seizures accompanied by acquired aphasia).[42]

Detailed genetic and neurological evaluations for isolated speech and language impairments are of low yield, and an underlying etiology will be determined in less than 5% of cases. If hypernasality is noted with suspected velopharyngeal insufficiency, then further investigation for chromosome 22q11.2 deletion syndrome is indicated, including referral to otorhinolaryngology and chromosomal microarray analysis. Language (expressive language, verbal fluency, phonological processing, comprehension, and word retrieval) and language-related learning (reading and spelling) problems occur in 70% to 80% of individuals with Klinefelter syndrome (47, XXY) and should be considered in males, especially those with hypogonadism or gynecomastia.[43] If a child has dysmorphic features or is found to have global developmental delay, then a full evaluation by a clinical geneticist is recommended. This evaluation varies with the risk factors and findings and may include brain imaging, electroencephalogram, genetic testing, and/or metabolic testing.[44]

Treatment

Even when there is a question regarding the underlying diagnosis, all children suspected of having speech or language impairment should be referred promptly to their local early intervention program. Early intervention programs enrich a child's language experience through both parent training and provision of language-stimulating preschool environments. If a child is suspected of having a language disorder and fails a language screening test, in addition to hearing testing, referral to an early intervention program for immediate evaluation by a speech-language pathologist is recommended. Speech and language therapy may prevent further delays, improve auditory comprehension and phonological disorders, and help reduce behavior difficulties associated with frustrated attempts to communicate.[45,46]

Treatment of speech-language disorders includes 3 components: causal, habilitative, and supportive. Causal treatment is focused on repairing defects, correcting dysfunction, or eliminating factors that contribute to the language problem (eg, cleft palate repair or hearing aids). Habilitative treatment is designed to directly improve the child's language skills (ie, speech-language therapy and counseling of parents to actively engage in the child's language development). Supportive treatment aims to boost language acquisition (eg, training programs for speech-related skills and increasing social contacts).

Children aged 0 to 3 years can obtain services through the Individuals with Disabilities Education Act, Part C.[47] School-aged children may receive services through the public school system. If additional services are needed, or if the child lives in an area where there is a shortage of therapists in the school system, therapy is also available on an outpatient basis. A child may receive speech therapy privately in addition to in school if the goals of therapy are different; for example, after-school outpatient therapy may work more on social aspects of language whereas speech therapy in school may focus more on grammatical errors and vocabulary. Augmentative and alternative communication (AAC) intervention approaches address the communication needs of children who are unable to use speech consistently for functional communication. The overall goal is to improve communication with others, whether by spoken language or nonverbally through the use of sign language or communication systems such as the Picture Exchange Communication System or an augmentative communication device. Some parents may voice concerns that early use of sign language or another communication system will impair a child's ability to speak, but there is evidence that using these systems may actually enhance a child's speech and language development.[48]

In addition to therapy, parent education that focuses on language stimulation activities is essential. Structured and stimulating child care centers, preschool programs, or "Mother's Day Out" programs are also beneficial, particularly in children with isolated nonpathological speech-language delay reflecting developmental variation or lack of a stimulating home environment.

Interventions for APD are directed toward improving the listening environment, the acoustic signal, and auditory skills, and using bypass strategies. There is moderate support for the use of frequency modulation devices (amplification devices) in children who have auditory processing difficulties.[22] More research is needed to clearly identify APD problems and the best intervention for each child.

While therapy may improve the degree of impairment and prognosis, many children do not "outgrow" speech and language disorders, although these disorders manifest in different ways over time. A child who has early language delays may have difficulty in reading, written expression, learning a foreign language, or learning appropriate social interactions.[49,50] Developmental promotion of language and early identification and intervention for speech and language disorders are vital to providing the greatest long-term functional benefits.

References

1. Glascoe FP. Can clinical judgment detect children with speech-language problems? *Pediatrics.* 1991;87(3):317–322

2. Law J, Boyle J, Harris F, Harkness A, Nye C. Prevalence and natural history of primary speech and language delay: findings from a systematic review of the literature. *Int J Lang Commun Disord.* 2000;35(2):165–188

3. US Department of Education, US Department of Health and Human Services. *Workshop Summary. Childhood Bilingualism: Current Status and Future Directions, April 22-23, 2004;* Washington, DC: Rose Li and Associates; 2005

4. Leaper C, Smith TE. A meta-analytic review of gender variations in children's language use: talkativeness, affiliative speech, and assertive speech. *Dev Psychol.* 2004;40(6):993–1027

5. Dale PS, Price TS, Bishop DVM, Plomin R. Outcomes of early language delay: I. Predicting persistent and transient language difficulties at 3 and 4 years. *J Speech Lang Hear Res.* 2003;46(3):544–560

6. Bashir AS, Scavuzzo A. Children with language disorders: natural history and academic success. *J Learn Disabil.* 1992;25(1):53–65

7. Cohen NJ, Barwick MA, Horodezky NB, Vallance DD, Im N. Language, achievement, and cognitive processing in psychiatrically disturbed children with previously identified and unsuspected language impairments. *J Child Psychol Psychiatry.* 1998;39(6):865–877

8. Cohen NJ, Menna R, Vallance DD, Barwick MA, Im N, Horodezky NB. Language, social cognitive processing, and behavioral characteristics of psychiatrically disturbed children with previously identified and unsuspected language impairments. *J Child Psychol Psychiatry.* 1998;39(6):853–864

9. Werker JF, Tees RC. Speech perception as a window for understanding plasticity and commitment in language systems of the brain. *Dev Psychobiol.* 2005;46(3):233–251

10. Eisenberg RB. *Auditory Competence in Early Life: The Roots of Communicative Behavior.* Baltimore, MD: University Park Press; 1976

11. Coplan J. Normal speech and language development: an overview. *Pediatr Rev.* 1995;16(3):91–100

12. Flipsen P. Measuring the intelligibility of conversational speech in children. *Clin Linguist Phon.* 2006;20(4):202–312

13. Nyhout A, O'Neill DK. Mothers' complex talk when sharing books with their toddlers: book genre matters. *First Language.* 2013;33(2):115–131

14. American Speech-Language-Hearing Association. Definitions of communication disorders and variations (Relevant Paper). *ASHA Suppl.* 1993 Mar;35(3 Suppl 10):40–41

15. Johnson CP, Myers SM; American Academy of Pediatrics Council on Children With Disabilities. Identification and evaluation of children with autism spectrum disorders. *Pediatrics.* 2007;120(5):1183–1215

16. Rescorla LA, Dale PS, eds. *Late Talkers: Language Development, Interventions, and Outcomes.* 1st ed. Baltimore, MD: Paul H. Brookes; 2013. Fey ME KA, ed. Communication and Language Intervention Series

17. Van Mourik M, Catsman-Berrevoets CE, Paquier PF, Yousef-Bak E, Van Dongen HR. Acquired childhood dysarthria: review of its clinical presentation. *Pediatr Neurol.* 1997;17(4):299–307

18. Yoss KA, Darley FL. Developmental apraxia of speech in children with defective articulation. *J Speech Hear Res.* 1974;17(3):399–416

19. Murray E, McCabe P, Ballard KJ. A systematic review of treatment outcomes for children with childhood apraxia of speech. *Am J Speech Lang Pathol.* 2014;23(3):486–504

20. Gray SD, Smith ME, Schneider H. Voice disorders in children. *Pediatr Clin North Am.* 1996;43(6):1357–1384

21. Ward D. The aetiology and treatment of developmental stammering in childhood. *Arch Dis Child.* 2008;93(1):68–71

22. Tew B. The "cocktail party syndrome" in children with hydrocephalus and spina bifida. *Br J Disord Commun.* 1979;14(2):89–101

23. American Psychiatric Association. *Diagnostic and Statistical Manual of Mental Disorders.* 5th ed. Arlington, VA: American Psychiatric Association; 2013

24. Moore DR. The diagnosis and management of auditory processing disorder. *Lang Speech Hear Serv Sch.* 2011;42(3):303–308

25. Rapin I. Practitioner review: developmental language disorders: a clinical update. *J Child Psychol Psychiatry.* 1996;37(6):643–655

26. Russell RL. Social communication impairments: pragmatics. *Pediatr Clin North Am.* 2007;54(3):483–506

27. Norbury CF. Practitioner review: social (pragmatic) communication disorder conceptualization, evidence and clinical implications. *J Child Psychol Psychiatry.* 2014;55(3):204–216

28. Green BC, Johnson KA, Bretherton L. Pragmatic language difficulties in children with hyperactivity and attention problems: an integrated review. *Int J Lang Commun Disord.* 2014;49(1):15–29

29. Snowling MJ, Hayiou-Thomas ME. The dyslexia spectrum: continuities between reading, speech, and language impairments. *Top Lang Disord.* 2006;26(2):110–126

30. Bishop DVM. The role of genes in the etiology of specific language impairment. *Journal of Communication Disorders.* 2002;35(4):311–328

31. American Academy of Pediatrics, Council on Children With Disabilities, Section on Developmental and Behavioral Pediatrics; Bright Futures Steering Committee; Medical Home Initiatives for Children with Special Needs Project Advisory Committee. Identifying infants and young children with developmental disorders in the medical home: an algorithm for developmental surveillance and screening. *Pediatrics.* 2006;118(1):405–420

32. Glascoe F. *Parents' Evaluation of Developmental Status (PEDS).* Nashville, TN: Ellsworth and Vandermeer Press; 2005

33. Glascoe F. *Parents' Evaluation of Developmental Status: Developmental Milestones (PEDS:DM).* Nashville, TN: Ellsworth and Vandermeer Press; 2007

34. Squires J, Bricker D, Twombly E, et al. *Ages & Stages Questionnaires (ASQ-3): A Parent-Completed Child Monitoring System.* 3rd ed. Baltimore, MD: Paul H. Brookes Publishing Co; 2009

35. Bzock KR, League R, Brown VL. *REEL-3: Receptive-Expressive Emergent Language Test.* 3rd ed. Austin, TX: Pro-Ed; 2003

36. Fenson L, Marchman VA, Thal DJ, et al. *MacArthur Communicative Development Inventories: User's Guide and Technical Manual,* 2nd ed. Baltimore, MD: Brookes Publishing; 2006

37. Rescorla L. The language development survey: a screening tool for delayed language in toddlers. *J Speech Hear Disor.* 1989;54(4):587–599

38. Weatherby AM, Prizant BM. *Communication and Symbolic Behavior Scales Developmental Profile Infant/Toddler Checklist.* Baltimore, MD: Paul H. Brookes Publishing Company; 2001

39. Accardo PJ, Capute A, Bennett A, et al. *The Capute Scales: Cognitive Adaptive Test and Clinical Linguistic and Auditory Milestones Scales.* Baltimore, MD; Brookes Pub 2005

40. Coplan J. The Early Language Milestone Scale (Revised). Austin, TX: Pro-Ed; 1993

41. Gordon-Brannan M, Hodson BW. Intelligibility/severity measurements of prekindergarten children's speech. *Am J Speech Lang Pathol.* 2000;9:141–150

42. Rogers SJ. Developmental regression in autism spectrum disorders. *Ment Retard Dev Disabil Res Rev.* 2004;10(2):139–143

43. Skakkebaek A, Walletin M, Gravholt CH. Neuropsychology and socioeconomic aspects of Klinefelter syndrome: new developments. *Curr Opin Endocrinol Diabetes Obes.* 2015;22 (3):209–216

44. Shevell MI, Majnemer A, Rosenbaum P, Abrahamowicz M. Etiologic determination of childhood developmental delay. *Brain Dev.* 2001;23(4):228–235

45. Almost D, Rosenbaum P. Effectiveness of speech intervention for phonological disorders: a randomized controlled trial. *Dev Med Child Neurol.* 1998;40(5):319–325

46. Glogowska M, Roulstone S, Enderby P, Peters TJ. Randomised controlled trial of community based speech and language therapy in preschool children. *BMJ.* 2000;321(7266):923–926

47. United States Federal Government. Individuals with Disabilities Education Act (IDEA). https://sites.ed.gov/idea/statuteregulations/. Accessed November 2, 2017

48. Millar DC, Light JC, Schlosser RW. The impact of augmentative and alternative communication intervention on the speech production of individuals with developmental disabilities: a research review. *J Speech Lang Hear Res.* 2006;49(2):248–264

49. Catts HW, Fey ME, Tomblin JB, Zhang X. A longitudinal investigation of reading outcomes in children with language impairments. *J Speech Lang Hear Res.* 2002;45(6):1142–1157

50. Robertson SB, Weismer SE. Effects of treatment on linguistic and social skills in toddlers with delayed language development. *J Speech Lang Hear Res.* 1999;42(5):1234–1248

CHAPTER 17

Learning Disabilities

Jason M. Fogler, MA, PhD

William J. Barbaresi, MD, FAAP

Definition of "Learning Disability" and Scope of the Problem

The terms *learning disability* (LD) and *learning disorder* are often used interchangeably. The *Diagnostic and Statistical Manual of Mental Disorders,* Fifth Edition (*DSM-5*) uses the term *Specific Learning Disorder* and states that learning disorders are diagnosed when difficulties in learning and academic skills "are substantially and quantifiably below those expected for the individual's chronological age, and cause significant interference with academic or occupational performance, or with activities of daily living, as confirmed by individually administered standardized achievement measures and comprehensive clinical assessment."[1] This differs from the previous (*DSM-IV-TR*) definition of learning disorders, which specified that academic achievement must fall "substantially below that expected given the individual's chronological age, measured intelligence, and age-appropriate education."[2] In other words, according to *DSM-5,* the child must demonstrate a significant discrepancy between achievement scores in reading (fluency or comprehension), writing (spelling or written expression), or math (number sense or mathematical reasoning) in comparison to his or her chronological age. The *DSM-5* definition further emphasizes that specific learning problems in reading, mathematics, or written language must be distinguished from situations in which low academic achievement is better accounted for by overall lower cognitive ability as measured by an IQ test. It is important to emphasize that the shift away from an explicit statement about a discrepancy between academic achievement and IQ does not preclude the diagnosis of specific learning disorder in a child who, for example, has IQ scores in the "gifted" range (>120) with academic achievement in the "average" range (eg, standard score of 100 on an academic achievement test). Similarly, children with borderline IQ scores may manifest unexpected, severe academic underachievement in comparison to their cognitive ability. Rather, the *DSM-5* encourages a broader consideration of the many factors that can influence academic achievement, such as cognitive ability, exposure to appropriate instruction, and genetic and environmental factors. The new wording in *DSM-5* should not be interpreted in ways that diminish the appropriate application of the diagnosis and provision of special educational supports for children who have significant academic achievement difficulties compared to their learning potential, including children with very strong or borderline cognitive ability. The child must demonstrate an impact of these discrepant measures on academic achievement in the classroom. Furthermore, according to *DSM-5,* learning disorders should not be diagnosed when delays in academic achievement are primarily attributable to impaired hearing or vision, intellectual disability, other mental or neurological disorders, psychosocial adversity, lack of proficiency in the language of academic instruction, or inadequate educational instruction.[1] A child may meet the diagnostic criteria for a specific learning disorder in one or more academic skill sets (reading, mathematics, and/or written language).

Discrepancy Versus Low Achievement Definitions of Learning Disability

Previous federal special education laws emphasized the concept of a "significant discrepancy" between measurements of academic achievement and cognitive ability, typically defined as a 1– to 2–standard deviation or more difference in academic achievement and full-scale IQ scores.[1] However, recently there has been a trend toward LD definitions that emphasize low academic achievement among children with at least low-average cognitive skills.[3] This is a particularly important concept for children who may, for example, have IQ scores in the low-average range (80–90). In order to meet a discrepancy-based definition of LD, such a child would have to have academic achievement standard scores of 50 to 60, representing delays of several grade levels or more, in comparison to peers. In contrast, a child with an IQ of 100 or more would be required to have an achievement score of 70 in order to meet a discrepancy-based LD definition. In both instances, the child would be underachieving to a degree that would significantly impact his or her ability to succeed in school, yet the child with low-average intelligence would be required to have far lower achievement scores in order to be eligible to receive special education assistance, if only discrepancy definitions of LD are employed. For this and other reasons, Kavale and Forness caution against conflating learning disorder, a distinct neurodevelopmental entity with enduring neuropsychological correlates, with "low achievement," a remediable multidimensional phenomenon stemming from psychosocial adversity and/or lack of adequate educational resources.[3]

Legal Definition of Learning Disability as Per the Individuals with Disabilities Education Act

The reauthorization of the Individuals with Disabilities Education Act (IDEA), the federal legislation that governs special education services in public schools, reflects the trend away from discrepancy-based definitions of LD. In fact, the legislation states that LD criteria "must not require the use of a severe discrepancy for determining whether a child has a specific learning disability…."[4] Further, the law states that the presence of LD may also be defined by a child's failure to improve academic achievement "in response to scientific, research-based intervention" while also continuing to allow other "research-based procedures" to determine LD status.[4] Thus the law continues to allow children to qualify for LD services if they manifest a discrepancy between academic achievement and intellectual ability, but it now also allows children who meet "low achievement" definitions of LD to receive special educational assistance. This should help to ensure that more children who are struggling with academic achievement will receive appropriate services. It is also possible that these new regulations will diminish the number of children who fulfill medical diagnostic criteria for LD yet who do not qualify for LD services in public schools. Most importantly, a child is deemed to have a specific LD if he or she "does not achieve adequately" for age or meet grade-level standards, assuming that appropriate instruction has been provided. Specific LDs can be reflected in problems with the following specific academic tasks: oral expression, listening comprehension, written expression, basic reading skills, reading fluency skills, reading comprehension, mathematics calculation, and mathematics problem-solving.[3] It is important for primary pediatric health care professionals to be familiar with the terminology in the reauthorization of IDEA, particularly *Response to Intervention* (RTI). Special education services must be supported by "scientifically based research…accepted by a peer-reviewed journal or approved by a panel of independent experts through a comparably rigorous, objective, and scientific review."[4] Outlined in sections 34 CFR 300.35 and 20 U.S.C. 1411(e(2)(C)(xi)] [sec. 9101(37) of the Elementary and Secondary Education Act (ESEA)], a proposed intervention must meet standards for clear and replicable methodology and analytic methods, appropriate experimental/quasi-experimental study design with control subjects (eg, randomized controlled trial), and sufficient clarity of reporting to be accepted by a peer-reviewed journal or approved by a panel of independent experts.[5] (For further information on RTI, see also Chapter 20, Interpreting Psychoeducational Testing Reports, Individualized Family Service Plans [IFSP], and Individualized Education Program [IEP] Plans.)

This higher standard for methodological rigor and replication should help to ensure that unproven, non-evidence-based practices are gradually eliminated from special educational programs. The federal law requires that each state enact special education laws that are consistent with the federal law. This leaves the states considerable latitude in special education laws, which is likely to continue the historic tendency for significant state-by-state variations in criteria required to receive special educational services, as well as the nature of the services themselves. Unfortunately, despite the fact that this legislation was passed in 2004, many states have yet to operationalize IDEA by changing relevant state laws. In 2007, states were given "report cards" on their ability to implement IDEA and offered two levels of aid (assistance and intervention) if they fell below their self-imposed requirements.[6] It is concerning to note that, as of 2009, only 13 states and one US territory have met their own self-imposed requirements for educating children with disabilities. Twelve states met criteria for "Needs Assistance," with an additional 13 states and 4 US territories meeting that classification for two consecutive years. One state met criteria for "Needs Intervention," the highest level of concern, and 3 states have held this worrisome status for 2 consecutive years.[7]

Epidemiology of Learning Disability

Learning disorders are among the most common neurodevelopmental disorders in childhood, and it is therefore essential for primary pediatric health care professionals to understand the important role that they play in identification, diagnosis, intervention, and advocacy for their patients with LD. The *DSM-5* includes prevalence estimates of "5–15% (across all LD types) among school-aged children across different languages and cultures."[1] Estimates for the incidence (likelihood of developing LD during childhood) of reading disorder range from 5.3% to 11.8% and for mathematics disorder from 5.9% to 13.8%.[8,9] For each type of LD, the highest incidence rates are obtained with "low achievement" definitions, while discrepancy-based definitions lead to considerably lower estimates. It is also important to recognize that epidemiological studies demonstrate that boys are 2 to 3 times more likely than girls are to manifest any type of LD.[8-10]

Identifying Children With Learning Disability

Children at Risk for Learning Disability

As with other neurodevelopmental disorders, primary pediatric health care professionals play a crucial role in the early identification of children with LDs. This begins with recognition of medical, genetic, and psychosocial conditions that place children at greater risk for development of an LD. They also have a unique opportunity to contribute to early identification of children at risk for LD based on their knowledge of their patient's family, medical, and psychosocial histories. Learning disabilities are clearly familial, with genetics contributing substantially to a child's risk for LD.[11] The family history should include information about learning and other developmental disorders.

Two categories of medical risk factors for LD deserve special attention: prematurity and cyanotic congenital heart disease. Premature infants are at significantly higher risk not only for global developmental delays, but also for LD.[12,13] In particular, children born at less than 32 weeks' gestation or who experience perinatal and postnatal complications such as prolonged ventilation, intracranial hemorrhage, sepsis, seizures, prolonged acidosis, or hypoglycemia are at higher risk for neurodevelopmental sequelae. Similarly, children now surviving previously fatal congenital cardiac anomalies are another group at high risk for LDs.[14,15] Children living in poverty and other adverse circumstances that would fall under the category of *toxic stress* are at risk for academic underachievement and premature dropout, while their risk for LD may be less clear.[16] Nevertheless, such children certainly warrant increased vigilance for not only developmental delays but also LD.

Several genetic disorders have been linked to risks for various forms of LD. In particular, children with Klinefelter syndrome, Turner syndrome, velocardiofacial syndrome, or spina bifida with shunted hydrocephalus have all been shown to be at significant risk for LD.[17,18] Some studies have suggested that children with Turner syndrome and children with spina bifida and shunted hydrocephalus may be specifically at risk for problems with visuospatial cognitive skills and math achievement.[17,19] However, given the limitations in the available literature, it is more appropriate to view these children as being at risk for LD in general, rather than for a specific type of learning problem.

Male gender is also a risk factor for LD. While some authors have suggested that boys and girls are at equal risk for certain types of LD, epidemiological studies have consistently demonstrated that boys are at greater risk for all LDs.[8-10] Girls certainly deserve to be monitored for LD as part of routine care, but boys are at significantly higher risk for LD.

When one of these risk factors is identified, the child should be monitored more carefully, with a low threshold for referral for comprehensive assessment, either privately or through public early intervention and school-based programs.

Early Development and Risk for Learning Disability

The importance of careful developmental surveillance and screening cannot be overestimated, not only in order to identify developmental delays that should be addressed in the toddler or preschool-aged child, but also to identify children at risk for later problems with language-based learning. In addition to formal developmental surveillance and screening, certain "red flags" suggest that a child may be at increased risk for later reading problems. These include delays in receptive and expressive language and speech articulation in toddlers and young preschoolers. Later, children may have difficulty learning simple songs or rhymes.[20] Unfortunately, less is known about early indicators of risk for math LD.

– The Prekindergarten Checkup

Aside from immunizations and hearing and vision testing, primary pediatric health care professionals may question the utility of the prekindergarten preventive care visit. However, this visit provides an ideal opportunity to identify children at risk for LD. Milder delays in language development and speech articulation, which would not have been detectable using standardized developmental screens in the birth to 3 year age group, should be apparent at this age. At the prekindergarten visit, identification of at least 4 random letters that are not in alphabetical order is strongly associated with appropriate phonological processing skills needed for reading decoding. Early indicators of risk for math LD, such as difficulty learning to count or understanding the concept of one-to-one correspondence, may be detected. Children who have difficulty drawing simple shapes (a circle at 3 years, a square at 4 years, or a triangle at 5 years) at the prekindergarten checkup may be at risk for difficulties with writing. In addition, several good developmental screens that include early academic learning skills are available, including the parent-completed Ages & Stages Questionnaires (ASQ) and the directly administered Brigance Screens—II and Parents' Evaluation of Developmental Status: Developmental Milestones (PEDS:DM). Children who appear to be at risk for LD may be scheduled for reassessment during or toward the end of the kindergarten year. At that time, if problems are noted with acquisition of basic number and letter identification or counting, or if teacher concerns are reported, it may be appropriate to refer the child for further assessment (see below).

– School Age: The Report Card Visit

While schools are mandated to evaluate children whose academic performance suggests the presence of an LD, children often "fall through the cracks" and are not assessed until their academic achievement lags far behind their same-aged peers. Alternatively, secondary behavioral and psychosocial problems may develop, and these may be the presenting concern when children are brought to their primary pediatric health care professional. During school-age well-child visits, primary pediatric health care professionals have an opportunity to assess academic progress and identify children who warrant referral for more comprehensive assessment. This requires that a few, brief questions are asked about progress in reading, math, and writing: (1) Has the first-grade child learned all of the letters and letter sounds, numbers, and beginning addition and subtraction facts? (2) Does the child have poor memory for spelling words or numbers? (3) Has the teacher expressed any concerns about academic progress? Parents should be encouraged to bring copies of their child's report card to these visits. At times, academic concerns may be masked by behaviorally acting out in the classroom or while doing homework. LD should be considered among the leading differential diagnoses when the child's acting out occurs around a specific academic subject (eg, only reading or math).

Federal educational policy requires frequent, standardized assessment of student progress. Often the results of these standardized tests are used to gauge the overall performance of a school or school district. However, standardized tests can also help to identify children at risk for LD who require further assessment, but only if parents understand how to interpret the tests. Parents can be instructed to bring their child's standardized test reports to every well-child visit. The primary pediatric health care professional can then quickly identify children who score low on math, reading, and written language tests and who warrant further assessment. Similarly, parents can be instructed to bring their child's most recent report card to every well-child visit. Again, a quick review of the report card can assist in identifying worrisome academic performance and teacher comments that suggest a possible LD. All school-age well-child visits could be greatly enhanced by this brief review of standardized test scores and report cards as a routine practice.

Referring Children for Evaluation by Local School or Private Agency

While it is the responsibility of the school to determine whether or not a child qualifies for special education services, primary pediatric health care professionals can guide parents to formally request an evaluation for their child. Once a formal, written request for evaluation is made, the applicable state special education rules take effect, and the evaluation process begins. Often a brief note from the pediatric health care professional outlining the concerns that prompted the referral will be helpful in getting the evaluation process started. If the quality or result of the school-based assessment is not satisfactory, the professional can assist the family by requesting additional assessment at school or making a referral to a qualified psychologist to complete additional testing. This may be especially important for children who have more complex learning problems or who have not demonstrated adequate progress with school-based services. It should be noted that schools are not required to accept the findings from private assessments, although some school districts will accept such assessment reports. However, by elucidating patterns of strength and weakness in a child's learning profile, and outlining evidence-based strategies that are likely to help, private assessment may still help to ensure that a child's needs are appropriately addressed—even if the school chooses to complete their own testing to verify the findings from private assessments. In these situations, families will need to consider the cost of private assessments because they are typically not covered by health insurance unless there are medical conditions that are directly related to the child's learning difficulties (eg, a diagnosed neurological disorder such as epilepsy).

Comprehensive Assessment for Learning Disability

Primary pediatric health care professionals have an important role to play not only in early identification and referral but also in the evaluation of children with suspected LD. This begins with a complete medical history, physical examination (including formal hearing and vision testing, and lead and iron deficiency screening), and a thorough neurological examination. Primary pediatric health care professionals will also be familiar with the child's family and psychosocial history. The latter is particularly relevant, as stressful or frankly neglectful home environments can lead to academic underachievement and school failure.[21] A medical assessment can also identify behaviors suggestive of emotional and behavioral problems, such as depression or oppositional behavior, that can interfere with school performance. Finally, problems with attention and concentration associated with attention-deficit/hyperactivity disorder (ADHD) should be assessed as potential primary contributors to academic underachievement or as a comorbid condition with LD.[22] Of course, assessment for LD requires psychometric testing, including administration of individual standardized measures of cognitive ability (intelligence tests) and academic achievement. These assessments may be completed by school psychologists as part of an assessment of eligibility for special education services or by private psychologists.

What Causes Learning Disability?

A lengthy review of the genetic, neurological, and neuropsychological factors that underlie LD is beyond the scope of this chapter. However, it is important for primary pediatric health care professionals to have some basic information on these topics.

First, and most important, is an understanding that LD is in large measure genetically determined.[11] This does not diminish the important contribution of environment to a child's developmental progress, including the development of preacademic and academic skills. Nevertheless, it does highlight the importance of the family history in identifying young children at risk for LD. A thorough family history, obtained at the time of an infant or young child's first well-child visit, is therefore an essential component of early identification of LD in primary care pediatric practice.

Recently, functional magnetic resonance imaging (fMRI) technology has helped researchers begin the process of understanding the neurological underpinnings of LD. This has been particularly true for reading LD, with studies showing clear differences in fMRI activation patterns between individuals with normal reading skills and those with reading LD.[23]

These differences in central nervous system function correlate with deficits in phonological processing, a skill that has been shown to be essential for efficient reading decoding and that is impaired in individuals with classic dyslexia.[24] Phonological processing refers to "awareness that words can be broken down into smaller segments of sound."[23,24] While children may have deficits in reading that are caused by a variety of other issues (eg, poor reading comprehension due to problems with receptive language deficits), impaired phonological processing seems to be the most common underlying problem for children who experience difficulty with the basic process of decoding (ie, "reading") written words.

Studies of the neurophysiological and neuropsychological deficits associated with underachievement in math and written language are few in comparison to the reading LD literature. Math LD presents a particular challenge because learning math is dependent on a number of factors, including visual information processing, language, and memory, among others. Hopefully, future research will provide much-needed new information on the etiology of math and written language LDs.

Learning Disability Subtypes/Comorbidities

Multiple Learning Disabilities

While reading LD (or dyslexia) tends to get the most attention in both the research literature and the classroom, it is important to recognize that many children have more than one type of LD. A recent study of math LD demonstrated that, depending on how LD is defined, 35% to 56.7% of children with math LD also had reading LD.[15] The key for primary pediatric health care professionals is to recognize that children who are found to have problems in one area of academic achievement often have problems in other areas; hence, such children should be carefully assessed in all areas of academic achievement to ensure that they receive appropriate intervention. The new *DSM-5* diagnostic categories of Other Specified Neurodevelopmental Disorder (formerly Cognitive Disorder—Not Otherwise Specified under *DSM-IV*) and Unspecified Neurodevelopmental Disorder (formerly Learning Disorder—Not Otherwise Specified)[1,2] are intended to capture learning problems that do not fit easily or neatly into discrete categories. Other Specified NDD is intended to implicate a known biomedical etiology to the learning problems, such as fetal alcohol exposure or anoxia, whereas Unspecified Neurodevelopmental Disorder is intended to capture problems in learning, such as nonverbal learning disabilities, in which the etiology is unknown or unclear.

Learning Disability and Attention-Deficit/Hyperactivity Disorder

Epidemiological studies have demonstrated that children with ADHD experience multiple school-related problems, including academic underachievement, as well as increased rates of absenteeism, grade retention, and school dropout.[22] Comorbid LDs account for at least some of the observed academic underachievement in children with ADHD. This association is so common that every child with LD should be considered to be at risk for ADHD and vice versa. Primary pediatric health care professionals should at least screen for ADHD among their patients with known LD by asking about symptoms of ADHD and considering obtaining ADHD-specific rating scales from the child's parents and teachers. Children with learning problems often exhibit secondary attention deficits or attention problems secondary to the underlying learning disorder. That is, it can be very difficult for a student to maintain focus on tasks that are difficult for him or her to understand. It is sometimes difficult to distinguish "secondary" attention deficits from primary attention deficits.

Language-based Versus Nonverbal Learning Disorders

Most children with LD have problems with language-based learning. This is evident in the "classic" profile of psychometric test results in children with LD, with verbal cognitive measures typically being lower than nonverbal measures. Children with language-based LDs can be expected to have the greatest difficulty in reading and written expression. Teachers and special educators understandably tend to be most experienced in meeting the needs of children with language-based LDs.

In contrast, a smaller, though uncertain, proportion of children manifest nonverbal LD.[17] Such children have nonverbal cognitive measures that are significantly lower than their verbal scores. Children with nonverbal LD experience problems with math computation, organization (particularly in middle and high school), and higher-order math and science concepts. In addition, these children often manifest significant problems with social perception and social interaction that contributes to their negative experiences in educational settings. It is important to distinguish between language-based and nonverbal LDs, both because of the differing profile of academic challenges and differences in associated problems and intervention strategies. School personnel tend to be less familiar with approaches that are successful for children with nonverbal LD, in part due to ongoing controversies about whether nonverbal LD should be considered a diagnosis in its own right or secondary to related conditions such as autism spectrum disorder and social communication disorder. (In clinical settings, nonverbal LD is acknowledged under the broad diagnostic category of Unspecified Neurodevelopmental Disorder in the *DSM-5* but has yet to be formally identified as a "diagnosis under consideration" by any of the *DSM* Workgroups.) Hence, primary pediatric health care professionals can play an important role in advocating for these children.

Intervention and Advocacy

Understanding Special Education Laws

As described earlier, LD is defined in the federal special education law. Each state, in turn, must enact laws that are consistent with the federal statute. As a result, the precise definition of LD varies from state to state, making it important for professionals to familiarize themselves with their own state's special education laws. Individual states' department of education Web sites will typically provide a summary of relevant laws to enable primary pediatric health care professionals to understand the system in their state and thus to be knowledgeable advocates for their patients.

In addition to the terminology described earlier, several other important abbreviations are worth noting.[4] The federal law stipulates that a child's special education plan will be described in detail in an Individualized Education Program (IEP) plan. Primary pediatric health care professionals can play a critical role for families as an independent resource to review school-based psychometric testing reports and IEPs with families to ensure that the IEP provides services appropriate to meet each child's needs.[25] In preparing an IEP, schools must adhere to the principle of a free and appropriate public education (FAPE). This means that children must be provided with an appropriate array of accommodations and services to meet their basic educational needs. This raises an important distinction between services provided under the federal special education law and services that may be available on a private basis. According to the FAPE principle, the child's intervention plan must be appropriate, but it is not required to be "optimal." States have a great deal of latitude in defining an appropriate level of service, and pediatric health care professionals can play an important role in assessing the extent to which school services are sufficient or should be supplemented by privately available educational services.

The law also requires that educational programs be provided in the *least restrictive environment* (LRE). For example, a child with an LD may be able to receive sufficient support in a regular classroom to allow him or her to succeed, while another child may require more intensive services in a separate special education classroom for a certain period of the day or for certain academic subjects. The law requires that the services are always provided in the setting that most closely matches the typical setting for a child of that age and grade placement.

Interventions: School-based and Private Services

One of the greatest challenges in the LD field has been to ensure access to evidence-based interventions for children with LDs. Recently, multiple studies have clearly demonstrated that reading curricula that include explicit teaching of phonics are more effective. This is not surprising because phonological awareness has emerged as a critically important prerequisite for the development of good, basic reading skills. Functional magnetic resonance imaging has evolved as a powerful new research tool for the study of brain activation patterns during reading. This technique has revealed differences between dyslexic and nondyslexic readers.[24, 26] Reading skills in young children are positively correlated with activation in the left occipitotemporal area, a region of the brain that seems to be responsible for the most rapid, efficient reading skills.[24] Furthermore, when dyslexic children were exposed to an empirically validated educational intervention, they demonstrated increased activation of left-sided, occipitotemporal systems, making them functionally more similar to nondyslexic children.[26] These studies illustrate the potential application of functional imaging techniques to elucidate the underlying neurophysiology of learning disorders and to assess, in a direct manner, the impact of intervention on brain function. Unfortunately, far less is known about the most effective interventions for children with math or writing LD. It should be noted that functional imaging is not a clinically useful approach at this time.

For children who qualify for special educational services, the IEP must list specific learning goals, as well as the nature and intensity of services to be provided. Some children may require direct, individual, or small-group instruction with a special education teacher in a special education resource room. In other cases, support from the regular or special education teacher, or a paraprofessional assistant, may be provided in the regular classroom. According to federal law, interventions must be provided in the LRE (see above) while still meeting the child's educational needs. In addition to direct instructional services, IEPs can include accommodations, such as shortened assignments, increased time to complete tests (so as not to penalize children for slower reading of questions), or oral administration of tests for children with reading problems. The key is to ensure that services and accommodations specifically match the demonstrated needs of the child based on the results of individual assessment of learning strengths and weaknesses.

Some children who lag behind their peers in math or reading may not fulfill state and federal criteria to receive formal special educational services through an IEP. For such children, another option may be Title 1 reading and math support. Title 1 is a federal program, originally enacted in 1965 and revised in the No Child Left Behind Act of 2001, designed to provide additional support in reading and math for economically disadvantaged children.[27] Title 1 services are available to all students in a school building only if a sufficient percentage of students who attend that building are economically disadvantaged, based on receipt of federally subsidized free-lunch services.

Some children may have delays or deficits in academic achievement that are significant but not severe enough to qualify for any additional services in the school. In these instances, the only options are private services provided by individual teachers, tutors, or tutoring agencies. The primary pediatric health care professional can play an important role in directing families to high-quality tutoring services in the community.

Unfortunately, unproven, ineffective "interventions" and treatments for LD are available, often at significant cost in both time and money. The issue of nonstandard therapies for children with developmental and behavioral disorders is addressed in detail elsewhere in this book (see Chapter 24, Complementary Health Approaches in Developmental and Behavioral Pediatrics). However, one specific, supposed "intervention" for reading LD deserves mention. Although there is no empirical evidence to support it, "vision therapy" is available in many communities and is typically provided by optometrists. This intervention is based on the non–evidence-based belief that reading problems can be corrected by "eye exercises" aimed at somehow improving the child's ability to process the written word. This clearly contradicts all of the research evidence that demonstrates that reading skills depend on language-based cognitive processes, such as phonological awareness. In a joint policy statement, both the American Academy of Pediatrics and the American Academy of Ophthalmology concluded that scientific evidence does not support the efficacy of eye exercises, behavioral vision therapy, or specially tinted filters or lenses for improving the long-term educational performance in children with reading LD, and thus, these vision therapies are not endorsed and should not be recommended for children with reading LD.[28]

Consequences of Failure to Intervene

The most recent changes in the federal special education laws were intended, in part, to prevent situations in which children were "required" to fall so far behind their peers before qualifying to receive special educational services that intervention was available too late to make a meaningful difference in learning outcomes. Children who do not receive timely intervention are at risk not only of academic failure but also for school dropout and the psychosocial morbidities that accompany limited academic achievement, such as unemployment, substance abuse, and juvenile delinquency.[29-31]

For reading LD, research has clearly demonstrated that intervention must be provided early, at least before third grade, in order to provide an opportunity to remediate reading problems.[32] Thus, early identification and timely access to evidence-based reading intervention is essential to ensure the best possible outcome. For math LD, the critical age by which problems must be identified is not yet known, although it is reasonable to assume that there may be a similarly limited window of opportunity to ensure adequate academic outcomes in math.

Historically, children who demonstrated inadequate academic achievement were often retained a grade, based on the assumption that another year at the same grade level would allow the child to "catch up" to his or her peers. For many children, repeating a grade led to a delay in assessment that would have revealed an LD and initiated appropriate remediation. We now know that grade retention is almost universally unsuccessful and is in fact associated with poorer long-term school outcomes.[33] If there is a role for grade retention, it is only for a limited number of children in the very early school years (kindergarten and first grade) and should be considered only after a thorough evaluation for specific LDs or other conditions that may account for the child's academic underachievement.

Advocacy

Throughout this chapter, the role that the primary pediatric health care professional can play to ensure that children with LD are identified in a timely fashion, referred for appropriate assessments, and offered evidence-based intervention has been highlighted (Box 17.1)

– Starting the Assessment Process

If primary pediatric health care professionals incorporate early identification and ongoing monitoring for LD into their routine practices, they will be in a position to direct their patients to timely assessments, either through the local school or through private psychologists. This is particularly important for families who may lack the resources to monitor and understand information about their child's academic progress.

– Reviewing Evaluation Reports and Individualized Education Programs

Similarly, the primary pediatric health care professional can assist the family by serving as an objective reviewer of assessment reports and making referrals for additional private evaluations when school assessments have not adequately addressed the child's needs. Once the evaluation is complete, the pediatric health care professional can meet with the family to review the IEP to ensure that goals match the demonstrated learning needs of the child.

– Get to Know Local Resources

Primary pediatric health care professionals are respected members of the community and recognized advocates for children under their care. It helps to develop a direct working relationship with local special education directors, school principals, and superintendents when possible. These relationships will help to ensure that the professional's input is considered when concerns arise with regard to school services. Similarly, it is helpful for the professional to become familiar with local providers and agencies that offer high-quality assessment and intervention for children who require private services to supplement programs that are provided in the public school.

– Advocating for Evidence-based Interventions and Curricula

Finally, the primary pediatric health care professional is in a position to help ensure that special educational and private interventions employ evidenced-based interventions, particularly for children with reading LD.

Box 17-1. Key Points

> ▸ Know your state's special education laws and local school district policies and procedures.
>
> ▸ Advise parents to request an evaluation if concerns are present.
>
> ▸ Write a brief note to the school requesting an evaluation.
>
> ▸ Get to know private psychologists who can evaluate the child if necessary.
>
> ▸ Psychosocial adversity and chronic illnesses can affect academic achievement (uncontrolled asthma is an excellent example).
>
> ▸ Rule out hearing and vision impairment.
>
> ▸ Rule out neurological disorders.
>
> ▸ Rule out common comorbidities of LD (especially attention-deficit/hyperactivity disorder).
>
> ▸ Be aware of services available at school and in the community (for kids who do not qualify for special education services at school).
>
> ▸ Refer parents to local advocates to review special education decisions and plans (Individualized Education Program [IEP]). The Learning Disabilities Association of America (https://ldaamerica.org) and the National Center for Learning Disabilities (www.ncld.org) are great sources of information and support.
>
> ▸ Be aware of the impact of LD on the child and family and look for areas of strength to help minimize the impact of LD on self-esteem.
>
> ▸ Counsel families to avoid unproven approaches for LD (diet, vitamins, visual training, or EEG biofeedback).
>
> ▸ Advocate for good reading instruction in your community, specifically, programs that include direct teaching of phonological awareness skills.
>
> ▸ Promote literacy in your practice and your community.

Abbreviations: LD, learning disability; EEG, electroencephalogram.

References

1. American Psychiatric Association. *Diagnostic and Statistical Manual of Mental Disorders*. 5th ed. Arlington, VA: American Psychiatric Association; 2013

2. American Psychiatric Association. *Diagnostic and Statistical Manual of Mental Disorders*. 4th ed. Text rev. Washington, DC: American Psychiatric Association; 2000

3. Kavale KA, Forness SR. What definitions of learning disability say and don't say: a critical analysis. *J Learn Disabil.* 2000;33(3):239–256

4. United States Department of Education. Assistance to states for the education of children with disabilities and preschool grants for children with disabilities: final rule. 34 CFR Parts 300 and 301. *Fed Regist.* 2006;71(156)

5. United States Department of Education, Office of Special Education Programs. (February 2007). Building the Legacy: IDEA 2004—Alignment with the No Child Left Behind Act. http://idea.ed.gov/uploads/Alignment_with_NCLB_2-2-07.pdf. Accessed November 27, 2017

6. Wright P. IDEA Report Cards: Did your state pass or fail? http://www.wrightslaw.com/news/07/idea.report.cards.htm. Updated June 26, 2007. Accessed November 27, 2017

7. United States Department of Education Determination Letters on State Implementation of the IDEA. http://www2.ed.gov/policy/speced/guid/idea/monitor/factsheet.html. Updated February 4, 2009. Accessed November 27, 2017

8. Katusic SK, Colligan RC, Barbaresi WJ, Schaid DJ, Jacobsen SJ. Incidence of reading disability in a population-based cohort, 1976–1982, Rochester, Minn. *Mayo Clin Proc.* 2001;76(11):1081–1092

9. Barbaresi WJ, Katusic SK, Colligan RC, Weaver AL, Jacobsen SJ. Math learning disorder: incidence in a population-based birth cohort, 1976–82, Rochester, Minn. *Ambul Pediatr.* 2005;5(5):281–289

10. Rutter M, Caspi A, Fergusson D, et al. Sex differences in developmental reading disability: new findings from 4 epidemiological studies. *JAMA.* 2004;291(16):2007–2012

11. Pennington BF. Genetics of learning disabilities. *J Child Neurol.* 1995;10:69–77

12. Rais-Bahrami K, Short BL. Premature and small-for-dates infants. In: Batshaw ML, Pellegrino L, Roizen NJ, eds. *Children with Disabilities.* 6th ed. Baltimore, MD: Paul H. Brookes Publishing; 2007:107–122

13. Institute of Medicine (US) Committee on Understanding Premature Birth and Assuring Healthy Outcomes. *Preterm Birth: Causes, Consequences, and Prevention.* Behrman RE, Stith Butler A, eds. Washington, DC: National Academies Press (US); 2007

14. Bellinger DC, Wypij D, duPlessis AJ, et al. Neurodevelopmental status at eight years in children with dextro-transposition of the great arteries: the Boston Circulatory Arrest Trial. *J Thorac Cardiovasc Surg.* 2003;126(5):1385–1396

15. Wernovsky G, Shillingford AJ, Gaynor JW. Central nervous system outcomes in children with complex congenital heart disease. *Curr Opin Cardiol.* 2005;20(2):94–99

16. Shonkoff, JP, Garner, AS, American Academy of Pediatrics Committee on Psychosocial Aspects of Child and Family Health, Committee on Early Childhood, Adoption, and Dependent Care, and Section on Developmental and Behavioral Pediatrics. The lifelong effects of early childhood adversity and toxic stress. *Pediatrics.* 2012;129(1):e232–e246

17. Rourke BP, Ahmad SA, Collins DW, Hayman-Abello BA, Hayman-Abello SE, Warriner EM. Child clinical/pediatric neuropsychology: some recent advances. *Ann Rev Psychol.* 2002;53:309–339

18. Rovet J, Netley C, Keenan M, Bailey J, Stewart D. The psychoeducational profile of boys with Klinefelter syndrome. *J Learn Disabil.* 1996;29(2):180–196

19. Wills KE, Holmbeck GN, Dillon K, McLone DG. Intelligence and achievement in children with myelomeningocele. *J Pediatr Psychol.* 1990;15(2):161–176

20. Learning Disabilities Association of America. Support and Resources for Parents. https://ldaamerica.org/parents/. Accessed November 27, 2017

21. Panel on Research on Child Abuse and Neglect, Commission on Behavioral and Social Sciences and Education, National Research Council. Chapter 6: Consequences of child abuse and neglect. In: *Understanding Child Abuse and Neglect.* Washington, DC: National Academies Press. 1993:208–252

22. Barbaresi WJ, Katusic SK, Colligan RC, Weaver AL, Jacobsen SJ. Long-term school outcomes for children with attention-deficit/hyperactivity disorder: a population-based perspective. *J Dev Behav Pediatr.* 2007;28(4):265–273

23. Shaywitz BA, Shaywitz SE, Pugh KR, et al. Disruption of posterior brain systems for reading in children with developmental dyslexia. *Biol Psychiatry.* 2002;52(2):101–110

24. Shaywitz BA, Skudlarski P, Holahan JM, et al. Age-related changes in reading systems of dyslexic children. *Ann Neurol.* 2007;61(4):363–370

25. American Academy of Pediatrics Committee on Children With Disabilities. The pediatrician's role in development and implementation of an individual education plan (IEP) and/or an individual family service plan (IFSP). *Pediatrics.* 1999;104(1 pt 1):124–127

26. Shaywitz BA, Shaywitz SE, Blachman BA, et al. Development of left occipitotemporal systems for skilled reading in children after a phonologically-based intervention. *Biol Psychiatry.* 2004;55(9):926–933

27. No Child Left Behind Act of 2001, 20 USC §6301

28. American Academy of Pediatrics Section on Ophthalmology and Council on Children With Disabilities, American Academy of Ophthalmology, American Association for Pediatric Ophthalmology and Strabismus, American Association of Certified Orthoptists. Learning disabilities, dyslexia and vision. *Pediatrics.* 2009;124(2):837–844

29. Beitchm an JH, Young AR. Learning disorders with a special emphasis on reading disorders; a review of the past 10 years. *J Am Acad Child Adolesc Psychiatry.* 1997;36(8):1020–1032

30. Esser G, Schmidt MH. Children with specific reading retardation—early determinants and long-term outcome. *Acta Paedopsychiatr.* 1994;56(3):229–237

31. Maughan B. Annotation: long-term outcomes of developmental reading problems. *J Child Psychol Psychiatry.* 1995;36(3):357–371

32. Shaywitz SE, Fletcher JM, Holahan JM, et al. Persistence of Dyslexia: the Connecticut Longitudinal Study at adolescence. *Pediatrics.* 1999;104(6):1351–1359

33. Jimerson SR. Meta-analysis of grade retention research: implications for practice in the 21st century. *School Psych Rev.* 2001;30(3):420–437

CHAPTER 18

Attention-Deficit/Hyperactivity Disorder

Michael I. Reiff, MD, FAAP

Martin T. Stein, MD, FAAP

Introduction

Overactive children were described in the medical literature over a century ago. In 1902, George Still observed a pattern of behavior in children that consisted of restlessness, inattentiveness, and over-arousal with an inability to internalize rules and limits. As a reflection of the Victorian era, he attributed the condition to a defect in moral character.[1] Children who recovered from influenza encephalitis following the endemic of 1917–1918 often displayed symptoms of restlessness, inattention, impulsivity, easy arousability, and hyperactivity. This was described as a postencephalitic behavior disorder.[2] Research in neuropsychology, coupled with clinical observations, led to progressive changes in the name of the condition from hyperkinetic impulse disorder to attention deficit disorder and, most recently, to attention-deficit/hyperactivity disorder (ADHD).

The core symptoms of ADHD are inattention, hyperactivity, and impulsivity. Attention-deficit/hyperactivity disorder is one of the most common and most extensively studied behavioral disorders in school-aged children. It is a chronic condition of childhood and adolescence and can persist into adulthood.[3]

Demographics/Epidemiology

The prevalence rate of ADHD varies depending on diagnostic criteria, the population studied, and the number of sources used to establish a diagnosis. The absence of biological markers to establish a diagnosis of ADHD and the need to depend on parent and teacher reports of behavior is a challenge to epidemiological research. In a national study, 7% of children met the *Diagnostic and Statistical Manual of Mental Disorders* (*DSM*) criteria for ADHD.[4] In this study, fewer than half of children identified with ADHD received either a diagnosis or regular treatment for ADHD. Poor children were more likely to meet criteria for ADHD, whereas wealthier children were more likely to receive regular medication treatment.

In studies that use clinical samples, there is a male predominance of ADHD with a male-to-female ratio of 3:1 for the combined type and 2:1 for the predominantly inattentive type.[5] In community samples, predominantly inattentive ADHD is the most prevalent subtype (about 1.5 times more common than the combined type).[5] School-aged and adolescent girls are more likely to comprise the inattentive subtype.[6] Attention-deficit/ hyperactivity disorder does occur in preschool children, although the diagnosis is more challenging.[7] The *International Classification of Diseases*, 10th Revision (*ICD-10*),[8] uses the term *hyperkinetic disorder*. According to this classification, the diagnosis requires the presence of both impaired attention and activity problems; because of this, there is a lower prevalence of ADHD according to the *ICD-10* criteria than according to the *DSM-5* criteria.

Etiology

Attention-deficit/hyperactivity disorder is a heterogeneous disorder with a multifactorial etiology. A diverse set of biobehavioral pathways can lead to the behavioral expression of the core symptoms of ADHD.[9] Genetic, epigenetic, and environmental factors interact to give rise to the ADHD phenotypes. A multifactorial model integrates genetic, neural, cognitive, and behavioral mechanisms. Behavioral disinhibition has been proposed as the major core deficit in ADHD.[10] In this model, children with ADHD are found to have difficulty mobilizing delayed gratification, the ability to interrupt ongoing responses (eg, stopping playing a video game because it is time for homework), and interference control (eg, not reacting to a friend walking past the classroom door while concentrating on a math problem).

Meta-analyses of candidate-gene association studies have found strong associations between ADHD and multiple genes involved in dopamine and serotonin pathways.[11] The gene most strongly implicated in ADHD is the human dopamine receptor *D4* gene.[12] In support of this observation, stimulant medications are primarily dopamine reuptake inhibitors. Imbalances in dopaminergic and noradrenergic regulation mediate the core symptoms of ADHD.[13-15] These neurotransmitters may increase the inhibitory influences of frontal cortical activity on subcortical structures. Stimulant medications and other medications found effective in ADHD treatment increase the inhibitory influences of frontal lobe activity through these dopaminergic and noradrenergic influences.[16,17]

Deficits in frontal lobe functioning and subcortical connections with the frontal lobes—particularly the caudate, putamen, and globus pallidus—have been found in neurobiological and neuroimaging studies.[18] Neuroimaging studies have also found ADHD to be associated with delays in cortical maturation. Cortical development in children with ADHD lags behind typically developing children by years but follows the normal sequence of brain development. This observation has led to the conclusion that ADHD represents a delay rather than a deviance in cortical brain maturation.[19,20] Cortical delay is most prominent in the lateral prefrontal cortex, an area that supports the ability to suppress inappropriate responses, executive control of attention, evaluation of reward contingencies, higher-order motor control, and working memory. These are the domains of neuropsychological functioning that have been found to be impaired in children with ADHD. Measures of brain structure and function in children diagnosed with ADHD overlap significantly with those of the general population and, because of this, are not useful in diagnosis.

Attention-deficit/hyperactivity disorder has strong familial associations. Parents and siblings of a child with ADHD carry a 2- to 8-fold increase in the risk for ADHD. Twin studies have found that 75% of the variance in ADHD phenotype can be attributed to genetic factors. If one identical twin has ADHD, the other twin has a greater than 50% chance of having ADHD.[21]

Biological and psychosocial factors also contribute to meeting criteria for the ADHD diagnosis. Prenatal exposure to alcohol, cocaine, and nicotine are associated with ADHD phenotypes.[22] Psychosocial adversity is also an important risk factor. Chronic family conflict, decreased family cohesion, and parental psychopathology have been found to occur more commonly in families of children with ADHD than in controls.

Functional Impairment

The diagnosis of ADHD and subsequent treatment require *evidence of impairment in functioning*. Children with ADHD have been found to have significant functional impairment in the areas of academic achievement, family relationships, peer relationships, self-esteem and self-perception, and overall adaptive function.[23–25] Although ADHD increases the risk for impairments in learning, social relationships, and adult outcomes, there is a wide variation in how it affects each individual. ADHD is associated with:

- Underachievement in school/work
- Learning disabilities
- Special education classes
- Repeating a grade
- More suspensions
- School drop-out
- Parenting distress
- Perceived incompetence in parenting
- Impairment in parental harmony
- Parent-child interaction problems
- Negative peer ranking of social problems
- Low self-esteem/self-perception
- Difficult peer relationships
- Immature social skills
- Suboptimal participation in community life
- Increased accidental injuries
- Increased automobile accidents

Core symptoms of ADHD challenge school-related activities and tasks, relationships, and other functions. Cognitive impairments are mediated by lack of impulse control and deficits in attention, memory, organization, time management, and judgment. Activity limitations include difficulties in learning and applying knowledge (eg, reading, writing, and mathematics), and problems with carrying out single or multiple tasks, studying, and self-managing behavior. Attention-deficit/hyperactivity disorder also impacts interpersonal interactions; communication and self-care; adjusting to and succeeding in educational programs; leaving school to enter work; and establishing a community, social, and civic life. *It is these broad functional disabilities, rather than the core diagnostic criteria, that should become targets for intervention in individuals with ADHD.*[26]

Coexisting Conditions

The majority of children and adolescents meeting diagnostic criteria for ADHD also have coexisting problems and conditions. The most prevalent conditions include other disruptive behavior disorders (oppositional defiant disorder [ODD] and conduct disorder), anxiety disorder, depressive disorders, and learning disabilities. Sleep disturbances are also common. Each of these conditions adds its own elements to the functional impairment of individuals with ADHD (Table 18.1).

Table 18.1. Prevalence of Conditions in Community Samples With and Without Attention-Deficit/Hyperactivity Disorder (ADHD)		
Condition	**Coexisting With ADHD**[a]	**In Non-ADHD Populations**[b]
Oppositional defiant disorder	35%	2%–16% (males)
Conduct disorder	25%	6%–16% (males); 2%–9% (females)
Anxiety disorder	25%	5%–10%
Depressive disorder	18%	2% (child); 5% (adolescent)
Reading disability[c]	51% boys 47% girls	14.5% boys 7.7% girls

[a] Green M, Wong M, Atkins D, et al. *Diagnosis of Attention Deficit/Hyperactivity Disorder. Technical Review 3.* Rockville, MD: US Department of Health and Human Services; 1999. Agency for Health Care Policy and Research (AHCPR) publication 99–0050.
[b] Lewis MB, ed. *Child and Adolescent Psychiatry: A Comprehensive Textbook. 3rd ed.* Philadelphia, PA: Lippincott Williams & Wilkins; 2002.
[c] Yoshimasu K, Barbaresi WJ, Colligan RC, et al. Gender, ADHD, and reading disability in a population-based birth cohort. *Pediatrics.* 2010;126(4):e788–e795.

In addition to coexisting with ADHD, many disorders can mimic ADHD, with presenting concerns about inattention, including learning disabilities, intellectual disabilities, autism spectrum disorder, anxiety, depression, seizure disorders, sleep disorders, central nervous system trauma or infection, hyperthyroidism, sexual abuse, and substance abuse. ADHD criteria can also be met as part of the presentations of fragile X syndrome, fetal alcohol spectrum disorder, and Tourette disorder.[27]

The presence of a coexisting condition can substantially change predictors of outcomes and influence the targets for treatment. For example, children with ADHD and coexisting ODD are at risk for developing conduct disorder, which can be a gateway to adolescent substance abuse.[28] Children with ADHD and coexisting mood disorders may have a poorer outcome during adolescence than children with ADHD alone. Children with coexisting anxiety disorders may differ in their response to stimulant medication and, in some cases, may respond just as well to behavioral treatments as to medication management.[29] Children and adolescents with ADHD and coexisting academic problems may benefit from accommodative services under Section 504 of the Rehabilitation Act or for more intensive special education services under the Individuals with Disabilities Education Act (IDEA), depending on the extent of their academic problems.[30]

Prognosis

The long-term outcome for children with ADHD is related to the severity and type of symptoms, coexisting conditions (eg, mental health disorders and learning disabilities), cognitive abilities (IQ), family situation, and treatment. Nearly one-third of children with ADHD will continue to fulfill norm-referenced criteria for ADHD as adults, and the majority will have at least one mental health disorder in adulthood.[31] Hyperactivity tends to diminish over time, but impulsivity and inattention often persist. Adolescents with ADHD often display immature peer interactions.[32]

It is important to recognize that most follow-up studies of children with ADHD do not evaluate the effects of treatment strategies. The longest systematic evidence based follow-up to date is the 14-month outcome Multimodal Treatment Study of Children with ADHD (MTA).[33] This study found that carefully crafted medication management was superior to behavioral treatment and to routine community care that included medication. At 14 months, 68% of students who had received the extensive behavioral and medication interventions in the study protocol appeared "normalized" on behavior rating scales filled out by their teachers. This was contrasted with 56% receiving only the strict medication component and 34% receiving only the extensive behavioral interventions in the study protocol. The combined therapy was also superior for treating children with low socioeconomic status and with coexisting anxiety.[33]

Follow-up of the MTA cohort 6 to 8 years after the trial, when the original participants were 13 to 18 years of age, showed that the original study groups had not continued to receive their randomly assigned treatment and did not differ significantly from each other with respect to any variables, including grades, arrests, and psychiatric hospitalizations. The study participants were actually found to demonstrate worse outcomes than local age-matched, normative comparison groups. The best predictors of functioning in these subjects, now that they were adolescents, were the severity of symptoms at enrollment, the socioeconomic status of the participant's family, and the degree of the individuals' response to any of the initial assigned study treatments.[34]

The adult follow-up study of the children in the MTA cohort (mean age 25 years) showed that functional outcomes (educational, occupational, legal, emotional, substance use disorder, and sexual behavior) among the children treated for ADHD compared to community controls varied; outcomes were generally worse when ADHD symptoms persisted. Initial ADHD symptom severity, parental mental health, and childhood comorbidity affected persistence of ADHD symptoms into adulthood.[35] One possible interpretation of these results is that in the absence of systematic, regular, follow-up, gains from an optimal treatment plan may deteriorate.

Adolescents with ADHD have more driving violations and more motor vehicle accidents, including accidents with fatalities. They also initiate intercourse sooner, with more sexual partners, and use birth control less often; they have more sexually transmitted infections and more teenage pregnancy. Teenagers with ADHD smoke at a younger age and have a higher prevalence of smoking. Those with conduct disorders are at increased risk for substance abuse. The risk of substance use disorders over the lifespan is up to twice as great in individuals with ADHD. Adolescent girls with ADHD have more depression, anxiety, poor teacher relationships, and impaired academic performance compared with their peers. Compared with boys with ADHD, they are more impaired by self-reported anxiety, distress, depression, and an external locus of control.[36]

Attention-deficit/hyperactivity disorder is associated with academic underachievement in reading and impaired school functioning.[37] Children and adolescents with ADHD have greater rates of school absenteeism, grade retention, and school dropout. They are more frequent users of school-based services and have increased rates of detention and expulsion.[23] Coexisting learning disabilities and psychiatric disorders add to the magnitude of poor school outcomes. Although students may be doing well on stimulant medications, medication treatment does not necessarily improve standardized test scores or ultimate educational attainment. Stimulant treatment has been associated with a significant decrease in the rate of substance abuse disorder,[37] although some recent studies have challenged this effect of treatment.[38]

Studies of adults with ADHD suggest that they have lower socioeconomic status, more work difficulties, and more frequent job changes, as well as fewer years of education and lower rates of professional employment. Adults with ADHD also report more psychological maladjustment, more speeding violations and suspension of drivers' licenses, poorer work performance, and more frequent quitting or being fired from jobs.[39]

Diagnosis and Evaluation

Hyperactivity, impulsivity, and inattention are observed in many children and adolescents during typical development. Attention-deficit/hyperactivity disorder is considered only when the symptoms are persistent and pervasive (present in multiple environments) and impair critical functions of learning and social development consistent with a child's developmental age. Most studies of children meeting criteria for ADHD include only school-aged children and adolescents. The diagnostic challenge to define ADHD in preschool children is significant in that, to some degree, all behaviors associated with ADHD are part of normal development in the preschool age group.

Unlike most medical conditions, but similar to other behaviorally defined disorders, there are no biological tests or imaging studies that can be used to diagnose ADHD. Instead, the diagnostic criteria from the *DSM,* an empirically based classification system of behavior disorders, are recommended as the framework for primary pediatric health care professionals' clinical assessment of ADHD. The *DSM* facilitates communication among professionals and patients, provides information relevant to treatment and prevention, and encourages research in understanding behavioral problems that impact development.

Diagnostic criteria for ADHD in school-aged children and adolescents include documentation of the following:

1. Several symptoms present *before age 12 years.*
2. Symptoms present in 2 or more major settings.
3. Symptoms cause significant difficulty in *functioning.*
4. Adolescents can *meet less criteria* than children.
5. Criteria consider *functioning* by asking for *severity.* (The *DSM,* however, is not helpful regarding how to determine level of functioning at any developmental stage.)
6. Significant impairments in learning and/or social interactions.
7. Symptoms are not attributable to another mental health condition.

Eighteen specific behaviors must be ascertained as a part of the diagnostic process using the *DSM-5.* Three subtypes of ADHD (predominantly hyperactive-impulsive type, predominantly inattentive type, and combined type) are delineated.[3]

The diagnostic process must include ascertainment of how many of the 18 ADHD-associated behaviors occur frequently and in most situations. The *DSM for Primary Care* is a guide to distinguish normal developmental variation from the behaviors associated with ADHD.[40] Documenting that the behaviors occur frequently is the first step toward good practice. One significant shortfall of the *DSM,* with the exception of allowing adolescents to meet diagnostic standards with only 5 inattentive and/or hyperactive/impulsive criteria instead of the 6 required for children, is that it is not developmentally sensitive. In contrast, preschoolers may display many more of these criteria as part of their normal development.

A clinician must establish whether the behaviors are limited to a particular environment or situations only, or whether the behaviors are present in a variety of situations. *There must be evidence that core ADHD behaviors occur across a child's major environments, including home and school.* Knowledge about behaviors in social activities outside of school and home (eg, during sports, camp, scouting, or religious activities) may also be useful. If a child is exhibiting ADHD symptoms only at school but not at home or in any other settings, the symptoms may not represent ADHD but might be secondary to a primary language, learning, or intellectual disability. Alternatively, if the child is exhibiting the ADHD symptoms only at home, not at school or any other setting, a parental-child interaction problem, developmentally inappropriate parental expectations or limit-setting, or parental psychopathology may be the primary cause of these symptoms. Inattentive behaviors may also be the result of problems with hearing, vision, anxiety, depression, allergic rhinitis, or obstructive sleep disorders. Ascertaining that the duration of symptoms is longer than 6 months is crucial. Many of the 18 ADHD symptoms may occur in response to life event changes (eg, marital discord, divorce, economic stress, a family move, a new school, or an illness in a family member) or during the early stages of a disease process (eg, posttraumatic encephalopathy, petit mal seizures, acquired hearing loss, or adrenoleukodystrophy). Chronic problems, such as living in poverty or enduring ongoing physical abuse or significant emotional neglect, may also produce symptoms indistinguishable from ADHD.

Symptoms of ADHD that are not associated with impairments in schoolwork or with successful social relationships do not meet the diagnostic criteria for ADHD. An inadequate assessment of functional impairment is a common cause of overdiagnosis. For example, the hyperactivity, impulsivity, or inattentiveness in some school-aged children is either not severe enough or is situational in an educational or social environment but not at home. *Overactivity and situational inattentiveness in a school-aged child who is doing well in the classroom, achieving academically, and socially engaging is not ADHD.* Clinical judgment is important in assessing the effect of the core ADHD symptoms on academic achievement, classroom performance, family life, social skills, independent functioning, self-esteem, leisure activities, and self-care. Asking a parent or teacher, "Do you think that Billy's inattention and hyperactivity are impairing his school performance or peer interactions?" can help to establish the presence of functional impairment.

An evidence-based practice guideline for the diagnosis of school-aged children with ADHD has been published by the American Academy of Pediatrics (AAP).[41] Following is a summary of the guidelines.

Recommendation 1: In a child 6 to 12 years old who presents with inattention, hyperactivity, impulsivity, academic underachievement, or behavior problems, primary care clinicians should initiate an evaluation for ADHD.

Early recognition of ADHD by primary pediatric health care professionals is ensured when screening for core symptoms and problems in school and social relationships occurs during health supervision visits. The AAP practice guideline suggests the following screening questions:

1. How is your child doing in school?
2. Are there any problems with learning that you or the teacher have seen?
3. Is your child happy in school?
4. Are you concerned with any behavioral problems in school, at home, or when your child is playing with friends?
5. Is your child having problems completing classwork or homework?

Recommendation 2: The diagnosis of ADHD requires that a child meet *DSM-5* criteria.

> **AUTHORS' CLINICAL COMMENTARY**
>
> This recommendation can pose a problem for the clinician. Consider the child or adolescent who is experiencing significant functional disability in significant areas but falls short of meeting full criteria for the ADHD diagnosis. The authors suggest that clinical judgment of the presence of significant functional disabilities should override strict adherence to *DSM* criteria in these situations because access to treatments, such as medication management, are contingent on receiving the ADHD diagnosis, as is likely the family's insurance coverage for the visit.

Recommendation 3: The assessment of ADHD requires evidence directly obtained from parents or caregivers regarding the core symptoms of ADHD in various settings, age of onset, duration of symptoms, and degree of functional impairment. Use of ADHD-specific scales is a clinical option when evaluating children for ADHD. A toolkit for clinicians, *ADHD: Caring for Children With ADHD: A Resource Toolkit for Clinicians,*[42] contains one of the available scales. It can be downloaded from the AAP Web site for use in the office or clinic. The traditional pediatric clinical interview with a child and a parent (together and separately) provides rich information, some of which may not be apparent or emphasized on a behavioral rating scale. The clinical interview also begins the therapeutic alliance between the clinician, parent, and child, a process that is crucial to later adherence to a treatment plan.

> **AUTHORS' CLINICAL COMMENTARY**
>
> Keep in mind that the core criteria for ADHD diagnosis may not describe the major functional disabilities of a particular child or adolescent. As clinicians, we treat children and adolescents, not diagnostic criteria. What we need to consider are problems and functional disabilities related to ADHD, as well as coexisting conditions and other additional individual concerns falling outside the formal diagnostic criteria.

Recommendation 4: The assessment of ADHD requires evidence directly obtained from the classroom teacher (or other school professional) regarding the core symptoms of ADHD, duration of symptoms, degree of functional impairment, and coexisting conditions. This can be accomplished with an ADHD-specific rating scale complemented by a teacher narrative, in which a clinician requests a written response to the following: "Tell me about _____ in your classroom. Tell me about his/her learning style and behaviors."

AUTHORS' CLINICAL COMMENTARY

A simple "ADHD questionnaire" is not sufficient to be able to understand the student. A multifaceted questionnaire like the Vanderbilt scales[43] may be more helpful but still may not be adequate to understand some of the student's additional struggles. Unfortunately, none of the scales we generally use consider the student's strengths, which can be a powerful guide to successful interventions after diagnosis. Open-ended items on a questionnaire (as suggested above), a brief chat with the teacher, or a few direct questions about these issues on a questionnaire may be helpful and quite revealing.

Recommendation 5: Evaluation of the child with ADHD should include assessment for coexisting conditions. The AAP toolkit[42] includes a scale specific for ADHD behaviors that also ascertains coexisting ODD, conduct disorder, symptoms of anxiety and depression, learning problems, and level of impairment. Primary pediatric health care professionals may have difficulty diagnosing some coexisting conditions and may need to consult with a developmental-behavioral pediatrician, neurodevelopmental pediatrician, psychologist, or psychiatrist. In this regard, a primary care toolkit, *Addressing Mental Health Concerns in Primary Care: A Clinician's Toolkit,* is available from the AAP.

Recommendation 6: Other diagnostic tests are not routinely indicated to establish the diagnosis of ADHD. These include hematocrit, blood lead, thyroid hormone levels, brain imaging studies, electroencephalography, and computerized continuous performance tests.

A physical examination can be done to rule out findings that might produce symptoms mimicking ADHD or that suggest syndromes with a high prevalence of ADHD behaviors. Depending on whether these have already been a part of a recent, routine primary care visit, the examination can include visual acuity, an audiogram, measurements for height, weight, head circumference, heart rate, and blood pressure. A neurological examination should also be done. An observation for dysmorphic features may suggest a syndrome with a high prevalence of ADHD (eg, fetal alcohol syndrome or fragile X syndrome).

Expanding the traditional neurological examination is an option for primary pediatric health care professionals. This can include some neurodevelopmental screening items that can informally assess a variety of components of neurological function that may be associated with ADHD or coexisting conditions. Examples of some informal neurodevelopmental screening tasks that can be easily incorporated into a primary care office visit can be found in Table 18.2.[44] Although these neurodevelopmental screening tasks are not standardized, they can provide clues to a specific learning disability or language disorder that requires further standardized assessment. The mild stress induced by these tasks may be associated with hyperactivity (fidgetiness, getting up from seat, constant motion, etc.) and inattentiveness (distractibility, not on task, daydreaming), signs that emerge in the office only during this part of the examination.

Another method to engage a younger child during the evaluation is to ask the child to "draw a picture of their family doing something." These kinetic family drawings within the context of a primary pediatric health care professional's office visit can be valuable in several ways. They may reduce the stress of the visit by giving the child something enjoyable to do while the clinician is talking to a parent. The drawing can be used to assess fine motor and visual-perceptual skills that are important in learning. They also provide an opportunity to do surveillance regarding emotional and behavioral concerns and to open new areas of communication with both parents and children. Ask the child, "Tell me about the drawing? What's going on? Where is _____?" Then give the parent an opportunity to comment. One cautionary note: The drawings should not be overly interpreted; they are best used in the primary care pediatric practice for a source for enhanced communication with a child and parent.[45]

Table 18.2. Informal Neurodevelopmental Screening Tasks	
Task	**Function**
Ask child to write a sentence.	Written expression and dysgraphia
Ask child to tell you about a movie or video seen recently.	Oral expression, memory, sequencing
Ask child to read a paragraph.	Reading fluency and comprehension appropriate for age (Grey Oral Reading Test, 5th edition)[a]
Ask child to copy geometric figures or do a draw-a-person test.	Fine motor and visual-spatial skills
Ask child to repeat a series of random numbers in both a forward and reversed manner.	Attention, short-term memory, sequencing, working memory
Ask child a multiple-step task to complete in order given.	Attention, memory, auditory processing

[a] Wiederholt JL, Bryant BR. *Gray Oral Reading Test.* 5th ed. San Antonio, TX: Pearson Psychological Corporation; 2012.

Similar to other chronic conditions, the diagnosis of ADHD often requires more than a single visit to a primary pediatric health care professional. Data gathering, a clinician interview and examination, and a summary of results for parents and child require a significant time commitment. An adaptation to schedule restrictions in primary care is to schedule several 30-minute visits in order to assess each patient accurately.

Treatment and Follow-up

Medication and behavioral therapy techniques based on behavior modification have been found to be effective treatments for children and adolescents with ADHD. Educating the family (including the child and caregivers) about ADHD is the first step to ensuring a good outcome. A discussion should include an understanding that ADHD is "brain based" and not due to poor parenting or intentional misbehavior, is amenable to change through medication and behavioral therapy, and is responsive to accommodations in the home and classroom. Most parents appreciate an empathetic clinician who makes a clear statement about how difficult it must be to raise a child with ADHD and clarifies the primary pediatric health care professional's role as a partner in the coordination of care between the family, school, and medical office. The AAP clinical guideline on the evaluation and treatment of children with ADHD supports this approach.[41]

AUTHORS' CLINICAL COMMENTARY

Primary pediatric health care professionals should keep in mind that they are first and foremost treating the child and not the diagnosis. The treatment for ADHD includes addressing the core symptoms, the coexisting conditions, and the individual's functional disabilities. Practitioners need to address more than the ADHD criteria and select the major treatment targets. To do this successfully, the clinician must also be familiar with the child or adolescent and the family's strengths and barriers to care to establish a multilayered, longitudinal treatment plan. The clinical job over time is to progressively empower the child and adolescent. The treatment plan and follow-up visits should dwell not only on problems but on progress and accomplishments. This can avoid pathologizing the visits and turn the child's perceptions of the visit from "blaming and shaming" to problem-solving.

Salient clinical points from the clinical guidelines follow.

Recommendation 1: Primary care clinicians should establish a management program that recognizes ADHD as a chronic condition. The chronic disease model of care includes parent/patient education, continuous availability for questions and counseling, coordination with other services, setting specific goals, and monitoring.

The care of ADHD is best achieved by establishing a medical home model—the provision of comprehensive primary care in a high-quality and cost-effective manner. In a medical home for a patient with ADHD, a primary pediatric health care professional works in partnership with the family and patient to ensure that all of the medical and nonmedical needs of the child are met. Through this partnership, the primary pediatric health care professional can help the family access and coordinate specialty care, educational services, out-of-home care, family support, and other public and private community services that are important to the overall outcome (see Chapter 25, Social and Community Services for Children With Developmental Disabilities and/or Behavioral Disorders and Their Families).[46]

Recommendation 2: The treating clinician, parent, and child, in collaboration with school personnel, should specify appropriate *target outcomes* to guide management. For the child with ADHD, target outcomes should reflect key behaviors that the child manifests and the specific impairments these symptoms cause. Impairments and problem behaviors differ greatly from child to child. Establishing target outcomes individualizes the treatment plan.

ESTABLISH TREATMENT TARGETS

Treat the presenting chief concerns/ functional disabilities . . .	NOT the core symptoms/diagnostic criteria
– Homework does not come home	– Inattention
– Missing assignments	– Hyperactive/impulsive behaviors
– Poor self-esteem	
– Depressive symptoms	
– Difficulty keeping friends	

Target outcomes are reflections of the functional impairment that are the result of core behaviors. It is these functional impairments that should be the foci for specific interventions.

Recommendation 3: The clinician should recommend medication and/or behavior therapy as appropriate to improve target outcomes in children with ADHD.

In general, medication management alone has been found to be a stronger intervention than behavioral treatment alone, particularly for the core diagnostic criteria for ADHD. There are particular circumstances, such as ADHD with comorbid anxiety disorders, where the 2 interventions (medication and/or cognitive behavioral therapy) may be equally effective, and other circumstances, such as difficult parent-child interactions, where the combined treatment with both medication and behavioral therapy is more effective than either intervention alone.

Recommendation 4: When the selected management for a child with ADHD has not met target outcomes, clinicians should evaluate the original diagnosis, use of all appropriate treatments, adherence to the treatment plan, and the presence of coexisting conditions.

Recommendation 5: The clinician should periodically provide a systematic follow-up for the child with ADHD. Monitoring of the ongoing treatment plan should be directed to target outcomes and adverse effects of medication by obtaining specific information from parent, teacher, and child.

AUTHORS' CLINICAL COMMENTS

Follow-up visits should be used to select and prioritize target behaviors and devise measures for assessing outcome of interventions. Different targets may require different doses of medication. Follow-up goals include empowering the child or adolescent and building a treatment plan around his or her individual needs. Providers should monitor self-esteem and use patients' strengths to enhance outcomes. It is important to balance the visit and celebrate successes as well as problem-solve around persistent barriers to optimal outcomes. Systematic follow-up visits can be used as vehicles for building relationships and establishing trust.

Medication

Methylphenidate (MPH), amphetamine, atomoxetine, and extended-release guanfacine are approved by the US Food and Drug Administration (FDA) for use in children and adolescents with ADHD on the basis of evidence-based safety and efficacy studies. Other medications with limited evidence from randomized, controlled studies, but without FDA approval for use in ADHD, include bupropion, clonidine, guanfacine, and tricyclic antidepressants.

– Stimulants

The most widely prescribed medications for children and adolescents with ADHD are the psychostimulants, including preparations derived from both MPH and amphetamine.[45] Well over 200 scientific studies support their value for children with ADHD. Stimulants act as dopamine and norepinephrine reuptake inhibitors by increasing the available dopamine and norepinephrine in the caudate nucleus and prefrontal cortex.[47]

Stimulant medications are currently available in short-acting (3–6 hours), intermediate-acting (6–8 hours), and long-acting (10–12 hours) preparations (Table 18.3). Behavioral effects are seen within 30 to 45 minutes. Some parents report an intense wear-off period (rebound) as the behavioral effects decline. Children and adolescents do not develop tolerance to stimulants. Stimulant dosing is not based on milligrams per kilogram but rather on the dose that works best without significant side effects up to the FDA-recommended maximum doses (see Table 18.3 and Chapter 23, Basics of Psychopharmacological Management).[48] Primary pediatric health care professionals often settle for stimulant doses that are helpful but suboptimal. Stimulants should be titrated in dose to achieve the best response, rather than using the dose that produces the first noticeable changes. Pharmacodynamic effects differ with specific targets. Disruptive behaviors are affected rapidly following a dose of stimulants, while increased attention to subjects like math may take up to 1.5 hours after administration. Stimulants work at school to increase on-task behavior and decrease interrupting and fidgeting. At home, they improve on-task behavior, parent-child interactions, and compliance.

Table 18.3. Stimulant Medications: First-Line Treatments[a]			
Generic Class (Brand Name)	**Daily Dosage Schedule**	**Duration of Behavioral Effects, Hours**	**Prescribing Schedule**
Methylphenidate			
Short-acting			
Ritalin, Metadate, Methylin	BID to TID	3–5	2.5–20 mg BID to TID
Focalin	BID to TID	3–5	2.5–10 mg BID to TID
Intermediate-acting			
Ritalin SR, Metadate ER, Methylin ER, Ritalin LA	QD to BID	3–8	10–40 mg QD or 40 mg in the morning and 20 mg early afternoon
Long-acting			
Concerta, Metadate CD	QD	10–12	18–72 mg
Focalin XR	QD	10–12	5–30 mg QD
Daytrana (transdermal patch)	QD	9	10–30 mg QD
QuilliChew ER (chewable long acting)	QD	10–12	20–60 mg QD
Quillivant XR suspension (25 mg/5 mL)	QD	10–12	20–60 mg QD
Amphetamines			
Short-acting			
Dexedrine, Dextrostat	BID to TID	4–6	5–15 mg BID or 5–10 mg TID
Intermediate-acting			
Adderall, Dexedrine Spansules	QD to BID	6–8	5–30 mg QD or 5–15 BID
Long-acting			
Adderall XR	QD	10–12	10–40 mg QD
Lisdexamfetamine	QD	12	30–70 mg QD
Adzenys XR-ODT	QD	12	6.3–18.8 mg QD (6–12 years) 6.3–12.5 mg QD (13–17 years)

Abbreviations: BID, twice a day; QD, every day; TID, 3 times a day.

[a] Adapted with permission from American Academy of Pediatrics Subcommittee on Attention-Deficit/Hyperactivity Disorder and Committee on Quality Improvement. Treatment of the school-aged child with attention-deficit/hyperactivity disorder. *Pediatrics.* 2001;108:1033–1044.

They also improve peer perceptions of social standing and increase attention while playing sports. Stimulant medications are also effective in preschool children with ADHD; however, in this age group, side effects are more frequent and severe.[49]

The most frequent side effects of stimulants include stomachaches and headaches (these symptoms typically resolve spontaneously after the first week), decreased appetite, difficulty with sleep initiation, and jitteriness. Motor tics may also occur in some children. These side effects often occur early in treatment, are usually mild, and can often be ameliorated by alterations in dose, timing, or the use of alternate stimulant medications. There are no differences in potential side effects among stimulants. However, a child or adolescent with a specific side effect on one stimulant medication may not experience it on another. The 3-year follow-up of the Multimodal Treatment Study of Children with ADHD (MTA)[50] reported that growth in newly treated children averaged 2.0 cm less in height and 2.7 kg less in weight than growth in unmedicated children. The reduced growth occurred mostly in the first year of treatment and was not seen in the third year.[51] A recent long-term study concluded that adult height did not differ between children who were treated and those not treated with stimulant medication; there was no correlation with duration of treatment.[52]

Treatment of adolescent patients with ADHD with stimulant medication has been associated with a reduction in risk for subsequent drug and alcohol use disorders.[53] Use of stimulants is contraindicated in cases of previous sensitivity, glaucoma, or drug abuse; in patients who are taking a monoamine oxidase inhibitor; and in patients who are actively psychotic. Stimulants are not contraindicated in cases of tics, and stimulants seem to pose a minimal risk for lowering the seizure threshold.[54] Stimulant medications are associated with a modest and typically clinically insignificant increase in heart rate and blood pressure. Most studies do not support an association between the use of stimulant medication and sudden cardiac death. The AAP recommends a careful assessment of children starting stimulants. Screening should include a targeted cardiac history, including a patient history of previously detected cardiac disease, palpitations, syncope, or seizures; a family history of sudden death in children or young adults, hypertrophic cardiomyopathy, or long QT syndrome; and a cardiovascular physical examination.[49] In general, stimulants are considered quite safe and effective for treatment of ADHD. Height and weight should be monitored regularly. Blood pressure and heart rate should be checked before and during treatment with stimulant medications. If the family history or child's history includes severe heart palpitations, exercise intolerance, fainting spells, chest pain, or sudden unexplained death, a cardiology consultation is recommended before initiating stimulant medications. Routine electrocardiograms are not indicated prior to stimulant use.[55]

The development of long-acting stimulants was a response to problems observed by parents, teachers, and clinicians. Gaps in the behavioral effects of multiple, daily doses of 4-hour preparations (immediate-release stimulants) occur at some of the least structured times of the day (bus rides, lunch time, and recess). In addition, many children feel embarrassed taking medication in school under the scrutiny of the school nurse and their peers, and compliance then becomes an issue. In some cases, homework time remains uncovered and may require an afternoon dose of an immediate-release stimulant.

– Nonstimulants

Stimulants remain the first-line psychopharmacological treatment for ADHD. It is estimated that at least 80% of children will respond to one of the stimulants, if they are used in a systematic way. Nonstimulants remain an option for children and adolescents for whom stimulants are not effective or cause significant adverse side effects or exacerbation of other coexisting disorders, or where nonstimulants are a preferred option for treating ADHD and a coexisting disorder with a single medication.

Atomoxetine (Strattera) is a nonstimulant medication that is approved for use in school-aged children, adolescents, and adults with ADHD. It is a norepinephrine reuptake inhibitor and blocks the presynaptic norepinephrine transporter in the prefrontal cortex. It has been found to have a beneficial effect on children and adolescents with ADHD but to have lower efficacy than stimulants.[56-59] Atomoxetine may provide symptom relief during the evening and early morning hours. Motor and verbal tics associated with atomoxetine have not been reported. In addition, atomoxetine may have less effect on delayed sleep onset compared with stimulants. The side effects are otherwise similar to those of stimulants, but atomoxetine may be associated with more fatigue and nausea compared with stimulants, and there have also been rare reports of liver toxicity in association with atomoxetine use. Atomoxetine may be effective in children with ADHD and coexisting anxiety. The initial studies of atomoxetine reported a twofold increase compared with control subjects in suicidal ideation, usually occurring in the first month of treatment; actual suicide attempts were not increased. Dosing of atomoxetine is on a per-kilogram basis, in contrast to stimulants.

Methylphenidate, amphetamine, and atomoxetine have somewhat different efficacies. Reported effect sizes of atomoxetine are moderate (about 0.7 in children and 0.4 in adults compared with stimulants, which have approximately 1.0 effect sizes in clinical trials).[60] Among those who do not respond sufficiently or who develop intolerable side effects to the first ADHD medication tried, about half will respond to one of the other medicines. There is variability in dose response between patients; it is recommended to begin with a small dose of stimulants and titrate upward every 2 to 4 weeks to reach the optimal effect while monitoring side effects. Most children are treated with medication daily, including weekends.[61]

Clonidine and guanfacine are presynaptic, central-acting alpha-2 adrenergic agonists that work by affecting norepinephrine discharge rates in the locus ceruleus, which may indirectly affect dopamine. Long-acting forms of guanfacine (Intuniv) and clonidine (Kapvay) are also approved by the FDA for the treatment of ADHD. These medications are considered second-line treatments for ADHD and should be considered, along with norepinephrine reuptake inhibitors, when stimulants are not effective or contraindicated. Clonidine (as well as melatonin) has been used clinically to counteract the stimulant side effect of delayed sleep initiation and for children and adolescents with ADHD who also have significant aggressive behavior. Guanfacine may also be effective in children with ADHD, tics, and aggression.

Behavioral Treatment

Effective psychosocial treatment for ADHD employs the principles of behavior therapy. These principles include the use of behavior modification techniques and social learning theory. They emphasize contingency management and shaping children's behaviors through observing and modeling appropriate behaviors, attitudes, and emotional reactions of others. Parents and teachers can be trained in these behavior management principles, and there is good evidence that behavioral interventions are effective for children with ADHD. The goals of parent training are (1) to help parents learn to achieve consistent and positive interactions with their children, (2) to gain a better understanding of what behaviors are developmentally normal, (3) to help parents cut down on negative interactions with their children (eg, arguing or constantly having to repeat commands), (4) to teach parents to provide appropriate consequences for their child's behaviors and to become more empathetic to their child's viewpoint, and (5) to help children to improve their abilities to manage their own behaviors.[62] Many parents have fallen into the trap of almost solely providing negative attention in response to negative behaviors. Using behavior therapy principles, parents learn to conceptualize discipline as teaching self-control rather than as punishing negative behaviors. They are taught what behaviors can be reinforced by praise and extinguished by actively ignoring the behavior, using appropriate punishments only for intolerable or dangerous behaviors[63] (see Chapter 7, Basics of Child Behavior and Primary Care Pediatric Management of Common Behavioral Problems). A sound parent training program teaches parents how to:

- Deliver and follow through on clear commands
- Shape behaviors in gradual increments
- Use daily contingency charts (stars or "happy-face" charts)
- Institute procedures such as time-out, token economies (earning rewards and privileges contingent on performing desired behaviors), and a response cost (losing tokens or privileges for noncompliance)

The same principles of clinical behavioral therapy have been used effectively in training teachers in classroom behavior management. Once parents and teachers have been trained, they can learn to implement systems that provide continuity from home to school, such as daily behavioral report cards that can be used to report on specific target behaviors that are monitored daily and allow parents to provide either positive reinforcement or consequences at home.

Behavioral interventions alone may be insufficient for effective treatment of core ADHD behaviors. For parents who are hesitant to use prescribed medications to treat their child, initiating treatment with a behavior therapy program alone should be supported with frequent monitoring.

A novel form of behavioral therapy utilized small groups of parents in pediatric practices, focusing on encouraging parents to share challenges with their child with ADHD and reflect on their child's strengths.[64] The children met in separate groups to identify feelings and manage negative emotions. ADHD behaviors decreased in the group cohort compared to traditional care, but the difference was not significant. Intervention families reported significantly improved adaptive functioning in their children.[64]

Combined Medication and Psychosocial Treatments: The MTA Study

The short-term benefits of medications and behavioral therapy have been well established. Few studies have also looked at medication treatment and behavioral therapies in head-to-head comparisons. The National Institute of Mental Health's MTA study followed 579 children, aged 7 to 9 years, in 6 sites over a 14-month period. The children were randomly assigned to 1 of 4 groups: (1) intensive medication management (MedMgt), (2) intensive behavioral treatments (Beh), (3) combined MedMgt and Beh (Comb), and (4) study diagnostic procedures and then routine care in the community (CC). Medication management was initiated with MPH, using alternative stimulants or nonstimulants for MPH nonresponders.[29] The intensive behavioral treatments included 8 sessions of parent training with concurrent teacher consultation and an intensive child-focused treatment consisting of an 8-week, daily summer school treatment program. In addition, a school-based treatment program was carried out involving 10 to 16 teacher behavior management consultation sessions, 12 weeks of a part-time paraprofessional aide working with the child, and daily home/school report cards.

For the core symptoms of ADHD (inattention, impulsivity, hyperactivity) the MTA intensive MedMgt was superior to routine CC, in spite of the fact that more than two-thirds of the children receiving CC were being treated with stimulant medication. It was determined that children in the MedMgt group were on significantly higher doses of stimulant medication, as after a month of blind trials of different doses, they were assigned to the dose that led to the optimal symptom control without limiting side effects.

The Comb treatment did not yield significantly greater benefits than the MedMgt alone for the core symptoms of ADHD, but outcomes in the Comb group could sometimes be achieved at lower medication doses than in the group that received only MedMgt alone. Combined treatment was superior to MedMgt alone for many non-ADHD domains of functioning, including oppositional or aggressive symptoms, symptoms of depression and anxiety, parent-child relations, and reading achievement. Based on a composite of parent and teacher ratings, 68% of the Comb children "normalized" by the end of the 14-month study, compared with 56% of the MedMgt alone, 34% of the Beh management alone, and only 25% of the CC children. The benefit seen in the medication groups persisted at 24 months but not at 36 months, regardless of original treatment assignment.[50] Factors associated with worse outcomes at 36 months were initial symptom severity, male gender, oppositional/disruptive behaviors, public assistance, and ADHD in a parent. The 8-year and adult follow-up MTA studies are reviewed in the "Prognosis" section above. Results of the MTA study are limited by the absence of a control group and the use of short-acting stimulant medications (long-acting formulations were not available). For clinicians, an important implication of the study results is that *systematic monitoring with a plan for follow-up office visits is a critical component of successful treatment for children with ADHD.*

School Interventions

Comprehensive pediatric care for children and adolescents with ADHD is achieved when the primary pediatric health care professional communicates effectively with the school. With the parents' approval, it begins with informing the teacher about the diagnosis and treatment. A monitoring system for transferring information to the clinical office about the patient's school behavior and educational achievement should be in place. Effective communication between teachers and pediatricians has been a challenge. A preliminary study suggests that when a pediatrician has an Internet portal to connect with the teacher and parent, teacher and parent behavior rating scales are accessed more frequently at the time of diagnosis and follow-up visits.[65] Communication works best when parents partner with the school and the medical home.

Federal laws support school interventions for children with ADHD. For mild cases, Section 504 of the Rehabilitation Act requires that a school provide classroom accommodations to improve learning. These accommodations can include preferential seating, reduced assignments and homework, assisting the teacher in formulating a classroom behavioral program, and providing an "ADHD coach" to assist students in organizing, planning, homework completion, homework flow, and getting assignments submitted in a timely manner. For more severe cases, the IDEA recognizes ADHD under the "Other Health Impairment" category and requires schools to provide comprehensive educational testing followed by an Individualized Education Program (IEP) plan with measurable behavioral and academic achievement goals. Periodic monitoring and reassessment is incorporated into the IEP (see Chapter 20, Interpreting Psychoeducational Testing Reports, Individualized Family Service Plans [IFSP], and Individualized Education Program [IEP] Plans).

Daily home-school report cards are an effective method to monitor classroom behaviors. Parents and teachers decide on 3 to 5 behaviors that impair success in school. Each behavior is monitored daily and a daily home-school report card is sent home with the child. The daily report card is attached to an award system (eg, privileges or prizes) to encourage compliance. This system allows for frequent, immediate feedback that can be motivating to the child, parents, and teacher. An example of a daily report card with directions can be downloaded from **https://ccf.fiu.edu/_assets/pdfs/how_to_establish_a_school_drc.pdf.**

Complementary and Alternative Therapies

Many parents seek complementary or alternative therapies either alone or in combination with evidence-based medication and behavioral management.[66] Most of these treatments have not undergone randomized, controlled trials and cannot be recommended (see Chapter 24, Complementary Health Approaches in Developmental and Behavioral Pediatrics). Some alternative therapies have side effects and may be harmful to children; others are safe. For the parent who is set on trying an alternative treatment or who has already found it helpful, many clinicians incorporate the alternative plan with the more evidence-based proven treatments. If the treatment is not dangerous and does not interfere with other aspects of primary pediatric health care, collaborative management is the most effective strategy. It is best not to alienate a parent, as the goal should be one of partnership in doing what is best for the child. Recent studies provide preliminary support for 2 complementary therapies for children with ADHD: neurofeedback and physical activity.[67,68]

Conclusion

Attention-deficit/hyperactivity disorder is a common, chronic neurobehavioral condition associated with functional impairments in educational achievement and social development. The diagnosis of ADHD in children and adolescents can be established with confidence by primary pediatric health care professionals with the use of the AAP evidence-based guideline. Inclusion of screening procedures for coexisting psychological conditions, learning disabilities, and psychosocial stressors is an important component of the diagnostic process. Effective treatment strategies include parent/patient education about ADHD, FDA-approved medications, and behavior management techniques. Ongoing communication with teachers, a system of communication with the medical home that parents can access with ease, a care plan that systematically empowers parents, children, and adolescents, and a plan for follow-up office visits ensure effective monitoring of a treatment plan for a child or adolescent with ADHD. This approach promotes the best opportunity to ameliorate or prevent academic, social, and occupational sequelae associated with ADHD.

References

1. Still GF. The Goulstonian lectures on some abnormal psychical conditions in children. Lectures I–III. *Lancet.* 1902;159:1008–1012, 1077–1082, 1163–1168
2. Hochman LB. Post-encephalitic behavior disorder in children. *Bull Johns Hopkins Hosp.* 1922;33:372–375
3. American Psychiatric Association. *Diagnostic and Statistical Manual of Mental Disorders.* 5th ed. Arlington, VA: American Psychiatric Association; 2013
4. Biederman J. Attention-deficit/hyperactivity disorder: a selective overview. *Biol Psychiatry.* 2005;57(11):1215–1220
5. Froehlich TE, Lanphear BP, Epstein JN, et al. Prevalence, recognition, and treatment of attention-deficit/hyperactivity disorder in a national sample of US children. *Arch Pediatr Adolesc Med.* 2007;161(9):857–864
6. Carlson C, Mann M. Attention-deficit/hyperactivity disorder, predominantly inattentive subtype. *Child Adolesc Psychiatr Clin N Am.* 2000;9(3):499–510
7. Connor DF. Preschool attention deficit hyperactivity disorder: a review of prevalence, diagnosis, neurobiology and stimulant treatment. *J Dev Behav Pediatr.* 2002;23(1 suppl):S1–S9

8. *International Statistical Classification of Diseases and Related Health Problems (ICD-10). 10th Rev. World Health Organization;* 2010

9. Coghill D, Nigg J, Rothenberger A, Sonuga-Barke E, Tannock R. Whither causal models in the neuroscience of ADHD? *Dev Sci.* 2005;8(2):105–114

10. Barkley R. *ADHD and the Nature of Self-Control.* New York, NY: Guilford Press; 1997

11. Faraone SV, Mick E. Molecular genetics of attention deficit hyperactivity disorder. *Psychiatr Clin North Am.* 2010;33(1):159–180

12. Smalley SL, Bailey JN, Palmer CT, et al. Evidence that the dopamine D4 receptor is a susceptibility gene in attention deficit hyperactivity disorder. *Mol Psychiatry.* 1998;3(5):427–430

13. Barr CL, Wigg KG, Bloom S, et al. Further evidence from haplotype analysis for linkage of the dopamine D4 receptor gene and attention-deficit hyperactivity disorder. *Am J Med Genet.* 2000;96(3):262–267

14. Volkow ND, Wang GJ, Fowler JS, et al. Effects of methylphenidate on regional brain glucose metabolism in humans: relationship to dopamine D2 receptors. *Am J Psychiatry.* 1997;154(1):50–55

15. Swanson J, Castellanos FX, Murias M, LaHoste G, Kennedy J. Cognitive neuro-science of attention deficit hyperactivity disorder and hyperkinetic disorder. *Curr Opin Neurobiol.* 1998;8(2):263–271

16. Arnsten AD, Steere JC, Hunt RD. The contribution of alpha 2-noradrenergic mechanisms of prefrontal cortical cognitive function: potential significance for attention-deficit hyperactivity disorder. *Arch Gen Psychiatry.* 1996;53(5):448–455

17. Pliszka SR, McCracken JT, Mass JW. Catecholamines in attention-deficit hyperactivity disorder: current perspectives. *J Am Acad Child Adolesc Psychiatry.* 1996;35(3):264–272

18. Swanson JM, Castellanos FX. Biological bases of ADHD—neuroanatomy, genetics, and pathophysiology. In: Jensen PS, Cooper JR, eds. *Attention Deficit Hyperactivity Disorder: State of the Science, Best Practices.* Kingston, NJ: Civic Research Institute, Inc.; 2002:7–1–7–20

19. Castellanos FX, Lee PP, Sharp W, et al. Developmental trajectories of brain volume abnormalities in children and adolescents with attention-deficit/hyperactivity disorder. *JAMA.* 2002;288(14):1740–1748

20. Shaw P, Eckstrand K, Sharp W, et al. Attention-deficit/hyperactivity disorder is characterized by a delay in cortical maturation. *Proc Natl Acad Sci U S A.* 2007;104(49):19649–19654

21. Barkley RA. Attention-deficit hyperactivity disorder. *Sci Am.* 1998;279(3):66–71

22. Swanson JM, Castellanos FX. Biological bases of ADHD: neuroanatomy, genetics and pathophysiology. Paper presented at: NIH Consensus Development Conference on Diagnosis and Treatment of Attention Deficit Hyperactivity Disorder; November 1998; Bethesda, MD

23. Hinshaw SP. Is ADHD an impairing condition in childhood and adolescence? In: Jensen PS, Cooper JR, eds. *Attention Deficit Hyperactivity Disorder: State of the Science: Best Practices.* Kingston, NJ: Civic Research Institute; 2002:5–1–5–12

24. Matza LS, Rentz AM, Secnik K, et al. The link between health-related quality of life and clinical symptoms among children with attention-deficit hyperactivity disorder. *J Dev Behav Pediatr.* 2004;25(3):166–174

25. Üstün T. Using the International Classification of Functioning, Disease and Health in attention-deficit/hyperactivity disorder: separating the disease from its epiphenomena. *Ambul Pediatr.* 2007;7(1 suppl):132–139

26. Stein MT, Reiff MI. Hyperactivity and inattention: over-activity and distractibility. In: Rudolph CD, Rudolph AM, eds. *Rudolph's Pediatrics.* 22nd ed. New York, NY: McGraw Hill; 2011:321–326

27. Feldman HM and Reiff MI. Attention deficit–hyperactivity disorder in children and adolescents. *N Engl J Med.* 2014;370(9):838–846

28. Loeber R, Lahey BB, Winters A, et al. Oppositional defiant and conduct disorder: a review of the past 10 years, part 1. *J Am Acad Child Adolesc Psychiatry.* 2000;40(12):1393–1400

29. Jensen PS, Hinshaw SP, Swanson JM, et al. Findings from the NIMH multimodal treatment study of ADHD (MTA): implications and applications for primary care providers. *J Dev Behav Pediatr.* 2001;22(1):60–73

30. Stein MT, Lounsbury B. A child with a learning disability; navigating school-based services. *J Dev Behav Pediatr.*2001;22(3):188–192

31. Barbaresi WJ, Colligan RC, Weaver AL, Voigt RG, Killian JM, Katusic SK. Mortality, ADHD, and psychosocial adversity in adults with childhood ADHD: a prospective study. *Pediatrics.* 2013;131(4):637–644

32. Loe IM, Feldman HM. Academic and educational outcomes of children with ADHD. *Ambul Pediatr.* 2007;7(1 suppl):82–90

33. A 14-month randomized clinical trial of treatment strategies for attention-deficit/hyperactivity disorder. The MTA Cooperative Group. Multimodal Treatment Study of Children with ADHD. A 14-month randomized clinical trial of treatment strategies for attention-deficit/hyperactivity disorder. *Arch Gen Psychiatry.* 1999;56(12):1073–1086

34. Molina BS, Hinshaw SP, Swanson JM, et al. MTA Cooperative Group. The MTA at 8 years: prospective follow-up of children treated for combined-type ADHD in a multisite study. *J Am Acad Child Adolesc Psychiatry.* 2009;48(5):484–500

35. Hechtman L, Swanson JM, Sibley MH et al. Functional adult outcomes 16 years after childhood diagnosis of attention-deficit/hyperactivity disorder: MTA Results. *J Am Acad Child Adolesc Psychiatry.* 2016;55(11):945–952

36. Wolraich ML, Bibblesman CJ, Brown TE, et al. Attention-deficit/hyperactivity disorder among adolescents: a review of the diagnosis, treatment, and clinical implications. *Pediatrics.* 2005;115(6):1734–1746

37. Barbaresi WJ, Katusic SK, Colligan RC, Weaver AL, Jacobsen SJ. Modifiers of long-term school outcomes for children with attention-deficit/hyperactivity disorder: does treatment with stimulant medication make a difference? Results from a population-based study. *J Dev Behav Pediatr.* 2007;28(4):274–287

38. Biederman J, Monuteaux MC, Spencer T, Wilens TE, MacPherson HA, Faraone SV. Stimulant therapy and risk for subsequent substance use disorders in male adults with ADHD: a naturalistic controlled 10-year follow up study. *Am J Psychiatry.* 2008;165(5):597–603

39. Murphy K, Barkley RA. Attention deficit hyperactivity disorder adults: comorbidities and adaptive impairments. *Compr Psychiatry.* 1996;37(6):393–401

40. Wolraich ML, Felice ME, Drotar D, eds. *The Classification of Child and Adolescent Mental Diagnoses in Primary Care—Diagnostic and Statistical Manual for Primary Care (DSM-PC) Child and Adolescent Version.* Elk Grove Village, IL: American Academy of Pediatrics; 1996

41. American Academy of Pediatrics Committee on Quality Improvement and Subcommittee on Attention-Deficit/ Hyperactivity Disorder. ADHD: Clinical practice guideline for the diagnosis, evaluation, and treatment of attention-deficit/hyperactivity disorder in children and adolescents. *Pediatrics.* 2011;128(5):1007–1022

42. American Academy of Pediatrics. *ADHD: Caring for Children With ADHD: A Resource Toolkit for Clinicians.* 2nd ed. Elk Grove Village, IL: American Academy of Pediatrics; 2011

43. Bard DE, Wolraich ML, Neas B, et al. The psychometric properties of the Vanderbilt attention-deficit hyperactivity disorder diagnostic parent rating scale in a community population. *J Dev Behav Pediatr.* 2013;34(2):72–82

44. Reiff MI, Stein MT. Attention-deficit/hyperactivity disorder: diagnosis and treatment. *Adv Pediatr.* 2004;51:289–327

45. Dixon SD, Stein MT. *Encounters with Children: Pediatric Behavior and Development.* 4th ed. Philadelphia, PA: Mosby-Elsevier; 2006

46. American Academy of Pediatrics Medical Home Initiatives for Children with Special Health Care Needs Project Advisory Committee. The medical home. *Pediatrics.* 2002;110(1 Pt 1):184–186

47. Soltano MV. Neuropsychopharmacological mechanisms of stimulant drug action in attention-deficit hyperactivity disorder. *Behav Brain Res.* 1998;94(1):127–152

48. Pliiszka SR, Greenhill LL, Crismon MN, et al. The Texas Children's Medication Algorithm Project: report of the Texas Consensus Conference Panel on Medication treatment of childhood attention-deficit/hyperactivity disorder. Part II: tactics. Attention-deficit/hyperactivity disorder. *J Am Acad Child Adolesc Psychiatry.* 2000;39(7):920–927

49. Greenhill L, Kollins S, Abikoff H, et al. Efficacy and safety of immediate-release methylphenidate treatment for preschoolers with ADHD. *J Am Acad Child Adolesc Psychiatry.* 2006;45(11):1284–1293

50. Jensen PS, Arnold LE, Swanson JM, et al. 3-year follow-up of the NIMH MTA study. *J Am Acad Child Adolesc Psychiatry.* 2007;46(8):989–1002

51. Swanson JM, Elliott GR, Greenhill LL, et al. Effects of stimulant medication on growth rates across 3 years in the MTA follow-up. *J Am Acad Child Adolesc Psychiatry.* 2007;46(8):1015–1027

52. Harstad EB, Weaver AL, Katusic SK et al. ADHD stimulant treatment, and growth: A longitudinal study. *Pediatrics.* 2014;134(4):e935–e944

53. Wilens TE, Faraone SV, Biederman J, Gunawardene S. Does stimulant therapy of attention-deficit/hyperactivity disorder beget later substance abuse? A meta-analytic review of the literature. *Pediatrics.* 2003;111(1):179–185

54. Hemmer SA, Pasternak JF, Zecker SG, Trommer BL. Stimulant therapy and seizure risk in children with ADHD. *Pediatr Neurol.* 2001;Feb:24(2):99–102

55. Perrin JM, Friedman RA, Knilans TK, Black Box Working Group, American Academy of Pediatrics Section on Cardiology and Cardiac Surgery. Cardiovascular monitoring and stimulant drugs for attention-deficit/ hyperactivity disorder. *Pediatrics.* 2008;122(2):451–453

56. Michelson D, Faries D, Wernicke J, et al. Atomoxetine in the treatment of children and adolescents with attention-deficit/hyperactivity disorder: a randomized, placebo-controlled, dose-response study. *Pediatrics.* 2001;108(5):e83

57. Spencer T, Biederman J. Non-stimulant treatment for attention-deficit/hyperactivity disorder. *J Atten Disord.* 2002;6(suppl 1):S109–S119

58. Kratochvil CJ, Heiligenstein JH, Dittmann R, et al. Atomoxetine and methylphenidate treatment in children with ADHD: a prospective, randomized, open-label trial. *J Am Acad Child Adolesc Psychiatry.* 2002;41(7):776–784

59. Michelson D, Allen AJ, Busner J, et al. Once-daily atomoxetine treatment for children and adolescents with attention deficit hyperactivity disorder: a randomized, placebo-controlled study. *Am J Psychiatry.* 2002;159(11):1896–1901

60. Lock TM, Worley KA, Wolraich ML. Attention-deficit/hyperactivity disorder. In: Wolraich ML, Drotar DD, Dworkin PH, Perrin EC, eds. *Developmental Behavioral Pediatrics: Evidence and Practice.* Philadelphia, PA: Mosby/Elsevier; 2008:579–601

61. Wender EH. Managing stimulant medication for attention-deficit/hyperactivity disorder. *Pediatr Rev.* 2002;23(7):234–236

62. American Academy of Pediatrics. *ADHD: What Every Parent Needs to Know.* Reiff MI, ed. Elk Grove Village, IL: American Academy of Pediatrics; 2011

63. Anastopoulos AD, Rhoads LH, Farley SE. Counseling and training parents. In: Barkley RA, ed. *Attention-Deficit/Hyperactivity Disorder: A Handbook for Diagnosis and Treatment.* 3rd ed. New York, NY: Guilford Press; 2006:453–479

64. Bauer NS, Szczepaniak D, Sullivan PD et al. Group visits to improve pediatric attention-deficit hyperactivity disorder chronic care management. *J Dev Behav Pediatr.* 2015;36(8):553–561

65. Epstein JN, Langberg JM, Lichtenstein PK, et al. Use of an Internet portal to improve community-based pediatric ADHD: a cluster randomized trial. *Pediatrics.* 2011;128(5):e1201–e1208

66. Chan E, Rappaport LA, Kemper K. Complementary and alternative therapies in childhood attention and hyperactivity problems. *J Dev Behav Pediatr.* 2003;24(1):4–8

67. Steiner NJ, Frenette EC, Rene KM, et al. Neuro-feedback and cognitive attention training for children with attention-deficit hyperactivity disorder in schools. *J Dev Behav Pediatr.* 2014;35(1):18

68. Vanheist J, Beghin L, Duhamel A. Physical activity is associated with attention capacity in adolescents. *J Pediatr.* 2016;168:126–131

CHAPTER 19

Autism Spectrum Disorder

Scott M. Myers, MD, FAAP

Thomas D. Challman, MD, FAAP

In 1943 Leo Kanner eloquently described 11 children with innate "autistic disturbances of affective contact" characterized by profound lack of reciprocal social engagement and interaction; disturbances in communication ranging from mutism to echolalia, pronoun reversal, and literalness; and unusual responses to the environment, including insistence on sameness that was not explained by general cognitive impairment.[1] More than 7 decades later, diagnostic criteria and assessment instruments remain remarkably influenced by Kanner's original description.

Definition and Classification: *DSM-5*

In the American Psychiatric Association *Diagnostic and Statistical Manual of Mental Disorders,* Fifth Edition (*DSM-5*), published in 2013, the *DSM-IV* umbrella term *pervasive developmental disorders* and diagnostic classifications *autistic disorder, Asperger's disorder, childhood disintegrative disorder, Rett's disorder,* and *pervasive developmental disorder not otherwise specified* (PDD-NOS) were replaced by a single diagnostic term, *autism spectrum disorder* (ASD).[2] These changes were prompted by research demonstrating that the subclassifications had little scientific justification and were not used reliably, even by experts.[3] The *International Classification of Diseases* (ICD) criteria, the 11th revision of which are scheduled to be published in 2018, are expected to also include these changes and to be very similar to the *DSM-5* criteria.[4]

The *DSM-5* diagnostic criteria for ASD are presented in Box 19.1, and the severity level classification, which is new to the *DSM*, is described in Box 19.2.[2] ASD diagnosis requires meeting all 3 of the social communication and interaction criteria and at least 2 of 4 restricted and repetitive behavior criteria. The symptoms must cause clinically significant impairment in current functioning and must have been present in the early developmental period, although they may not become fully manifest until social demands exceed limited capacities, or they may be masked by learned strategies in later life. To make a diagnosis of ASD in an individual with intellectual disability (ID), social communication and interaction skills must be below what would be expected based on general developmental level.

Box 19.1. *DSM-5* **Diagnostic Criteria for Autism Spectrum Disorder**[a] **(299.00; F84.0)**

A. **Persistent deficits in social communication and social interaction across multiple contexts, as manifested by the following, currently or by history (examples are illustrative, not exhaustive, see text):**
  1. Deficits in social-emotional reciprocity, ranging, for example, from abnormal social approach and failure of normal back-and-forth conversation; to reduced sharing of interests, emotions, or affect; to failure to initiate or respond to social interactions.

  2. Deficits in nonverbal communicative behaviors used for social interaction, ranging, for example, from poorly integrated verbal and nonverbal communication; to abnormalities in eye contact and body language or deficits in understanding and use of gestures; to a total lack of facial expressions and nonverbal communication.

  3. Deficits in developing, maintaining, and understanding relationships, ranging, for example, from difficulties adjusting behavior to suit various social contexts; to difficulties in sharing imaginative play or in making friends; to absence of interest in peers.

  Specify **current severity: Severity is based on social communication impairments and restricted, repetitive patterns of behavior (see Box 19.2).**

B. **Restricted, repetitive patterns of behavior, interests, or activities, as manifested by at least two of the following, currently or by history (examples are illustrative, not exhaustive; see text):**
  1. Stereotyped or repetitive motor movements, use of objects, or speech (e.g., simple motor stereotypies, lining up toys or flipping objects, echolalia, idiosyncratic phrases).

  2. Insistence on sameness, inflexible adherence to routines, or ritualized patterns of verbal or nonverbal behavior (e.g., extreme distress at small changes, difficulties with transitions, rigid thinking patterns, greeting rituals, need to take same route or eat food every day).

  3. Highly restricted, fixated interests that are abnormal in intensity or focus (e.g, strong attachment to or preoccupation with unusual objects, excessively circumscribed or perseverative interest).

  4. Hyper- or hypo-reactivity to sensory input or unusual interests in sensory aspects of the environ-ment (e.g., apparent indifference to pain/temperature, adverse response to specific sounds or textures, excessive smelling or touching of objects, visual fascination with lights or movement).

  Specify **current severity : Severity is based on social communication impairments and restricted, repetitive patterns of behavior (see Box 19.2).**

C. **Symptoms must be present in the early developmental period (but may not become fully manifest until social demands exceed limited capacities, or may be masked by learned strategies in later life).**

D. **Symptoms cause clinically significant impairment in social, occupational, or other important areas of current functioning.**

E. **These disturbances are not better explained by intellectual disability (intellectual developmental disorder) or global developmental delay. Intellectual disability and autism spectrum disorder frequently co-occur; to make comorbid diagnoses of autism spectrum disorder and intellectual disability, social communication should be below that expected for general developmental level.**

Note: Individuals with a well-established *DSM-IV* diagnosis of autistic disorder, Asperger's disorder, or pervasive developmental disorder not otherwise specified should be given the diagnosis of autism spectrum disorder. Individuals who have marked deficits in social communication, but whose symptoms do not otherwise meet criteria for autism spectrum disorder, should be evaluated for social (pragmatic) communication disorder.

Specify if:
With or without accompanying intellectual impairment
With or without accompanying language impairment
Associated with a known medical or genetic condition or environmental factor
Associated with another neurodevelopmental, mental, or behavioral disorder
With catatonia (refer to the criteria for catatonia associated with another mental disorder for definition)

Box 19.2. *DSM-5* **Severity Levels for Autism Spectrum Disorder**[a]

Severity Level	Social Communication	Restricted, Repetitive Behaviors
Level 3 "Requiring very substantial support"	Severe deficits in verbal and nonverbal social communication skills cause severe impairments in functioning, very limited initiation of social interactions, and minimal response to social overtures from others. For example, a person with few words of intelligible speech who rarely initiates interaction and, when he or she does, makes unusual approaches to meet needs only and responds to only very direct social approaches	Inflexibility of behavior, extreme difficulty coping with change, or other restricted/repetitive behaviors markedly interfere with functioning in all spheres. Great distress/difficulty changing focus or action.
Level 2 "Requiring substantial support"	Marked deficits in verbal and nonverbal social communication skills; social impairments apparent even with supports in place; limited initiation of social interactions; and reduced or abnormal responses to social overtures from others. For example, a person who speaks simple sentences, whose interaction is limited to narrow special interests, and how has markedly odd nonverbal communication.	Inflexibility of behavior, difficulty coping with change, or other restricted/repetitive behaviors appear frequently enough to be obvious to the casual observer and interfere with functioning in a variety of contexts. Distress and/or difficulty changing focus or action.
Level 1 "Requiring support"	Without supports in place, deficits in social communication cause noticeable impairments. Difficulty initiating social interactions, and clear examples of atypical or unsuccessful response to social overtures of others. May appear to have decreased interest in social interactions. For example, a person who is able to speak in full sentences and engages in communication but whose to-and-fro conversation with others fails, and whose attempts to make friends are odd and typically unsuccessful.	Inflexibility of behavior causes significant interference with functioning in one or more contexts. Difficulty switching between activities. Problems of organization and planning hamper independence.

[a] Reprinted with permission from the *Diagnostic and Statistical Manual of Mental Disorders,* Fifth Edition, (Copyright © 2013). American Psychiatric Association. All Rights Reserved.

Social (pragmatic) communication disorder (SCD) was introduced as a diagnostic classification in *DSM-5*.[2,4] The goal was to more accurately recognize individuals who have early-onset, persistent difficulty using verbal and nonverbal communication for social purposes, leading to significant functional limitations in effective communication, social participation, development and maintenance of social relationships, academic achievement, and/or occupational performance.[2] The diagnostic criteria for SCD are provided in Box 19.3.[2] By definition, the communication deficits in SCD are not explained by low general cognitive ability or low abilities in the domains of word structure and grammar, and they occur in the absence of the repetitive and restricted behaviors and interests that characterize ASD; in fact, ASD must be ruled out for SCD to be diagnosed. Diagnosis of SCD with other communication disorders is permitted. However, it is expected that diagnosis of SCD would seldom be made before the age of 4 to 5 years, when structural

Box 19.3. *DSM-5* **Diagnostic Criteria for Social (Pragmatic) Communication Disorder (315.39; F80.89)**

A. **Persistent difficulties in the social use of verbal and nonverbal communication as manifested by all of the following:**
   1. Deficits in using communication for social purposes, such as greeting and sharing information, in a manner that is appropriate for the social context.
   2. Impairment of the ability to change communication to match context or the needs of the listener, such as speaking differently in a classroom than on the playground, talking differently to a child than to an adult, and avoiding use of overly formal language.
   3. Difficulties following rules for conversation and storytelling, such as taking turns in conversation, rephrasing when misunderstood, and knowing how to use verbal and nonverbal signals to regulate interaction.
   4. Difficulties understanding what is not explicitly stated (e.g., making inferences) and nonliteral or ambiguous meanings of language (e.g., idioms, humor, metaphors, multiple meanings that depend on the context for interpretation).

B. **The deficits result in functional limitations in effective communication, social participation, social relationships, academic achievement, or occupational performance, individually or in combination.**

C. **The onset of the symptoms is in the early developmental period (but deficits may not become fully manifest until social communication demands exceed limited capacities).**

D. **The symptoms are not attributable to another medical or neurological condition or to low abilities in the domains of word structure and grammar, and are not better explained by autism spectrum disorder, intellectual disability (intellectual developmental disorder), global developmental delay, or another mental disorder.**

language abilities are often adequate to determine that deficits in pragmatic language are discrepant from structural language abilities.[4]

SCD is likely to apply to some individuals who would have been classified as having PDD-NOS by *DSM-IV-TR* criteria but do not meet the *DSM-5* criteria for ASD due to lack of restricted repetitive behaviors.[4,5] The *DSM-5 SCD* concept expands upon research on pragmatic language impairment by including nonverbal communication, and further evaluation of the validity of the diagnosis is needed.[4] Preliminary evidence suggests that this diagnosis identifies individuals who have marginally subthreshold autistic traits, rather than being qualitatively distinct from ASD.[5]

Epidemiology

The Centers for Disease Control and Prevention (CDC) Autism and Developmental Disabilities Monitoring Network (ADDM) 2012 estimate of ASD prevalence in 8-year-old children was 1.46%, or 1 in 68.[6] Analysis of a general population cohort of more than 3 million children using a commercial managed health care administrative database yielded a similar prevalence of 1.25% in the United States.[7] Somewhat higher prevalence estimates have been described in survey studies, which are based on parent report of ASD diagnosis. For example, parents reported a current diagnosis of ASD in 2.0% of children aged 6 to 17 years in the 2011–2012 National Survey of Children's Health,[8] and the rate of parent-reported lifetime diagnosis of ASD was 2.24% of children aged 3 to 17 years in the 2014 National Health Interview Survey.[9] The estimated global prevalence of ASD is lower: 0.76% in the Global Burden of Disease Study 2010,[10] although recent estimates based on national registry data in Sweden, Denmark, and Iceland were greater than 1%,[11–13] and the highest recent prevalence estimate, 2.64% for 7- to 12-year-old children in 2005–2009, was from South Korea.[14] Males are more commonly affected than females, by a ratio of 4:1 to 4.5:1 in most studies,[6] although a 2017 meta-analysis of studies conducted since the introduction of *DSM-IV* and *ICD-10* criteria concluded that the true ratio is closer to 3:1.[15]

Substantial increases in the estimated prevalence of ASD in the United States over the last 3 decades have been found in studies using special education and developmental services administrative data,[16–18] national family surveys,[8,9,19] and active public health surveillance conducted by the CDC ADDM Network.[6] Similarly, studies using registry data in Denmark,[20] Norway,[21] Iceland,[12] Sweden,[11,22] Israel,[23] and other countries have reported an increase in ASD prevalence. However, incidence data adequate for determining time trends are scarce, and there is controversy about whether the available prevalence data actually establish that there has been an increase in ASD.[10,24–26] For example, a 2015 systematic review of epidemiological studies with Bayesian meta-regression analysis found that after accounting for methodological variations, there was no clear evidence of a change in estimated worldwide prevalence of *DSM-IV-TR–*defined autism spectrum disorders (autistic disorder, Asperger disorder, and PDD-NOS) between 1990 and 2010.[10]

If there has been an increase in prevalence, it is not clear whether there has been a true secular increase in incidence due to etiologic factors in addition to the clear contribution of nonetiologic factors such as changes in identification and diagnostic practices, variation in study methods, and increased public awareness and availability of services.[6,10,20,22,25] Some studies provide evidence of diagnostic recategorization toward ASD and away from other diagnoses such as ID and language disorders.[18,27–31]

Etiology/Pathophysiology

ASD is etiologically heterogeneous and, perhaps unsurprisingly, a unifying pathophysiology has not been identified for either the disorder as a whole or its core behavioral components. Although research aimed at elucidating the biological basis of ASD and related neurodevelopmental disorders is in its early stages, much progress has been made in the areas of genetics, neuroimaging, neurophysiology, and neuropathology.

Genetics and Genomics

Although clinically and etiologically heterogeneous, ASD is heritable, as demonstrated by family studies showing increased risk of ASD in siblings of affected individuals and twin studies documenting substantially higher concordance rates for monozygotic twins than for dizygotic twins.[32-36] For example, a large population-based family study involving more than 2 million Swedish children, including 14,516 diagnosed with ASD, yielded a heritability estimate of 0.83.[36] Heritability estimates range from 64% to 91%, according to a meta-analysis of twin studies involving 6,413 twin pairs.[35]

The complex genetic architecture of ASD is currently thought to involve the following[37-42]:

1. A large number of rare variants, each conferring significant risk

2. Polygenic risk conferred primarily by a large number of common variants, or polymorphisms, which individually confer very small risk but collectively contribute substantially to the phenotype and to heritability

3. Some combination of genotype-by-genotype interactions (epistasis), genotype-by-environment interactions, and epigenetic effects

Although common variants, epistasis, and environmental modification of genotype effects are thought to be important, these aspects of the genetics of ASD are still poorly understood.[39,42,43] Genome-wide association studies and candidate gene association studies have not yet implicated replicable risk loci, likely due to small effect sizes and lack of statistical power.[38,41,43] Epistasis is difficult to detect because of the need for very large sample sizes, and there is little evidence so far for environmental modification of genotype effects.[39]

In contrast, advances such as the development of microarray and next-generation sequencing technologies have resulted in identification of large-effect variants that appear to be causally associated with ASD, including copy number variants (CNVs), which are microdeletions or microduplications ≥1,000 base pairs in size that alter the dosage of genes, short insertions and deletions (indels), and single-nucleotide variants (SNVs).[40-42,44] Pathogenic rare variants may arise de novo or be inherited as autosomal dominant, autosomal recessive, or X-linked mutations. Microarray and exome sequencing studies have established that although de novo and inherited rare variants of large effect size are collectively common, no individual pathogenic variant accounts for more than 1% of nonsyndromic cases of ASD.[37,45-48]

It is important to note that no specific mutation has been identified that is unique to ASD. Chromosomal microarray analysis (CMA) and whole exome sequencing (WES) studies in ASD cohorts and other populations have made it clear that there is substantial genetic overlap between ASD and other neurodevelopmental disorders, including ID, epilepsy, and schizophrenia. These disorders all are associated with increased CNV and single gene loss-of-function mutation burden, and individual pathogenic variants are not specific to one categorical diagnostic phenotype—the same pathogenic CNVs and SNVs have been detected in individuals with ASD, ID, epilepsy, schizophrenia, and other clinical presentations.[49-55]

In clinical practice, a genetic etiologic diagnosis may be suspected clinically and confirmed by targeted genetic testing, or, more commonly, it may be revealed by CMA or WES completed as a routine part of the evaluation of a patient with ASD in the absence of a clinically recognizable syndrome. Examples of some of the most common genetic syndromes and mutations, including SNVs and recurrent CNVs, that are causally associated with ASD are presented in Table 19.1.[40,42,44,56–60] Proteins encoded by genes that have been implicated in ASD have a variety of biological functions, but a pattern of convergence on functional pathways involved in synaptic structure and function and transcription regulation/chromatin remodeling has emerged.[38,40,42,59]

Increased maternal and paternal age are independently associated with ASD risk, and there is evidence for a combined parental age effect as well; ASD risk increases when the difference between the parental ages is 10 years or more.[61–63] At least part of the ASD

Table 19.1. Genetic Etiologies: Examples of Clinical Syndromes, Copy Number Variants, and Single-Nucleotide Variants Associated With Autism Spectrum Disorder[40,42,44,54,56–60]

Genetic syndromes often suspected clinically and confirmed by genetic testing (implicated genes in parentheses)	**Recurrent CNVs** commonly identified by whole genome chromosomal microarray analysis	**Single gene mutations,** including SNVs and small insertions or deletions identified by whole exome sequencing[a]
Angelman syndrome (*UBE3A*) CHARGE syndrome (*CHD7*) Cohen syndrome (VPS13B) Cornelia de Lange syndrome (*NIPBL, RAD21, SMC3, HDAC8, SMC1A*) Down syndrome/trisomy 21 Fragile X syndrome (*FMR1*) Neurofibromatosis type 1 (*NF1*) *PTEN* hamartoma tumor syndrome (*PTEN*) Rett syndrome (*MECP2*) Smith-Lemli-Opitz (*DHCR7*) Timothy syndrome (*CACNA1C*) Tuberous sclerosis (*TSC1, TSC2*)	1q21.1 deletion 1q21.1 duplication 3q29 deletion 7q11.23 duplication 15q11.2-q13.1 (BP2-BP3) duplication 15q13.2-q13.3 (BP4-BP5) deletion 16p11.2 deletion 16p11.2 duplication 16p13.11 deletion 17q12 deletion 22q11.2 deletion 22q11.2 duplication	*ADNP* *ANK2* *ARID1B* *ASH1L* *CHD2* *CHD8* *DYRK1A* *GRIN2B* *KATNAL2* *NRXN1a* *POGZ* *SCN2A* *SHANK3* *SUV420H1* *SYNGAP1* *TBR1*

[a] In the case of *NRXN1*, a very large gene (1.1 Mb, 24 exons), large intragenic deletions may be detected by chromosomal microarray analysis.

Abbreviations: CNV, copy number variant; SNV, single-nucleotide variant.

Gene names: *ADNP*, activity-dependent neuroprotector homeobox; *ANK2*, ankyrin 2; *ARID1B*, AT rich interactive domain 1B (SWI1-like); *ASH1L*, ASH1 (absent, small, or homeotic)-like; *CACNA1C*, calcium channel, voltage-dependent, L-type, alpha-1c subunit; *CHD2*, chromodomain helicase DNA binding protein 2; *CHD7*, chromodomain helicase DNA binding protein 7; *CHD8*, chromodomain helicase DNA binding protein 8; *DHCR7*, 7-dehydrocholesterol reductase; *DYRK1A*, dual-specificity tyrosine-(Y)-phosphorylation regulated kinase 1A; *FMR1*, fragile X mental retardation 1; *GRIN2B*, glutamate receptor, ionotropic, N-methyl-D-aspartate 2B; *HDAC8*, histone deacetylase 8; *KATNAL2*, katanin p60 subunit A-like 2; *MECP2*, methyl-CpG-binding protein 2; *NF1*, neurofibromatosis 1; *NIPBL*, nipped-B-like; *NRXN1*, neurexin 1; *POGZ*, pogo transposable element with ZNF domain; *PTEN*, phosphatase and tensin homolog; *RAD21*, double-strand-break repair protein rad21 homolog; *SCN2A*, sodium channel, voltage-gated, type II, alpha subunit; *SHANK3*, SH3 and multiple ankyrin repeat domains 3; *SMC1A*, structural maintenance of chromosomes protein 1A; *SMC3*, structural maintenance of chromosomes protein 3; *SUV420H1*, suppressor of variegation 4–20 homolog 1; *SYNGAP1*, synaptic Ras GTPase activating protein 1; *TBR1*, T-box brain, 1; TSC1, tuberous sclerosis 1; TSC2, tuberous sclerosis 2; *UBE3A*, ubiquitin protein ligase E3A.

risk associated with advancing paternal age is explained by an age-related increase in the rate of de novo loss-of-function mutations in the male germ cell; potential mechanisms mediating the effect of advancing maternal age are under investigation.[64]

Environment

There is evidence that aspects of the prenatal environment such as exposure to maternal medications (eg, valproate), short interpregnancy interval, multiple gestation, maternal obesity, gestational diabetes, gestational bleeding, and infections (eg, rubella, cytomegalovirus, influenza) may be associated with increased risk of ASD.[65-67] The case for in utero selective serotonin reuptake inhibitor exposure as a causal risk factor independent of the maternal conditions (eg, depression and anxiety) for which they are prescribed has not yet been proven.[67] Perinatal factors such as prematurity, low birth weight, fetal growth restriction, intrapartum hypoxia, and neonatal encephalopathy also may be associated ASD risk.[67-69] However, more research is required to determine whether these are independent risk factors because genetic susceptibility may be associated with both obstetric suboptimality and neonatal encephalopathy.

Although toxic environmental chemicals have not been proven to cause ASD, associations between some compounds such as organophosphates and certain other pesticides, metals, and volatile organic compounds and ASD risk at the population level have been published.[66,67,70] Several US studies have suggested an association between ASD and prenatal exposure to traffic-related air pollutants,[70-72] but it is difficult to exclude confounding from sociodemographic or other factors; a Swedish twin study and a collaborative study of 4 European population-based cohorts found no such association.[73,74]

Epidemiological studies have definitively refuted the idea that toxic effects of either the measles-mumps-rubella vaccine, mercury exposure via thimerosal-containing vaccines, or excessive burden on the immune system caused by a larger number of vaccines is responsible for the increased prevalence of ASD, and the weight of all of the available scientific evidence overwhelmingly favors rejection of the hypothesis that there is a causal association between immunizations and ASD.[70,75-80]

Epigenetics

The potential role of epigenetic factors in the etiology of ASD is also an active area of investigation and speculation.[81,82] Epigenetic modifications, such as DNA cytosine methylation and posttranslational histone modification, produce heritable changes in gene expression that do not involve a change in the DNA sequence. Abnormal patterns of DNA methylation and chromatin structure can result in altered morphology, physiology, and behavior, and some genetic disorders associated with ASD involve dysregulation of epigenetic processes during development. Examples include syndromes caused by mutations in genes encoding epigenetic regulators (eg, MECP2 in Rett syndrome and CHD7 in CHARGE syndrome) and syndromes caused by mutations in genes that are sensitive to alterations in their epigenetic regulation (eg, 15q duplication, Angelman,

Prader-Willi, and fragile X).[81,83] Epigenetic mechanisms are responsible for genomic imprinting, the process whereby certain genes are epigenetically marked during gametogenesis in a parent of origin specific manner so that gene expression is restricted to only one of the parental alleles.[83,84] Imprinted genes tend to be particularly sensitive to changes in their epigenetic status, and alteration of the gene dosage often results in pathology.[84] One of the most common cytogenetic abnormalities in patients with ASD is maternally derived duplication of the imprinted domain on chromosome 15q11-q13.[85]

It has been speculated that epigenetic alteration of gene expression by environmental factors may play a role in the etiology of ASD, but replicated examples of environmental epigenetic marks and evidence of causality are currently lacking.[82,83] A small number of candidate gene studies and genome-wide analyses of DNA methylation in a variety of brain regions and peripheral tissues have provided preliminary evidence of alteration of DNA methylation in association with ASD or ASD-related traits. However, methodological issues and the absence of replication studies limit the conclusions that can be drawn from the existing literature.[82,86,87]

Because epigenetic modifications can be influenced by environmental factors, such as prenatal exposures and postnatal experience, they represent one interface between genes and environment. Although appealing because they provide a tangible link between genes and environment, changes to the epigenome are not the only mechanism by which environmental effects are mediated, and epigenetics should not be conflated with the broader category of environmental effects.[83,88] In fact, biochemical cause-and-effect should be demonstrated to establish epigenetics as the mechanism of a proposed gene by environment interaction.[83,88] Despite the limitations of the existing evidence, exploration of the role of epigenetic and other nongenetic modifications that alter gene activity without changing the DNA sequence is likely to be an increasingly active and potentially important area of etiologic research in ASD.

Neuropathology

No uniform neuropathology has been identified, which is not surprising given the etiologic and phenotypic heterogeneity of ASD. The systematic neuropathological studies of postmortem brain tissue from individuals with ASD have been summarized in Supplemental Table 1 of the 2015 review by Chen and colleagues,[38] available at **http://www.annualreviews.org.** Dysplasia, altered neurogenesis, and neuronal migration abnormalities have been described within the cerebral neocortex, limbic system structures including the hippocampus and amygdala, basal ganglia, thalamus, brainstem, and cerebellum.[38,89] The vast majority of abnormalities described originate prenatally.[89,90]

Focal disruption of the normal laminar architecture, minicolumnar abnormalities, and variations in neuronal density are among the most common cerebral cortical abnormalities described.[89,90] Reduced neuronal number and/or size, increased cell-packing density, and decreased complexity of the neuropil have been found in the hippocampus and amygdala, although not in all individuals.[38] Microglial infiltration and activation and astrocytosis have been observed in cerebral cortex and cerebellum, and postmortem transcriptome studies have reported upregulation of genes enriched in activated microglia and astrocytes, implicating dysregulation of neuron-glia signaling and neuroinflammation.[38,42] However, it is not yet clear whether these findings represent primary pathology or a reactive or secondary process.

Biomarkers

Biomarkers are objectively measured biological characteristics that influence or predict the incidence or outcome of disease. Proposed biomarkers of ASD include head circumference growth trajectory; structural and functional magnetic resonance imaging (MRI) markers; electroencephalographic characteristics; eye tracking markers; genetic and biochemical markers in blood, urine, or brain tissue; placental pathology; and maternal autoantibody profiles. However, no biomarker has yet been shown to be clinically valuable.[91–93] Despite the limitations of the existing data, the future of biomarker research in ASD is promising due to increasing availability of bioresources linked to phenotypic data, advances in laboratory and neuroimaging technology and data management, and increasingly collaborative discovery and validation efforts.[93]

– Early Brain Overgrowth and Neuroimaging Markers

Cross-sectional and longitudinal studies suggest that as a group, children later diagnosed with ASD have average or below-average head circumferences at birth, with abnormal acceleration in brain growth during the first 1 to 2 years of life leading to significantly above-average head circumferences and MRI brain volumes in toddlers, followed by a plateau in brain growth resulting in brain volumes that are not significantly different from controls in adolescence and adulthood.[94,95] Although this raises the possibility that atypical patterns of brain growth might be used for early identification, rate of head growth did not predict which infants developed ASD in the first 3 years of life in a large, prospective study of high-risk infants.[96]

True brain overgrowth, defined as abnormally large brain size and abnormally rapid rate of brain growth, occurs in a minority of children with ASD. A systematic literature review and meta-analysis of 27 studies concluded that the prevalence of macrocephaly, defined as head circumference above the 97th percentile, in individuals with ASD was 15.7%.[95] Some recent studies have suggested that when individuals with ASD are compared to locally recruited controls rather than commonly used historical growth reference norms such as those provided by the CDC, the data are equivocal with regard to the finding of early brain overgrowth.[97] Additional research is needed to clarify the relationship between early brain overgrowth and ASD, whether it distinguishes ASD from other neurodevelopmental disorders, and to what extent it is part of generalized somatic overgrowth.[97,98]

Although there are many conflicting findings, structural MRI volumetric studies of infants and young children have most consistently demonstrated increases in total brain volume, cortical gray and white matter volume (particularly frontal, temporal, and cingulate cortex), extra-axial cerebral spinal fluid volume, and amygdala volume in groups of young children with ASD relative to controls.[99–101] Longitudinal studies suggest that neuroimaging findings are dynamic, and most of these volumetric differences do not persist into adolescence or adulthood.[100,101] Mean cortical thickness is somewhat increased in childhood in ASD but declines more rapidly than the typical decline that occurs in adolescence, resulting in decreased mean cortical thickness in adulthood, particularly in the frontal lobes.[101,102] Diffusion tensor imaging studies suggest age-dependent abnormalities of white matter microstructure, organization, and integrity based on metrics such as fractional anisotropy and mean diffusivity.[99,101] Cross-sectional studies suggest that reduced fractional anisotropy and other measures of white matter microstructure persist into adolescence and adulthood, particularly in the corpus callosum, cingulum, and white matter tracts connecting aspects of the temporal lobe.[100,103]

Functional MRI (fMRI) studies have shown that ASD is associated with differences in activation of various brain regions relative to controls on tasks assessing motor skills, visual processing, executive functions, language, and basic and complex social processing skills.[99,104] The authors of a meta-analysis and systematic review noted some common themes across task domains, including lack of preference for social stimuli, lack of modulation in response to task demands or intensity of stimuli, and decreased activation of areas of the prefrontal cortex generally recruited for executive functions (visual-spatial systems are favored instead).[104] Most studies have identified evidence of task-dependent and resting state functional hypoconnectivity across a wide variety of brain areas in association with ASD, but other studies provide evidence of short range hyperconnectivity, particularly between subcortical regions and sensory cortices.[104,105] The evidence for functional underconnectivity is strongest for long-range, frontal-posterior networks.[99,104,105]

Machine learning strategies including multivariate pattern classification have demonstrated that individuals can be classified categorically as having ASD with statistically significant accuracy using structural MRI and fMRI, and there is some evidence that they can predict the severity of symptoms (a quantitative or dimensional classification), but these methods have not yet been validated for clinical use.[106,107]

– Electrophysiological Markers and Eye Tracking

Electrophysiological techniques such as auditory brainstem response, electroencephalography (EEG), and event-related potentials allow precise temporal discrimination, and magnetoencephalography allows fine resolution in both time and space. Although the evidence has not yet established the utility of any marker in clinical practice, studies using these techniques have identified electrophysiological correlates of abnormalities in low-level and higher cognitive auditory and visual processing (including language processing and face processing), somatosensory response, multisensory integration, recognition memory, selective attention, attentional shifting, and neural connectivity in association with ASD.[108–111]

Resting-state and task-related quantitative EEG measures such as spectral power, complexity, and coherence are continuous and relate to typical development, making them good candidates for biomarker status.[109,110,112] EEG spectral coherence loading patterns, for example, have been shown to differentiate between children with ASD and typically developing children with a high degree of success, but their ability to discriminate ASD from other neurodevelopmental disorders and their clinical relevance remain to be investigated.[113]

ASD is characterized by early emerging impairments in social attention, and eye tracking technologies have been used to demonstrate decreased fixation on the eyes' region of the face and increased fixation on the mouth and background elements, as well as preliminary evidence that infants later diagnosed with ASD exhibit a decline in eye fixation between the ages of 2 and 6 months.[114–117]

– Biochemical, Gene Expression, and Other Tissue Markers

The biochemical markers most consistently reported to differentiate groups of individuals with ASD from controls include increased platelet serotonin level, decreased plasma melatonin and urine melatonin sulphate, indicators of increased oxidative stress or altered redox status, and markers of altered immune response such as irregular cytokine profiles and central nervous system microglial activation.[91,92,93,118] Unlike variations in DNA sequence, which are largely fixed across tissues throughout the life span, the amount of RNA transcribed from each gene is tissue specific and varies developmentally and in response to environmental changes. Studies of gene expression in ASD are in their infancy and the results have varied widely, but several have reported upregulation of genes involved in immune and inflammatory responses in blood and postmortem brain tissue.[119,120] Efforts to classify ASD risk based on gene expression profiling are preliminary, and it has been noted that the genes included in the classification panels derived by 2 different research groups do not overlap.[121,122]

Increased frequency of trophoblast inclusions relative to controls has been documented retrospectively in the placentas of children with ASD and prospectively in the placentas of children at risk for ASD based on having an affected sibling.[123,124] However, trophoblast inclusions also have been identified in association with chromosome aneuploidy and placenta accreta, and further investigation is needed to determine the predictive value in regard to ASD and other neurodevelopmental outcomes.[93,125] The pathogenic role of circulating maternal antibodies directed to fetal brain tissue and the potential value of maternal antibody panels as biomarkers of ASD also are active areas of investigation, but clinical value has not been established.[92,126–130]

Clinical Features

ASD is defined clinically by the core impairments, which contribute to the *DSM-5* diagnostic criteria in Box 19.1. However, no single specific behavior or deficit is pathognomonic for ASD and, although not part of the diagnostic criteria, other features such as cognitive and motor deficits, maladaptive behaviors, and associated medical problems have a dramatic impact on adaptive functioning and are also important aspects of the clinical presentation.

Core Impairments

ASD is characterized by early onset, clinically significant impairment in social communication and other reciprocal social behavior and restricted and repetitive patterns of behavior, interests, and activities (Box 19.1).[2] By definition, these symptoms interfere substantially with functioning and do not simply reflect coexisting ID. Clinical features of ASD, as elaborated in Boxes 19.4 and 19.5, vary with age, developmental level/intellectual ability, and severity of the condition.

– Social Communication and Social Interaction

Pervasive and persistent impairment in reciprocal social behavior that is not accounted for by developmental level (or mental age) is a defining feature of ASD; deficits in the development and understanding of social and emotional reciprocity, nonverbal communicative behaviors, and interpersonal relationships are required for diagnosis[2] (Box 19.1).

As infants and toddlers, children with ASD may not smile responsively or adopt a posture conveying anticipation and readiness or desire to be picked up. Young children with ASD typically lack developmentally appropriate joint attention (JA), which is coordinating attention with another individual to an external focus, showing social engagement and awareness of the partner's mutual interest.[131,132] JA behaviors can be receptive, (eg, responding by following the direction of eye gaze and gestures of others) or expressive (eg, initiating JA by using eye contact and gestures to direct the attention of others to an object or event of interest for the purpose of sharing their experience). Both are commonly delayed in children with ASD; however, initiation of JA for the purpose of sharing interest and enjoyment/positive affect rather than requesting is particularly atypical.[131] JA ability is an important precursor and predictor of language and theory of mind, an important component of empathy.[131,133] Reciprocal social behaviors such as seeking to share enjoyment with others, recognizing and reacting to the mental states of others, and forming reciprocal friendships that go beyond classroom or parent-arranged interactions are limited, even in older children.[134] Even highly functioning adolescents and adults with ASD typically have difficulty navigating social interactions when it is necessary to make accurate inferences about other people's beliefs, motivations, goals, and emotional states.[135,136]

Wing and Gould[137] described 3 types of social impairment exhibited by individuals with ASD: *aloof, passive,* and *active but odd*. Individuals in the first group, whose social impairment is most easily recognized, are generally aloof and indifferent to others, especially peers, but may accept physical affection from familiar people and enjoy physical play. Those in the passive group do not socially interact spontaneously but passively accept and even appear to enjoy approaches from others. The active but odd group includes people who make active social approaches that are naïve, odd, inappropriate, and one-sided. Stability of the social interaction subgroup classification varies with level

Box 19.4. Clinical Presentation of Autism Spectrum Disorder: Social Communication and Interaction Impairment

Younger or More Severely Impaired Children	Older or Less Severely Impaired Children
Poor eye contact, gaze aversion	Decreased or atypical eye contact
Limited or absent responsive smiling	Difficulty forming developmentally appropriate friendships that involve a mutual sharing of interests, activities, and emotions
Decreased sharing of joyful affect	
Marked lack of interest in other people	Socially immature and less independent than peers
▷ Often aloof and indifferent, may prefer to be alone	▷ May be viewed as odd, eccentric, or "weird" by peers
▷ More interested in objects than people	▷ May initiate interactions in inappropriate, awkward, or stilted ways
▷ May bump into people as if the child did not see them or climb on them as if they were furniture	▷ Lack of awareness of personal space
▷ Rather than being distant, some children display indiscriminate affection	▷ Gullible, naïve, lacking "common sense"
Deficits in joint attention	▷ Lack of modulation of behavior according to social context
▷ Lack of response when name is called	Poor perspective-taking ability that may contribute to inappropriate, offensive behavior
▷ Failure to follow the gaze and pointing gestures of others	▷ Difficulty anticipating how another person will feel or what he or she might think
▷ Failure to spontaneously alternate gaze between an object and another person	▷ Lack of cognitive aspects of empathy
▷ Absent or limited attempts to draw the attention of others to objects or events for the purpose of sharing experiences (including lack of pointing for the purpose of showing, commenting, or sharing interest or enjoyment)	▷ Difficulty knowing how to react to another person's behavior or emotions
	▷ Difficulty accepting that there might be multiple perspectives, not just a single correct perspective
Lack of adjustment of behavior according to environment or social context	Unusual vocabulary for age and/or social group
May not have any meaningful speech	Difficulty answering open-ended questions
Greater proportion of syllables with atypical phonation (eg, squeals, growls, and yells)	Dysprosody (atypical intonation, inflection, rhythm of voice)
Delayed receptive and expressive language milestones	▷ Singsong or cartoonish
	▷ Monotone
Increased idiosyncratic or inappropriate means of communication	Difficulty with initiation and closure of conversation and topic changes
▷ Self-injurious behavior, aggression, tantrums	▷ Failure to provide enough background information
▷ Immediate echolalia (eg, in response to questions)	▷ Tangential remarks
Pronoun reversal (often "you" for "I" or "me")	▷ Abrupt topic changes
May label objects or actions but not use those words to make requests or answer questions	▷ Difficulty maintaining conversation by elaborating or requesting more information
Delayed, decreased, or absent use of symbolic gestures (eg, waving, pointing, shaking head for "no," nodding head for "yes," depicting actions)	

Box 19.4. Clinical Presentation of Autism Spectrum Disorder: Social Communication and Interaction Impairment (*continued*)

Younger or More Severely Impaired Children	Older or Less Severely Impaired Children
Persistent use of primitive motor gestures to communicate (eg, contact gesture of leading or pulling another's hand)	One-sided conversations that revolve almost exclusively around the individual's intense interest or include irrelevant details
Nonsequential acquisition of milestones (eg, early labeling of letters and numbers despite having a small vocabulary and not using words to make requests)	▸ Lack of reciprocal exchange (monologue-like)
	▸ Inadequate clarification, vague references
	▸ Topic preoccupation, perseveration
Early lack of interest in toys	▸ Scripted, stereotyped discourse
Subsequent preoccupation with elementary sensory features of toys	Overly literal; difficulty understanding nonliteral forms of communication, such as idioms, metaphors, humor/jokes, sarcasm, and irony
▸ Feeling, mouthing, lining, spinning, arranging, hoarding, and carrying	Difficulty recognizing and resolving communication breakdowns; unresponsive to partner's cues
Later appreciation of symbolic meaning, appropriate functional use	Difficulty adapting style of communication to social situation
▸ Sequences of appropriate actions	▸ Inability to infer expected degree of formality
▸ Impoverished, lacks typical creativity or variability	▸ Excessively formal or pedantic style
▸ Repetitious, mechanical	Good memory for details, difficulty understanding themes
▸ Often precisely imitated from videos	
Solitary and parallel play, often some interactive physical play	Lack of appropriate use of facial expression, gestures, and body postures to facilitate communication
Difficulty with turn-taking in play	Difficulty with flexible cooperative imaginative play, such as interactive role-playing with peers
Delayed and impaired development of pretend play	May have difficulty tolerating losing at games or sports
	May lack creativity and imagination

of cognitive ability. Children with higher levels of cognitive ability may move, for example, from the aloof group in early childhood to the passive or active but odd group in adolescence, whereas those with severe or profound ID are more likely to remain aloof and indifferent to others.

The severity of language impairment ranges from profound (eg, verbal auditory agnosia) to relatively mild (eg, pragmatic impairment), and the clinical features vary with age and developmental level (Box 19.4). [138–140] Communicative speech is often delayed or absent in young children with ASD, and comprehension is impaired.[139] Nonverbal communication is also impaired, so there is often little or no attempt to compensate by using facial expressions, gestures, or pantomime, especially in young children with ASD. Approximately 20% to 30% of individuals remain nonverbal or minimally verbal.[139,141]

Box 19.5. Clinical Presentation of Autism Spectrum Disorder: Repetitive Behavior/ Restricted Interests and Activities

Younger or More Severely Impaired Children	Older or Less Severely Impaired Children
Stereotyped, repetitive movements ▸ Hand-flapping, finger-flicking, rocking, spinning, jumping or prancing on toes; whole body twisting or posturing, etc. ▸ Incorporation of objects (eg, lining, flipping, or tapping various objects; dangling and jiggling or twirling strings or cords) ▸ Self-injurious behavior (independent of situation, automatically reinforced) Stereotyped, repetitive speech ▸ Delayed echolalia (scripted verses, reciting memorized phrases) ▸ Greeting rituals Insistence on sameness ▸ Excessive distress with deviation from routines or small changes in environment ▸ Difficulty with transitions ▸ Extreme dietary selectivity Very limited range of interests and activities Strong, preoccupying attachment to unusual objects (often hard rather than soft) Unusual sensory interests ▸ Visual fascination with lights or objects that move or spin ▸ Atypical visual inspection, lateral eye gaze ▸ Excessive smelling, licking, or touching of objects Aversion or hyperreactivity to sensory stimuli Distress, avoidance, ear-covering in response to certain sounds Gagging in response to smells or tastes or even the sight of foods with certain textures Tactile defensiveness, aversion to social touch or certain textures Hyporeactivity to sensory stimuli ▸ Lack of response to certain sounds, especially human voice ▸ Apparent indifference to pain or temperature ▸ Increased tolerance of spinning or being upside down	Repetitive movements and compulsions ▸ Complex stereotyped motor mannerisms ▸ Touching, tapping, rubbing ▸ Ordering, hoarding Repetitive speech ▸ Telling or asking ▸ Reciting of memorized dialogue ▸ Idiosyncratic phrases Strong desire to maintain sameness ▸ Inflexible adherence to routines or rituals ▸ Rigid thinking patterns ▸ Difficulty accepting unexpected change ▸ Difficulty with transitions ▸ Overly selective diet Excessively narrow or circumscribed scope of interests and activities ▸ Special interests of abnormal intensity and/or focus ▸ Unusual preoccupations ▸ Obsession with facts, details, or collections Aversion to and avoidance of certain sensations ▸ Sounds ▸ Smells ▸ Touch/textures (eg, tags in clothing, social touch) Excessive smelling or touching of objects or people

Although structural language skills are extremely variable and may be normal in some individuals, echolalia, jargon, neologisms, and other unusual semantic and syntactic error patterns are more frequent among children with ASD than typically developing children or children with ID.[139,142] Even among individuals with higher verbal skills, the language profile that emerges in childhood and persists into adulthood is characterized by unevenness, including poor comprehension relative to expressive language, persistence of certain morphological errors, semantic processing anomalies despite normal performance on vocabulary tests, and idiosyncratic word usage despite relatively intact articulation and syntax.[139,142]

Deficits in pragmatics, which is the ability to use language in context for social purposes, are universal in individuals with ASD.[139,140] Even the most able communicators with ASD typically exhibit significant atypicality in conversational discourse, including poor topic maintenance, difficulty with turn-taking, failure to respond adequately to questions or comments, inclusion of non-contextual or socially inappropriate utterances, and difficulty recognizing and repairing a misunderstanding or unclear referent.[139] Other common deficits involve understanding figurative and metaphorical language, making inferences, and resolving ambiguous language.[139,140]

Children with ASD typically exhibit deficits in functional and symbolic play, including delayed onset, decreased frequency, reduced diversity, and qualitative atypicality.[143] Qualitatively, the play of children with ASD tends to be solitary, repetitive, stereotyped, and excessively focused on sensorimotor manipulation of objects rather than interactive, varied, flexible, imaginative, and creative (Box 19.4).

– Restricted, Repetitive Behavioral Repertoire

Restricted and repetitive behaviors (RRBs) include repetitive sensorimotor actions (eg, stereotyped motor mannerisms and repetitive manipulation of objects), insistence on sameness/behavioral rigidity (eg, resistance to change, compulsive adherence to nonfunctional rituals or routines), and circumscribed interests (eg, fascination/preoccupation with one subject or activity that is abnormal in intensity or focus; Box 19.5).[144,145] It is important to recognize that repetitive behaviors, including stereotyped movements and behaviors related to desire for sameness, occur in normal development and in individuals with other developmental disabilities or psychiatric conditions, although most are more prevalent and/or severe in children with ASD.[146,147]

In general, younger children are more likely to engage in repetitive sensorimotor actions, whereas older children are more likely to exhibit repetitive behaviors based on insistence on sameness/behavioral rigidity and circumscribed interests.[144,145,148] As a group, RRBs commonly decline in adolescence and adulthood, although there is considerable variability.[135] Stereotyped movements are more persistent in adolescents and adults with ASD who also have ID, whereas behaviors based on insistence on sameness and circumscribed interests tend to be more independent of age and IQ.[144,149] However, even in highly functioning individuals, unusual preoccupations and circumscribed interests often interfere with social interaction. Conversely, in addition to being sources of pleasure and motivation, special interests may provide themes around which social activities can be developed and, potentially, opportunities for employment.[150]

Atypical reactivity to sensory input and unusual interest in sensory aspects of the environment were incorporated into the *DSM* diagnostic criteria for ASD for the first time in *DSM-5*; symptoms in this category can fulfil 1 of the 4 restricted and repetitive behavior criteria, 2 of which are required for diagnosis (Box 19.1).[2] Sensory modulation symptoms have been defined as difficulties in regulating and organizing the type and intensity of behavioral responses to sensory input to match environmental demands and are categorized as follows: (a) over-responsivity, which is exaggerated, rapid onset, and/or prolonged reactions to sensory stimulation; (b) under-responsivity, which is unawareness or slow response to sensory input; and (c) maladaptive sensation seeking, which describes craving of and interest in sensory experiences that are prolonged or intense. Examples include apparent indifference to pain or temperature (under-responsivity), distress and ear-covering in response to certain sounds (over-responsivity), and atypical fascination with visual inspection of lights or spinning objects (sensation-seeking), as well as others (Box 19.5). Unusual sensory responses are described more commonly in children with ASD than in typically developing children; the effect size of the difference is greatest for under-responsivity, followed by over-responsivity and then sensation seeking.[151] Although they may diminish in later childhood and adolescence, atypical reactivity to and/or interest in environmental sensory input may persist through adulthood.[151,152]

Autistic Regression

Population-based studies suggest that approximately 20% of children with ASD experience loss of previously established language skills and/or social interest and engagement skills at a mean age of 21 to 24 months.[153,154] Clinic-based samples and survey studies yield higher rates of reported regression (35%–40%).[153] However, even the more accurate population-based studies are plagued by problems with variable and sometimes vague case definition and reliance on parent-reported skill loss without verification by rigorous clinical information gathering, and the prevalence of true regression may be substantially lower.[155]

Autistic regression may be gradual or sudden and may occur following typical development or be superimposed on preexisting atypical development.[153,156] Some studies suggest that regression is associated with increased likelihood of ID and higher rates of certain RRBs (eg, stereotyped speech, insistence on sameness, sensory interests and/or behaviors), but there is no definitive consensus.[154,156] Although there is evidence that epilepsy is more common in individuals with ASD who have a history of regression, this association appears to be driven by lower IQ.[157,158]

Neuropsychological Features

Historically, ID was thought to be present in 70% to 75% of children with ASD, but many recent studies suggest that the prevalence of ID among individuals with ASD is substantially lower (32%–55%).[6,11,12,159] A systematic review and meta-analysis of male to female ratio in ASD included 24 epidemiological studies published between 1996 and 2015 that provided sufficient information to determine that the mean proportion of participants with IQ <70 was 48%.[15]

Individuals with ASD often display an unusual degree of unevenness in cognitive abilities, frequently including a significant discrepancy between verbal and nonverbal abilities, which can be in either direction (verbal<nonverbal or verbal>nonverbal), and/or isolated strengths that significantly exceed not only their own general level of ability but general population norms as well.[160] A strong correlation between uneven intellectual development and autistic-like symptoms, including those outside of the clinical range for ASD, has also been reported.[161] Although a high degree of variability between domains and subtests is common, a prototypical profile of cognitive strengths and weaknesses does not exist.[160,162]

IQ testing to identify verbal and nonverbal cognitive abilities and specific strengths and weaknesses is useful in educational planning for children with ASD, as it is for children with other disabilities. Although IQ is one of the most robust predictors of outcome for individuals with ASD, it is important to recognize that low IQ is more reliably predictive of a poorer outcome than high IQ is of a better outcome and that IQ, especially among higher-ability individuals, often significantly exceeds adaptive functioning in the community.[160]

Performance profiles also vary on standardized measures of academic achievement. Skills requiring primarily rote, mechanical, or procedural abilities are typically intact, but skills requiring more abstract reasoning, conceptualization, or interpretive analysis are often deficient.[163,164] For example, a child with ASD may have very good phonological awareness and decoding abilities but poor reading comprehension. Because the types of skills emphasized in the early elementary grades play to their strengths in memorization and concrete tasks, such as decoding and numerical operations, young children with ASD may perform well academically. In later elementary and middle school grades, when comprehension, analytic interpretation, and abstract reasoning skills are emphasized, these children often struggle academically and require more supports.[164,165] Even high-functioning children with ASD often have weaknesses in graphomotor skills, attention, and processing speed that interfere substantially with academic performance.[164,166]

Neuropsychological theories that help to explain the behavior and cognitive performance profile of individuals with ASD are described in Table 19.2.[167–171] Some neuropsychological theories suggest that cognitive impairments or biases, such as executive functioning and information-processing differences, underlie the behavioral manifestations of ASD throughout development.[167] In contrast, social motivation and social cognition theories emphasize early emerging, core social deficits that precipitate a developmental cascade of disrupted social and communicative development. Although no single theory adequately explains all aspects of ASD, recognition of the fundamental deficits in social motivation, perspective-taking, cognitive flexibility, and the ability to

Table 19.2. Major Neuropsychological Theories[133,167–169]	
Theory[a]	**Description[a]**
Executive Functioning Impairment	Key impairment in higher-level cognitive skills (eg, working memory, planning, inhibition, cognitive flexibility, self-monitoring) that underlie independent, goal-oriented behavior important for social and adaptive functioning.
	Deficit in using executive functions to go beyond automatic activities and plan and carry out an integrated course of action. – Difficulty with creating strategies for behavior, making plans, shifting topics, maintaining a representation in working memory, solving tasks requiring ability to be flexible and innovative. – Deficits on tasks such as the Tower of London, Tower of Hanoi, and Wisconsin Card Sorting Test.
Information Processing Impairment	Differential ability to process information that differs in kind (global/featural) or level of complexity.
	Atypicality at the level of whole-brain processing.
1. Weak central coherence	Limited drive for "central coherence" (meaningful wholes). – Tendency to focus on details/featural elements and overlook broader contexts and global meaning. – As a group, children with ASD are good at finding figures embedded in larger forms, completing jigsaw puzzles, and reproducing patterns with blocks. – Approximately 20% have islets of special ability, or splinter skills. – Intact local processing, impaired global processing.
2. Complex information processing impairment	Overall information processing is reduced relative to general cognitive ability level.
	Abilities and tasks most impacted are those that place the highest demands on information processing. – Difficulty with memory for complex information – Difficulty with higher-order integrative and interpretative aspects of language and concept formation – Intact basic attention, sensory perception, associative memory, and language encoding and decoding abilities
	The information processing disturbance is generalized and includes nonsocial cognition.
	Many things that come naturally to typically developing children must be cognitively discovered by or explicitly taught to those with ASD using compensatory strategies.
Social Motivation Impairment	Innate, biologically based attenuation of responsiveness to social stimuli and motivation for social engagement is theorized to limit the child's early social experiences, which negatively impacts normal experience-expectant neurodevelopmental processes that underlie the emergence of a wide variety of social communicative behaviors that are known to be impaired in ASD (eg, face processing, joint attention, social information processing). – Failure to orient to social stimuli, such as human sounds, and to prefer human to nonhuman speech in infancy – Impaired face recognition, emotion recognition from faces and from voices, and matching facial and vocal expressions of emotions

Table 19.2. Major Neuropsychological Theories[133,167–169] *(continued)*	
Theory[a]	**Description**[a]
Social Cognition Impairment	Impairments in the capacity to represent and reason about the thoughts, beliefs, and emotional states of others
1. Theory of mind (ToM) deficit (mindblindness, mentalizing deficit)	Impaired ability to take the perspective of others and understand that other people have intentions, knowledge, and beliefs that may differ from their own. – Delays and deficiencies in developmental tasks such as understanding relationships between mental states (eg, seeing leads to knowing), knowing that people can have "false beliefs" and "beliefs about beliefs," recognizing faux pas, and understanding subtle and figurative aspects of speech such as idioms, irony, metaphor, and sarcasm – Necessary for developing the ability to identify other people's intentions based on their gestures, expressions, and speech and for understanding deception – The cognitive component of empathy
2. "Extreme male" empathizing-systemizing profile	Empathizing: Capacity to predict and respond to the behavior of agents (usually people) by inferring their mental states (ie, cognitive empathy or ToM) *and* to respond with an appropriate emotion (affective empathy). Systemizing: Capacity and drive to analyze or construct systems, which are governed by rules. Systemizing involves trying to identify the rules that govern the system to predict how that system will behave. In both males and females with ASD, there is a profile of relatively low empathizing (explaining social communication and interaction deficits) and high systemizing (explaining the narrow interests, repetitive behavior, and insistence on sameness)—a more extreme form of the typical male pattern.

Abbreviation: ASD, autism spectrum disorder.

[a]These theories and features are overlapping, not mutually exclusive.

process complex information and form a coherent global picture is very helpful for understanding the behavior of children with ASD and explaining it to parents and teachers.

Associated Impairments

In addition to the core impairments that define ASD and its neuropsychological characteristics, there are other common medical and behavioral features that impact clinical presentation and management.

– Motor Impairments

In addition to motor stereotypies, children with ASD often exhibit less distinctive motor abnormalities, including impairment in basic aspects of motor coordination (eg, postural control, gait, attainment of gross and fine motor skills), performance of skilled motor gestures (dyspraxia), and motor learning activities.[172–174] A core feature of motor dysfunction in ASD seems to be excessive reliance on proprioceptive feedback and weak integration of visual feedback.[174] Clinically, parents may be concerned about delayed attainment of motor milestones, clumsiness, toe-walking, or difficulty with handwriting. Neurological examination may reveal hypotonia, decreased postural stability, poor motor imitation abilities, and other subtle, neurological signs, such as slow speed, dysrhythmia, and increased overflow movements on timed movements of the hands and feet and stressed gait maneuvers. Tic disorders, including Tourette disorder, also occur with increased frequency in children with ASD and in their siblings.[175–177]

– Epilepsy

ASD is associated with increased risk of epilepsy, with bimodal peaks in age of onset in early childhood and adolescence.[158,178] All seizure types occur in individuals with ASD, but complex partial seizures, with or without secondary generalization, are reported to be more common than primary generalized seizures.[178] The reported prevalence of epilepsy in ASD ranges widely, with the largest studies reporting ranges of 12.5% to 37% in clinic-based samples[157,179,180] and 6.6% to 22.5% in population-based samples.[181–183] In a large cross-sectional study combining 3 clinical samples and 1 population-based sample (n=5,815), the best estimate of the cumulative prevalence of epilepsy in ASD through age 17 years was 26%.[157]

The most robust risk factors for epilepsy in children and adolescents with ASD are low IQ and older age.[158,178,184] Although the prevalence is highest in individuals with severe ID and those with identified genetic etiologies, even the subgroup with idiopathic, high-functioning autism has a rate of epilepsy that is substantially higher than the rate in the general population.[178] The rate of medically refractory epilepsy may be increased in this population as well.[185] In addition, many children with ASD have interictal epileptiform activity on EEG, especially during sleep, even though they have not had definite clinical seizures.[178,186] The clinical significance of the increased rate of interictal EEG abnormalities is unclear, however, and very little information has been published to support the idea that epilepsy or epileptiform EEG abnormalities cause ASD or have treatment implications.[158,178,186,187]

– Neurobehavioral Symptoms/Coexisting Psychiatric Disorders

Neurobehavioral features that are commonly associated with ASD and cause significant impairment and distress include irritability, anger outbursts, aggression, self-injurious behavior, property destruction, elopement or wandering, sleep disturbance, mood instability, anxiety, hyperactivity, impulsivity, inattention, and other disruptive behaviors or manifestations of emotional dysregulation. Although these problem behaviors are not core features of ASD, they commonly interfere with functioning in school, at home, and in the community, and they contribute substantially to the burden on families.[188–194] In some cases, the diagnosis of a coexisting psychiatric disorder can be reasonably made, although modifications of the diagnostic criteria may be necessary when there is significant intellectual impairment. Psychiatric diagnoses reported to co-occur with ASD in children and adults include attention-deficit/hyperactivity disorder (ADHD) (28%–44%), anxiety (42%–56%), depression (12%–70%), psychotic disorders (12%–17%), tic disorders (14%–38%), and oppositional defiant disorder (16%–28%).[194]

Sleep problems are reported in 40% to 80% of children with ASD (versus 25%–40% of typical controls), and they are common at all ages and levels of intellectual ability.[195]

Sleep disturbances are burdensome to children with ASD and their family members due to their prevalence, chronicity, and impact on emotional and behavioral problems. Insufficient sleep is associated with exacerbation of core ASD symptoms (RRBs and social communication and interaction difficulties) as well as tantrums, self-injurious behavior, aggression, and other disruptive behaviors.[195] Children with ASD experience a variety of sleep problems, including bedtime resistance, prolonged sleep-onset latency, decreased sleep efficiency, increased waking after sleep onset, reduced total sleep time, and daytime sleepiness.[195,196] Behavioral factors, including inadequate sleep hygiene, maladaptive sleep-onset associations (eg, being held until asleep), and problems with limit-setting, are common, but ASD-associated melatonin or GABA abnormalities, coexisting neurological or psychiatric disorders (eg, epilepsy, ADHD, and anxiety), other medical problems (eg, gastroesophageal reflux), and adverse effects of medications may also contribute to disordered sleep.[195,196] Occasionally, other sleep disorders, such as obstructive sleep apnea, parasomnias, and periodic limb movements of sleep, are identified.

– Gastrointestinal and Feeding Problems

A meta-analysis of 15 methodologically suitable studies involving 2,215 children indicated that children with ASD experience significantly more general gastrointestinal (GI) symptoms, diarrhea, constipation, and abdominal pain than comparison groups.[197] The available data were not sufficient to determine whether symptoms often suggestive of organic GI pathology, such as gastroesophageal reflux, gastroenteritis, inflammatory bowel disease, or food allergies, occur more frequently in children with ASD than in controls, and there is no evidence suggesting a unique GI pathophysiology in ASD.[197,198] The contribution of behavioral factors such as delayed bowel training, rigidity about toileting routine, sensorimotor issues, and food selectivity to the observed higher prevalence of symptoms in children with ASD is unclear but plausibly substantial.[197]

These symptoms may impact behavior substantially. For example, in a well-characterized sample of children who participated in 2 Research Units on Pediatric Psychopharmacology Autism Network medication trials, the subgroup of children with GI problems (23%) had greater symptom severity on measures of irritability, anxiety, and social withdrawal than those without GI problems, and their irritability was less likely to respond to treatment with risperidone.[199] GI problems may not be obvious in some children with ASD due to communication deficits and/or under-responsivity to sensory input but should be considered in cases of unexplained irritability/agitation, food refusal, self-injury, aggression, sleep disturbance, or other problem behavior that is new or represents a significant exacerbation of baseline status.[197,198]

Feeding problems, including food selectivity (often based on texture, color, or temperature), rituals around food presentation, and compulsive eating of certain foods, are common, as are behaviors associated with food refusal (eg, holding food in the mouth, volitional gagging, emesis), rumination, and pica.[200–202]

Identification

Surveillance and Screening

Surveillance is the ongoing process of actively identifying children who may be at risk for developmental disorders, and screening is the use of standardized tools at specific intervals to support and refine risk. The American Academy of Pediatrics (AAP) has established guidelines for developmental surveillance and screening (see Chapter 9, Developmental and Behavioral Surveillance and Screening Within the Medical Home).[203] Surveillance is a continuous process that should occur at every preventive care visit during childhood and include the following components: eliciting and attending to the parents' concerns, maintaining a developmental history, making accurate and informed observations of the child, identifying the presence of risk factors and protective factors, and documenting the process and findings.[203]

The AAP recommends general developmental screening using a broadband measure for all children at ages 9, 18, and 24 to 30 months or at any time concerns are raised by a caregiver or primary pediatric health care professional.[203] In addition, specific screening for ASD is recommended at the 18- and 24-month visits and whenever parents' concerns are raised or other risk factors are identified through general developmental surveillance and screening.[138] The 2007 recommendation for universal screening for ASD in toddlers was based on the recognition that symptoms can be observed in very young children and mounting evidence that early identification leads to early intervention and improved outcomes.[138,204] The US Preventive Services Task Force (USPSTF) completed a literature review and concluded that the current evidence is insufficient to assess the balance of benefits and harms of screening for ASD in young children (ages 18–30 months) for whom no concerns of ASD have been raised.[205] This is not a recommendation against universal screening in this age group, but it is also not a recommendation for the practice. The AAP has affirmed its recommendation for universal screening for ASD at the ages of 18 and 24 months, and several strong commentaries have supported the approach and criticized aspects of the USPSTF interpretation of the data.[206–209]

A variety of general developmental (broadband), language-specific, and autism-specific screening tools have been shown to identify children of different ages who are at risk for ASD. Some examples of parent-completed screening measures that may be appropriate for use in primary care are described in Table 19.3. The Infant-Toddler Checklist, which is part of the Communication and Symbolic Behavior Scales Developmental Profile, is a screen for communication deficits in 6- to 24-month-olds that has been shown to identify ASD, language delay, and other developmental delay at age 12 months.[210] The Modified Checklist for Autism in Toddlers, Revised, with Follow-Up (M-CHAT-R/F) is the most commonly used tool for screening toddlers for ASD. It consists of a 20-question caregiver form as the first stage and, when the score is elevated, a brief, structured interview administered by a health care professional. Among children who fail the M-CHAT-R/F in community primary care settings, 50% are ultimately diagnosed with

Table 19.3. Examples of Parent/Caregiver-Completed Screening and Assessment Instruments		
	Age Range	**Time to Complete (min)**
Screening Instruments (potentially appropriate for use in unselected populations)		
Infant-Toddler Checklist (ITC)[a]	9–24 mo	5–10
Modified Checklist for Autism in Toddlers (M-CHAT-R/F)[b]	16–30 mo	5
Parent's Observations of Social Interactions (POSI)[c]	18–35 mo	5
Pervasive Developmental Disorders Screening Test-II Primary Care Screener (PDDST-II PCS)	18–48 mo	10–15
Autism Spectrum Quotient-Children's Version (AQ-Child)	4–11 y	10
Childhood Autism Spectrum Test (CAST)	4–11 y	10
Social Communication Questionnaire (SCQ)	4–18 y	10–15
Autism Spectrum Screening Questionnaire (ASSQ)	6–17 y	10
Assessment Instruments (commonly used in diagnostic evaluations and for monitoring purposes)		
Autism Spectrum Rating Scales (ASRS)	2–18 y	15–20
Children's Communication Checklist (CCC-2)	4–16 y	5–10
Gilliam Autism Rating Scale (GARS-3)	3–22 y	10
Social Responsiveness Scale (SRS-2)	2.5–99 y	15–20

[a] The ITC is part of the Communication and Symbolic Behavior Scales Developmental Profile (CSBS-DP).
[b] The original M-CHAT is a parent/caregiver form. The M-CHAT, Revised, with Follow-Up (M-CHAT-R/F) includes a caregiver form as the first stage and, in some cases, a structured survey administered by a health care professional.
[c] The POSI is part of a comprehensive primary care screening instrument, the Survey of Wellbeing of Young Children (SWYC).

ASD and 98% have an actionable developmental concern.[207,211] If a screening test is positive ("failed"), suggesting risk of ASD, the child should be simultaneously referred to the early intervention program or school evaluation team for services and to a specialist or team for comprehensive diagnostic evaluation.[138] Audiological evaluation is often warranted, particularly in a young child with delayed receptive and expressive language development.

Diagnostic Evaluation

The diagnostic evaluation will vary depending on the availability of local resources and clinician preferences. An interdisciplinary team specializing in ASD and other developmental disabilities may be ideal, but often these are not available outside of major medical centers, and waiting lists may be very long because of high demand. Many communities will have at least one expert who is capable of interpreting and integrating information from various disciplines and comfortable with making the diagnosis of ASD even if there is not an interdisciplinary team that meets in person. This may be a developmental-behavioral or neurodevelopmental pediatrician, child and adolescent psychiatrist, pediatric neurologist, or pediatric psychologist, for example.

The clinical standard of care for ASD diagnosis is expert clinician evaluation and application of the current *DSM* or *ICD* criteria (*DSM-5, ICD-10; ICD-11* [2018]). There is considerable overlap in symptoms among developmental and behavioral diagnoses, especially in very young children and those with ID or language impairment, and it is important for the diagnostician to consider the alternate explanations for observed symptoms. Standardized rating scales, such as the assessment instruments presented in Table 19.3, which are completed by parents, teachers, or other intervention professionals, may be used to gather and quantify information. In the hands of trained clinicians, diagnostic instruments such as those presented in Table 19.4 help to operationalize the *diagnostic* criteria and inform clinical judgment.[138,212,213]

Table 19.4. Diagnostic Evaluation Tools	
Instrument	**Format**
Autism Diagnostic Interview—Revised (ADI-R)	Structured caregiver interview
Diagnostic Interview for Social and Communication Disorders (DISCO)	Structured caregiver interview
Autism Diagnostic Observation Schedule (ADOS)	Semi-structured direct observation/elicitation
Childhood Autism Rating Scale (CARS)	Combination interview and unstructured observation/elicitation

The diagnostic evaluation should ideally incorporate the following elements[138,212–214]:

1. **Caregiver interview.** This includes a thorough developmental and behavioral history (including milestone attainment and report of current abilities), medical history, social history, and family history (at least 3 generations). Structured interview tools (eg, Autism Diagnostic Interview-Revised, Diagnostic Interview for Social and Communication Disorders) are informative but are often impractical in clinical settings because of time constraints. Standardized rating scales completed by parents/caregivers and teachers or other professionals, such as the assessment instruments described in Table 19.3, are commonly used to quantify ASD symptoms and compare them to normative populations.

2. **Review of pertinent existing data.** The pertinent medical and educational records should be reviewed, especially any available standardized testing completed by psychologists, speech-language pathologists, occupational therapists, early intervention evaluators, or others. Although not necessary for categorical diagnosis, it is helpful to note the results of any previous etiologic investigations and other pertinent tests that have been completed (eg, genetic testing, audiometry, central nervous system imaging).

3. **Direct clinical assessment.** This includes standardized developmental and psychological testing (appropriate for age and level of ability) and neurobehavioral observation/elicitation. Receptive and expressive language, nonverbal intellectual ability, and functional adaptive behavior should be measured. Administration of standardized ASD-specific direct observation/elicitation instruments (eg, Autism Diagnostic

Observation Schedule, Childhood Autism Rating Scale) is desirable. When the evaluating diagnostician is a physician or advanced care practitioner, physical examination targeting the neurological examination and evaluation for dysmorphic features and other clues to etiology should be included.

4. **Integration of information and determination of *DSM-5* (or *ICD-10/11*) categorical diagnoses.** Clinical judgment is informed by the caregiver interview and direct clinical assessment, often including information from ASD-specific diagnostic instruments and by input from other sources (eg, narrative reports or standardized rating scales completed by a teacher, paraprofessional aide, or therapist).

The goal should not be to simply decide whether the child has ASD or not but to determine the child's developmental diagnoses, whatever they may be, and the diagnostic summary should include domain-specific information regarding the child's level of functioning/severity of impairment.[212,213] Children who have been diagnosed with ASD also require periodic formal reevaluation because their strengths, weaknesses, and educational needs often change even if the ASD diagnosis does not.[212]

Management

The role of primary pediatric health care professionals does not end with diagnosis. Comprehensive management of patients after the diagnosis of ASD includes conducting an etiologic investigation; providing genetic counseling; promoting general health and well-being through effective longitudinal health care within a medical home; guiding families to effective educational, behavioral, and medical interventions; and alleviating family distress by providing support, education, and access to resources.[214,215] Primary pediatric health care professionals may take part in any or all of these duties in addition to making referrals and coordinating subspecialty care and other services.

Etiologic Evaluation

Currently, there is no single consensus approach to etiologic evaluation for children newly diagnosed with ASD. In recent years the availability of new methods of genetic testing has progressed so rapidly that the publication of state-of-the-art guidelines by professional organizations lags behind. Therefore, the recommendations in this chapter reflect the authors' assessment of the current literature rather than strict adherence to guidelines published previously by various professional organizations.

– Genetic Testing

Identifying a genetic etiologic diagnosis may allow clinicians to provide more accurate prognostication and recurrence risk counseling, identify and treat or prevent medical comorbidities, guide patients and families to condition-specific resources and supports, and, in some cases, refine treatment options.[216–224] For these reasons, there is consensus agreement that a genetic evaluation should be offered to every person with ASD.[225–228] However, surveys suggest that that only about 33% of children with ASD in the United States have undergone any genetic testing.[229–233]

Chromosomal Microarray Analysis and Next-Generation Sequencing

CMA reveals a definitively pathogenic CNV in 5% to 14% (median 9%) of individuals with ASD in clinical cohorts.[46,234–242] These numbers do not reflect variants of uncertain significance, many of which are likely to subsequently be determined to be pathogenic; when variants of uncertain significance are included, the reported CNV detection rate in these studies is 17% to 24%. Large, clinical whole exome sequencing studies have consistently identified a molecular diagnosis in 26% to 29% of individuals for whom neurodevelopmental disorders were the primary indication for testing.[243–245] Studies restricted to clinically ascertained samples of patients with ASD and analyses of ASD subgroups within the large, laboratory-based samples have reported WES yields of 8% to 20%.[46,48,245] There is emerging evidence that WES is not only diagnostically useful but also cost-efficient in the etiologic evaluation of children with neurodevelopmental disorders, including ASD.[246–249]

Fragile X Testing

The combined yield of fragile X testing in 6 recent large studies was 9 full mutations in 1,984 individuals tested (0.45%), and 22% of those found to have fragile X syndrome were female.[237,238,241,250–252] Because males and females with fragile X syndrome are identified fairly frequently in ASD cohorts, testing is relatively inexpensive, and the condition has important genetic counseling implications due to always being inherited, it is reasonable to routinely test both males and females with ASD for fragile X syndrome, at least until more data become available to clarify the issue. DNA testing for fragile X syndrome is ordered as a separate test because pathogenic repeat expansions such as the CGG trinucleotide repeat expansion that is responsible for fragile X syndrome are not detected on CMA or WES.

Approach to the Genetic Etiologic Evaluation

When the diagnosis of ASD is made by a physician or a diagnostic team that includes a physician, the physician may also take responsibility for the etiologic evaluation. If the diagnosis is made by a psychologist or by a physician who does not provide this service, referral to a medical geneticist is appropriate. In some cases, the primary pediatric health care professional may take on this role. In any case, clinicians should only order tests that they are capable of explaining (ie, providing pretest counseling and obtaining informed consent) and interpreting, although full interpretation of abnormal or equivocal results may involve referral to an appropriate subspecialist (eg, a medical geneticist). Pretest counseling involves describing the nature of the test, including potential outcomes, and addressing points such as possible impact on other family members. Most pediatric subspecialists who diagnose ASD, and many general pediatricians, are comfortable with explaining, ordering, and interpreting fragile X testing and CMA. WES is typically ordered by a medical geneticist or, in some cases, another pediatric subspecialist with the appropriate expertise, and a genetic counselor is likely to be involved in the vast majority of cases.

An etiologic search begins with a careful medical and family history and physical examination. Important aspects of the physical examination include assessment for abnormal growth (including head circumference), major and minor congenital anomalies, evidence of visceral storage, skin manifestations of neurocutaneous disorders or mosaicism, and neurological abnormalities.[228] When a specific syndrome or metabolic disorder is suspected, the next step is to proceed with the appropriate targeted testing or refer to medical genetics. For example, a child presenting with ASD and micro-cephaly, ptosis, anteverted nares, and cutaneous 2–3 toe syndactyly should have a 7-dehydrocholesterol level measured to test for Smith-Lemli-Opitz syndrome. Similarly, marked macrocephaly and pigmented macules on the glans penis in a child diagnosed with ASD would warrant *PTEN* sequencing and deletion/duplication analysis. If there is no strong suspicion of a particular diagnosis or testing for suspected diagnoses has been completed and is negative, CMA and fragile X DNA analysis are recommended. If these are unrevealing, clinical WES is recommended. These steps are outlined in Box 19.6.

Box 19.6. Genetic/Genomic Etiologic Investigation in Patients With Autism Spectrum Disorder

1. History, including 3-generation family history, and physical examination
   — If a specific syndrome diagnosis or metabolic disorder is suspected, proceed with targeted testing.
   — Otherwise, proceed to step 2.
2. Whole-genome chromosomal microarray analysis (CMA) and fragile X analysis
   — If these studies do not reveal the etiology, proceed to step 3.
3. Whole exome sequencing (WES)

Genomic testing technology is evolving rapidly and the current recommendations about methods of testing for mutations will surely have to change with these technological advances. For example, it is anticipated that steps 2 and 3 in Box 19.6 will be combined due to improvements in accurate identification of CNVs using exome or genome sequence data and that sequencing of the exome will be replaced by sequencing of the entire genome as the issues with interpretation and cost become more manageable.[46,253]

– Metabolic Testing

There is genetic and biochemical evidence implicating a wide variety of metabolic disorders, including mitochondrial disorders, in the pathogenesis of ASD in a small subset of children.[229,253–259] Several studies have suggested that the yield of routine metabolic testing in patients with ASD is very low.[228,254,260–263] For example, Campistol[263] found no biochemical evidence of a metabolic disorder in any of 406 patients with nonsyndromic ASD (ages 3–22 years) whose urine samples were analyzed for evidence of cerebral creatine deficiency syndromes, purine and pyrimidine disorders, amino acid metabolism defects, mucopolysaccharidoses, and organic acidurias. However, large population-based studies are lacking, so accurate prevalence and diagnostic yield esti-mates are not available.

Although metabolic disorders are uncommon causes of ASD, the potential impact is high because of potential treatment and high recurrence risk.[228,256,264] Metabolic disor-ders associated with ASD phenotype are most commonly autosomal recessive disorders that present early in life with symptoms such as acute or intermittent decompensation and neurodevelopmental regression, lethargy, seizures, extrapyramidal movement disorders, severe hypotonia, ataxia, oculomotor abnormalities, ptosis, hearing loss, cyclic vomiting, failure to thrive, and multisystem organ dysfunction (eg, cardiac, hepatic, and renal).[228,255,265] At this time, based on the available evidence, no metabolic tests are routinely recommended for all children with ASD.[228] However, clinical findings such as these should raise the level of suspicion of an inborn error of metabolism.

– Neuroimaging

The published research to date has not demonstrated that any specific clinical neuroimaging findings are more prevalent in ASD than in other neurodevelopmental disorders or that any specific abnormalities are correlated with clinical, etiologic, or pathophysiological aspects of the disorder.[266-270] For example, Vasa and colleagues[268] found that the prevalence of brain MRI abnormalities in 7- to 13-year-olds with ASD and full scale IQ of 80 or higher (11%) was not different from that of typically developing controls (11%) or children with ADHD (12%), and that no neuroradiological findings were preferentially associated with ASD. The abnormalities detected in this study did not constitute etiologic diagnoses and would not be expected to affect clinical care. A study comparing children with ASD and ID (mean IQ 50) to children with nonsyndromic ID (mean IQ 52) and typically developing children (mean IQ 106) found higher rates of MRI abnormalities (44%, 54%, and 22%, respectively), but the abnormalities were not specific to either ASD or ID.[270] Although some of the MRI abnormalities, such as hypoplastic corpus callosum and mega cisterna magna, were considered to be markers of atypical brain development, they were minor and not etiologic or clinically actionable findings.

Although neuroimaging research has identified volumetric and other abnormalities in groups of patients with ASD relative to controls, reliable markers for diagnosis or clinical subtyping have not been identified, and currently evidence is insufficient to recommend routine clinical neuroimaging for all individuals with ASD. However, MRI of the brain should be considered for a subset of children with ASD based on features such as focal seizures or intractable epilepsy, neurocutaneous findings, significantly abnormal neurological examination (eg, cranial nerve abnormalities, spasticity, rigidity, ataxia), unexplained microcephaly, or history of neurodevelopmental regression.[138,228,271-273]

– Electroencephalography

Although discussed here within the Approach to the Genetic Etiologic Evaluation section, very little information has been published to support the idea that epilepsy or epileptiform EEG abnormalities cause ASD.[158,178,186,187,274] Therefore, when a clinical EEG is undertaken in a child with ASD, it is typically not truly an etiologic study but an evaluation for evidence of a coexisting condition (ie, epilepsy).

Based on the available evidence, an EEG is not routinely indicated for all children with ASD but is recommended when seizures are suspected clinically.[158,178,187,271] However, evidence suggests that even when children with ASD are evaluated for episodes of staring and reduced responsiveness, the yield of significant interictal EEG findings on routine EEG is low.[275] Hughes et al[275] found interictal epileptiform abnormalities on routine EEG in 13% of 92 children with ASD and episodes of staring, but only 3% were considered to be potentially clinically significant in the context of the presenting problem. In this series, no children had absence or focal dyscognitive (partial complex) seizures confirmed on EEG, and the authors recommended judicious use of EEG when evaluating children with ASD and staring episodes.[275] Although the evidence is mixed, many authorities consider unexplained developmental regression, especially involving language, to warrant a sleep-deprived EEG with appropriate sampling of slow-wave sleep, preferably an overnight study.[158,271,276]

Primary pediatric health care professionals should discuss the increased risk and the signs and symptoms of seizures with the families of children diagnosed with ASD, maintain a high index of clinical suspicion for seizures, and obtain an EEG and/or refer to a pediatric neurologist when concerned about the possibility of seizures.[158,178,187]

Genetic Counseling and Recurrence Risk

The parents of a child with ASD should be counseled regarding recurrence risk in subsequent pregnancies. When a specific genetic etiology has been determined, the family can be provided with accurate information about the risk of recurrence in each subsequent pregnancy. For example, the chance of each subsequent child having the mutation may range from as high as 50% in the case of an inherited maternally derived chromosome 15q11-q13 interstitial duplication to 25% in the case of an autosomal recessive disorder such as Smith-Lemli-Opitz syndrome to the baseline population rate of approximately 1.5% if the affected child has a de novo pathogenic CNV or SNV. These numbers reflect the chance of the child having the mutation, but the penetrance and exact phenotypic expression may vary.

When the etiology is unknown because genetic testing did not identify a causal variant or has not yet been completed, recurrence risk counseling is based on group averages derived from the existing literature. Published recurrence risk rates for full siblings of a child with ASD range from 4% to almost 19%.[277-286] Very large studies in Sweden, Denmark, and Finland have found recurrence rates in full siblings ranging from 9% to 13%.[284-286] The highest reported recurrence risk, 18.7%, was from a large, prospective study of younger siblings of children with ASD who were recruited in infancy and monitored closely[283]; however, when families that already had 2 or more children with ASD (multiplex families) were excluded, the recurrence rate was 13.5% in this study. Studies that recruit families with one or more children with ASD and include in the analysis all siblings born before and after the index case have reported ASD recurrence rates of 6% to 10%,[279-281] but they also may underestimate recurrence risk due to stop-page effect. Studies that include only families with later-born siblings to avoid the stop-page effect have reported higher recurrence rates of 8.6% to 18.7%.[277,282,283] Regardless of whether the analyses are restricted to later-born siblings, studies of families with at least one affected child are at risk for bias introduced by increased parental awareness and differential participation.

Overall, for a couple with one child with ASD of unknown cause, the current best estimate of recurrence in a subsequent child is approximately 10% based on information from a variety of study designs. If a couple already has 2 or more children with idiopathic ASD, the chance of a subsequent child having ASD may be as high as 32% to 36%.[277,283,287] Because of the increased risk of ASD, all younger siblings of an affected child should be monitored through routine administration of ASD screening tools to facilitate early identification and intervention. However, the risk is not limited to ASD. A large Finnish epidemiological study found that among siblings of a child with ASD, the prevalence of ASD was 10.5%, but the risk of tic disorders, ADHD, ID, learning or coordination disorders, conduct or oppositional disorders, and childhood-onset emotional disorders was also increased, and a total of 29.7% of these siblings had some type of childhood-onset neurodevelopmental or psychiatric disorder (versus 11.6% of controls, adjusted risk ratio 3.0).[286] Other studies have suggested that 20% to 25% of siblings who do not meet criteria for ASD do have a history of language impairment or delay.[283,288] For this reason, it has been suggested that recurrence risk counseling should address not only the chance of recurrence of ASD but also the broader risk of neurodevelopmental and psychiatric disorders.[289]

Evidence-Based Educational, Developmental, and Behavioral Interventions

Treatment goals include remediating or minimizing the core deficits (social communication and interaction impairment and restricted, repetitive behavioral repertoire) and associated deficits; maximizing functional independence by facilitating skill development; and eliminating or minimizing aberrant, maladaptive behaviors that interfere with functioning (Box 19.7).[290-294] Nonpharmacological, psychosocial interventions such as behavioral, developmental, and educational interventions are the primary means of achieving these goals. Although most primary pediatric health care professionals are not experts on interventions for ASD, they are often in a position in their role in the patient-centered medical home to make referrals, provide resources, guide families to empirically supported interventions, participate in the development of comprehensive care plans, and communicate with educators and other service providers about treatment plans and progress.[215,290]

A wide variety of methods have been used in intervention programs for children and adolescents with ASD. All interventions, including behavioral and developmental interventions, traditional habilitative therapies, and educational practices, should be based on sound theoretical constructs, rigorous methodologies, and objective scientific evidence of effectiveness. In addition to randomized controlled trials, experimental methods such as single-subject experimental designs and quasi-experimental group comparisons contribute to the scientific evidence of effectiveness.[291,292,295-298] The vast majority of studies of psychosocial interventions for ASD focus on children between

Box 19.7. Targets of Autism Spectrum Disorder Intervention[291–294]

---

1. Building developmentally appropriate skills

- ▶ Learning readiness skills (not directly related to task content)
- ▶ Verbal and nonverbal communication
- ▶ Interpersonal social skills needed to interact with others
- ▶ Higher cognitive functions
- ▶ Motor skills (fine motor, gross motor, visual-motor coordination)
- ▶ Play and leisure skills
- ▶ Preacademic, academic, and vocational/employment preparation skills
- ▶ Personal responsibility/self-care skills needed for functional independence
- ▶ Self-regulation/management of one's own behaviors to meet a goal

2. Reducing maladaptive behavior

- ▶ General symptoms (directly associated with autism spectrum disorder or related psychoeducational needs)
- ▶ Problem behaviors that can harm the individual or others, result in property damage, or interfere with learning and expected routines in the community
- ▶ Restricted, repetitive, nonfunctional patterns of behavior, interest, or activity
- ▶ Difficulties with sensory and emotional regulation (ability to flexibly modify one's level of arousal or response to function effectively in the environment)

---

the ages of 3 and 12 years, and the evidence base is strongest for this age range.[291–293] Few studies have rigorously assessed intervention approaches for adolescents or adults with ASD, so the available evidence of efficacy is limited.[291,299–305]

In recent years, the volume, theoretical range, and scientific rigor of published intervention studies has increased substantially.[291–293,303,306,307] Several large-scale, systematic literature reviews have assessed the evidence base using specific, valid, predetermined criteria to determine effectiveness. Interventions that were found to meet criteria for "evidence-based" (National Professional Development Center criteria)[292,293] or "established" (National Standards Project criteria)[291] are presented in Table 19.5. Although not a cure, these interventions have been shown to facilitate development of important cognitive, adaptive, behavior regulation, and social communication and interaction skills in children with ASD.

The ASD intervention literature reflects substantial variation in underlying theoretical principles (eg, behavior analytical, developmental social-pragmatic, combined), study design (eg, randomized controlled trials, within-subject experimental designs), and practice elements such as scope (focused/targeted, comprehensive), delivery modality (eg, individual versus group/classroom, delivered by professional versus trained parent), and specific intervention targets.[291,306,307] For example, comprehensive treatment models (CTMs) are a set of theory-driven practices designed to achieve a broad impact on the core deficits of ASD and associated impairments,[308,309] whereas focused intervention

Table 19.5. Empirically Supported Interventions for Autism Spectrum Disorder: Two Large-Scale Systematic Reviews Employing Strictly Defined Evaluation Criteria[a]

	National Professional Development Center on Autism Spectrum Disorder	National Standards Project
Reference(s)	Wong et al (2014)[292,b] and Wong et al (2015)[293,b]	National Autism Center (2015)[291]
Publication Years	1990–2011	1957–2007 (Phase 1), 2007–2012 (Phase 2)
Age Range	<22 y	<22 y	≥22 y
Designation	Evidence-based practice	Established	Established
Interventions	Antecedent-based intervention Cognitive behavioral intervention Differential reinforcement of alternative, incompatible, or other behavior Discrete trial training/teaching Exercise Extinction Functional behavior assessment Functional communication training Modeling Naturalistic intervention Parent-implemented intervention Peer-mediated instruction and intervention Picture Exchange Communication System Pivotal response training Prompting Reinforcement Response interruption/redirection Scripting Self-management Social narratives Social skills training Structured play group Task analysis Technology-aided instruction and intervention Time delay Video modeling Visual support	Behavioral interventions Cognitive behavioral intervention package Comprehensive behavioral treatment for young children Language training (production) Modeling Natural teaching strategies Parent training Peer training package Pivotal response training Schedules Scripting Self-management Social skills package Story-based intervention	Behavioral interventions

[a] These reviews included studies with experimental group designs and studies with single-subject research designs

[b] Wong et al (2014)[292] and Wong et al (2015)[293] included only focused interventions, not comprehensive treatment models.

practices are designed to address a single or limited number of key skills or behavioral goals.[292,293,306,308] These practices are operationally defined, address specific outcomes, and are delivered over a shorter time than CTMs to achieve the specific goals. In many cases, these focused interventions are important components of the comprehensive models. A focused intervention may address a core component of ASD, such as increasing social communication or decreasing ritualistic behavior, or may focus on building functional, adaptive skills such as personal hygiene tasks or compliance with medical and dental procedures. Alternatively, the primary goal may be to decrease an undesired behavior such as aggression or property destruction. However, even when reduction of problem behavior is the primary goal, interventions include a skill-building component to increase appropriate alternative behaviors/skills. Some focused intervention practices, especially those appropriate for school-aged children, are provided as outpatient therapies delivered individually (eg, cognitive behavioral therapy [CBT]) or in groups (eg, social skills training) and have been evaluated in recent years using group design studies. For example, there is strong evidence from randomized controlled trials supporting the use of CBT for anxiety symptoms in school-aged children with ASD who have average to above average IQ.[291–293,303,310]

The 2 predominant theoretical approaches to ASD intervention, particularly for young children, are applied behavior analysis (ABA) and developmental social-pragmatic (DSP) models.[294,306,311,312] Although there are important distinctions, some of which are outlined in Table 19.6, there is also significant overlap. Intervention models for very young children, for example, have increasingly incorporated developmental orientations and naturalistic behavioral approaches.[294,313,319] Some empirically supported models explicitly integrate ABA and DSP elements and have been referred to as *naturalistic developmental behavioral interventions* (NDBI).[294,306] Treatment and Education of Autistic and Related Communication-Handicapped Children (TEACCH) is a widely adopted, structured teaching intervention that does not fit within the ABA, DSP, or NDBI classifications (Table 19.6).[308,309,314,315,320]

– Applied Behavior Analysis and Naturalistic Developmental Behavioral Interventions

ABA and NDBI approaches are described in Table 19.6. There is a vast literature demonstrating the efficacy of focused ABA interventions for a wide variety of outcomes from all of the skill-building and maladaptive behavior reduction categories described in Box 19.7, and most of the empirically supported interventions identified by the systematic reviews summarized in Table 19.5 are interventions that are fundamental ABA techniques (antecedent-based intervention, reinforcement, prompting, modeling, scripting, and extinction), assessment and analytic techniques that are the basis for ABA interventions (functional behavior assessment and task analysis), or combinations of primarily behavioral practices packaged for systematic use as a replicable procedure (discrete trial training, functional communication training, and pivotal response training).[291–294,306] For example, individually delivered, focused ABA interventions such as pivotal response training and the Picture Exchange Communication System (PECS) are effective for spoken communication and alternative and augmentative

Table 19.6. Common Intervention Methods[294,306,309,313–318]

General Category[a]	Examples	Comments
Applied Behavior Analysis (ABA)	Antecedent-based interventions, applied verbal behavior-based approaches, chaining procedures, differential reinforcement procedures, discrete trial training, errorless teaching, extinction procedures, functional analysis, functional behavior assessment, functional communication training, incidental teaching, modeling procedures including video modeling, natural environment teaching (or naturalistic teaching approaches), pivotal response training, positive behavioral support, various prompting and prompt-fading procedures, respondent procedures (eg, systematic desensitization), scripting and script fading, shaping, task analysis, and many others Comprehensive models, such as the Lovaas Institute model, also known as *early and intensive behavioral intervention* (EIBI); UCLA Young Autism Project; comprehensive behavioral treatment for young children (CBTYC); Learning Experiences—An Alternative Programs for Preschoolers and Their Parents (LEAP)	The defining assumption of ABA is that most behavior is learned and controlled by contingencies within the environment, and application of ABA to the treatment of ASD is based on the view that deficits associated with ASD represent learning difficulties, and the behaviors exhibited are consistent with the laws of operant learning.[317] ABA interventions are empirically based practices that are built on operant conditioning procedures, and they include strategies ranging from highly structured, adult-directed approaches (eg, discrete trial training and verbal behavioral applications) to naturalistic teaching approaches that may be child-led and may be implemented in the context of play activities or daily routines and activities. Most of the empirically supported interventions identified by the systematic reviews summarized in Table 19.5 are interventions that are fundamental ABA techniques, assessment and analytical techniques that are the basis for ABA interventions (eg, functional behavior assessment, task analysis), or combinations of primarily behavior practices packaged for systematic use as a replicable procedure (eg, discrete trial training, functional communication training, pivotal response training). In addition to their importance in teaching and maintaining new skills and desirable behaviors, behavioral analytic methods are the primary treatment for problematic maladaptive behaviors such as self-injury and aggression.
Developmental Social-Pragmatic (DSP)	Denver model; Hanen; responsive interaction; responsive teaching; Relationship Development Intervention (RDI); Developmental, Individual Differences, Relationship-Based Approach/Floortime (DIR/Floortime); PLAY: Play and Language for Autistic Youngsters; Preschool Autism Communication Trial (PACT)	DSP models focus on increasing adult (ie, interventionist or parent/caregiver) responsiveness by imitating, expanding on, or joining into child-initiated play activities and on remediation of fundamental deficits in pivotal developmental skills such as joint attention, imitation, and affective social engagement, which are thought to affect the development of language, reciprocal social behavior, emotional relationships, and cognitive abilities such as theory of mind. DSP models have also been referred to as *developmental, transactional, interpersonal, child-oriented,* and *relationship-based.*

Table 19.6. Common Intervention Methods[294,306,309,313–318] (*continued*)

General Category[a]	Examples	Comments
Naturalistic Developmental Behavioral Intervention (NDBI; ABA + DSP components)	Early Achievements, Early Start Denver Model (ESDM), enhanced milieu teaching (EMT), Incidental Teaching (IT), Joint Attention Symbolic Play Engagement and Regulation (JASPER), pivotal response training (PRT), Project ImPACT (Improving Parents As Communication Teachers), reciprocal imitation training (RIT), Social Communication/Emotional Regulation/Transactional Supports (SCERTS)	Empirically supported subset of natural teaching strategies that incorporate developmental principles such as emphasis on developmentally based learning targets and foundational social learning skills, intervention in the context of naturally occurring social activities within natural environments, and use of child-initiated teaching episodes, natural contingencies, and turn-taking interactions within play routines (balanced turns) as well as ABA elements, including systematic use of adult prompts to promote new skills, delivery of contingent reinforcement, and ongoing data collection and analysis to address intervention goals that are socially significant. Schreibman et al[294] assert that evidence-based NDBIs are based upon well-established principles of ABA and, therefore, fall under the umbrella of ABA intervention.
Structured Teaching	Treatment and Education of Autistic and Related Communication-Handicapped Children (TEACCH) is a widely-adopted structured teaching intervention that does not fit within the ABA, DSP, or NDBI classifications.	The TEACCH approach to skill acquisition includes assessment-based curriculum development and an emphasis on structure, including predictable organization of activities and use of visual schedules, organization of the physical environment to optimize learning and avoid frustration (eg, minimizing distractions and/or sensory dysregulation), and adaptation and organization of materials and tasks to promote independence from adult directions or prompts.

[a] Categories are not mutually exclusive; in practice, there is significant overlap.

Abbreviation: ASD, autism spectrum disorder.

communication.[291–293,306,321–323] Focused ABA and NDBI (ABA plus DSP) interventions, such as pivotal response training, Joint Attention Symbolic Play Engagement and Regulation, reciprocal imitation training, and others, are effective for improving specific social communication outcomes such as joint attention, imitation, social engagement, and functional and symbolic play in young children with ASD, whether delivered individually by therapists or within classroom settings by teachers.[303,306,316,321,323,324]

Examples of well-known CTMs include clinic- or home-based ABA programs such as the Lovaas Institute model (often referred to as *early and intensive behavioral intervention* [EIBI], and in the National Standards Project Phase 2 as *comprehensive behavioral treatment for young children* [CBTYC]) and classroom-based ABA programs such as Learning Experiences—An Alternative Program for Preschoolers and Their Parents (LEAP). For young children with ASD, the efficacy of intensive (20–40 hours per week), individually delivered comprehensive ABA intervention (EIBI/CBTYC) for outcomes such as IQ, adaptive functioning, language, social skills, academic achievement, and play/leisure skills has been established by numerous individual studies and comprehensive systematic reviews and meta-analyses.[291–293,306,325–330] Although the Lovaas EIBI model is delivered individually by an interventionist, another ABA intervention model, LEAP, was specifically designed as a classroom intervention that blends ABA and common aspects of early childhood education and integrates children with ASD with typically developing peers.[331,332] A large, cluster randomized controlled trial involving 294 preschool children showed that LEAP was associated with improvement in socialization, cognition, language, and challenging behavior and was superior to a treatment-as-usual control group.[332] However, another large study with a quasi-experimental design demonstrated no significant differences in outcome among LEAP, TEACCH, and treatment as usual in non–model-specific special education classrooms; children in all 3 groups improved significantly during the school year.[315]

There is also substantial evidence supporting the Early Start Denver Model (ESDM), a comprehensive NDBI program for very young children with ASD that combines ABA strategies (especially pivotal response training) with relationship-based approaches (Denver Model) and targets all aspects of development, with a special focus on social reciprocity, affective engagement, and social attention and motivation.[333,334] In a randomized controlled trial involving 48 toddlers with ASD, 2 years of ESDM initiated at age 18–30 months was superior to treatment as usual in the community on measures of cognitive, language, social, and adaptive behavior.[333] A prospective follow-up study demonstrated that the gains associated with ESDM were maintained 2 years after the intervention ended, and core ASD symptoms improved relative to the control group.[335] Emerging evidence suggests that ESDM may be effective in a group/classroom delivery model.[336–338] However, in a multisite randomized controlled trial, a low-intensity ESDM parent training program (1 hour per week) initiated at ages 14 to 24 months was not superior to treatment as usual.[339]

Interventions based on the principles of ABA are generally acknowledged to have the most robust empirical support in the literature at this time.[291,293,303,306,340–343] However, there is large variation in outcomes across children, and the strength of the evidence supporting ABA-based interventions for children with ASD reported in systematic literature reviews and meta-analyses varies substantially depending on the evaluation criteria.[292,293,298,306,314] The vast majority of the evidence supporting the efficacy of ABA-based interventions comes from small studies that use within-subject experimental designs rather than randomized clinical trials. Therefore, reviews that include studies utilizing within-subject experimental designs generally conclude that there is strong evidence supporting ABA-based treatments,[291,292,306,329,330,344] whereas those that emphasize randomized clinical trials and exclude within-subject experimental analyses report low to moderate strength of evidence.[303,330,345]

– Developmental Social-Pragmatic Interventions and Structured Teaching

DSP and structured teaching (TEACCH) approaches are described in Table 19.6. The empirical support for DSP models (without a major ABA component) and structured teaching is far more limited than for ABA and NDBI interventions.[291–293,303,306,308,309,330,346,347] For example, Relationship Development Intervention and Developmental, Individual-Difference, Relationship-Based (DIR)/Floortime approaches lack evidence of efficacy from studies with strong experimental designs.[348–354] There is evidence supporting the efficacy of several models that involve training parents to deliver interventions, including DSP interventions. For example, Play and Language for Autistic Youngsters (commonly known as PLAY), a manualized approach based on DIR/Floortime, has been evaluated as an adjunct to community interventions in a randomized controlled trial of 112 preschoolers with ASD.[355] After the intervention, parents who received the instruction were less directive in their interactions and their children were rated as more socially responsive, although there were no differences between groups in IQ or language scores.

Stronger support comes from a well-designed study, the Preschool Autism Communication Trial (PACT), which evaluated a parent training program that consisted of twelve 2-hour therapy sessions over 6 months, followed by monthly support and extension sessions for another 6 months.[356] At the end of the intervention, children in the parent training group initiated communication more often than children in the treatment-as-usual control group, but there was only a small estimated group difference in ASD symptoms in favor of the PACT intervention and no significant difference in standardized measures of language (although parent ratings of language and social communication were significantly higher).[356] More impressively, follow-up 6 years after completion of the intervention revealed significant treatment effects on ASD symptom severity in both social-communication and repetitive behavior domains as well as child social communicative initiations.[357]

A meta-analysis of published studies evaluating TEACCH suggested beneficial effects of small magnitude on perceptual, motor, verbal, and cognitive skills.[314] Effects on adaptive behavior ratings, including communication skills, activities of daily living, and motor functioning were negligible to small. Improvements in social and maladaptive behavior were larger in terms of effect size but require further replication. The authors cautioned that although it provided limited support for the TEACCH program, their meta-analysis should be considered exploratory due to the small pool of studies available, small sample sizes, and methodological limitations complicating empirical assessment.[314]

– Traditional Habilitative Therapies

Children with ASD also commonly receive traditional habilitative therapies, especially speech-language therapy and occupational therapy.

Speech-language pathologists use a variety of treatment approaches, including many of the empirically supported focused intervention practices listed in Table 19.5. Developmental sequences and processes of language development provide a framework for determining appropriate intervention goals and priorities and matching the treatment with intervention goals that are appropriate for the child's developmental stage. A variety of communication modalities (eg, spoken language, gestures, sign language, picture communication, speech-generating devices, written language) may be utilized in a program that is individualized based on the child's abilities and the contexts of communication. In addition to providing direct intervention, speech-language pathologists should train, support, and collaborate with teachers, educational support staff, parents/caregivers, and the child's peers to increase communication in all settings.

Meta-analyses have demonstrated significant benefits of interventions to improve structural language and pragmatic language competence in children with ASD and suggest that larger effect sizes are obtained when a systematic parent training component is included.[358,359] There is also substantial evidence supporting the role of augmentative and alternative communication strategies, including PECS and speech-generating devices for establishing and advancing communication.[360–364]

Occupational therapy addresses fine motor deficits and associated adaptive deficits that interfere with attaining academic, self-care, or prevocational goals. Targets of therapy may include self-care skills (eg, dressing, manipulating fasteners, using utensils, personal hygiene) and academic skills (eg, cutting with scissors, writing).[290,365] Occupational therapists also may assist in promoting development of play skills, modifying classroom materials and routines to improve attention and organization, and providing prevocational training. However, ASD-specific research regarding the efficacy of traditional occupational therapy is lacking.

Sensory processing interventions, which can be divided into sensory-based interventions and sensory integration therapy, are also commonly delivered by occupational therapists to children with ASD.[366] Sensory integration therapies (SITs) are characterized as clinic-based interventions that use sensory-rich, child-directed activities to improve a child's adaptive responses to sensory experiences, whereas sensory-based interventions (SBIs) are classroom-based, adult-directed interventions that use single-sensory strategies, or combinations of strategies such as brushing, massage, swinging, bouncing on a therapy ball, or wearing a weighted vest, to improve behaviors attributed to sensory modulation disorders. Evidence of efficacy of SBI is lacking. Some positive effects of SIT have been observed in small randomized controlled trials, but rigorous trials using manualized protocols are needed. Overall, the efficacy of sensory interventions has not been objectively demonstrated.[366–369] The AAP has recommended that parents be informed that the research regarding the effectiveness of sensory processing interventions is limited and inconclusive.[369]

– Unestablished Interventions

The National Standards Project also identified some interventions as unestablished, meaning that there is insufficient evidence in the scientific literature to determine effectiveness or to rule out the possibility that they are harmful.[291] These interventions cannot be recommended at this time. In the case of facilitated communication, the intervention has been proven ineffective and potentially harmful.[370–372] Other psycho-social interventions that have been classified as unestablished include animal-assisted therapy, auditory integration training, concept mapping, DIR/Floortime, movement-based intervention, SENSE Theatre intervention, sensory intervention package, social behavioral learning strategy, social cognition intervention, and social thinking intervention.[291]

– Common Characteristics/Principles of Effective Intervention

Although there are differences, there are also common elements among empirically supported interventions, and it has been suggested that these "best practices" should routinely be included in treatment programs for children with ASD (Box 19.8).[290,294,306,307, 315,373–375] Treatment programs should be assessment based, individualized, and intensive, with a focus on achieving the competence in social communication, functional adaptive skills, and emotional and behavioral regulation necessary for independence. The most important evidence of effectiveness at the individual student level is the progress the student makes when the intervention is instituted, so it is very important for practitioners to implement the practice with fidelity, collect student performance data relevant to treatment goals, and use the data to evaluate and adjust intervention strategies.[292,293,376]

Early intervention and school-based programs can be built upon evidence-based focused intervention practices that are selected to meet the needs of groups and individual students. Odom and colleagues refer to this as a "technical eclectic approach" and describe programs using this approach as "evidence-supported" because evidence-based focused interventions are integral features; however, the efficacy of the program model as a whole has not been validated experimentally.[292,293,376,377] The National Professional Development Center on ASD developed a process to help professionals to systematically apply best practices for children with ASD using this approach.[293,378]

Medical Management

Children with ASD have the same basic health care needs as other children and benefit from the same health promotion and disease prevention activities, including immunizations. Some have additional health care needs related to associated medical problems,

Box 19.8. "Best Practices" in Autism Spectrum Disorder Treatment: Common Elements of Empirically Supported Autism Spectrum Disorder Interventions[290,294,306,307,315,373–375]

1. Systematic assessment of existing skills. Selection of individualized measurable goals and instructional procedures based on objective assessment of each child.

2. Use of assessment-based, empirically supported instructional methods (see Table 19.6) to build, generalize, and maintain skills and reduce problem behaviors. Inclusion of specific intervention content to address the impairments in social communication and restricted and repetitive behavioral repertoire.

3. Individualization of services and supports. Use of the child's interests and preferences in determining reinforcement systems and incorporation of preferred activities to increase engagement in activities. A low student to teacher ratio may be necessary to allow sufficient amounts of 1:1 time and small group instruction to meet specific individualized goals.

4. Comprehensible, structured environments, including elements such as predictable routine, visual activity schedules and other methods to help children to anticipate transitions between activities, and organized workspaces with features such as physical boundaries to minimize distractions and facilitate task completion. Arrangement of environments to control access to materials of interest and set up communicative temptations to facilitate child initiation and interaction.

5. Functional assessment of problem behaviors to identify the functions or outcomes of the behaviors and selection of treatment strategies based on the assessment (eg, interventions designed to change the outcomes of the problem behaviors and procedures to teach and differentially reinforce alternative, acceptable behaviors to serve the original functions).

6. Systematic measurement and documentation of the individual child's progress and adjustment of instructional strategies as necessary to enable acquisition of target skills.

7. Family education and involvement to promote consistency of implementation of the interventions across settings (enhancing generalization and increasing learning opportunities) and to gain the benefit of their knowledge of the child.

8. Explicit transition planning (eg, from home-based early intervention to preschool services, preschool to elementary school, elementary school to middle school, middle school to high school, high school to work or postsecondary education, home to community living).

such as epilepsy, or to underlying etiologic conditions. Efforts to optimize medical care are likely to have a positive impact on educational progress and quality of life, and it is important for primary pediatric health care professionals to provide longitudinal general health care, anticipatory guidance, and chronic disease management within a medical home.[215,290,375]

More time is often required for office visits, which may be challenging due to the patients' deficits in social interaction and communication, difficulty accepting novelty, and sensory aversions. Strategies such as familiarizing the patient with the office environment, staff, and routine during a "practice" visit; slowing down the pace of the visit; allowing ample time for talking before touching the patient; allowing the child to manipulate instruments and materials; keeping instructions simple; using visual cues and supports; exaggerating social cues; and having family and/or familiar staff available may be helpful in reducing resistance to physical examination and increasing family and patient comfort with the provider.[215,290,379]

Currently, medical therapies are directed to specific symptoms or coexisting conditions rather than ASD itself. For example, children with ASD who have seizures are treated with anticonvulsant medications based on the same criteria that are used for other children with epilepsy, including accurate diagnosis of the particular seizure type and consideration of medication tolerability.[178,380] There have been no randomized controlled trials, cohort studies, or systematic reviews of case-control studies of anticonvulsant medications for seizure management focusing on the ASD population. Similarly, those who present with common GI problems such as constipation, diarrhea, or abdominal pain should be evaluated and treated just as any other child with these symptoms would be evaluated and treated, with some adaptations as necessary to existing guidelines related to ability to tolerate certain tests.[198,381] Children with pica or persistent mouthing of objects or fingers should be evaluated for elevated blood lead concentrations, particularly if the history suggests potential environmental exposure, and measurement of iron and zinc levels should also be considered in the case of pica, because deficiency of either of these minerals can drive the behavior. Evaluation of sleep problems in children with ASD also follows the standard approach, and when intervention for insomnia is necessary, it should begin with parent education in the use of behavioral approaches.[382]

– Psychopharmacology

Psychotropic medications have not been demonstrated to correct the core social and communication impairments that characterize ASD, and their impact on restricted and repetitive behaviors is limited,[383–386] but they are commonly used to target coexisting psychiatric disorders (eg, ADHD, mood disorders, anxiety disorders) or associated problem behaviors or symptoms that cause significant impairment and distress.

There is significant variation in prescription rates among different countries.[387,388] In the United States, psychotropic medication use by individuals with ASD is common and has increased over time, as has polypharmacy (concurrent use of 2 or more psychotropic medications).[389–391] Data from the Autism Speaks Autism Treatment Network (ATN) and Interactive Autism Network (IAN) registries suggest that the prevalence of use of one or more psychotropic medications among children is approximately 0% to 1% in those younger than 3 years, 10% to 11% at ages 3 to 5 years, 38% to 46% at ages 6 to 11 years, and 64% to 67% at ages 12 to 17 years.[392,393] The total prevalence of psychotropic medication use was 27% in the ATN registry cohort and 35% in the IAN cohort.[392,393] Similarly, the 2-year rate of psychotropic medication use in a Medicaid-eligible, population-based ASD cohort in South Carolina was 40%,[394] and parents reported that 41.7% of children with ASD in the Simons Simplex Collection research cohort had ever used psychotropic medication.[395] Higher rates have been described in large national studies utilizing claims data from Medicaid and commercial insurance plans (56%–65%).[391,396,397]

Psychotropic medication use increases with increased age, lower IQ/presence of intellectual disability, and higher prevalence levels of challenging behavior or coexisting psychiatric diagnoses.[392,393,395–398] The likelihood of psychotropic medication use also appears to be affected by factors external to the clinical presentation, such as geographic characteristics and race/ethnicity.[392,396,399] Reported polypharmacy rates range from 12% in the ATN registry cohort[393] to 29% to 35% in large studies of Medicaid claims data,[391,397] and rates of concurrent use of 3 or more psychotropic medications range from 5% to 15%.[392–394,396,397]

Examples of problem behaviors/symptoms associated with ASD that may interfere with functioning and contribute substantially to the burden on families include irritability, aggression, self-injurious behavior, property destruction, perseveration, behavioral rigidity, compulsions, repetitive stereotyped movements, sleep disturbance, depression, mood lability, anxiety, hyperactivity, impulsivity, inattention, and other disruptive behaviors or manifestations of emotional dysregulation.[188–194] These behaviors/symptoms can be categorized for clinical purposes into 5 symptom clusters: ADHD symptoms, irritability/severe disruptive behavior, repetitive behavior, anxiety, and sleep problems.[290,400]

Although a detailed discussion of psychotropic medication management is beyond the scope of this chapter, a clinical approach is outlined in Box 19.9. The Autism Intervention Research Network on Physical Health (AIR-P) and the ATN have combined as the AIR-P/ATN to develop and publish several evidence-informed clinical practice guidelines that are pertinent to ASD-related psychopharmacological management.[401] These focus on ADHD symptoms,[402] sleep,[382] irritability and related problem behavior,[403]

Box 19.9. An Approach to Clinical Psychopharmacological Management[a]

> **Evaluation of Target Symptoms**
>
> ▶ Identify and assess target behaviors.
>   – Parent/caregiver interview, input from school staff and other caregivers.
>   • Frequency
>   • Intensity
>   • Duration
>   • Exacerbating factors/triggers (time, setting/location, demand situations, denials, transitions, etc)
>   • Ameliorating factors and response to behavioral interventions
>   • Time trends (increasing, decreasing, stable)
>   • Degree of interference with functioning
>
>   – Baseline behavior rating scales and/or baseline direct observational data (eg, collect data on number of episodes of aggression or self-injury in a given time period).
>   – Consider formal functional analysis of behavior.
>
> ▶ Search for medical factors that may be causing or exacerbating target behavior(s).
>   – Consider sources of pain or discomfort (see Table 19.7).
>   – Consider other medical causes or contributors (obstructive sleep apnea, seizures, menstrual cycle, etc).
>
> ▶ Assess existing and available supports.
>   – Behavioral supports and services
>   – Educational program, habilitative therapies
>   – Family psychosocial supports, respite care
>
> ▶ Complete any medical tests that may have a bearing on treatment choice (eg, electroencephalography if possible seizures).

Box 19.9. An Approach to Clinical Psychopharmacological Management[a] (*continued*)

Initiation and Monitoring of Psychopharmacological Therapy

▶ Consider psychotropic medication based on the presence of
  – Evidence that the target symptoms are interfering substantially with learning/academic prog-ress, socialization, health/safety, or quality of life
  – Suboptimal response to appropriate available behavioral interventions and environmental modifications
  – Research evidence that the target behavioral symptoms or coexisting psychiatric diagnoses are potentially amenable to pharmacological intervention

▶ Choose a medication on the basis of
  – Likely efficacy for the specific target symptoms
  – Potential adverse effects
  – Practical considerations, such as formulations available, dosing schedule, cost, and require-ment for laboratory or electrocardiographic monitoring
  – Patient's other medical conditions (eg, obesity, asthma) that might be exacerbated by certain medications
  – Informed consent (verbal or written) from parent/guardian and, when possible, assent from the patient

▶ Establish a plan for monitoring of effects.
  – Identify outcome measures for the target behaviors/symptoms.
  – Discuss course of expected effects and appropriate timing of follow-up telephone contact, completion of rating scales, reassessment of behavioral data, and office visits.
  – Outline a plan regarding what might be tried next if there is a negative or suboptimal response or to address additional target symptoms.
    • Change to a different medication.
    • Add another medication to augment a partial or suboptimal therapeutic response to the initial medication (same target symptoms).
    • Add a different medication to address additional target symptoms that remain problematic.
  – Obtain baseline laboratory data if necessary for the drug being prescribed and plan appropri-ate future lab monitoring.

▶ Explore the reasonable dose range for a single medication for an adequate length of time before changing to or adding a different medication; titrate to optimal effect without intolerable side effects.

▶ Monitor for adverse effects systematically.

▶ Consider careful withdrawal of the medication after 6–12 months of therapy to determine whether it is still needed.

[a] Adapted from Myers SM, Johnson CP; American Academy of Pediatrics Council on Children With Disabilities. Management of children with autism spectrum disorders. *Pediatrics*. 2007;120:1162–1182; and Myers SM. Management of autism spectrum disorders in primary care. *Pediatr Ann*. 2009;38:42–49.

and anxiety.[404] The AIR-P/ATN practice pathway for the evaluation and management of irritability-related problem behavior in ASD includes a stepwise approach and detailed checklist that can be applied to other behavioral symptoms as well.[403]

Evaluation of problem behaviors begins with characterizing the specific behaviors, prioritizing based on severity and threat to the safety of the individual with ASD and others, and identifying potential contributing factors such as medical problems, adverse effects of current medications, coexisting psychiatric disorders, mismatch between demands or other aspects of the environment and the patient's abilities, functional com-munication deficits, psychosocial stressors (including parental stress), and maladaptive reinforcement patterns.[290,403,405] In most cases, problem-focused behavioral interventions informed by functional behavioral assessment are an important and effective component of treatment.[403,406-409]

In some cases, medical factors may cause or exacerbate maladaptive behaviors, and recognition and treatment of medical conditions may eliminate or reduce the need for psychotropic medications or other interventions (Table 19.7).[376,403,410-415] For example, an individual may present with disrupted sleep due to obstructive sleep apnea or gastro-esophageal reflux or an acute onset or exacerbation of self-injurious behavior due to an occult source of discomfort such as otitis media, constipation, a dental abscess, or menstruation-related pain or dysphoria. Maintaining a relatively high index of suspicion and completing a careful history and physical examination may enhance the ability of the clinician to detect these and other medical conditions in a patient who has limited ability to communicate and who may exhibit aberrant behaviors at baseline. Some behaviors may have their basis in a painful condition that has resolved. The challenging behavior can take on an operant, or learned, function that persists after resolution of the initial medical condition. In these cases, behavioral intervention may also be required.

After treatable medical causes and modifiable behavioral and environmental factors have been ruled out or addressed, a therapeutic trial of medication directed at specific target symptoms or behaviors may be considered. Literature reviews have summarized the evidence pertaining to psychopharmacological management, the details of which are beyond the scope of this chapter.[399,405,416-419] However, selected options for 5 common target symptom clusters are outlined in Table 19.8, including supporting references. Clinicians should carefully weigh potential risks and benefits, use psychotropic medications as part of a comprehensive treatment approach, and only prescribe medications with which they have sufficient expertise, including knowledge of indications and contraindications, dosing, potential adverse effects, drug-drug interactions, and monitoring requirements.[290]

– Complementary Health Approaches

The National Center for Complementary and Integrative Health now uses the term *complementary health approaches* (CHAs) when referring to treatments that fall outside the mainstream of standard medical care, and *integrative health* to convey the idea of using standard and nonstandard therapies in a coordinated manner[459] (see Chapter 24, Complementary Health Approaches in Developmental and Behavioral Pediatrics). CHAs commonly used for children with ASD include "natural products" such as special diets, vitamins, minerals, and omega-3 fatty acids; mind-body practices such as auditory integration training, chiropractic acupuncture, and therapeutic touch; and nonstandard biomedical interventions such as hyperbaric oxygen, antifungal agents, and heavy metal chelation therapy.[460]

Potential risks of CHA treatments include direct toxic effects of biological agents, adverse physical effects of manipulative techniques, presence of contaminants, interactions with prescribed medications, interference with appropriate nutrition, and

Table 19.7. Examples of Treatable Medical Conditions That May Cause or Exacerbate Maladaptive Behaviors[a]

Medical Condition	Potential Treatment (Examples)
Allergies – Atopic dermatitis – Environmental (rhinitis, conjunctivitis) – Food	Antihistamine therapy, antileukotriene therapy, topical or systemic steroid therapy, environmental interventions, dietary elimination
Dental discomfort – Abscess – Caries – Impaction – Trauma	Antimicrobial therapy, analgesia, extraction or dental repair
Endocrine disorders – Hyperthyroidism, hypothyroidism – Premenstrual discomfort or dysphoria	Antithyroid medication, thyroid hormone replacement, analgesia, oral or injectable contraceptive therapy
Gastrointestinal disorders – Constipation – Diarrhea, cramping – Esophagitis, gastroesophageal reflux – Gastritis	Laxative therapy, fiber, acid-inhibiting therapy (proton pump inhibitors, histamine antagonists), antibiotic treatment of infectious causes (eg, *Helicobacter pylori* gastritis)
Infectious diseases – Otitis media – Otitis externa – Sinusitis – Pharyngitis	Antimicrobial therapy, analgesia
Medication side effects – Dietary supplements – Prescription medications – Over-the counter medications	Discontinuation of the offending agent
Musculoskeletal problems – Arthralgia – Strain or sprain – Occult fracture	Analgesia, anti-inflammatory agent, casting, splinting, rest, surgical intervention
Neurological disorders – Headache (including migraine) – Seizures	Analgesia, abortive therapies, prophylactic therapies, anticonvulsant medication
Nutritional deficiencies – Iron deficiency – Protein-calorie malnutrition – Zinc deficiency	Nutritional supplementation
Ophthalmological problems – Corneal abrasion – Retinal detachment	Analgesia, foreign body removal, temporary patching, surgical intervention
Sleep disorders – Obstructive sleep apnea – Other sleep disordered breathing	Weight reduction, tonsillectomy and adenoidectomy, continuous positive airway pressure

[a]Adapted from Myers SM. Management of autism spectrum disorders in primary care. *Pediatr Ann.* 2009;38: 42–49. Reprinted by permission of Slack, Inc.

Table 19.8. Psychotropic Medication Options for Common Target Symptoms[382,402–405,420–458]

Target Symptoms	Published Clinical Pathway/ Treatment Recommendations (AIR-P/ATN)	Medication Class	Examples[a]	Selected References
ADHD symptoms – Hyperactivity, impulsivity, inattention, distractibility	Mahajan[402]	Psychostimulants	Methylphenidate	Quintana et al[420] Handen et al[421] RUPP Autism Network[422,b] Pearson et al[423] Posey et al[424]
		Selective norepinephrine reuptake inhibitors	Atomoxetine	Arnold et al[425] Harfterkamp et al[426]
		Alpha-2 adrenergic agonists	Clonidine Guanfacine	Fankhauser et al[427] Jaselskis et al[428] Handen et al[429] Scahill et al[430]
		Atypical Antipsychotics[b] (second-generation antipsychotics)	Aripiprazole Risperidone	McCracken et al[431] Shea et al[432] Marcus et al[433] Owen et al[434]
Irritability and related problem behavior (also referred to as *severely disruptive behavior*) – Vocal and motoric outbursts of anger, frustration, and distress – Acts of aggression, self-injury, property destruction – Sometimes referred to by caregivers as *agitation, tantrums, meltdowns,* or *rages*	McGuire et al[403]	Atypical antipsychotics (second-generation antipsychotics)	Aripiprazole[c] Risperidone[c]	McCracken et al[431] Shea et al[432] Pandina et al[435] Aman et al[436] Arnold et al[437] Kent et al[438] Marcus et al[433] Owen et al[434] Ghanizadeh et al[439] RUPP Autism Network[440,a] Troost et al[441] Marcus et al[442] Findling et al[443]

Table 19.8. Psychotropic Medication Options for Common Target Symptoms[382,402-405,420-458] (continued)

Target Symptoms	Published Clinical Pathway/Treatment Recommendations (AIR-P/ATN)	Medication Class	Examples[a]	Selected References
Irritability and related problem behavior (also referred to as *severely disruptive behavior*), continued	McGuire et al[403] (*continued*)	Glutamatergic modulator/antioxidant	N-acetylcysteine	Hardan et al[444] Ghanizadeh et al[439,d] Nikoo et al[446,d]
		Alpha-2 adrenergic agonists	Clonidine	Jaselskis et al[428]
		Selective serotonin reuptake inhibitors[e]	Fluvoxamine (adults)	McDougle et al[447]
		Anticonvulsant mood stabilizers	Valproic acid/divalproex sodium	Hollander et al[448]
		Serotonin-norepinephrine reuptake inhibitor	Venlafaxine[f]	Niederhofer[449,f]
Repetitive behavior — Stereotyped motor mannerisms, compulsions, behavioral rigidity/insistence on sameness		Atypical antipsychotics (second-generation antipsychotics)	Aripiprazole Risperidone	McDougle et al[450] McCracken et al[431] Shea et al[432] Marcus et al[433] Owen et al[434]
		Anticonvulsants	Valproic acid/divalproex sodium	Hollander et al[448]
		Selective serotonin reuptake inhibitors	Fluoxetine Fluvoxamine	Hollander et al[452] (adults) McDougle et al[447] (adults)
Anxiety	Vasa et al[404,g]	Selective serotonin reuptake inhibitors	None	Strawn et al[453]
		Atypical antipsychotics (second-generation antipsychotics)	Risperidone (adults)	McDougle et al[450]

Table 19.8. Psychotropic Medication Options for Common Target Symptoms[382,402-405,420-458] *(continued)*

Target Symptoms	Published Clinical Pathway/ Treatment Recommendations (AIR-P/ATN)	Medication Class	Examples[a]	Selected References
Sleep problems/insomnia	Malow et al[382]	Endogenous indoleamine chronobiotic and hypnotic	Melatonin	Cortesi et al[454] Wright et al[455] Wirojanan et al[456] Garstang and Wallis[457]

Abbreviations: ADHD, attention-deficit/hyperactivity disorder; AIR-P, Autism Intervention Research Network on Physical Health; ATN, Autism Speaks Autism Treatment Network; RUPP, Research Units on Pediatric Psychopharmacology.

[a] For all examples listed, there is at least one double-blind, placebo-controlled trial supporting efficacy in patients with autism spectrum disorder.

[b] Hyperactivity and related behaviors were secondary outcomes in randomized controlled trials assessing atypical antipsychotics for the treatment of irritability; atypical antipsychotics have not been evaluated for the treatment of ADHD symptoms in patients without significant irritability.

[c] Risperidone and aripiprazole are currently the only medications with US Food and Drug Administration–approved labeling specific to autism (for the symptomatic treatment of irritability, including aggressive behavior, deliberate self-injury, and temper tantrums in children and adolescents with autism).

[d] Adjunctive to risperidone (N-acetylcysteine plus risperidone versus placebo plus risperidone).

[e] Irritability also improved on citalopram relative to placebo in one controlled trial, but this was a secondary finding of small effect size that was judged by the authors not to be clinically significant.[458]

[f] Effect size of improvement associated with venlafaxine was small, and irritability was not the primary outcome measured.

[g] Due to the lack of data regarding the pharmacological treatment of anxiety in children and adolescents with autism spectrum disorder, the medication component of the treatment recommendations is based on data in typically developing pediatric populations and expert consensus.[404]

interruption or postponement of empirically validated therapies, as well as unwarranted expenditure of time, effort, and financial resources.[460,461] The AAP has stated that pediatricians should (1) critically evaluate the scientific evidence of efficacy and risk of harm of various treatments and convey this information to families, (2) help families understand how to evaluate scientific evidence and recognize unsubstantiated treatments and pseudoscience, and (3) insist that studies that examine CHA treatments be held to the same scientific standards as all clinical research.[290] The use of CHA in children with disabilities despite the general paucity of scientific support is addressed in Chapter 24, Complementary Health Approaches in Developmental and Behavioral Pediatrics, of this volume, and specific approaches used with children with ASD have been reviewed by Levy and Hyman.[460]

Outcomes

Although specific features change over time and outcomes vary, most children diagnosed with ASD using *DSM* criteria remain within the spectrum as adolescents and adults. Regardless of their level of intellectual functioning, these individuals continue to experience difficulty with social relationships, independent living, employment, and mental/behavioral health.[135]

ASD is associated with increased morbidity, mortality, and health care utilization and costs. Mortality risk among individuals with ASD is approximately twice that of the general population (standardized mortality ratio 2.8 [95% CI 1.8–4.2]).[184] Moderate to profound ID, epilepsy, and female sex are associated with increased risk of death in this population. Much of the substantial direct and indirect economic effect of ASD is due to the cost of special education in childhood and to costs associated with residential accommodation, medical care, and productivity losses in adulthood.[462]

Approximately 10% to 20% of children with well-documented ASD ultimately lose the diagnosis because they no longer fulfill diagnostic criteria and are reported to function within the range of normal cognitive and adaptive functioning.[135,149] As a group, individuals with this type of "optimal outcome" or "very positive outcome" have a different pattern of developmental trajectories on standardized measures than most individuals with ASD and similar average IQ. It is not clear whether this is attributable to interventions, the nature of the original clinical presentation, intrinsic/genetic predisposition to a highly atypical developmental trajectory, or perhaps resolution of an interfering process. Despite the excellent outcomes in this group, there is a high rate of persisting difficulties in social understanding, pragmatic language, attention, emotional maturity and self-control, and psychiatric symptoms and diagnoses.[135,191,463]

Although most studies, including those focusing on high-functioning individuals, have reported limited social integration and employment prospects, poorer outcomes on quality of life measures, and high rates of mental health problems, the research findings are highly variable and sometimes contradictory.[135,136] The intrinsic factors most consistently associated with prognosis are early language abilities and IQ. Useful speech by age 5 to 6 years, verbal IQ greater than 70, and nonverbal IQ greater than 70 are associated with better prognosis, but these factors alone are not enough to ensure a positive outcome.[136,464] Much more systematic research is needed to describe the range of outcomes and determine the intrinsic characteristics and extrinsic factors (ie, educational, behavioral, vocational, and social supports) that influence developmental trajectories, enhance resilience, and promote good outcomes.[135]

Conclusion

ASD is a clinically and etiologically heterogeneous, behaviorally defined condition characterized by distinctive impairments in reciprocal social interaction and social communication that do not simply reflect associated ID, and by the presence of a restricted, repetitive behavioral repertoire. Primary pediatric health care professionals play an important role in identification and management of children with this common neurodevelopmental disorder. Although no clinically useful biological markers have been identified, substantial advances have been made in characterizing the genetics, neurobiology, and neuropsychology of this heterogeneous disorder. There is a growing body of evidence demonstrating that certain educational, behavioral, and medical interventions and community supports ameliorate symptoms and improve functioning in children with ASD. However, there is much research to be done to determine which interventions are most effective for children with ASD, what variables moderate treatment effects and predict outcomes, and how much improvement can reasonably be expected. By providing their patients affected by ASD with high-quality longitudinal medical care and guiding them to effective psychosocial interventions, primary pediatric health care professionals can help to maximize important outcomes, including functional independence and quality of life.

References

1. Kanner L. Autistic disturbances of affective contact. *Nerv Child.* 1943;2:217–250
2. American Psychiatric Association. *Diagnostic and Statistical Manual of Mental Disorders.* 5th ed. Arlington, VA: American Psychiatric Association; 2013
3. Lord C, Petkova E, Hus V, et al. A multisite study of the clinical diagnosis of different autism spectrum disorders. *Arch Gen Psychiatry.* 2012;69(3):306–313
4. Baird G, Norbury CF. Social (pragmatic) communication disorders and autism spectrum disorder. *Arch Dis Child.* 2016;101:745–751
5. Mandy W, Wang A, Lee I, Skuse D. Evaluating social (pragmatic) communication disorder. *J Child Psychol Psychiatry.* 2017;58(10):1166–1175
6. Christensen DL, Baio J, Braun KV, et al. Prevalence and characteristics of autism spectrum disorder among children aged 8 years—autism and developmental disabilities monitoring network, 11 sites, United States, 2012. *MMWR Surveill Summ.* 2016;65(No. SS-3):1–23
7. Palmer N, Beam A, Agniel D, et al. Association of sex with recurrence of autism spectrum disorder among siblings. *JAMA Pediatr.* 2017;171(11):1107–1112
8. Blumberg SJ, Bramlett MD, Kogan MD, et al. Changes in prevalence of parent-reported autism spectrum disorder in school-aged U.S. children: 2007 to 2011–2012. *Natl Health Stat Report.* 2013;(65):1–11
9. Zablotsky B, Black LI, Maenner MJ, Schieve LA, Blumberg SJ. Estimated prevalence of autism and other developmental disabilities following questionnaire changes in the 2014 National Health Interview Survey. *Natl Health Stat Report.* 2015;(87):1–20
10. Baxter AJ, Brugha TS, Erskine HE, Scheurer RW, Vos T, Scott JG. The epidemiology and global burden of autism spectrum disorders. *Psychol Med.* 2015;45(3):601–613

11. Idring S, Rai D, Dal H, et al. Autism spectrum disorders in the Stockholm Youth Cohort: design, prevalence and validity. *PLoS One.* 2012;7(7):e41280

12. Saemundsen E, Magnússon P, Georgsdóttir I, Egilsson E, Rafnsson V. Prevalence of autism spectrum disorders in an Icelandic birth cohort. *BMJ Open.* 2013;3(6):1–6

13. Atladottir HO, Gyllenberg D, Langridge A, et al. The increasing prevalence of reported diagnoses of childhood psychiatric disorders: a descriptive multinational comparison. *Eur Child Adolesc Psychiatry.* 2015;24(2):173–183

14. Kim YS, Leventhal BL, Koh, et al. Prevalence of autism spectrum disorders in a total population. *Am J Psychiatry.* 2011;168(9):904–912

15. Loomes R, Hull L, Mandy WPL. What is the male-to-female ratio in autism spectrum disorder? A systematic review and meta-analysis. *J Am Acad Child Adolesc Psychiatry.* 2017;56(6):466–474

16. Newschaffer CJ, Falb MD, Gurney JG. National autism prevalence trends from United States special education data. *Pediatrics.* 2005;115(3):e277–e282

17. Cavagnaro AT. Autistic spectrum disorders: changes in the California caseload: an update: June 1987–June 2007. California Department of Developmental Services. http://www.dds.ca.gov/AUTISM/docs/AutismReport_2007.pdf. Accessed February 12, 2018

18. Polyak A, Kubina RM, Girirajan S. Comorbidity of intellectual disability confounds ascertainment of autism: implications for genetic diagnosis. *Am J Med Genet B Neuropsychiatr Genet.* 2015;168(7):600–608

19. Schieve LA, Rice C, Yeargin-Allsopp M, et al. Parent-reported prevalence of autism spectrum disorders in US-born children: an assessment of changes within birth cohorts from the 2003 to the 2007 National Survey of Children's Health. *Matern Child Health J.* 2012;16(suppl 1):S151–S157

20. Hansen SN, Schendel DE, Parner ET. Explaining the increase in the prevalence of autism spectrum disorders: the proportion attributable to changes in reporting practices. *JAMA Pediatr.* 2015;169(1):56–62

21. Isaksen J, Diseth TH, Schjølberg S, Skjeldal OH. Observed prevalence of autism spectrum disorders in two Norwegian counties. *Eur J Paediatr Neurol.* 2012;16(6):592–598

22. Lundström S, Reichenberg A, Anckarsäter H, Lichtenstein P, Gillberg C. Autism phenotype versus registered diagnosis in Swedish children: prevalence trends over 10 years in general population samples. *BMJ.* 2015;350:1961

23. Raz R, Weisskopf MG, Davidovitch M, Pinto O, Levine H. Differences in autism spectrum disorders incidence by sub-populations in Israel 1992–2009: a total population study. *J Autism Dev Disord.* 2015;45(4):1062–1069

24. Brugha TS, McManus S, Bankart J, et al. Epidemiology of autism spectrum disorders in adults in the community in England. *Arch Gen Psychiatry.* 2011;68(5):459–465

25. Rice CE, Rosanoff M, Dawson G, et al. Evaluating changes in the prevalence of the autism spectrum disorders (ASDs). *Public Health Rev.* 2012;34(2):1–22

26. Isaksen J, Diseth TH, Schjølberg S, Skjeldal OH. Autism spectrum disorders—are they really epidemic? *Eur J Paediatr Neurol.* 2013;17(4):327–333

27. Shattuck PT. Diagnostic substitution and changing autism prevalence. *Pediatrics.* 2006;117(4):1438–1439

28. Newschaffer CJ. Investigating diagnostic substitution and autism prevalence trends. *Pediatrics.* 2006;117(4):1436–1437

29. Bishop DV, Whitehouse AJ, Watt HJ, et al. Autism and diagnostic substitution: evidence from a study of adults with a history of developmental language disorder. *Dev Med Child Neurol.* 2008;50(5):341–345

30. Coo H, Ouellette-Kuntz H, Lloyd JE, Kasmara L, Holden JJ, Lewis ME. Trends in autism prevalence: diagnostic substitution revisited. *J Autism Dev Disord.* 2008;38:1036–1046

31. Miller JS, Bilder D, Farley M, et al. Autism spectrum disorder reclassified: a second look at the 1980s Utah/UCLA Autism Epidemiologic Study. *J Autism Dev Disord.* 2013;43:200–210

32. Georgiades S, Szatmari P, Zwaigenbaum L, et al. A prospective study of autistic-like traits in unaffected siblings of probands with autism spectrum disorder. *JAMA Psychiatry.* 2013;70:42–48

33. Grønborg TK, Schendel DE, Parner ET. Recurrence of autism spectrum disorders in full- and half-siblings and trends over time: a population-based cohort study. *JAMA Pediatr.* 2013;167:947–953

34. Sandin S, Lichtenstein P, Kuja-Halkola R, Larsson H, Hultman CM, Reichenberg A. The familial risk of autism. *JAMA.* 2014;311:1770–1777

35. Tick B, Bolton P, Happé F, Rutter M, Rijsdijk F. Heritability of autism spectrum disorders: a meta-analysis of twin studies. *J Child Psychol Psychiatry.* 2016;57:585–595

36. Sandin S, Lichtenstein P, Kuja-Halkola R, Hultman C, Larsson H, Reichenberg A. The heritability of autism spectrum disorder. *JAMA.* 2017;318:1182–1184

37. Liu X, Takumi T. Genomic and genetic aspects of autism spectrum disorder. *Biochem Biophys Res Commun.* 2014;452(2):244–253

38. Chen JA, Penagarikano O, Belgard TG, Swarup V, Geschwind DH. The emerging picture of autism spectrum disorder: genetics and pathology. *Annu Rev Pathol.* 2015;10:111–144

39. Kim YS, Leventhal BL. Genetic epidemiology and insights into interactive genetic and environmental effects in autism spectrum disorders. *Biol Psychiatry.* 2015;77:66–74

40. Bourgeron T. From the genetic architecture to synaptic plasticity in autism spectrum disorder. *Nat Rev Neurosci.* 2015;16:551–563

41. De Rubeis S, Buxbaum JD. Recent advances in the genetics of autism spectrum disorder. *Curr Neurol Neurosci Rep.* 2015;15:36

42. de la Torre-Ubieta L, Won H, Stein JL, Geschwind DH. Advancing the understanding of autism disease mechanisms through genetics. *Nat Med.* 2016;22:345–361

43. Gaugler T, Klei L, Sanders SJ, et al. Most genetic risk for autism resides with common variation. *Nat Genet.* 2014;46:881–885

44. Sanders SJ, He X, Willsey J, et al. Insights into autism spectrum disorder genetic architecture and biology from 71 risk loci. *Neuron.* 2015;87:1215–1233

45. Jeste SS, Geschwind DH. Disentangling the heterogeneity of autism spectrum disorder through genetic findings. *Nat Rev Neurol.* 2014;10(2):74–81

46. Tammimies K, Marshall CR, Walker S, et al. Molecular diagnostic yield of chromosomal microarray analysis and whole-exome sequencing in children with autism spectrum disorder. *JAMA.* 2015;214:895–903

47. Lee H, Deignan JL, Dorrani N, et al. Clinical exome sequencing for genetic identification of rare Mendelian disorders. *JAMA.* 2014;312(18):1880–1887

48. Retterer K, Juusola J, Cho MT, et al. Clinical application of whole-exome sequencing across clinical indications. *Genet Med.* 2016;18:696–704

49. Coe BP, Girirajan S, Eichler EE. The genetic variability and commonality of neurodevelopmental disease. *Am J Med Genet C Semin Med Genet.* 2012;160C:118–129

50. Malhotra D, Sebat J. CNVs: harbingers of a rare variant revolution in psychiatric genetics. *Cell.* 2012;148:1223–1241

51. Moreno-De-Luca A, Myers SM, Challman TD, Moreno-De-Luca D, Evans DW, Ledbetter DH. Developmental brain dysfunction: revival and expansion of old concepts based on new genetic evidence. *Lancet Neurol.* 2013;12:406–414

52. Pescosolido MF, Gamsiz ED, Nagpal S, Morrow EM. Distribution of disease-associated copy number variants across distinct disorders of cognitive development. *J Am Acad Child Adolesc Psychiatry.* 2013;52:414–430

53. Buxbaum JD. DSM-5 and psychiatric genetics—round hole, meet square peg. *Biol Psychiatry.* 2015;77:766–768

54. Gonzalez-Mantilla AJ, Moreno-De-Luca A, Ledbetter DH, Martin CL. A cross-disorder method to identify novel candidate genes for developmental brain disorders. *JAMA Psychiatry.* 2016;73:275–283

55. Li J, Cai T, Jiang Y, et al. Genes with de novo mutations are shared by four neuropsychiatric disorders discovered from NPdenovo database. *Mol Psychiatry.* 2016;21:290–297

56. Moreno-De-Luca D, Sanders SJ, Willsey AJ, et al. Using large clinical data sets to infer pathogenicity for rare copy number variants in autism cohorts. *Mol Psychiatry.* 2013;18:1090–1095

57. Kirov G. CNVs in neuropsychiatric disorders. *Hum Mol Genet.* 2015;24(R1):R45–R49

58. Richards C, Jones C, Groves L, Moss J, Oliver C. Prevalence of autism spectrum disorder phenomenology in genetic disorders: a systematic review and meta-analysis. *Lancet Psychiatry.* 2015;2:909–916

59. Stessman HA, Turner TN, Eichler EE. Molecular subtyping and improved treatment of neurodevelopmental disease. *Genome Med.* 2016;8(1):22

60. Geisinger. Developmental Brain Disorder Genes Database. http://geisingeradmi.org/care-innovation/studies/dbd-genes. Accessed February 12, 2018

61. Sandin S, Hultman CM, Kolevzon A, Gross R, MacCabe JH, Reichenberg A. Advancing maternal age is associated with increasing risk for autism: a review and meta-analysis. *J Am Acad Child Adolesc Psychiatry.* 2012;51(5):477–486

62. Sandin S, Schendel D, Magnusson P, et al. Autism risk associated with parental age and with increasing difference in age between the parents. *Mol Psychiatry.* 2016;21(5):693–700

63. Lee BK, McGrath JJ. Advancing parental age and autism: multifactorial pathways. *Trends Mol Med.* 2015;21(2):118–125

64. McGrath JJ, Petersen L, Agerbo E, et al. A comprehensive assessment of parental age and psychiatric disorders. *JAMA Psychiatry.* 2014;71(3):301–309

65. Christensen J, Grønborg TK, Sørensen MJ, et al. Prenatal valproate exposure and risk of autism spectrum disorders and childhood autism. *JAMA.* 2013;309:1696–1703

66. Lyall K, Schmidt RJ, Hertz-Picciotto I. Environmental factors in the preconception and prenatal periods in relation to risk for ASD. In: Volkmar FR, Rogers SJ, Paul R, Pelphrey KA, eds. *Handbook of Autism and Pervasive Developmental Disorders.* 4th ed. Vol I. Hoboken, NJ: John Wiley & Sons; 2014:424–456

67. Mandy W, Lai MC. Annual Research Review: the role of the environment in the developmental psychopathology of autism spectrum condition. *J Child Psychol Psychiatry.* 2016;57:271–292

68. Gardener H, Spiegelman D, Buka SL. Perinatal and neonatal risk factors for autism: a comprehensive meta-analysis. *Pediatrics.* 2011;128:344–355

69. Sandin S, Kolevzon A, Levine SZ, Hultman CM, Reichenberg A. Parental and perinatal risk factors for autism: epidemiological findings and potential mechanisms. In: Buxbaum JD, Hof PR, eds. *The Neuroscience of Autism Spectrum Disorders.* Oxford, United Kingdom: Elsevier; 2013:195–202

70. Kalkbrenner AE, Schmidt RJ, Penlesky AC. Environmental chemical exposures and autism spectrum disorders: a review of the epidemiological evidence. *Curr Probl Pediatr Adolesc Health Care.* 2014;44:277–318

71. Becerra TA, Wilhelm M, Olsen J, Cockburn M, Ritz B. Ambient air pollution and autism in Los Angeles County, California. *Environ Health Perspect.* 2012;121:380–386

72. Volk HE, Lurmann F, Penfold B, Hertz-Picciotto I, McConnell R. Traffic related air pollution, particulate matter, and autism. *JAMA Psychiatry.* 2013;70:71–77

73. Gong T, Almqvist C, Bolte S, et al. Exposure to air pollution from traffic and neurodevelopmental disorders in Swedish twins. *Twin Res Hum Genet.* 2014;17:553–562

74. Guxens M, Ghassabian A, Gong T, et al. Air pollution exposure during pregnancy and childhood autistic traits in four European population-based cohort studies: the ESCAPE Project. *Environ Health Perspect.* 2016;124(1):133–140

75. Uno Y, Uchiyama T, Kurosawa M, Aleksic B, Ozaki N. Early exposure to the combined measles-mumps-rubella vaccine and thimerosal-containing vaccines and autism spectrum disorder. *Vaccine.* 2015;33:2511–2516

76. Taylor LE, Swerdfeger AL, Eslick GD. Vaccines are not associated with autism: an evidence-based meta-analysis of case-control and cohort studies. *Vaccine.* 2014;32:3623–3629

77. Maglione MA, Das L, Raaen L, et al. Safety of vaccines used for routine immunization of U.S. children: a systematic review. *Pediatrics.* 2014;134:325–327

78. DeStefano F, Price CS, Weintraub ES. Increasing exposure to antibody-stimulating proteins and polysaccharides in vaccines is not associated with risk of autism. *J Pediatr.* 2013;163:561–567

79. Demicheli V, Rivetti A, Debalini MG, Di Pietrantonj C. Vaccines for measles, mumps and rubella in children. *Cochrane Database Syst Rev.* 2012;15(2):CD004407

80. Gerber JS, Offit PA. Vaccines and autism: a tale of shifting hypotheses. *Clin Infect Dis.* 2009;48:456–461

81. Tordjman S, Somogyi E, Coulon N, et al. Gene x environment interactions in autism spectrum disorders: role of epigenetic mechanisms. *Front Psychiatry.* 2014;5:53

82. Loke YJ, Hannan AJ, Craig JM. The role of epigenetic change in autism spectrum disorders. *Front Neurol.* 2015;6:107

83. Isles AR. Neural and behavioral epigenetics; what it is, and what is hype. *Genes Brain Behav.* 2015;14:64–72

84. Peters J. The role of genomic imprinting in biology and disease: an expanding view. *Nat Rev Genet.* 2014;15:517–530

85. McNamara GI, Isles AR. Dosage-sensitivity of imprinted genes expressed in the brain: 15q11-q13 and neuropsychiatric illness. *Biochem Soc Trans.* 2013;41:721–726

86. Ladd-Acosta C, Hansen KD, Briem E, Fallin MD, Kaufmann WE, Feinberg AP. Common DNA methylation alterations in multiple brain regions in autism. *Mol Psychiatry.* 2014;19:862–871

87. Wong CCY, Meabum EL, Ronald A, et al. Methylomic analysis of monozygotic twins discordant for autism spectrum disorder and related behavioural traits. *Mol Psychiatry.* 2014;19:495–503

88. Bohacek J, Mansuy IM. Molecular insights into transgenerational non-genetic inheritance of acquired behaviours. *Nat Rev Genet.* 2015;16:641–652

89. Casanova MF. The neuropathology of autism. In: Volkmar FR, Rogers SJ, Paul R, Pelphrey KA, eds. *Handbook of Autism and Pervasive Developmental Disorders.* 4th ed. Vol I. Hoboken, NJ: John Wiley & Sons; 2014:497–531

90. Stoner R, Chow ML, Boyle MP, et al. Patches of disorganization in the neocortex of children with autism. *N Engl J Med.* 2014;370:1209–1219

91. Goldani AAS, Downs SR, Widjaja F, Lawton B, Hendren RL. Biomarkers in autism. *Front Psychiatry.* 2014;5:1–13

92. Anderson GM. Autism biomarkers: challenges, pitfalls and possibilities. *J Autism Dev Disord.* 2015;45:1103–1113

93. Ruggeri B, Sarkans U, Schumann G, Persico A. Biomarkers in autism spectrum disorder: the old and the new. *Psychopharmacology (Berl).* 2014;231:1201–1216

94. Courchesne E, Campbell K, Solso S. Brain growth across the lifespan in autism: age-specific changes in anatomical pathology. *Brain Res.* 2011;1380:138–145

95. Sacco R, Gabriele S, Persico AM. Head circumference and brain size in autism spectrum disorder: a systematic review and meta-analysis. *Psychiatry Res.* 2015;234:239–251

96. Zwaigenbaum L, Young GS, Stone WL, et al. Early head growth in infants at risk of autism: a Baby Siblings Research Consortium study. *J Am Acad Child Adolesc Psychiatry.* 2014;53:1053–1062

97. Raznahan A, Wallace GL, Antezana L, et al. Compared to what? Early brain overgrowth in autism and the perils of population norms. *Biol Psychiatry.* 2013;74:563–575

98. Chaste P, Klei L, Sanders SJ, et al. Adjusting head circumference for covariates in autism: clinical correlates of a highly heritable continuous trait. *Biol Psychiatry.* 2013;74:576–584

99. Mahajan R, Mostofsky SH. Neuroimaging endophenotypes in autism spectrum disorder. *CNS Spectr.* 2015;20:412–426

100. Blackmon K. Structural MRI biomarkers of shared pathogenesis in autism spectrum disorder and epilepsy. *Epilepsy Behav.* 2015;47:172–182

101. Lainhart JE. Brain imaging research in autism spectrum disorders: in search of neuropathology and health across the lifespan. *Curr Opin Psychiatry.* 2015;28:76–82

102. Zielinski BA, Prigge MB, Nielsen JA, et al. Longitudinal changes in cortical thickness in autism and typical development. *Brain.* 2014;137:1799–1812

103. Travers BG, Adiuru N, Ennis C, et al. Diffusion tensor imaging in autism spectrum disorder: a review. *Autism Res.* 2012;5:289–313

104. Philip RCM, Dauvermann MR, Whalley HC, et al. A systematic review and meta-analysis of the fMRI investigation of autism spectrum disorders. *Neurosci Biobehav Rev.* 2012;36:901–942

105. Cerliani L, Mennes M, Thomas RM, et al. Increased functional connectivity between subcortical and cortical resting-state networks in autism spectrum disorder. *JAMA Psychiatry.* 2015;72:767–777

106. Ecker C, Bookheimer SY, Murphy DGM. Neuroimaging in autism spectrum disorder: brain structure and function across the lifespan. *Lancet Neurol.* 2015;14:1121–1134

107. Plitt M, Barnes KA, Martin A. Functional connectivity classification of autism identifies highly predictive brain features but falls short of biomarker standards. *Neuroimage Clin.* 2015;7:359–366

108. Jeste SS, Nelson CA. Event related potentials in the understanding of autism spectrum disorders: an analytical review. *J Autism Dev Disord.* 2009;39:495–510

109. Jeste SS, Frohlich J, Loo SK. Electrophysiological biomarkers of diagnosis and outcome in neurodevelopmental disorders. *Curr Opin Neurol.* 2015;28:110–116

110. Boutros NN, Lajiness-O'Neill R, Zillgitt A, Richard AE, Bowyer SM. EEG changes associated with autistic spectrum disorders. *Neuropsychiatr Electrophysiol.* 2015;1:3

111. Port RG, Anwar AR, Ku M, Carlson GC, Siegel SJ, Roberts TPL. Prospective MEG biomarkers in ASD: pre-clinical evidence and clinical promise of electrophysiological signatures. *Yale J Biol Med.* 2015;88:25–36

112. Billeci L, Sicca F, Maharanta K, et al. On the application of quantitative EEG for characterizing autistic brain: a systematic review. *Front Hum Neurosci.* 2013;7:1–15

113. Duffy FH, Als H. A stable pattern of EEG spectral coherence distinguishes children with autism from neuro-typical controls—a large case control study. *BMC Med.* 2012;10:64

114. Dawson G, Bernier R, Ring RH. Social attention: a possible early indicator of efficacy in autism clinical trials. *J Neurodev Disord.* 2012;4(1):11

115. Klin A, Lin DJ, Gorrindo P, Ramsay G, Jones W. Two-year-olds with autism fail to orient towards human biological motion but attend instead to non-social, physical contingencies. *Nature.* 2009;459:257–261

116. Rice K, Moriuchi JM, Jones W, Klin A. Parsing heterogeneity in autism spectrum disorders: visual scanning of dynamic social scenes in school-aged children. *J Am Acad Child Adolesc Psychiatry.* 2012;51:238–248

117. Jones W, Klin A. Attention to eyes is present but in decline in 2–6-month-old infants later diagnosed with autism. *Nature.* 2013;504:427–421

118. Gabriele S, Sacco R, Persico AM. Blood serotonin levels in autism spectrum disorder: a systematic review and meta-analysis. *Eur Neuropsychopharmacol.* 2014;24:919–929

119. Maurer MH. Genomic and proteomic advances in autism research. *Electrophoresis.* 2012;33:3653–3658

120. Voineagu I. Gene expression studies in autism: moving from the genome to the transcriptome and beyond. *Neurobiol Dis.* 2012;45:69–75

121. Glatt SJ, Tsuang MT, Winn M, et al. Blood-based gene expression signatures of infants and toddlers with autism. *J Am Acad Child Adolesc Psychiatry.* 2012;51(9):934–944

122. Kong SW, Shimizu-Motohashi Y, Campbell MG, et al. Peripheral blood gene expression signature differentiates children with autism from unaffected siblings. *Neurogenetics.* 2013;14:143–152

123. Anderson GM, Jacobs-Stannard A, Chawarska K, Volkmar FR, Kliman HJ. Placental trophoblast inclusions in autism spectrum disorder. *Biol Psychiatry.* 2007;61:487–491

124. Walker CK, Anderson KW, Milano KM, et al. Trophoblast inclusions are significantly increased in the placentas of children in families at risk for autism. *Biol Psychiatry.* 2013;74:204–211

125. Adler E, Madankumar R, Rosner M, Reznik SE. Increased placental trophoblast inclusions in placenta accrete. *Placenta*. 2014;35:1075–1078

126. Braunschweig D, Van de Water J. Maternal autoantibodies in autism. *Arch Neurol*. 2012;69:693–699

127. Bressler JP, Gillin PK, O'Driscoll C, et al. Maternal antibody reactivity to lymphocytes of offspring with autism. *Pediatr Neurol*. 2012;47:337–340

128. Brimberg L, Sadiq A, Gregersen PK, Diamond B. Brain-reactive IgG correlates with autoimmunity in mothers of a child with an autism spectrum disorder. *Mol Psychiatry*. 2013;18:1171–1177

129. Braunschweig D, Krakowiak P, Duncanson P, et al. Autism-specific maternal autoantibodies recognize critical proteins in developing brain. *Transl Psychiatry*. 2013;3:e277

130. Bauman MD, Iosif A-M, Ashwood P, et al. Maternal autoantibodies from mothers of children with autism alter brain growth and social behavior development in the rhesus monkey. *Transl Psychiatry*. 2013;3:e278

131. Meindl JN, Cannella-Malone HI. Initiating and responding to joint attention bids in children with autism: a review of the literature. *Res Dev Disabil*. 2011;32:1441–1454

132. Murza KA, Schwartz JB, Hahs-Vaughn DL, Nye C. Joint attention interventions for children with autism spectrum disorder: a systematic review and meta-analysis. *Int J Lang Commun Disord*. 2016;51:236–251

133. Wheelwright S, Baron-Cohen S. Systemizing and empathizing. In: Fein D, ed. *The Neuropsychology of Autism*. New York, NY: Oxford University Press; 2011:317–337

134. Bauminger-Zviely N. School-age children with ASD. In: Volkmar FR, Rogers SJ, Paul R, Pelphrey KA, eds. *Handbook of Autism and Pervasive Developmental Disorders*. 4th ed. Vol I. Hoboken, NJ: John Wiley & Sons; 2014:148–175

135. Howlin P, Magiati I. Autism spectrum disorder: outcomes in adulthood. *Curr Opin Psychiatry*. 2017;30:69–76

136. Poon KK, Sidhu DJ. Adults with autism spectrum disorders: a review of outcomes, social attainment, and interventions. *Curr Opin Psychiatry*. 2017;30:77–84

137. Wing L, Gould J. Severe impairments of social interaction and associated abnormalities in children: epidemiology and classification. *J Autism Dev Disord*. 1979;9:11–29

138. Johnson CP, Myers SM; American Academy of Pediatrics Council on Children With Disabilities. Identification and evaluation of children with autism spectrum disorders. *Pediatrics*. 2007;120:1183–1215

139. Eigsti IM, de Marchena AB, Schuh JM, Kelley E. Language acquisition in autism spectrum disorders: a developmental review. *Res Autism Spectrum Disord*. 2011;2:681–691

140. Tager-Flusberg H, Caronna E. Language disorders: autism and other pervasive developmental disorders. *Pediatr Clin North Am*. 2007;54:469–481

141. Tager-Flusberg H, Kasari C. Minimally verbal school-aged children with autism spectrum disorder: the neglected end of the spectrum. *Autism Res*. 2013;6:468–478

142. Boucher J. Research review: structural language in autistic spectrum disorder—characteristics and causes. *J Child Psychol Psychiatry*. 2012;53:219–233

143. Kasari C, Chang Y. Play development in children with autism spectrum disorders: skills, object play, and interventions. In: Volkmar FR, Rogers SJ, Paul R, Pelphrey KA, eds. *Handbook of Autism and Pervasive Developmental Disorders*. 4th ed. Vol I. Hoboken, NJ: John Wiley & Sons; 2014:263–277

144. Richler J, Huerta M, Bishop SL, Lord C. Developmental trajectories of restricted and repetitive behaviors and interests in children with autism spectrum disorders. *Dev Psychopathol*. 2010;22:55–69

145. Bishop SL, Hus V, Duncan A, et al. Subcategories of restricted and repetitive behaviors in children with autism spectrum disorders. *J Autism Dev Disord*. 2013;43:1287–1297

146. Richler J, Bishop SL, Kleinke JR, Lord C. Restricted and repetitive behaviors in young children with autism spectrum disorders. *J Autism Dev Disord*. 2007;37:73–85

147. Kim SH, Lord C. Restricted and repetitive behaviors in toddlers and preschoolers with autism spectrum disorders based on the Autism Diagnostic Observation Schedule (ADOS). *Autism Res*. 2010;3:162–173

148. Esbensen AJ, Seltzer MM, Lam KSL, Bodfish JW. Age-related differences in restricted repetitive behaviors in autism spectrum disorders. *J Autism Dev Disord*. 2009;39:57–66

149. Lord C, Bishop S, Anderson D. Developmental trajectories as autism phenotypes. *Am J Med Genet C Semin Med Genet*. 2015;169:198–208

150. Kirchner JC, Dziobek I. Toward successful employment of adults with autism: a first analysis of special interests and factors deemed important for vocational performance. *Scand J Child Adolesc Psychiatr Psychol*. 2014;2:77–85

151. Ben-Sasson A, Hen L, Fluss R, Cermak SA, Engel-Yeger B, Gal E. A meta-analysis of sensory modulation symptoms in individuals with autism spectrum disorders. *J Autism Dev Disord*. 2009;39:1–11

152. Hazen EP, Stornelli JL, O'Rourke JA, Koesterer K, McDougle CJ. Sensory symptoms in autism spectrum disorders. *Harv Rev Psychiatry*. 2014;22:112–124

153. Barger BD, Campbell JM, McDonough JD. Prevalence and onset of regression within autism spectrum disorders: a meta-analytic review. *J Autism Dev Disord*. 2013;43:817–828

154. Bradley CC, Boan AD, Cohen AP, Charles JM, Carpenter LA. Reported history of developmental regression and restricted, repetitive behaviors in children with autism spectrum disorders. *J Dev Behav Pediatr.* 2016;37:451–456

155. Barbaresi WJ. The meaning of "regression" in children with autism spectrum disorder: why does it matter? *J Dev Behav Pediatr.* 2016;37:506–507

156. Meilleur AS, Fombonne E. Regression of language and non-language skills in pervasive developmental disorders. *J Intellect Disabil Res.* 2009;53:115–124

157. Viscidi EW, Triche EW, Pescosolido MF, et al. Clinical characteristics of children with autism spectrum disorder and co-occurring epilepsy. *PLoS One.* 2013;8:e67797

158. Jeste SS, Tuchman R. Autism spectrum disorder and epilepsy: two sides of the same coin? *J Child Neurol.* 2015;30:1963–1971

159. Charman T, Pickles A, Simonoff E, Chandler S, Loucas T, Baird G. IQ in children with autism spectrum disorders: data from the Special Needs and Autism Project (SNAP). *Psychol Med.* 2011;41:619–627

160. Joseph RM. The significance of IQ and differential cognitive abilities for understanding ASD. In: Fein D, ed. *The Neuropsychology of Autism.* New York, NY: Oxford University Press; 2011:281–294

161. Melling R, Swinson JM, Birak KS. The relationship between Autism Spectrum Quotient (AQ) and uneven intellectual development in school-age children. *Cogent Psychol.* 2016;3:1149136

162. Charman T, Jones CR, Pickles A, Simonoff E, Baird G, Happé F. Defining the cognitive phenotype of autism. *Brain Res.* 2011;1380:10–21

163. Prior M, Ozonoff S. Psychological factors in autism. In: Volkmar FR, ed. *Autism and Pervasive Developmental Disorders.* 2nd ed. Cambridge, United Kingdom: Cambridge University Press; 2007:69–128

164. Bauminger-Zviely N. School-age children with ASD. In: Volkmar FR, Rogers SJ, Paul R, Pelphrey KA, eds. *Handbook of Autism and Pervasive Developmental Disorders.* 4th ed. Vol I. Hoboken, NJ: John Wiley & Sons; 2014:148–175

165. Randi J, Newman T, Grigorenko EL. Teaching children with autism to read for meaning: challenges and possibilities. *J Autism Dev Disord.* 2010;40:890–902

166. Kushki A, Chau T, Anagnostou E. Handwriting difficulties in children with autism spectrum disorders: a scoping review. *J Autism Dev Disord.* 2011;41:1706–1716

167. Rozga A, Anderson SA, Robins DL. Major current neuropsychological theories of ASD. In: Fein D, ed. *The Neuropsychology of Autism.* New York, NY: Oxford University Press; 2011:97–120

168. Minshew NJ, Webb SJ, Williams DL, Dawson G. Neuropsychology and neurophysiology of autism spectrum disorders. In: Moldin SO, Rubenstein JLR, eds. *Understanding Autism: From Basic Neuroscience to Treatment.* Boca Raton, FL: Taylor & Francis; 2006:379–415

169. Sigman M, Spence SJ, Wang AT. Autism from developmental and neuropsychological perspectives. *Annu Rev Clin Psychol.* 2006;2:327–255

170. Baron-Cohen S. Empathizing, systemizing, and the extreme male brain theory of autism. *Prog Brain Res.* 2010;186:167–175

171. Baron-Cohen S, Cassidy S, Auyeung B, et al. Attenuation of typical sex differences in 800 adults with autism vs. 3,900 controls. *PLoS One.* 2014;9(7):e102251

172. Maski KP, Jeste SS, Spence SJ. Common neurological comorbidities in autism spectrum disorders. *Curr Opin Pediatr.* 2011;23:609–615

173. Fournier KA, Hass CJ, Naik SK, Lodha N, Cauraugh JH. Motor coordination in autism spectrum disorders: a synthesis and meta-analysis. *J Autism Dev Disord.* 2010;40:1227–1240

174. Bodison S, Mostofsky S. Motor control and motor learning processes in autism spectrum disorders. In: Volkmar FR, Rogers SJ, Paul R, Pelphrey KA, eds. *Handbook of Autism and Pervasive Developmental Disorders.* 4th ed. Vol I. Hoboken, NJ: John Wiley & Sons; 2014:354–377

175. Canitano R, Vivanti G. Tics and Tourette syndrome in autism spectrum disorders. *Autism.* 2007;11:19–28

176. Simonoff E, Pickles A, Charman T, Chandler S, Loucas T, Baird G. Psychiatric disorders in children with autism spectrum disorders: prevalence, comorbidity, and associated factors in a population-derived sample. *J Am Acad Child Adolesc Psychiatry.* 2008;47:921–929

177. Jokiranta-Olkoniemi E, Cheslack-Postava K, Sucksdorff D, et al. Risk of psychiatric and neurodevelopmental disorders among siblings of probands with autism spectrum disorders. *JAMA Psychiatry.* 2016;73:622–629

178. El Achkar CM, Spence SJ. Clinical characteristics of children and young adults with co-occurring autism spectrum disorder and epilepsy. *Epilepsy Behav.* 2015;47:183–190

179. Kohane IS, McMurry A, Weber G, et al. The comorbidity burden of children and young adults with autism spectrum disorders. *PLoS One.* 2012;7:e33224

180. Yasuhara A. Correlation between EEG abnormalities and symptoms of autism spectrum disorder (ASD). *Brain Dev.* 2010;32:791–798

181. Jokiranta E, Sourander A, Suominen A, Timonen-Soivio L, Brown AS, Sillanpaa M. Epilepsy among children and adolescents with autism spectrum disorders: a population-based study. *J Autism Dev Disord.* 2014;44:2547–2557

182. Suren P, Bakken IJ, Aase H, et al. Autism spectrum disorder, ADHD, epilepsy, and cerebral palsy in Norwegian children. *Pediatrics.* 2012;130:e152–e158

183. Mouridsen SE, Rich B, Isager T. A longitudinal study of epilepsy and other central nervous system diseases in individuals with and without a history of infantile autism. *Brain Dev.* 2011;33(5):361–366

184. Woolfenden S, Sarkozy V, Ridley G, Coory M, Williams K. A systematic review of two outcomes in autism spectrum disorder—epilepsy and mortality. *Dev Med Child Neurol.* 2012;54:306–312

185. Sansa G, Carlson C, Doyle W, et al. Medically refractory epilepsy in autism. *Epilepsia.* 2011;52:1071–1075

186. Ghacibeh GA, Fields C. Interictal epileptiform activity and autism. *Epilepsy Behav.* 2015;47:158–162

187. Kagan-Kushnir T, Roberts SW, Snead III OC. Screening electroencephalograms in autism spectrum disorders: evidence-based guidelines. *J Child Neurol.* 2005;20:197–206

188. Joshi G, Petty C, Wozniak J, et al. The heavy burden of psychiatric comorbidity in youth with autism spectrum disorders: a large comparative study of a psychiatrically referred population. *J Autism Dev Disord.* 2010;40:1361–1370

189. Simonoff E, Jones CR, Baird G, Pickles A, Happé F, Charman T. The persistence and stability of psychiatric problems in adolescents with autism spectrum disorders. *J Child Psychol Psychiatry.* 2013;54:186–194

190. Hill AP, Zuckerman KE, Hagen AD, et al. Aggressive behavior problems in children with autism spectrum disorders: prevalence and correlates in a large clinical sample. *Res Autism Spectr Disord.* 2014;8:1121–1133

191. Gotham K, Brunwasser SM, Lord C. Depressive and anxiety symptom trajectories from school age through young adulthood in samples with autism spectrum disorder and developmental delay. *J Am Acad Child Adolesc Psychiatry.* 2015;54:369–376

192. Orinstein A, Tyson KE, Suh J, et al. Psychiatric symptoms in youth with a history of autism and optimal outcome. *J Autism Dev Disord.* 2015;45:3703–3714

193. Verheij C, Louwerse A, van der Ende J, et al. The stability of comorbid psychiatric disorders: a 7 year follow up of children with pervasive developmental disorder-not otherwise specified. *J Autism Dev Disord.* 2015;45:3939–3948

194. Lai MC, Lombardo MV, Baron-Cohen S. Autism. *Lancet.* 2014;383:896–910

195. Cohen S, Conduit R, Lockley SW, Rajaratnam SM, Cornish KM. The relationship between sleep and behavior in autism spectrum disorder (ASD): a review. *J Neurodev Disord.* 2014;6:44

196. Hollway JA, Aman MG. Sleep correlates of pervasive developmental disorders: a review of the literature. *Res Dev Disabil.* 2011;32:1399–1421

197. McElhanon BO, McCracken C, Karpen S, Sharp WG. Gastrointestinal symptoms in autism spectrum disorder: a meta-analysis. *Pediatrics.* 2014;133:872–883

198. Buie T, Campbell DB, Fuchs GJ III, et al. Evaluation, diagnosis, and treatment of gastrointestinal disorders in individuals with ASDs: a consensus report. *Pediatrics.* 2010;125(suppl):S1–S18

199. Nikolov RN, Bearss KE, Lettinga J, et al. Gastrointestinal symptoms in a sample of children with pervasive developmental disorders. *J Autism Dev Disord.* 2009;39:405–413

200. Sharp WG, Berry RC, McCracken C, et al. Feeding problems and nutrient intake in children with autism spectrum disorders: a meta-analysis and comprehensive review of the literature. *J Autism Dev Disord.* 2013;43:2159–2173

201. Hubbard KL, Anderson SE, Curtin C, Must A, Bandini LG. A comparison of food refusal related to characteristics of food in children with autism spectrum disorder and typically developing children. *J Acad Nutr Diet.* 2014;114:1981–1987

202. Emond A, Emmett P, Steer C, Golding J. Feeding symptoms, dietary patterns, and growth in young children with autism spectrum disorders. *Pediatrics.* 2010;126:e337–e342

203. American Academy of Pediatrics Council on Children With Disabilities, Section on Developmental and Behavioral Pediatrics, Bright Futures Steering Committee, Medical Home Initiatives for Children With Special Needs Project Advisory Committee. Identifying infants and young children with developmental disorders in the medical home: an algorithm for developmental surveillance and screening. *Pediatrics.* 2006;118:405–420

204. Zwaigenbaum L, Bauman ML, Fein D, et al. Early screening of autism spectrum disorder: recommendations for practice and research. *Pediatrics.* 2015;136(suppl 1):S41–S59

205. Siu AL, US Preventive Services Task Force (USPSTF), Bibbins-Domingo K, et al. Screening for autism spectrum disorder in young children: US Preventive Services Task Force recommendation statement. *JAMA.* 2016;315:691–696

206. Fein D; Baby Sibs Research Consortium. Commentary on USPSTF final statement on universal screening for autism. *J Dev Behav Pediatr.* 2016;37:573–578

207. Robins DL, Casagrande K, Barton M, Chen CM, Dumont-Mathieu T, Fein D. Validation of the modified checklist for autism in toddlers, revised with follow-up (M-CHAT-R/F). *Pediatrics.* 2014;133:37–45

208. Dawson G. Why it's important to continue universal autism screening while research fully examines its impact. *JAMA Pediatr.* 2016;170:527–528

209. Veenstra-VanderWeele J, McGuire K. Rigid, inflexible approach results in no recommendation for autism screening. *JAMA Psychiatry.* 2016;73:327–328

210. Pierce K, Carter C, Weinfeld M, et al. Detecting, studying, and treating autism early: the one-year well-baby check-up approach. *J Pediatr.* 2011;159:458–465.e1–6

211. Chlebowski C, Robins DL, Barton ML, Fein D. Large-scale use of the modified checklist for autism in low-risk toddlers. *Pediatrics.* 2013;131:e1121–e1127

212. Huerta M, Lord C. Diagnostic evaluation of autism spectrum disorders. *Pediatr Clin North Am.* 2012;59:103–111

213. Steiner AM, Goldsmith TR, Snow AV, Chawarska K. Practitioner's guide to assessment of autism spectrum disorders in infants and toddlers. *J Autism Dev Disord.* 2012;42:1183–1196

214. Myers SM. Diagnosing developmental disabilities. In: Batshaw ML, Roizen NJ, Lotrecchiano GR, eds. *Children With Disabilities.* 7th ed. Baltimore, MD: Paul H. Brookes Publishing Co Inc; 2013:243–266

215. Hyman SL, Johnson JK. Autism and pediatric practice: toward a medical home. *J Autism Dev Disord.* 2012;42:1156–1164

216. ACMG Board of Directors. Clinical utility of genetic and genomic services: a position statement of the American College of Medical Genetics and Genomics. *Genet Med.* 2015;17:505–507

217. Sun F, Oristaglio J, Levy SE, et al. *Genetic Testing for Developmental Disabilities, Intellectual Disability, and Autism Spectrum Disorder: Technical Brief No. 23.* AHRQ Publication No.15-EHC024-EF. Rockville, MD: Agency for Healthcare Research and Quality. https://effectivehealthcare.ahrq.gov/topics/genetic-testing-developmental-disabilities/technical-brief. Published June 30, 2015. Accessed February 12, 2018

218. Iglesias A, Anyane-Yeboa K, Wynn J, et al. The usefulness of whole-exome sequencing in routine clinical practice. *Genet Med.* 2014;16:922–931

219. Riggs ER, Wain KE, Riethmaier D, et al. Chromosomal microarray impacts clinical management. *Clin Genet.* 2013;85:147–153

220. Srivastava S, Cohen JS, Vernon H, et al. Clinical whole exome sequencing in child neurology practice. *Ann Neurol.* 2014;76:473–483

221. Coulter ME, Miller DT, Harris DJ, et al. Chromosomal microarray testing influences medical management. *Genet Med.* 2011;13:770–776

222. Mroch AR, Flanagan JD, Stein QP. Solving the puzzle: case examples of array comparative genomic hybridization as a tool to end the diagnostic odyssey. *Curr Probl Pediatr Adolesc Health Care.* 2012;42:74–78

223. Ellison JW, Ravnan JB, Rosenfeld JA, et al. Clinical utility of chromosomal microarray analysis. *Pediatrics.* 2012;130:e1085–e1095

224. Bruno DL, Ganesamoorthy D, Schoumans J, et al. Detection of cryptic pathogenic copy number variations and constitutional loss of heterozygosity using high resolution SNP microarray analysis in 117 patients referred for cytogenetic analysis and impact on clinical practice. *J Med Genet.* 2009;46:123–131

225. Miller DT, Adam MP, Aradhya S, et al. Consensus statement: chromosomal microarray is a first-tier clinical diagnostic test for individuals with developmental disabilities or congenital anomalies. *Am J Hum Genet.* 2010;86:749–764

226. Manning M, Hudgins L. Array-based technology and recommendations for utilization in medical genetics practice for detection of chromosomal abnormalities. *Genet Med.* 2010;12:742–745

227. Michelson DJ, Shevell MI, Sherr EH, Moeschler JB, Gropman AL, Ashwal S. Evidence report: genetic and metabolic testing on children with global developmental delay: report of the Quality Standards Subcommittee of the American Academy of Neurology and the Practice Committee of the Child Neurology Society. *Neurology.* 2011;77:1629–1635

228. Schaefer GB, Mendelsohn NJ, Professional Practice and Guidelines Committee. Clinical genetics evaluation in identifying the etiology of autism spectrum disorders: 2013 guideline revisions. *Genet Med.* 2013;15:399–407

229. Vande Wydeven K, Kwan A, Hardan AY, Bernstein JA. Underutilization of genetics services for autism: the importance of parental awareness and provider recommendation. *J Genet Couns.* 2012;21:803–813

230. Narcisa V, Discenza M, Vaccari E, Rosen-Sheidley B, Hardan AY, Couchon E. Parental interest in a genetic risk assessment test for autism spectrum disorders. *Clin Pediatr (Phil).* 2013;52(2):139–146

231. Amiet C, Couchon E, Carr K, Caravol J, Cohen D. Are there cultural differences in parental interest in early diagnosis and genetic risk assessment for autism spectrum disorder? *Front Pediatr.* 2014;2:32

232. Cuccaro ML, Czape K, Alessandri M, et al. Genetic testing and corresponding services among individuals with autism spectrum disorder (ASD). *Am J Med Genet A.* 2014;164A:2592–2600

233. Kiely B, Vettam S, Adesman A. Utilization of genetic testing among children with developmental disabilities in the United States. *Appl Clin Genet.* 2016;9:93–100

234. Rosenfeld JA, Ballif BC, Torchia BS, et al. Copy number variations associated with autism spectrum disorders contribute to a spectrum of neurodevelopmental disorders. *Genet Med.* 2010;12(11):694–702

235. Schaefer GB, Starr L, Pickering D, Skar G, Dehaai K, Sanger WG. Array comparative genomic hybridization findings in a cohort referred for an autism evaluation. *J Child Neurol.* 2010;25(12):1498–1503

236. Bremer A, Giacobini M, Eriksson M, et al. Copy number variation characteristics in subpopulations of patients with autism spectrum disorders. *Am J Med Genet B Neuropsychiatr Genet.* 2011;156(2):115–124

237. Shen Y, Dies KA, Holm IA, et al. Clinical genetic testing for patients with autism spectrum disorders. *Pediatrics.* 2010;125:e727–e735

238. McGrew SG, Peters BR, Crittendon JA, Veenstra-Vanderweele J. Diagnostic yield of chromosomal microarray analysis in an autism primary care practice: which guidelines to implement? *J Autism Dev Disord.* 2012;42:1582–1591

239. Battaglia A, Doccini V, Berardini L, et al. Confirmation of chromosomal microarray as a first-tier clinical diagnostic test for individuals with developmental delay, intellectual disability, autism spectrum disorders, and dysmorphic features. *Eur J Pediatr Neurol.* 2013;17:589–599

240. Roberts JL, Hovanes K, Dasouki M, Manzardo AM, Butler MG. Chromosomal microarray analysis of consecutive individuals with autism spectrum disorders or learning disability presenting for genetic services. *Gene.* 2014;535:70–78

241. Eriksson MA, Lieden A, Westerlund J, et al. Rare copy number variants are common in young children with autism spectrum disorder. *Acta Paediatr.* 2015;104:610–618

242. Ho KS, Wassman ER, Baxter AL, et al. Chromosomal microarray analysis of consecutive individuals with autism spectrum disorders using an ultra-high resolution chromosomal microarray optimized for neurodevelopmental disorders. *Int J Mol Sci.* 2016;17(12):E2070

243. Yang Y, Muzny DM, Reid JG, et al. Clinical whole-exome sequencing for the diagnosis of Mendelian disorders. *N Engl J Med.* 2013;369:1502–1511

244. Yang Y, Muzny DM, Xia F, et al. Molecular findings among patients referred for clinical whole-exome sequencing. *JAMA.* 2014;312:1870–1879

245. Lee H, Deignan JL, Dorrani N, et al. Clinical exome sequencing for genetic identification of rare Mendelian disorders. *JAMA.* 2014;312:1880–1887

246. Soden SE, Saunders CJ, Willig LK, et al. Effectiveness of exome and genome sequencing guided by acuity of illness for diagnosis of neurodevelopmental disorders. *Sci Transl Med.* 2014;6:265ra168

247. Valencia CA, Husami A, Holle J, et al. Clinical impact and cost-effectiveness of whole exome sequencing as a diagnostic tool: a pediatric center's experience. *Front Pediatr.* 2015;3:67

248. Monroe GR, Frederix GW, Savelberg SMC, et al. Effectiveness of whole-exome sequencing and costs of the traditional diagnostic trajectory in children with intellectual disability. *Genet Med.* 2016;18:949–956

249. Nolan D, Carlson M. Whole exome sequencing in pediatric neurology patients: clinical implications and estimated cost analysis. *J Child Neurol.* 2016;31:887–894

250. Roesser J. Diagnostic yield of genetic testing in children diagnosed with autism spectrum disorders at a regional referral center. *Clin Pediatr.* 2011;50:834–843

251. Tassone F, Choudhary NS, Tassone F, et al. Identification of expanded alleles of the FMR1 gene in the Childhood Autism Risks from Genes and Environment (CHARGE) study. *J Autism Dev Disord.* 2013;43:530–539

252. Mordaunt D, Gabbett M, Waugh M, O'Brien K, Heussler H. Uptake and diagnostic yield of chromosomal microarray in an Australian child development clinic. *Children.* 2014;1:21–30

253. Jiang YH, Wang Y, Xiu X, et al. Genetic diagnosis of autism spectrum disorders: the opportunity and challenge in the genomics era. *Crit Rev Clin Lab Sci.* 2014;51:249–262

254. Manzi B, Loizzo AL, Giana G, Curatolo P. Autism and metabolic diseases. *J Child Neurol.* 2008;23:307–314

255. Zecavati N, Spence SJ. Neurometabolic disorders and dysfunction in autism spectrum disorders. *Curr Neurol Neurosci Rep.* 2009;9:129–136

256. Carter MT, Scherer SW. Autism spectrum disorder in the genetics clinic: a review. *Clin Genet.* 2013;83:399–407

257. Legido A, Jethva R, Goldenthal MJ. Mitochondrial dysfunction in autism. *Semin Pediatr Neurol.* 2013;20:163–175

258. Frye RE. Metabolic and mitochondrial disorders associated with epilepsy in children with autism spectrum disorder. *Epilepsy Behav.* 2015;47:147–157

259. Giulivi C, Zhang YF, Omanska-Klusek A, et al. Mitochondrial dysfunction in autism. *JAMA*. 2010;304:2389–2396

260. Herman GE, Henninger N, Ratliff-Schaub K, Pastore M, Fitzgerald S, McBride KL. Genetic testing in autism: how much is enough? *Genet Med*. 2007;9:268–274

261. Schiff M, Benoist JF, Aissaoui S, et al. Should metabolic diseases be systematically screened in nonsyndromic autism spectrum disorders? *PLoS One*. 2011;6:e21932

262. Hadjixenofontos A, Schmidt MA, Whitehead PL, et al. Evaluating mitochondrial DNA variation in autism spectrum disorders. *Ann Hum Genet*. 2013;77:9–21

263. Campistol J, Díez-Juan M, Callejón L, et al. Inborn error metabolic screening in individuals with nonsyndromic autism spectrum disorders. *Dev Med Child Neurol*. 2016;58:842–847

264. Brandler WM, Sebat J. From de novo mutations to personalized therapeutic interventions in autism. *Annu Rev Med*. 2015;66:487–507

265. Persico AM, Napolioni V. Autism genetics. *Behav Brain Res*. 2013;251:95–112

266. Zeegers M, Van Der Grond J, Durston S, et al. Radiological findings in autistic and developmentally delayed children. *Brain Dev*. 2006;28:495–499

267. Boddaert N, Zilbovicius M, Philipe A, et al. MRI findings in 77 children with non-syndromic autistic disorder. *PLoS One*. 2009;4:e4415

268. Vasa RA, Ranta M, Huisman TA, Pinto PS, Tillman RM, Mostofsky SH. Normal rates of neuroradiological findings in children with high functioning autism. *J Autism Dev Disord*. 2012;42:1662–1670

269. Erbetta A, Bulgheroni S, Contarino VE, et al. Neuroimaging findings in 41 low-functioning children with autism spectrum disorder: a single-center experience. *J Child Neurol*. 2014;29:1626–1631

270. Erbetta A, Bulgheroni S, Contarino VE, et al. Low-functioning autism and nonsyndromic intellectual disability: magnetic resonance imaging (MRI) findings. *J Child Neurol*. 2015;30:1658–1663

271. Filipek PA, Accardo PJ, Ashwal S, et al. Practice parameter: screening and diagnosis of autism: report of the Quality Standards Subcommittee of the American Academy of Neurology and the Child Neurology Society. *Neurology*. 2000;55:468–479

272. Volkmar F, Siegel M, Woodbury-Smith M, et al. Practice parameter for the assessment and treatment of children and adolescents with autism spectrum disorder. *J Am Acad Child Adolesc Psychiatry*. 2014;53:237–257

273. Moeschler JB, Shevell M; American Academy of Pediatrics Committee on Genetics. Comprehensive evaluation of the child with intellectual disability or global developmental delays. *Pediatrics*. 2014;134:e903–e918

274. Trauner D. Behavioral correlates of epileptiform abnormalities in autism. *Epilepsy Behav*. 2015;47:163–166

275. Hughes R, Poon W, Harvey AS. Limited role for routine EEG in the assessment of staring in children with autism spectrum disorder. *Arch Dis Child*. 2015;100:30–33

276. Besag FMC. Current controversies in the relationships between autism and epilepsy. *Epilepsy Behav*. 2015;47:143–146

277. Ritvo ER, Jorde LB, Mason-Brothers A, et al. The UCLA-University of Utah epidemiologic survey of autism: recurrence risk estimates and genetic counseling. *Am J Psychiatry*. 1989;146:1032–1036

278. Chakrabarti S, Fombonne E. Pervasive developmental disorders in preschool children. *JAMA*. 2001;285:3093–3099

279. Bolton P, Macdonald H, Pickles A, et al. A case-control family history study of autism. *J Child Psychol Psychiatry*. 1994;35:877–900

280. Chudley AE, Guitierrez E, Jocelyn LJ, Chodirker BN. Outcomes of genetic evaluation in children with pervasive developmental disorder. *J Dev Behav Pediatr*. 1998;19:321–325

281. Sumi S, Taniai H, Miyachi T, Tanemura M. Sibling risk of pervasive developmental disorder estimated by means of an epidemiologic survey in Nagoya, Japan. *J Hum Genet*. 2006;51:518–522

282. Constantino JN, Zhang Y, Frazier T, Abbacchi AM, Law P. Sibling recurrence and the genetic epidemiology of autism. *Am J Psychiatry*. 2010;167:1349–1356

283. Ozonoff S, Young GS, Carter A, et al. Recurrence risk for autism spectrum disorders: a Baby Siblings Research Consortium study. *Pediatrics*. 2011;128:e488–e495

284. Gronborg TK, Schendel DE, Parner ET. Recurrence of autism spectrum disorders in full- and half-siblings and trends over time: a population-based cohort study. *JAMA Pediatr*. 2013;167(10):947–953

285. Sandin S, Lichtenstein P, Kuja-Halkola R, Larsson H, Hultman CM, Reichenberg A. The familial risk of autism. *JAMA*. 2014;311:1770–1777

286. Jokiranta-Olkoniemi E, Cheslack-Postava K, Sucksdorff D, et al. Risk of psychiatric and neurodevelopmental disorders among siblings of probands with autism spectrum disorders. *JAMA Psychiatry*. 2016;73:622–629

287. Werling DM, Geschwind DH. Recurrence rates provide evidence for sex-differential, familial genetic liability for autism spectrum disorders in multiplex families and twins. *Mol Autism*. 2015;6:27

288. Lindgren KA, Folstein SE, Tomblin JB, Tager-Flusberg H. Language and reading abilities of children with autism spectrum disorders and specific language impairment and their first degree relatives. *Autism Res.* 2009;2:22–38

289. Finucane B, Myers SM. Genetic counseling for autism spectrum disorder in an evolving theoretical landscape. *Curr Genet Med Rep.* 2016;4:147–153

290. Myers SM, Johnson CP; American Academy of Pediatrics Council on Children With Disabilities. Management of children with autism spectrum disorders. *Pediatrics.* 2007;120:1162–1182

291. National Autism Center. *Findings and Conclusions: National Standards Project, Phase 2.* Randolph, MA: National Autism Center; 2015

292. Wong C, Odom SL, Hume K, et al. *Evidence-Based Practices for Children, Youth, and Young Adults with Autism Spectrum Disorder.* Chapel Hill, NC: The University of North Carolina, Frank Porter Graham Child Development Institute, Autism Evidence-Based Practice Review Group; 2014. http://autismpdc.fpg.unc.edu/sites/autismpdc.fpg.unc.edu/files/2014-EBP-Report.pdf. Accessed February 12, 2018

293. Wong C, Odom SL, Hume KA, et al. Evidence-based practices for children, youth, and young adults with autism spectrum disorder: a comprehensive review. *J Autism Dev Disord.* 2015;45:1951–1966

294. Schreibman L, Dawson G, Stahmer AC, et al. Naturalistic developmental behavioral interventions: empirically validated treatments for autism spectrum disorder. *J Autism Dev Disord.* 2015;45:2411–2428

295. Smith T, Scahill L, Dawson G, et al. Designing research studies on psychosocial interventions in autism. *J Autism Dev Disord.* 2007;37:354–366

296. Reichow B, Volkmar FR, Cicchetti DV. Development of the evaluative method for evaluating and determining evidence-based practices in autism. *J Autism Dev Disord.* 2008;38:1311–1319

297. Kratochwill TR, Hitchcock JH, Horner RH, et al. Single-case intervention research design standards. *Rem Spec Educ.* 2013;34:26–38

298. Smith T. What is evidence-based behavior analysis? *Behav Anal.* 2013;36:7–33

299. Howlin P, Moss P. Adults with autism spectrum disorders. *Can J Psychiatry.* 2012;57:275–283

300. Lounds Taylor J, Dove D, Veenstra-VanderWeele J, et al. *Interventions for Adolescents and Young Adults with Autism Spectrum Disorders.* Report No. 12-EHC063-EF. AHRQ Comparative Effectiveness Reviews. Rockville, MD: Agency for Healthcare Research and Quality; 2012

301. Taylor JL, McPheeters ML, Sathe NA, Dove D, Veenstra-Vanderwele J, Warren Z. A systematic review of vocational interventions for young adults with autism spectrum disorders. *Pediatrics.* 2012;130:531–538

302. Bishop-Fitzpatrick L, Minshew NJ, Eack SM. A systematic review of psychosocial interventions for adults with autism spectrum disorders. *J Autism Dev Disord.* 2013;43:687–694

303. Weitlauf AS, McPheeters ML, Peters B, et al. *Therapies for Children with Autism Spectrum Disorder: Behavioral Interventions Update.* Comparative Effectiveness Review No. 137. Rockville, MD: Agency for Healthcare Research and Quality. https://effectivehealthcare.ahrq.gov/topics/autism-update/research. Published August 6, 2014. Accessed February 12, 2018

304. Roth ME, Gillis JM, DiGennaro R. A meta-analysis of behavioral interventions for adolescents and adults with autism spectrum disorders. *J Behav Educ.* 2014;23:258–286

305. Murphy CM, Wilson CE, Robertson DM, et al. Autism spectrum disorder in adults: diagnosis, management, and health services development. *Neuropsychiatr Dis Treat.* 2016;12:1669–1686

306. Smith T, Iadarola S. Evidence base update for autism spectrum disorder. *J Clin Child Adolesc Psychol.* 2015;44:897–922

307. Zwaigenbaum L, Bauman ML, Choueiri R, et al. Early intervention for children with autism spectrum disorder under 3 years of age: recommendations for practice and research. *Pediatrics.* 2015;136(suppl 1):S60–S81

308. Odom SL, Boyd BA, Hall LJ, Hume K. Evaluation of comprehensive treatment models for individuals with autism spectrum disorders. *J Autism Dev Disord.* 2010;40:425–436

309. Odom SL, Boyd BA, Hall LJ, Hume KA. Comprehensive treatment models for children and youth with autism spectrum disorders. In: Volkmar FR, Rogers SJ, Paul R, Pelphrey KA, eds. *Handbook of Autism and Pervasive Developmental Disorders.* 4th ed. Vol 2. Hoboken, NJ: John Wiley & Sons; 2014:770–787

310. Sukhodolsky DG, Bloch MH, Panza KE, Reichow B. Cognitive-behavioral therapy for anxiety in children with high-functioning autism: a meta-analysis. *Pediatrics.* 2013;132:e1341–e1350

311. Ingersoll B, Dvortcsak A, Whalen C, Sikora D. The effects of a developmental, social-pragmatic language intervention on rate of expressive language production in young children with autistic spectrum disorders. *Focus Autism Other Dev Disabl.* 2005;20:213–222

312. Ingersoll BR. Teaching social communication: a comparison of naturalistic behavioral and developmental, social pragmatic approaches for children with autism spectrum disorders. *J Posit Behav Interv.* 2010;12:33–43

313. Roane HS, Fisher WW, Carr JE. Applied behavior analysis as treatment for autism spectrum disorder. *J Pediatr.* 2016;175:27–32

314. Virues-Ortega J, Julio FM, Pastor-Barriuso R. The TEACCH program for children and adults with autism: a meta-analysis of intervention studies. *Clin Psychol Rev.* 2013;33:940–953

315. Boyd BA, Hume K, McBee MT, et al. Comparative efficacy of LEAP, TEACCH and non-model-specific special education programs for preschoolers with autism spectrum disorders. *J Autism Dev Disord.* 2014;44:366–380

316. Bottema-Beutel K, Yoder P, Woynaroski T, Sandbank M. Targeted interventions for social communication symptoms in preschoolers with autism spectrum disorders. In: Volkmar FR, Rogers SJ, Paul R, Pelphrey KA, eds. *Handbook of Autism and Pervasive Developmental Disorders.* 4th ed. Vol 2. Hoboken, NJ: John Wiley & Sons; 2014:788–812

317. Smith T. Applied behavior analysis and early intensive intervention. In: Amaral DG, Dawson G, Geschwind DH, eds. *Autism Spectrum Disorders.* New York, NY: Oxford University Press; 2011:1037–1055

318. Leaf JB, Leaf R, McEachin J, et al. Applied behavior analysis is a science and, therefore, progressive. *J Autism Dev Disord.* 2016;46:720–731

319. Stahmer AC. Effective strategies by any other name. *Autism.* 2014;18:211–212

320. Reichow B, Barton EE. Evidence-based psychosocial interventions for individuals with autism spectrum disorders. In: Volkmar FR, Rogers SJ, Paul R, Pelphrey KA, eds. *Handbook of Autism and Pervasive Developmental Disorders.* 4th ed. Vol 2. Hoboken, NJ: John Wiley & Sons; 2014:969–992

321. Sham E, Smith T. Publication bias in studies of an applied behavior-analytic intervention: an initial analysis. *J Appl Behav Anal.* 2014;47:663–678

322. Schreibman L, Stahmer AC. A randomized trial comparison of the effects of verbal and pictorial naturalistic communication strategies on spoken language for young children with autism. *J Autism Dev Disord.* 2014;44:1244–1251

323. Murza KA, Schwartz JB, Hahs-Vaughn DL, Nye C. Joint attention interventions for children with autism spectrum disorder: a systematic review and meta-analysis. *Int J Lang Commun Disord.* 2016;51:236–251

324. Verschuur R, Didden R, Lang R, Sigafoos J, Huskens B. Pivotal response treatment for children with autism spectrum disorders: a review. *Rev J Autism Dev Disord.* 2014;1:34–61

325. Eldevik S, Hastings RP, Hughes JC, Jahr E, Eikeseth S, Cross S. Meta-analysis of early intensive behavioral intervention for children with autism. *J Clin Child Adolesc Psychol.* 2009;38:439–450

326. Eldevik S, Hastings RP, Hughes JC, Jahr E, Eikeseth S, Cross S. Using participant data to extend the evidence base for intensive behavioral intervention for children with autism. *Am J Intellect Dev Disabil.* 2010;115:381–405

327. Peters-Scheffer N, Didden R, Korzilius H, et al. A meta-analytic study on the effectiveness of comprehensive ABA based early intervention programs for children with autism spectrum disorders. *Res Autism Spectr Disord.* 2011;5:60–69

328. Makrygianni MK, Reed P. A meta-analytic review of the effectiveness of behavioural early intervention programs for children with autistic spectrum disorders. *Res Autism Spectr Disord.* 2010;4:577–593

329. Virués-Ortega J. Applied behavior analytic intervention for autism in early childhood: meta-analysis, meta-regression and dose-response meta-analysis of multiple outcomes. *Clin Psychol Rev.* 2010;30:387–399

330. Reichow B, Barton EE, Boyd BA, Hume K. Early intensive behavioral intervention (EIBI) for young children with autism spectrum disorders (ASD). *Cochrane Database Syst Rev.* 2012;10:CD009260

331. Strain PS, Hoyson M. On the need for longitudinal, intensive social skill intervention: LEAP follow-up outcomes for children with autism as a case-in-point. *Topics Early Child Spec Educ.* 2000;20:116–122

332. Strain PS, Bovey EH. Randomized, controlled trial of the LEAP model of early intervention for young children with autism spectrum disorders. *Topics Early Child Spec Educ.* 2011;31:133–154

333. Dawson G, Rogers S, Munson J, et al. Randomized, controlled trial of an intervention for toddlers with autism: the Early Start Denver Model. *Pediatrics.* 2010;125:e17–e23

334. Rogers SJ, Dawson G. *Early Start Denver Model for Young Children with Autism: Promoting Language, Learning, and Engagement.* New York,NY: Guilford Press; 2010

335. Estes A, Munson J, Rogers SJ, Greenson J, Winter J, Dawson G. Long-term outcomes of early intervention in 6-year-old children with autism spectrum disorder. *J Am Acad Child Adolesc Psychiatry.* 2015;54:580–587

336. Eapen V, Crncec R, Walter A. Clinical outcomes of an early intervention program for preschool children with autism spectrum disorder in a community group setting. *BMC Pediatr.* 2013;13:3

337. Vivanti G, Dissanayake C, Zierhut C, Rogers SJ; Victorian ASELCC Team. Brief report: predictors of outcomes in the Early Start Denver Model delivered in a group setting. *J Autism Dev Disord.* 2013;43:1717–1724

338. Vivanti G, Paynter J, Duncan E, et al. Effectiveness and feasibility of the Early Start Denver Model implemented in a group-based community childcare setting. *J Autism Dev Disord.* 2014;44:3140–3153

339. Rogers SJ, Estes A, Lord C, et al. Effects of a brief Early Start Denver model (ESDM)-based parent intervention on toddlers at risk for autism spectrum disorders: a randomized controlled trial. *J Am Acad Child Adolesc Psychiatry.* 2012;51:1052–1065

340. Vismara LA, Rogers SJ. Behavioral treatments in autism spectrum disorder: what do we know? *Annu Rev Clin Psychol.* 2010;6:447–468

341. Reichow B. Overview of meta-analyses on early intensive behavioral intervention for young children with autism spectrum disorders. *J Autism Dev Disord.* 2012;42:512–520

342. Dawson G, Bernier R. A quarter century of progress on the early detection and treatment of autism spectrum disorder. *Dev Psychopathol.* 2013;4:1455–1472

343. Suhrheinrich J, Hall LJ, Reed SR, Stahmer AC, Schreibman L. Evidence based interventions in the classroom. In: Wilkinson L, ed. *Autism Spectrum Disorder in Children and Adolescents: Evidence-based Assessment and Intervention in Schools.* Washington, DC: American Psychological Association; 2014:151–172

344. Young J, Corea C, Kimani J, Mandell D. *Autism Spectrum Disorders (ASDs) Services: Final Report on Environmental Scan.* https://www.medicaid.gov/medicaid/ltss/downloads/autism-spectrum-disorders.pdf. Published March 9, 2010. Accessed February 12, 2018

345. Maglione MA, Gans D, Das L, et al. Nonmedical interventions for children with ASD: recommended guidelines and further research needs. *Pediatrics.* 2012;130(suppl 2):S169–S178

346. Oono IP, Honey EJ, McConachie H. Parent-mediated early intervention for young children with autism spectrum disorders (ASD). *Cochrane Database Syst Rev.* 2013;(4):CD009774

347. Beaudoin AJ, Sébire G, Couture M. Parent training interventions for toddlers with autism spectrum disorder. *Autism Res Treat.* 2014;2014:839890

348. Zane T, Weiss MJ, Dunlop K, Southwick J. Relationship-based therapies for autism spectrum disorders. In: Foxx RM, Mulick JA, eds. *Controversial Therapies for Autism and Intellectual Disabilities: Fads, Fashion and Science in Professional Practice.* New York, NY: Routledge; 2016:357–371

349. Hobson JA, Tarver L, Beurkens N, Hobson RP. The relation between severity of autism and caregiver-child interaction: a study in the context of relationship development intervention. *J Abnorm Child Psychol.* 2016;44:745–755

350. Gutstein SE, Burgess AF, Montfort K. Evaluation of the relationship development intervention program. *Autism.* 2007;11:397–411

351. Casenhiser DM, Shanker SG, Stieben J. Learning through interaction in children with autism: preliminary data from a social-communication-based intervention. *Autism.* 2013;17:220–241

352. Pajareya K, Nopmaneejumruslers K. A pilot randomized controlled trial of DIR/Floortime™ parent training intervention for pre-school children with autistic spectrum disorders. *Autism.* 2011;15:563–577

353. Greenspan SI, Wieder S. Developmental patterns and outcomes in infants and children with disorders in relating and communicating: a chart review of 200 cases of children with autistic spectrum diagnoses. *J Dev Learn Disord.* 1997;1:87–141

354. Wieder S, Greenspan SI. Can children with autism master the core deficits and become empathetic, creative, and reflective? A ten to fifteen year follow-up of a subgroup of children with autism spectrum disorders (ASD) who received a comprehensive developmental, individual-difference, relationship-based (DIR) approach. *J Dev Learn Disord.* 2005;9:39–61

355. Solomon R, Van Egeren LA, Mahoney G, Quon Huber MS, Zimmerman P. PLAY Project Home Consultation intervention program for young children with autism spectrum disorders: a randomized controlled trial. *J Dev Behav Pediatr.* 2014;35:475–485

356. Green J, Charman T, McConachie H, et al. Parent-mediated communication-focused treatment in children with autism (PACT): a randomised controlled trial. *Lancet.* 2010;375(9732):2152–2160

357. Pickles A, Le Couteur A, Leadbitter K, et al. Parent-mediated social communication therapy for young children with autism (PACT): long-term follow-up of a randomised controlled trial. *Lancet.* 2016;388(10059):2501–2509

358. Hampton L, Kaiser A. Intervention effects on spoken-language outcomes for children with autism: a systematic review and meta-analysis. *J Intellect Disabil Res.* 2016;60:444–463

359. Parsons L, Cordier R, Munro N, Joosten A, Speyer R. A systematic review of pragmatic language interventions for children with autism spectrum disorder. *PLoS One.* 2017;12(4):e0172242

360. Ganz JB, Earles-Vollrath TL, Heath AK, Parker RI, Rispoli MJ, Duran JB. A meta-analysis of single case research studies on aided augmentative and alternative communication systems with individuals with autism spectrum disorders. *J Autism Dev Disord.* 2012;42:60–74

361. Ganz JB, Davis JL, Lund EM, Goodwyn FD, Simpson RL. Meta-analysis of PECS with individuals with ASD: investigation of targeted versus non-targeted outcomes, participant characteristics, and implementation phase. *Res Dev Disabil.* 2012;33:406–418

362. Ganz JB. AAC interventions for individuals with autism spectrum disorders: state of the science and future research directions. *Augment Altern Commun.* 2015;31:203–214

363. Schlosser RW, Koul RK. Speech output technologies in interventions for individuals with autism spectrum disorders: a scoping review. *Augment Altern Commun.* 2015;31:285–309

364. Iacono T, Trembath D, Erickson S. The role of augmentative and alternative communication for children with autism: current status and future trends. *Neuropsychiatr Dis Treat.* 2016;12:2349–2361

365. Shepherd J. Activities of daily living. In: Case-Smith J, O'Brien JC, eds. *Occupational Therapy for Children.* 6th ed. Maryland Heights, MO: Elsevier Mosby; 2010:474–517

366. Case-Smith J, Weaver LL, Fristad MA. A systematic review of sensory processing interventions for children with autism spectrum disorders. *Autism.* 2015;19:133–148

367. Barton EE, Reichow B, Schnitz A, Smith IC, Sherlock D. A systematic review of sensory-based treatments for children with disabilities. *Res Dev Disabil.* 2015;37:64–80

368. Lang R, O'Reilly M, Healy O, et al. Sensory integration therapy for autism spectrum disorders: a systematic review. *Res Autism Spectr Disord.* 2012;6:1004–1018

369. American Academy of Pediatrics Section on Complementary and Integrative Medicine, Council on Children With Disabilities. Sensory integration therapies for children with developmental and behavioral disorders. *Pediatrics.* 2012;129:1186–1189

370. Lilienfeld SO, Marshall J, Todd JT, Shane HC. The persistence of fad interventions in the face of negative scientific evidence: facilitated communication for autism as a case example. *Evid Based Commun Assess Interv.* 2014;8:62–101

371. Schlosser RW, Balandin S, Hemsley B, Iacono T, Probst P, von Tetzchner S. Facilitated communication and authorship: a systematic review. *Augment Altern Commun.* 2014;30:359–368

372. International Society for Augmentative and Alternative Communication. ISAAC position statement on facilitated communication. *Augment Altern Commun.* 2014;30:357–358

373. National Research Council, Committee on Educational Interventions for Children with Autism. *Educating Children with Autism.* Lord C, McGee JP, eds. Washington, DC: National Academies Press; 2001

374. Iovannone R, Dunlap G, Huber H, Kincaid D. Effective educational practices for students with autism spectrum disorders. *Focus Autism Other Dev Disabl.* 2003;18:150–165

375. Myers SM. Management of autism spectrum disorders in primary care. *Pediatr Ann.* 2009;38:42–49

376. Odom SL, Hume K, Boyd B, Stabel A. Moving beyond the intensive behavior therapy versus eclectic dichotomy: evidence-based and individualized program for students with autism. *Behav Modif.* 2012;36:270–297

377. Odom SL, Cox AW, Brock ME. Implementation science, professional development, and autism spectrum disorders. *Except Child.* 2013;79:233–251

378. Cox AW, Brock ME, Odom SL, et al. National Professional Development Center on ASD: an emerging national educational strategy. In: Doehring P, ed. *Autism Services Across America.* Baltimore, MD: Brookes; 2013:249–266

379. Volkmar FR, Wiesner LA, Westphal A. Healthcare issues for children on the autism spectrum. *Curr Opin Psychiatry.* 2006;19:361–366

380. Tuchman R, Alessandri M, Cuccaro M. Autism spectrum disorders and epilepsy: moving towards a comprehensive approach to treatment. *Brain Dev.* 2010;32:719–730

381. Buie T, Fuchs GJ III, Furuta GT, et al. Recommendations for evaluation and treatment of common gastrointestinal problems in children with ASDs. *Pediatrics.* 2010;125(suppl 1):S19–S29

382. Malow BA, Byars K, Johnson K, et al. A practice pathway for the identification, evaluation, and management of insomnia in children and adolescents with autism spectrum disorders. *Pediatrics.* 2012;130(suppl 2):S106–S124

383. Farmer C, Thurm A, Grant P. Pharmacotherapy for the core symptoms in autistic disorder: current status of the research. *Drugs.* 2013;73:303–314

384. Marrus N, Underwood-Riordan H, Randall F, Zhang Y, Constantino JN. Lack of effect of risperidone on core autistic symptoms: data from a longitudinal study. *J Child Adolesc Psychopharmacol.* 2014;24:513–518

385. McDougle CJ, Scahill L, Aman MG, et al. Risperidone for the core symptom domains of autism: results from the study by the autism network of the Research Units on Pediatric Psychopharmacology. *Am J Psychiatry.* 2005;162:1142–1148

386. Aman MG, Findling RL, Hardan AY, et al. Safety and efficacy of memantine in children with autism: randomized, placebo-controlled study and open-label extension. *J Child Adolesc Psychopharmacol.* 2017;27:403–412

387. Wong AY, Hsia Y, Chan EW, et al. The variation of psychopharmacological prescription rates for people with autism spectrum disorder (ASD) in 30 countries. *Autism Res.* 2014;7:543–554

388. Murray ML, Hsia Y, Glaser K, et al. Pharmacological treatments prescribed to people with autism spectrum disorder (ASD) in primary health care. *Psychopharmacology (Berl).* 2014;231:1011–1021

389. Aman MG, Lam KS, Van Bourgondien ME. Medication patterns in patients with autism: temporal, regional, and demographic influences. *J Child Adolesc Psychopharmacol.* 2005;15:116–126

390. Esbensen AJ, Greenberg JS, Seltzer MM, Aman MG. A longitudinal investigation of psychotropic and non-psychotropic medication use among adolescents and adults with autism spectrum disorders. *J Autism Dev Disord.* 2009;39:1339–1349

391. Schubart JR, Camacho F, Leslie D. Psychotropic medication trends among children and adolescents with autism spectrum disorder in the Medicaid program. *Autism.* 2014;18:631–637

392. Rosenberg R, Mandell DS, Farmer JE, Law JK, Marvin AR, Law PA. Psychotropic medication use among children with autism spectrum disorders enrolled in a national registry, 2007–2008. *J Autism Dev Disord.* 2010;40:342–351

393. Coury DL, Anagnostou E, Manning-Courtney P, et al. Use of psychotropic medication in children and adolescents with autism spectrum disorders. *Pediatrics.* 2012;130(suppl 2):S69–S76

394. Logan SL, Carpenter L, Leslie RS, et al. Aberrant behaviors and co-occurring conditions as predictors of psychotropic polypharmacy among children with autism spectrum disorders. *J Child Adolesc Psychopharmacol.* 2015;25:323–336

395. Mire SS, Nowell KP, Kubiszyn T, Goin-Kochel RP. Psychotropic medication use among children with autism spectrum disorders within the Simons Simplex Collection: are core features of autism spectrum disorder related? *Autism.* 2014;18:933–942

396. Mandell DS, Morales KH, Marcus SC, Stahmer AC, Doshi J, Polsky DE. Psychotropic medication use among Medicaid-enrolled children with autism spectrum disorders. *Pediatrics.* 2008;121:e441–e448

397. Spencer D, Marshall J, Post B, et al. Psychotropic medication use and polypharmacy in children with autism spectrum disorders. *Pediatrics.* 2013;132:833–840

398. Witwer A, Lecavalier L. Treatment incidence and patterns in children and adolescents with autism spectrum disorders. *J Child Adolesc Psychopharmacol.* 2005;15:671–681

399. Frazier TW, Shattuck PT, Narendorf SC, Cooper BP, Wagner M, Spitznagel EL. Prevalence and correlates of psychotropic medication use in adolescents with an autism spectrum disorder with and without caregiver-reported attention-deficit/hyperactivity disorder. *J Child Adolesc Psychopharmacol.* 2011;21:571–579

400. Accordino RE, Kidd C, Politte LC, Henry CA, McDougle CJ. Psychopharmacological interventions in autism spectrum disorder. *Expert Opin Pharmacother.* 2016;17:937–952

401. Perrin JM, Coury DL, Klatka K, et al. The Autism Intervention Research Network on Physical Health and the Autism Speaks Autism Treatment Network. *Pediatrics.* 2016;137(suppl 2):S67–S71

402. Mahajan R, Bernal MP, Panzer R, et al. Clinical practice pathways for evaluation and medication choice for attention-deficit/hyperactivity disorder symptoms in autism spectrum disorders. *Pediatrics.* 2012;130(suppl 2):S125–S138

403. McGuire K, Fung LK, Hagopian L, et al. Irritability and problem behavior in autism spectrum disorder: a practice pathway for pediatric primary care. *Pediatrics.* 2016;137(suppl 2):S136–S148

404. Vasa RA, Mazurek MO, Mahajan R, et al. Assessment and treatment of anxiety in youth with autism spectrum disorders. *Pediatrics.* 2016;137(suppl 2):S115–S123

405. Myers SM. The status of pharmacotherapy for autism spectrum disorders. *Expert Opin Pharmacother.* 2007;8:1579–1603

406. Hanley GP, Iwata BA, McCord BE. Functional analysis of problem behavior: a review. *J Appl Behav Anal.* 2003;36:147–185

407. Foxx RM. Applied behavior analysis treatment of autism: the state of the art. *Child Adolesc Psychiatr Clin N Am.* 2008;17:821–834

408. Harvey ST, Boer D, Meyer LH, Evans IM. Updating a meta-analysis of intervention research with challenging behaviour: treatment validity and standards of practice. *J Intellect Dev Disabil.* 2009;34:67–80

409. Doehring P, Reichow B, Palka T, Phillips C, Hagopian L. Behavioral approaches to managing severe problem behaviors in children with autism spectrum and related developmental disorders: a descriptive analysis. *Child Adolesc Psychiatr Clin N Am.* 2014;23:25–40

410. Bauman ML. Medical comorbidities in autism: challenges to diagnosis and treatment. *Neurotherapeutics.* 2010;7:320–327

411. Burke LM, Kalpakjian CZ, Smith YR, Quint EH. Gynecological issues of adolescents with Down syndrome, autism, and cerebral palsy. *J Pediatr Adolesc Gynecol.* 2010;23:11–15

412. Coury D. Medical treatment of autism spectrum disorders. *Curr Opin Neurol.* 2010;23(2):131–136

413. Maenner MJ, Arneson CL, Levy SE, Kirby RS, Nicholas JS, Durkin MS. Brief report: association between behavioral features and gastrointestinal problems among children with autism spectrum disorder. *J Autism Dev Disord.* 2012;42:1520–1525

414. Siegel M, Gabriels RL. Psychiatric hospital treatment of children with autism and serious behavioral disturbance. *Child Adolesc Psychiatr Clin N Am.* 2014;23:124–142

415. Guinchat V, Cravero C, Diaz L, et al. Acute behavioral crises in psychiatric inpatients with autism spectrum disorder (ASD): recognition of concomitant medical or non-ASD psychiatric conditions predicts enhanced improvement. *Res Dev Disabil.* 2015;38:242–255

416. King BH, de Lacy N, Siegel M. Psychiatric assessment of severe presentations in autism spectrum disorders and intellectual disability. *Child Adolesc Psychiatr Clin N Am.* 2014;23:1–14

417. Politte LC, Henry CA, McDougle CJ. Psychopharmacological interventions in autism spectrum disorder. *Harv Rev Psychiatry.* 2014;22:76–92

418. Ji N, Findling RL. An update on pharmacotherapy for autism spectrum disorder in children and adolescents. *Curr Opin Psychiatry.* 2015;28:91–101

419. Fung LK, Mahajan R, Nozzolillo A, et al. Pharmacologic treatment of severe irritability and problem behaviors in autism: a systematic review and meta-analysis. *Pediatrics.* 2016;137(suppl 2):S124–S135

420. Quintana H, Birmaher B, Stedge D, et al. Use of methylphenidate in the treatment of children with autistic disorder. *J Autism Dev Disord.* 1995;25:283–294

421. Handen BL, Johnson CR, Lubetsky M. Efficacy of methylphenidate among children with autism and symptoms of attention-deficit hyperactivity disorder. *J Autism Dev Disord.* 2000;30:245–255

422. Research Units on Pediatric Psychopharmacology Autism Network. Randomized, controlled, crossover trial of methylphenidate in pervasive developmental disorders with hyperactivity. *Arch Gen Psychiatry.* 2005;62:1266–1274

423. Pearson DA, Santos CW, Aman MG, et al. Effects of extended release methylphenidate treatment on ratings of attention-deficit/hyperactivity disorder (ADHD) and associated behavior in children with autism spectrum disorders and ADHD symptoms. *J Child Adolesc Psychopharmacol.* 2013;23:337–351

424. Posey DJ, Aman MG, McCracken JT, et al. Positive effects of methylphenidate on inattention and hyperactivity in pervasive developmental disorders: an analysis of secondary measures. *Biol Psychiatry.* 2007;61:538–544

425. Arnold LE, Aman MG, Cook AM, et al. Atomoxetine for hyperactivity in autism spectrum disorders: placebo-controlled crossover pilot trial. *J Am Acad Child Adolesc Psychiatry.* 2006;45:1196–1205

426. Harfterkamp M, van de Loo-Neus G, Minderaa RB, et al. A randomized double-blind study of atomoxetine versus placebo for attention-deficit/hyperactivity disorder symptoms in children with autism spectrum disorder. *J Am Acad Child Adolesc Psychiatry.* 2012;51:733–741

427. Fankhauser MP, Karumanchi VC, German ML, Yates A, Karumanchi SD. A double-blind, placebo-controlled study of the efficacy of transdermal clonidine in autism. *J Clin Psychiatry* 1992;53:77–82

428. Jaselskis CA, Cook EH Jr, Fletcher KE, Leventhal BL. Clonidine treatment of hyperactive and impulsive children with autistic disorder. *J Clin Psychopharmacol.* 1992;12:322–327

429. Handen BL, Sahl R, Hardan AY. Guanfacine in children with autism and/or intellectual disabilities. *J Dev Behav Pediatr.* 2008;29:303–308

430. Scahill L, McCracken JT, King BH, et al. Extended-release guanfacine for hyperactivity in children with autism spectrum disorder. *Am J Psychiatry.* 2015;172:1197–1206

431. McCracken JT, McGough J, Shah B, et al. Risperidone in children with autism and serious behavioral problems. *N Engl J Med.* 2002;347:314–321

432. Shea S, Turgay A, Carroll A, et al. Risperidone in the treatment of disruptive behavioral symptoms in children with autistic and other pervasive developmental disorders. *Pediatrics.* 2004;114:e634–e641

433. Marcus RN, Owen R, Kamen L, et al. A placebo-controlled, fixed-dose study of aripiprazole in children and adolescents with irritability associated with autistic disorder. *J Am Acad Child Adolesc Psychiatry.* 2009;48:1110–1119

434. Owen R, Sikich L, Marcus RN, et al. Aripiprazole in the treatment of irritability in children and adolescents with autistic disorder. *Pediatrics.* 2009;124:1533–1540

435. Pandina GJ, Bossie CA, Youssef E, Zhu Y, Dunbar F. Risperidone improves behavioral symptoms in children with autism in a randomized, double-blind, placebo-controlled trial. *J Autism Dev Disord.* 2007;37:367–373

436. Aman MG, McDougle CJ, Scahill L, et al. Medication and parent training in children with pervasive developmental disorders and serious behavior problems: results from a randomized clinical trial. *J Am Acad Child Adolesc Psychiatry.* 2009;48:1143–1154

437. Arnold LE, Aman MG, Li X, et al. Research Units of Pediatric Psychopharmacology (RUPP) autism network randomized clinical trial of parent training and medication: one-year follow-up. *J Am Acad Child Adolesc Psychiatry.* 2012;51:1173–1184

438. Kent JM, Kushner S, Ning X, et al. Risperidone dosing in children and adolescents with autistic disorder: a double-blind, placebo-controlled study. *J Autism Dev Disord.* 2013;43:1773–1783

439. Ghanizadeh A, Sahraeizadeh A, Berk M. A head-to-head comparison of aripiprazole and risperidone for safety and treating autistic disorders, a randomized double blind clinical trial. *Child Psychiatry Hum Dev* 2014;45:185–192

440. Research Units on Pediatric Psychopharmacology Autism Network. Risperidone treatment of autistic disorder: longer-term benefits and blinded discontinuation after 6 months. *Am J Psychiatry.* 2005;162:1361–1369

441. Troost PW, Lahuis BE, Steenhuis MP, et al. Long-term effects of risperidone in children with autism spectrum disorders: a placebo discontinuation study. *J Am Acad Child Adolesc Psychiatry.* 2005;44:1137–1144

442. Marcus RN, Owen R, Manos G, et al. Safety and tolerability of aripiprazole for irritability in pediatric patients with autistic disorder: a 52-week, open-label, multicenter study. *J Clin Psychiatry.* 2011;72:1270–1276

443. Findling RL, Mankoski R, Timko K, et al. A randomized controlled trial investigating the safety and efficacy of aripiprazole in the long-term maintenance treatment of pediatric patients with irritability associated with autistic disorder. *J Clin Psychiatry.* 2014;75:22–30

444. Hardan AY, Fung LK, Libove RA, et al. A randomized controlled pilot trial of oral N-acetylcysteine in children with autism. *Biol Psychiatry.* 2012;71:956–961

445. Ghanizadeh A, Moghimi-Sarani E. A randomized double blind placebo controlled clinical trial of N-acetylcysteine added to risperidone for treating autistic disorders. *BMC Psychiatry.* 2013;13:196

446. Nikoo M, Radnia H, Farokhnia M, Mohammadi MR, Akhondzadeh S. N-acetylcysteine as an adjunctive therapy to risperidone for treatment of irritability in autism: a randomized, double-blind, placebo-controlled clinical trial of efficacy and safety. *Clin Neuropharmacol.* 2015;38:11–17

447. McDougle CJ, Naylor ST, Cohen DJ, et al. A double-blind, placebo-controlled study of fluvoxamine in adults with autistic disorder. *Arch Gen Psychiatry.* 1996;53:1001–1008

448. Hollander E, Chaplin W, Soorya L, et al. Divalproex sodium vs placebo for the treatment of irritability in children and adolescents with autism spectrum disorders. *Neuropsychopharmacology.* 2010;35:990–998

449. Niederhofer H. Venlafaxine has modest effects in autistic children. *Therapy.* 2004;1:87–90

450. McDougle CJ, Holmes JP, Carlson DC, et al. A double-blind, placebo-controlled study of risperidone in adults with autistic disorder and other pervasive developmental disorders. *Arch Gen Psychiatry.* 1998;55:633–641

451. Hollander E, Soorya L, Wasserman S, Esposito K, Chaplin W, Anagnostou E. Divalproex sodium vs. placebo in the treatment of repetitive behaviours in autism spectrum disorder. *Int J Neuropsychopharmacol.* 2006;9:209–213

452. Hollander E, Soorya L, Chaplin W, et al. A double-blind placebo-controlled trial of fluoxetine for repetitive behaviors and global severity in adult autism spectrum disorders. *Am J Psychiatry.* 2012;169:292–299

453. Strawn JR, Welge JA, Wehry AM, Keeshin B, Rynn MA. Efficacy and tolerability of antidepressants in pediatric anxiety disorders: a systematic review and meta-analysis. *Depress Anxiety.* 2015;32:149–157

454. Cortesi F, Giannotti F, Sebastiani T, Panunzi S, Valente D. Controlled-release melatonin, singly and combined with cognitive behavioural therapy, for persistent insomnia in children with autism spectrum disorders: a randomized placebo-controlled trial. *J Sleep Res.* 2012;21:700–709

455. Wright B, Sims D, Smart S, et al. Melatonin versus placebo in children with autism spectrum conditions and severe sleep problems not amenable to behaviour management strategies: a randomised controlled crossover trial. *J Autism Dev Disord.* 2011;41:175–184

456. Wirojanan J, Jacquemont S, Diaz R, et al. The efficacy of melatonin for sleep problems in children with autism, fragile X syndrome, or autism and fragile X syndrome. *J Clin Sleep Med.* 2009;5:145–150

457. Garstang J, Wallis M. Randomized controlled trial of melatonin for children with autistic spectrum disorders and sleep problems. *Child Care Health Dev.* 2006;32:585–589

458. King BH, Hollander E, Sikich L, et al. Lack of efficacy of citalopram in children with autism spectrum disorders and high levels of repetitive behavior: citalopram ineffective in children with autism. *Arch Gen Psychiatry.* 2009;66:583–590

459. National Center for Complementary and Integrative Health Web site. https://nccih.nih.gov/health/integrative-health#term. Accessed February 12, 2018

460. Levy SE, Hyman SL. Complementary and alternative medicine treatments for children with autism spectrum disorders. *Child Adolesc Psychiatr Clin N Am.* 2015;24(1):117–143

461. Challman TD. Complementary and alternative medicine in autism: promises kept? In: Shapiro BK, Accardo PJ, eds. *Autism: Clinical and Research Frontiers.* Baltimore, MD: Brookes; 2008:177–190

462. Buescher AV, Cidav Z, Knapp M, Mandell DS. Costs of autism spectrum disorders in the United Kingdom and the United States. *JAMA Pediatr.* 2014;168:721–728

463. Orinstein AJ, Suh J, Porter K, et al. Social function and communication in optimal outcome children and adolescents with an autism history on structured test measures. *J Autism Dev Disord.* 2015;45:2443–2463

464. Magiati I, Tay XW, Howlin P. Cognitive, language, social and behavioural outcomes in adults with autism spectrum disorders: a systematic review of longitudinal follow-up studies in adulthood. *Clin Psychol Rev.* 2014;34:73–86

CHAPTER 20

Interpreting Psychoeducational Testing Reports, Individualized Family Service Plans (IFSP), and Individualized Education Program (IEP) Plans

Mary C. Kral, PhD

Introduction

According to the Centers for Disease Control and Prevention (CDC), 1 in 5 youth in the United States is diagnosed with a developmental disability.[1] Primary pediatric health care professionals are often first-line professionals who identify developmental, learning, social, and behavioral challenges and are uniquely poised to advocate for appropriate supports. To accomplish this goal, primary pediatric health care professionals need to work concertedly with a multidisciplinary team of school psychologists, special educators, social workers, and other allied health professionals to provide a road map for comprehensive care, including appropriate educational programming and referral for related services, such as occupational, physical, and speech/language therapies. In this context, it is critical that primary pediatric health care professionals understand psychoeducational evaluation procedures and federal guidelines concerning the provision of services to children and adolescents from birth through 21 years of age. This chapter provides an overview of psychoeducational evaluation and federally funded services for youth with developmental-behavioral disorders.

Evaluation of Cognitive Functioning and Academic Achievement

Many psychoeducational evaluation reports will cross the desks of primary pediatric health care professionals who need to understand how to interpret them in order to best advocate for the needs of their patients. This understanding includes up-to-date knowledge of commonly used instruments in psychoeducational evaluation, proficiency in the interpretation of quantitative data yielded by psychometric instruments, and communication of the results of psychoeducational evaluations in terms accessible to families.

Psychoeducational Evaluation

Psychoeducational evaluation involves the assessment of cognitive skills, academic achievement, social-emotional functioning, and behaviors that influence academic performance. Certified school psychologists and other licensed psychologists possess the necessary training, expertise, and credentialing to conduct psychoeducational evaluations. When concerns arise at school within the academic or behavioral domains, a child is referred to one of these professionals, who selects a battery of psychometric instruments to determine the source of these difficulties. Assessment of neurodevelopmental abilities may include intellectual functioning, language skills, and motor skills. Performance in these areas helps explain a child's academic achievement, which also is assessed in psychoeducational evaluation. Commonly used psychometric instruments in psychoeducational evaluation appear in Table 20.1. Often, parent- and teacher-completed behavior rating skills, clinical interviews, and classroom observations are also completed to assess functioning in adaptive behavioral, social-emotional, and behavioral domains.

Psychometrics 101

When selecting a battery of instruments to assess the cognitive, academic, social-emotional, and behavioral concerns for a particular child, the psychologist chooses an instrument with acceptable psychometric properties. The instrument's psychometric properties offer an objective indication that the observed sample of behavior obtained during the assessment is representative of the child's general behavior. Selection of psychometric instruments that are well standardized is key. *Standardization* refers to uniformity of content, administration, and scoring. Uniform administration of a psycho metric instrument includes adherence to detailed administration procedures, such as clearly delineated rules regarding presentation of test materials, time limits, specific oral directions, teaching or demonstration during sample items, queries permitted, and methods of handling questions. Standardization reduces measurement error.

Table 20.1. Examples of Commonly Used Instruments in Psychoeducational Evaluation		
Cognitive Domain	**Assessment Instrument**	**Age Range**
Intellectual Function	Assessment of Infant and Toddler Cognitive Development Bayley Scales of Infant Development, Third Edition[a] Mullen Scales of Early Learning[b]	1–42 months birth–68 months
	Assessment of Intelligence in Young Children Differential Ability Scales, Second Edition, Early Years Battery[c] Wechsler Preschool and Primary Scale of Intelligence, Fourth Edition[d]	2:6–6:11 years 2:6–7:7 years
	Assessment of Intelligence in School-aged Youth Differential Ability Scales, Second Edition, School-Age Battery[e] Stanford-Binet Intelligence Scales, Fifth Edition[f] Wechsler Adult Intelligence Scale, Fourth Edition[g] Wechsler Intelligence Scale for Children, Fifth Edition[h]	7:0–17:11 years 2:0–85+ years 16:0–90:11 years 6:0–16:11 years
	Assessment of Nonverbal Intellectual Functioning Leiter International Performance Scale, Third Edition[i]	3:0–75 years
Language Functions	Clinical Evaluation of Language Fundamentals, Fifth Edition[j] Comprehensive Test of Phonological Processing, Second Edition[k] Expressive Vocabulary Test, Second Edition[l] Oral and Written Language Scales, Second Edition[m] Peabody Picture Vocabulary Test, Fourth Edition[n] Preschool Language Scales, Fifth Edition[o]	5:0–21:11 years 4:0–24:11 years 2:6–90+ years 3:0–21:11 years 2:6–90+ years birth–7:11 years

479

Chapter 20: Interpreting Psychoeducational Testing Reports, Individualized Family Service Plans (IFSP), and Individualized Education Program (IEP) Plans

Table 20.1. Examples of Commonly Used Instruments in Psychoeducational Evaluation (*continued*)		
Cognitive Domain	**Assessment Instrument**	**Age Range**
Motor Functions	Developmental Test of Visual-Motor Integration, Sixth Edition[p] Bender Visual-Motor Gestalt Test, Second Edition[q] Peabody Developmental Motor Scales, Second Edition[r]	2:0–99:11 4:0–85+ years birth–5 years
Academic Achievement	Assessment of Academic Readiness Skills in Young Children Bracken Basic Concept Scale, Third Edition: Receptive and Expressive[s] Young Children's Achievement Test[t]	3:0–6:11 years 4:0–7:11 years
	Assessment of Academic Achievement in School-aged Youth Wechsler Individual Achievement Test, Third Edition[u] Woodcock-Johnson IV Tests of Achievement[v]	4:0–50:11 years 2:0–90+ years
Adaptive Behavioral Functioning	Adaptive Behavior Assessment System, Third Edition[w] Vineland Adaptive Behavior Scales, Third Edition[x]	birth–89+ years birth–90 years

[a] Bayley N. *Bayley Scales of Infant and Toddler Development.* 3rd ed. San Antonio, TX: Harcourt; 2006

[b] Mullen EM. *Mullen Scales of Early Learning.* Circle Pines, MN: American Guidance Service Inc.; 1995

[c] Elliott CD. *Differential Ability Scales, Second Edition, Early Years Battery.* San Antonio, TX: Psychological Corporation; 2007

[d] Wechsler D. *Wechsler Preschool and Primary Scales of Intelligence.* 4th ed. San Antonio, TX: Psychological Corporation; 2012

[e] Elliott CD. *Differential Ability Scales, Second Edition, School-Age Battery.* San Antonio, TX: Psychological Corporation; 2007

[f] Roid GH. *Stanford-Binet Intelligence Scales.* 5th ed. Itasca, IL: Riverside Publishing; 2003

[g] Wechsler D. *Wechsler Adult Intelligence Scale.* 4th ed. San Antonio, TX: Psychological Corporation; 2008

[h] Wechsler D. *Wechsler Intelligence Scale for Children.* 5th ed. San Antonio, TX: Psychological Corporation; 2014

[i] Roid GH, Miller L J, Pomplun M, Koch, C. *Leiter International Performance Scale.* 3rd ed. Wood Dale, IL: Stoelting Co.; 2013

[j] Wiig EH, Semel E, Secord WA. *Clinical Evaluation of Language Fundamentals.* 5th ed. San Antonio, TX: Pearson; 2013

[k] Wagner R, Torgesen J, Rashotte C, Pearson NA. *Comprehensive Test of Phonological Processing.* 2nd ed. Austin, TX: Pro-Ed, Inc.; 2013

[l] Williams KT. *Expressive Vocabulary Test.* 2nd ed. San Antonio, TX: Pearson; 2007

[m] Carrow-Woolfolk E. *Oral and Written Language Scales.* 2nd ed. San Antonio, TX: Pearson Assessments; 2011

[n] Dunn LM, Dunn D M. *Peabody Picture Vocabulary Test.* 4th ed. San Antonio, TX: Pearson Assessments; 2007

[o] Zimmerman IL, Steiner VG, Pond RE. *Preschool Language Scales.* 5th ed. San Antonio, TX: Psychological Corporation; 2011

[p] Beery KE, Buktenica NA, Beery NA. *The Beery-Buktenica Developmental Test of Visual-Motor Integration.* (BEERY VMI). 6th ed. Bloomington, MN: Pearson; 2010

[q] Brannigan GG, Decker SL. *Bender Visual-Motor Gestalt Test.* 2nd ed. Itasca, IL: Riverside; 2003

[r] Folio MR, Fewell RR. *Peabody Developmental Motor Scales.* 2nd ed. Austin: Pro-Ed; 2000

[s] Bracken BA. *Bracken Basic Concept Scale: Receptive and Expressive.* 3rd ed. San Antonio, TX: Pearson Assessments; 2006

[t] Hresko W, Peak P, Herron S, Bridges D. *Young Children's Achievement Test.* Austin: Pro-Ed; 2005

[u] Wechsler D. *Wechsler Individual Achievement Test.* 3rd ed. San Antonio, TX: Pearson; 2009

[v] Schrank FA, Mather N, McGrew KS. *Woodcock-Johnson IV Tests of Achievement.* Rolling Meadows, IL: Riverside; 2014

[w] Harrison PL, Oakland T. *Adaptive Behavior Assessment System.* 3rd ed. Torrance, CA: Western Psychological Services; 2015

[x] Sparrow SS, Cicchetti DV, Saulnier CA. *Vineland Adaptive Behavior Scales.* 3rd ed. Minneapolis, MN: Pearson; 2016

Selection of an instrument that is well normed also is critical. *Normatization* of a psychometric instrument involves the selection of a large, representative sample of individuals for whom the measure is designed. Adequate norms permit comparisons of an individual's performance to the representative group, or standardization sample, so that objective statements can be made about a child's level of performance in comparison to his or her peers. In addition, norm-referenced scores permit the comparison of a child's performance on one test or domain to their performance on another test or domain. When choosing a psychometric instrument, the examiner also considers whether the characteristics of the normatization sample are comparable to the demographic characteristics of the child.

A sound psychometric instrument also must be reliable and valid. *Reliability* means that the results a test yields are repeatable and consistent. For example, a child will obtain comparable scores on two different administrations of a test, barring compromise of cognitive functioning, if the measure is highly reliable. A psychometric instrument is reliable if it is free from measurement error and yields an individual's "true score." Some degree of measurement error is inevitably involved in psychoeducational evaluation. Therefore, scores are usually presented along with "confidence intervals." The confidence interval is based on the standard error of measurement (SEM) statistic. The SEM is an estimate of the amount of error associated with an obtained score and is directly related to a test's reliability (ie, the lower the reliability, the higher the SEM). Confidence intervals are usually reported as 90% or 95%, meaning a child's "true" score would be found 90% or 95% of the time within that range, or the statistical chances are 5 or 10 in 100 that a child's "true" score lies outside of the confidence interval.

Validity means that the psychometric instrument measures the construct (ie, specific cognitive ability) that it purports to assess. A valid psychometric instrument permits the examiner to draw inferences about a child's performance. For example, a well-validated measure of language enables the examiner to make statements about a child's ability to express ideas with words. Statistical procedures, such as confirmatory factor analysis, provide evidence for the validity of specific test instruments.

Psychoeducational evaluation involves quantifying behavioral samples by transforming raw test scores into norm-referenced scores. Raw scores have little meaning and cannot be used to compare a child's performance to typically developing peers. In contrast, norm-referenced scores permit comparison of a child's performance to the performance of children in the normatization sample. The collective performance of children in the normatization sample forms a distribution of scores that is typically bell-shaped. This normal distribution has a range of scores, the majority of which fall in the center of the distribution. In a normal distribution, one-half of the scores fall below the average, or mean, and one-half of the scores fall above the mean. Figure 20.1 provides a graphic depiction of the normal distribution.

The statistical properties of the normal distribution permit transformation of raw scores into norm-referenced scores such as percentile ranks, standard scores, and T-scores. Percentile ranks indicate the relative position of a child's performance when compared with the standardization sample. Percentile ranks provide results that are easily understood; however, percentile ranks may be confused with percentage correct. For example, a score at the 50th percentile does not mean the child achieved 50% of the items correctly; rather, the child performed as well or better than 50% of children in the standardization sample. In this case, the child's performance also could be described as falling in the

481

Chapter 20: Interpreting Psychoeducational Testing Reports, Individualized Family Service Plans (IFSP), and Individualized Education Program (IEP) Plans

average range. In addition, percentile ranks are problematic in as much as they over-emphasize differences in scores in the middle of the distribution and underemphasize differences in scores at the extremes of the distribution. Figure 20.1 provides a graphic illustration of this problem.

Standard scores and T-scores are norm-referenced transformations that express raw scores in terms of standard deviation units from the mean. The standard deviation refers to the amount of variability in the distribution of scores around the mean. When the average standard score is 100 with a standard deviation of 15, approximately 68% of children in the standardization population obtained scores within one standard deviation above and below the mean (ie, 85 to 115; see Figure 20.1). Standard scores also may be presented as "scaled scores" with a mean of 10 and a standard deviation of 3. T-scores are yet another norm-referenced transformation that is a common metric of behavior rating scales. T-scores have a mean of 50 and a standard deviation of 10. Because standard scores, scaled scores, and T-scores occur on an interval scale, one of these scores can be transcribed into another metric. For example, a standard score of 100 equals a scaled score of 10, which equals a T-score of 50. These equivalent scores

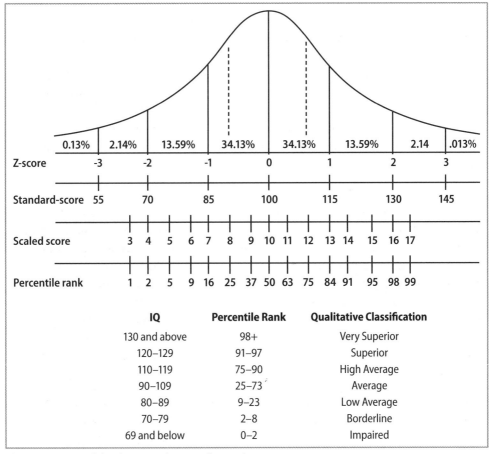

IQ	Percentile Rank	Qualitative Classification
130 and above	98+	Very Superior
120–129	91–97	Superior
110–119	75–90	High Average
90–109	25–73	Average
80–89	9–23	Low Average
70–79	2–8	Borderline
69 and below	0–2	Impaired

Figure 20.1. Normal distribution and norm-referenced scores.

facilitate comparison of performance across different tests and domains. Figure 20.1 graphically displays the relative position of various norm-referenced scores within the normal distribution.

Assessment of academic achievement also involves transformation of raw test scores into norm-referenced scores, such as standard scores and scaled scores. Some academic achievement instruments provide for transformation of raw test scores into age equivalents and grade equivalents. These equivalents reflect at what age or grade the average person in the standardization sample received the same score as the examinee. These scores are problematic because they do not suggest that the child has acquired all of the knowledge of a child in that grade or at that age. Also, age equivalents and grade equivalents are ordinally derived norm-referenced scores and cannot be used to assess progress. In general, if a child obtained a grade or age equivalent above his or her current grade or age, the child is probably performing better than other children of his or her age or grade in that particular area.

Interpreting Psychoeducational Test Results

Results of a psychoeducational evaluation are presented in the form of a written report. Reports often are divided into sections that present detailed information about (1) the referral question or presenting problem; (2) developmental, medical, and psychosocial histories; (3) educational history; (4) evaluation procedures, including a list of psychometric instruments administered; (5) general observations of behavior during the evaluation; (6) test results and interpretation; (7) summary and conclusions about eligibility for services; and (8) recommendations. In addition to a presentation of test scores, a report also may detail qualitative aspects of a child's performance during test administration. The use of particular problem-solving strategies, a slow cognitive tempo, and distractibility are examples of behaviors that may further explain a child's quantified performance (ie, test score).

Although test results and qualitative observations of behavior often are presented within separate domains in a psychoeducational evaluation, these various functions make interactive contributions to a child's daily functioning. In this regard, the summary section of the report integrates quantitative test scores and behavioral observations to present a profile of strengths and weaknesses. This profile may be characteristic of a specific developmental disability (eg, specific learning disorder in reading or attention-deficit/hyperactivity disorder) and informs the selection of recommended interventions, which may include specific therapies (eg, speech/language therapy or occupational therapy), educational or behavioral supports, and/or referral for medical interventions. Repeated (serial) evaluation may be recommended to monitor developmental progress and gauge the effectiveness of a specific intervention.

When communicating with families about the results of psychoeducational evaluations, the primary pediatric health care professional may find it most useful to summarize the findings qualitatively by using descriptive statements such as "average," "high

483

Chapter 20: Interpreting Psychoeducational Testing Reports, Individualized Family Service Plans (IFSP), and Individualized Education Program (IEP) Plans

average," or "borderline." Figure 20.1 provides qualitative descriptions that correspond to various ranges of standard scores and percentile ranks. This method of communication helps facilitate ready understanding of a child's strengths, weaknesses, and targets for intervention.

Early Intervention and Special Education Services

The results of psychoeducational evaluations are designed to determine eligibility for special education services. Two of the primary laws that determine eligibility for special education services and protect the rights of students with disabilities are the Individuals with Disabilities Education Act (IDEA),[2-4] most recently amended in 2004, and Section 504 of the Rehabilitation Act.[5-7] The IDEA was originally passed in 1975 to ensure that youth with disabilities have the opportunity to receive a "free and appropriate public education."[2] IDEA requires that special education and related services be made available to every eligible child or adolescent with a disability. Section 504, on the other hand, is a civil rights law that protects youth with disabilities from discrimination. Infants and toddlers (birth to 3 years of age) with disabilities receive early intervention services under IDEA Part C. Youth ages 3 through 21 years receive special education and related services under IDEA Part B.

Services for Infants and Toddlers. Part C of the IDEA governs the provision of early intervention services and helps improve service provision and outcomes for infants and toddlers with disabilities and their families. Part C is a federal program administered by states that serves infants and toddlers until age 3 years who have developmental delays or who have been diagnosed with physical or cognitive conditions that place them at high risk for developmental delays. The goal of early intervention is to ensure that children with disabilities are ready for preschool and kindergarten (See Chapter 6, Early Intervention).

Eligible infants and toddlers receive an *Individualized Family Service Plan (IFSP)*, which is a written statement that specifies provision of early intervention services. According to federal regulations, members of an IFSP team must include a service coordinator and at least one person involved in the eligibility evaluation. The IFSP includes the family's desired outcomes, at least two objectives, and specific early intervention services that may include:

- Assistive technology
- Audiology services
- Family training and counseling
- Health services
- Medical services for diagnosis and evaluation
- Nursing services
- Nutrition services
- Occupational therapy
- Physical therapy
- Psychological services
- Service coordination
- Sign language and cued language services
- Social work services
- Speech-language pathology
- Transportation and related costs
- Vision services

Services must be provided in the *least restrictive environment,* such as the child's home, child care facility, center-based early childhood special education classrooms (eg, preschool program), or community-based program (eg, Head Start). The least restrictive environment emphasizes a child's natural environment and ensures opportunity to be educated with nondisabled peers.

Many children benefit from early intervention services, and families often desire continued provision of services once their child turns 3 years of age. IDEA Part C specifies that IFSPs must address the transition to early childhood special education. Transition planning can begin 9 months prior to the child's third birthday but no later than 90 days before the third birthday. An *Individualized Education Program (IEP)* process and plan are developed to determine continued provision of special education services and related services when the child transitions to a public school setting at 36 months of age. For children with more complex needs, an *Individual Interagency Intervention Plan (IIIP)* may be developed, specifying a coordination of public school district services and services provided by another public agency (eg, mental health).

Services for School-aged Youth. Part B of the IDEA governs the provision of special education services and related services for youth ages 3 through 21 years. Each state determines regulations for implementation of IDEA. *Special education* is instruction that is specially designed to meet the needs of a child with a disability. This may include special education instruction in a resource or self-contained classroom, specialized transportation services to school, and vocational education. These services extend to the home setting when a child is placed on homebound instruction or a hospital or institution, such as an inpatient psychiatric facility. In order to meet eligibility for special education services, a child's educational performance must be adversely affected due to the disability. *Related services* are designed to help a child with a disability benefit from special education and include speech/language therapy and audiology services, interpreting services for youth who are deaf or hard of hearing, psychological services, and physical and occupational therapies.

According to the IDEA, eligibility is determined through an evaluation process that is requested by the child's parent, legal guardian, or a public agency. Before a child can receive special education and related services for the first time, a full and individual initial evaluation of the child must be conducted to determine eligibility. Informed written consent must be obtained from the child's parent or legal guardian before this evaluation may be conducted. When IDEA was reauthorized in 2004, a time frame was added, requiring completion of the initial evaluation within 60 days of receiving parental consent. An evaluation begins with a review of existing data, including functional, developmental, and academic information for the child; if sufficient, these data may be used to establish eligibility for special education services. If additional information is needed, data must be collected through a variety of approaches, such as classroom observation, structured interviews, psychometric instruments, and/or curriculum-based assessment to help determine a child's strengths and weaknesses.

485

Chapter 20: Interpreting Psychoeducational Testing Reports, Individualized Family Service Plans (IFSP), and Individualized Education Program (IEP) Plans

The evaluation must be conducted in the child's typical mode of communication in order to yield accurate and reliable data. For example, if the child has limited English proficiency, uses American Sign Language, or relies on assistive or alternative augmentative communication devices, the evaluation tools must be selected and administered to ensure fair and accurate measurement of the disability and special education needs. A description of the 14 categories of disability according to the IDEA is included in Table 20.2.

When a child with a disability is determined eligible to receive special education services, an IEP is developed. An IEP is a written statement for a student with a disability that is developed, reviewed, and revised in a multidisciplinary team meeting. Members of an IEP team must include the student's parent or legal guardian, at least one general education teacher, at least one special education teacher, the school psychologist or other specialist who can interpret the eligibility evaluation results, and a district representative with authority over special education services (eg, the director of special education or school principal). An IEP includes information about the student with a disability that must contain the following components:

- A statement of the child's present levels of academic achievement and functional performance, including how the disability affects progress in the general education curriculum
- A statement of measurable annual goals, including academic and functional goals
- A description of how the child's progress toward meeting the annual goals will be measured, and when periodic progress reports will be provided
- A statement of the special education and related services to be provided to the child
- An explanation of the extent, if any, to which the child will not participate with nondisabled children in the general education setting and in extracurricular and nonacademic activities
- A statement of any individual accommodations that are necessary to measure the academic achievement and functional performance of the child on state- and districtwide assessments
- The projected date for the beginning of the services and modifications and the anticipated frequency, location, and duration of those services and modifications

Under the IDEA, special education instruction must be provided to students with disabilities in the "least restrictive environment." This provision ensures that youth with disabilities have opportunities for education in contexts where youth without disabilities are served to the maximum extent appropriate. According to the IDEA, the least restrictive environment is the general education classroom. Provision of special education services in this setting is referred to as *inclusion resource services*. When more intensive educational interventions are required, a student may be served in a resource classroom, where provision of special education instruction is provided by a special education teacher in a specific academic area (eg, reading or math). A self-contained classroom is the most restrictive environment and involves instruction in all core academic areas (reading, writing, and math) in this setting.

Table 20.2. Categories of Disability According to the Individuals with Disabilities Education Act (IDEA 2004)

Autism Spectrum Disorder means a developmental disability significantly affecting verbal and nonverbal communication and social interaction, generally evident before 3 years of age, that adversely affects a child's educational performance. Other characteristics often associated with autism are engaging in repetitive activities and stereotyped movements, resistance to environmental change or change in daily routines, and unusual responses to sensory experiences. The term *autism* does not apply if the child's educational performance is adversely affected primarily because the child has an emotional disturbance.

Deaf-Blindness means concomitant [simultaneous] hearing and visual impairments, the combination of which causes such severe communication and other developmental and educational needs such that the child cannot be accommodated in special education programs solely for children with deafness or children with blindness.

Deafness means a hearing impairment so severe that a child is impaired, with or without amplification, in processing linguistic information through hearing such that it adversely affects a child's educational performance.

Developmental Delay means a delay in one or more of the following areas: physical development; cognitive development; communication; social or emotional development; or adaptive [behavioral] development, applying to children from birth to age 3 years (under IDEA Part C); and children from ages 3 through 9 years (under IDEA Part B).

Emotional Disturbance means a condition exhibiting one or more of the following characteristics over a long period of time and to a marked degree that adversely affects a child's educational performance: (a) an inability to learn that cannot be explained by intellectual, sensory, or health factors; (b) an inability to build or maintain satisfactory interpersonal relationships with peers and teachers; (c) inappropriate types of behavior or feelings under normal circumstances; (d) a general pervasive mood of unhappiness or depression; and (e) a tendency to develop physical symptoms or fears associated with personal or school problems. The term includes schizophrenia. The term does not apply to children who are socially maladjusted, unless it is determined that they have an emotional disturbance.

Hearing Impairment means an impairment in hearing, whether permanent or fluctuating, that adversely affects a child's educational performance but is not included under the definition of deafness.

Intellectual Disability means significantly subaverage general intellectual functioning, existing concurrently (at the same time) with deficits in adaptive behavior and manifested during the developmental period, that adversely affects a child's educational performance.

Multiple Disabilities means concomitant (simultaneous) impairments (eg, intellectual disability and blindness, intellectual disability and orthopedic impairment), the combination of which causes such severe educational needs that the child cannot be accommodated in a special education program solely for one of the impairments. The term does not include deaf-blindness.

487

Chapter 20: Interpreting Psychoeducational Testing Reports, Individualized Family Service Plans (IFSP), and Individualized Education Program (IEP) Plans

Table 20.2. Categories of Disability According to the Individuals with Disabilities Education Act (IDEA 2004) *(continued)*

Orthopedic Impairment means a severe orthopedic impairment that adversely affects a child's educational performance. The term includes impairments caused by a congenital anomaly, impairments caused by disease (eg, poliomyelitis, bone tuberculosis), and impairments from other causes (eg, cerebral palsy, amputations, and fractures or burns that cause contractures).

Other Health Impairment means having limited strength, vitality, or alertness, including a heightened alertness to environmental stimuli, that results in limited alertness with respect to the educational environment, that (a) is due to chronic or acute health problems such as asthma, attention-deficit/hyperactivity disorder, diabetes, epilepsy, a heart condition, hemophilia, lead poisoning, leukemia, nephritis, rheumatic fever, sickle cell anemia, and Tourette syndrome; and (b) adversely affects a child's educational performance.

Specific Learning Disability means a disorder in one or more of the basic psychological processes involved in understanding or in using language, spoken or written, that may manifest itself in the imperfect ability to listen, think, speak, read, write, spell, or to do mathematical calculations. The term includes such conditions as perceptual disabilities, brain injury, minimal brain dysfunction, dyslexia, and developmental aphasia. The term does not include learning problems that are primarily the result of visual, hearing, or motor disabilities; of intellectual disability; of emotional disturbance; or of environmental, cultural, or economic disadvantage.

Speech or Language Impairment means a communication disorder such as stuttering, impaired articulation, language impairment, or voice impairment that adversely affects a child's educational performance.

Traumatic Brain Injury means an acquired injury to the brain caused by an external physical force that results in total or partial functional disability, psychosocial impairment, or both, that adversely affects a child's educational performance. The term applies to open or closed head injuries resulting in impairments in one or more areas such as cognition; language; memory; attention; reasoning; abstract thinking; judgment; problem-solving; sensory, perceptual, and motor abilities; psychosocial behavior; physical functions; information processing; and speech. The term does not apply to brain injuries that are congenital or degenerative, or to brain injuries induced by birth trauma.

Visual Impairment Including Blindness means impairment in vision that, even with correction, adversely affects a child's educational performance. The term includes both partial sight and blindness.

Adapted from the Individuals with Disabilities Education Act, 20 USC §1400 et seq, 2004. Part B, Sec. Sec. 300.304 through 300.311; idea.ed.gov.

Beginning no later than 14 years of age, transition goals and objectives must be a part of the IEP process. *Transition* refers to activities that prepare students with disabilities for adult life. *Transition planning* helps the student identify career interests and select courses of study that will help him or her attain postsecondary or vocational goals. Beginning no later than 16 years of age, *transition services* are provided that focus on the student's functional needs and postsecondary interests. This coordination of services may include preparation for postsecondary education, vocational training, job shadowing or community-based apprenticeships, and/or training in independent living skills.

Response to Intervention

The reauthorization of IDEA in 2004 permits a new process of early identification of students at risk for academic and behavioral difficulties through universal screening and instructional interventions in the general education setting. This *Response to Intervention (RTI)* process specifies: (1) scientifically based instruction for all students in the general education setting, (2) early schoolwide screening of all students to identify those who are "at risk," (3) continuous progress monitoring of all "at risk" students to determine benefit from instructional supports, (4) implementation of scientifically based instruction with fidelity, and (5) procedural safeguards to ensure parents are aware of their rights within the education system. RTI is delivered in tiers, and a 3-tier model is most commonly implemented.

Tier 1 specifies high-quality, scientifically based instruction for all students that is provided by qualified personnel to ensure that academic or behavioral difficulties are not due to inadequate instruction. All students are screened on a periodic basis to establish an academic and behavioral baseline and to identify struggling learners who need additional support. Students identified as being "at risk" through universal screenings and/or results on state- or districtwide tests receive supplemental instruction during the school day in the regular education classroom. Student progress is closely monitored using a validated screening system, such as curriculum-based assessment (CBA). At the end of this period, students who show significant progress are returned to the general education curriculum. Students who do not show adequate progress are advanced to Tier 2. The current recommended time for measuring response to Tier 1 instruction is 8–10 weeks.

On the basis of levels of performance and rates of progress, Tier 2 specifies provision of increasingly intensive instruction matched to the needs of the struggling learner. These interventions are provided in small group settings in addition to instruction in the general education setting. Students who do not show adequate progress are considered for more intensive interventions as part of Tier 3.

Tier 3 specifies provision of individualized, intensive interventions that target the students' skills deficits. Students who do not achieve the desired level of progress in response to these targeted interventions are then referred for a comprehensive

489

Chapter 20: Interpreting Psychoeducational Testing Reports, Individualized Family Service Plans (IFSP), and Individualized Education Program (IEP) Plans

psychoeducational evaluation to determine eligibility for special education services under IDEA. The data collected during Tiers 1, 2, and 3 are included, along with the results of psychoeducational evaluation, and are used to make the eligibility decision.

Advantages of the RTI model include early identification, prompt intervention, and frequent progress monitoring for struggling learners. Advocates of RTI contend that the traditional IQ-achievement discrepancy model for determining eligibility for special education services is a "wait-to-fail" model because students, particularly during the early elementary years, often do not demonstrate a significant ability-achievement discrepancy until later in their education. Also, students described as "slower learners" (eg, those with borderline [IQ=70–79] or low average [IQ=80–89] intellectual functioning) who struggle academically, and who previously did not meet discrepancy models for receipt of special education services, may be identified earlier and more readily as "at risk" through universal screening.

Critics of the RTI model note that the selection of scientifically based instruction is determined by each school district, which is often dependent upon district funding and can vary significantly in quality from district to district. Another criticism of RTI is the use of CBA in universal screening and progress monitoring. Curriculum-based assessment utilizes local norms gathered from universal screening within a single school district. Benchmarks are established based on these local norms. For example, those students performing in the lower quartile on district-wide CBAs may comprise the "at risk" group. As such, the cutoff for inclusion in the "at risk" group may differ significantly from one district to another. In a related vein, underachieving gifted students may not perform below the benchmark on CBAs and may be underidentified through the RTI process. It also should be noted that at any point in the RTI process, IDEA indicates that parents may request a formal evaluation to determine eligibility for special education services. In other words, an RTI process cannot be used to deny or delay a formal evaluation for special education services.

504 Accommodation Plans

Section 504 of the Rehabilitation Act of 1973 is a federal law designed to protect the civil rights of individuals with disabilities in programs that receive federal funding. Those programs include public school districts, institutions of higher education, and other state and local education agencies. To qualify under Section 504, disability is defined broadly as a physical or mental impairment that substantially limits one or more major life activities. When a student is determined to be eligible for services under Section 504, the school must eliminate barriers to his or her access to full participation in school activities, including the general education curriculum. Barriers often are eliminated by providing accommodations to the student. Examples of accommodations may include testing in a quiet room, preferential seating, audio textbooks, modified homework assignments, or a sign language interpreter. It is important to note that 504 Accommodation Plans are not a "service," as would be specified in an IEP. This and other differences between an IEP and a 504 Accommodation Plan are detailed in Table 20.3.

Table 20.3. Differences between 504 Accommodation Plans and Individualized Education Programs (IEPs)		
	Individualized Education Program (IEP)	**504 Accommodation Plan**
Description	A written document specifying provision of special education services and related services to address a child's disability as eligible according to one of 14 IDEA classifications	A plan for environmental modifications and accommodations that eliminates barriers to the same participation in education as other students
Legal Basis	Individuals with Disabilities Education Act (IDEA 2004), a federal special education law for children with disabilities that is overseen by the US Department of Education, Office of Special Education and Rehabilitation Services	Section 504 of the Rehabilitation Act of 1973, a federal civil rights law protecting individuals with disabilities that is overseen by the US Department of Education, Office of Civil Rights
Eligibility	Special education services are granted to a child with a disability, *birth to age 21 years*, who meets criteria according to 14 specific classifications and whose disability adversely affects educational performance	Disability is broadly defined as a physical or mental impairment that substantially limits one or more major life activities for an individual of any age, including educational performance
Team Members	An IEP multidisciplinary team must be comprised of: • a parent or legal guardian • at least one general education teacher • at least one special education teacher • a school psychologist or other specialist who can interpret evaluation results • a district representative with authority over special education services	Criteria for 504 team members are less specific; they may include: • a parent or legal guardian • a school guidance counselor • a general education teacher (or teachers) • a school principal
Specific Supports	The IEP includes goals and objectives for a student with a disability and specifies services that will be provided to address these goals. An IEP must include: • a student's present levels of academic and functional performance • annual education goals and a plan for progress monitoring • specific services (eg, special education services, related services, extended school year services) • timing of services • accommodations • participation in standardized, statewide testing • inclusion in general education classes and school activities	A 504 Accommodation Plan is not a service. A 504 Accommodation Plan is implemented in the general education setting and generally includes: • a list of accommodations and/or environmental modifications • names of individuals who will implement the accommodations • the name of an individual who is responsible for ensuring that the plan is implemented

Adapted from US Department of Education. Protecting Students With Disabilities Web site. http://www2.ed.gov/about/offices/list/ocr/504faq.html. Accessed February 6, 2018.

491

Chapter 20: Interpreting Psychoeducational Testing Reports, Individualized Family Service Plans (IFSP), and Individualized Education Program (IEP) Plans

Special Considerations

English Language Learners

In January 2016, the United States Department of Education and the Department of Justice released guidelines to protect the civil rights of English language learners (ELLs) through Title III of the Elementary and Secondary Education Act (ESEA), as amended by the Every Student Succeeds Act (ESSA). A 10-chapter *English Learner Tool Kit*[8] followed that provided state and local educational agencies with guidelines to ensure that students who are English language learners receive the high-quality services they need to be college and career ready. The following are among these guidelines:

- Schools must identify, in a timely manner, students who are English learners in need of language assistance services by using valid and reliable assessment tools and communicate these results to parents or legal guardians.
- Schools must offer students who are English learners services and programs until they are proficient in English and can participate meaningfully in educational programs without English learner supports.
- Schools must provide appropriate special education services to students who are English learners with disabilities who are found to be eligible for special education and related services.

If a student who is an English learner is suspected of having a disability, schools must provide an evaluation in a timely manner to determine eligibility for special education services according to the IDEA, or appropriate environmental modifications according to Section 504. Disability determination may not be delayed due to a student's limited English proficiency; however, evaluations must consider the student's English proficiency and, whenever possible, administer special education evaluations in the student's native language. When a student who is an English learner is determined to be a child with a disability according to IDEA or a child with a disability according the broader definition of disability in Section 504, *both* the student's English learning needs and his or her disability-related educational needs must be met.

Gifted and Talented Students

Children who are gifted comprise 5% to 20% of the general school-age population, depending on how "gifted" is defined, or depending on the criteria being used to identify students who are gifted.[9] Although specific legislation recognizes the unique educational needs of students who are identified as gifted and talented (eg, the Jacob Javits Gifted and Talented Students Education Act, reauthorized in 2001 as part of the No Child Left Behind Act), the federal government does not mandate services for gifted students. Gifted and talented programming is not part of the IDEA. Rather, the majority of programs and services that gifted and talented students receive are determined by state laws and policies and funded at the state and local level. State laws that define gifted and talented programming and teacher training requirements, along with available funding for gifted education, vary widely. Most states and school districts use the following definition:[10]

> ❝Children and youth with outstanding talent perform or show the potential for performing at remarkably high levels of accomplishment when compared with others of their age, experience, or environment. These children and youth exhibit high capability in intellectual, creative, and/or artistic areas, possess an unusual leadership capacity, or excel in specific academic fields. They require services or activities not ordinarily provided by the schools. Outstanding talents are present in children and youth from all cultural groups, across all economic strata, and in all areas of human endeavor (p. 26).❞

Because identification of students eligible for gifted educational programming may vary from school district to school district, primary pediatric health care professionals are advised to become familiar with the policies relevant to the state in which they work, including educational options, such as magnet schools and charter schools. A searchable directory of state-specific information about gifted and talented educational programming can be found at the Web site of the National Association for Gifted Children (**http://www.nagc.org**). The primary pediatric health care professional also may consult with district school psychologists about the identification process and programming unique to a given school.

Educational Advocacy

Navigating the special education process is often overwhelming and confusing for families. A number of resources are available that provide information about disability eligibility, parents' and children's rights under the IDEA, and provision of early intervention and school-age services (see Chapter 25, Social and Community Services for Children With Developmental Disabilities and/or Behavioral Disorders and Their Families). The US Department of Education, Office of Special Education Programs funds Parent Training and Information Centers (PTIs). There is at least one PTI in each state that promotes opportunities for learning, inclusion, and empowerment for individuals with disabilities and their families through such means as education, advocacy, and outreach. Staffed primarily by parents of children with disabilities, PTIs conduct workshops, conferences, and seminars to inform families about the special education process. To locate PTIs, a searchable directory by state is available at **http://www.parentcenterhub.org/find-your-center/.** Excellent, reproducible materials also are available on the Web sites of the PACER Center (**http://www.pacer.org**) and the Center for Parent Information and Resources (**http: //parentcenterhub.org**)

493

Chapter 20: Interpreting Psychoeducational Testing Reports, Individualized Family Service Plans (IFSP), and Individualized Education Program (IEP) Plans

Conclusion

In summary, primary pediatric health care professionals are often the first-line professionals to identify the special needs of youth with developmental-behavioral disorders. By working concertedly with a multidisciplinary team of allied health professionals and encouraging family involvement, which is key to a child's success, the primary pediatric health care professional is poised to be a powerful advocate. Because school is central to the lives of youth with developmental-behavioral disorders, the primary pediatric health care professional who is knowledgeable about psychoeducational evaluation, special education, and related services will best be able to advocate for supports.

References

1. Boyle CA, Boulet S, Schieve LA, Cohen RA, et al. Trends in the prevalence of developmental disabilities in US Children, 1997–2008. *Pediatrics*. 2011;127(6):1034–1042
2. Individuals with Disabilities Education Act, 20 U.S.C. §1400 et seq., 2004
3. Individuals with Disabilities Education Improvement Act, 20 U.S.C. §1400–1485 et seq., 2005
4. US Department of Education, Office of Special Education Programs Web site. Building the Legacy: IDEA 2004. Washington, DC. http://idea.ed.gov. Accessed November 27, 2017
5. Section 504 of the Rehabilitation Act. 29 U.S.C. § 794, 1973. http://www.ed.gov/about/offices/list/ocr/504faq.html. Accessed November 27, 2017
6. Americans with Disabilities Act. 42 U.S.C. § 12101, 1990. https://www.ada.gov/pubs/adastatute08.htm. Accessed November 27, 2017
7. Americans with Disabilities Act Amendments of 2008. Public Law 110–325. https://www.ada.gov/pubs/ada.htm. Accessed November 27, 2017
8. US Department of Education, Office of English Language Acquisition. *English Learner Tool Kit*. Washington, DC: US Department of Education, Office of English Language Acquisition; 2016. http://www2.ed.gov/about/offices/list/oela/english-learner-toolkit/index.html. Accessed November 27, 2017
9. Pfeiffer SI, Stocking VB. Vulnerabilities of academically gifted students. *Special Services in the Schools*. 2000;16(1–2):83–93
10. Ross, PO. *National Excellence: A Case for Developing America's Talent*. Washington, DC: US Department of Education, Office of Educational Research and Improvement (ED). Programs for the Improvement of Practice; 1993

CHAPTER 21

Disruptive Behavior Disorders

Elizabeth B. Harstad, MD, MPH

William J. Barbaresi, MD, FAAP

Definition of Disruptive Behavior Disorders and Scope of the Problem

The term *disruptive behavior disorder* describes "socially disruptive behavior that is generally more disturbing to others than to the person initiating the behavior."[1] Disruptive and oppositional behaviors occur on a continuum, with normal toddler resistance and tantrums at one end and more severe, maladaptive behaviors warranting a medical diagnosis at the other end.[2] While it is very important for primary pediatric health care professionals to screen for and address any challenges related to disruptive behaviors, the focus of this chapter will primarily be on those behaviors significant enough to constitute a medical diagnosis.

In the *Diagnostic and Statistical Manual of Mental Disorders,* Fifth Edition (*DSM-5*),[3] disruptive behavior disorders are described in the chapter titled, "Disruptive, Impulse-Control, and Conduct Disorders." The diagnoses described include oppositional defiant disorder (ODD); conduct disorder (CD); intermittent explosive disorder; other specified disruptive, impulse-control and conduct disorder; unspecified disruptive, impulse-control and conduct disorder; pyromania; and kleptomania. This categorization is new for *DSM-5,* as the *Diagnostic and Statistical Manual of Mental Disorders,* Fourth Edition, Text Revision (*DSM-IV-TR*)[4] categorized ODD and CD in a chapter separately from intermittent explosive disorder. While all 3 of these disorders involve problems in both behavioral and emotional regulation, the criteria for CD focus mainly on poorly controlled behaviors, the criteria for intermittent explosive disorder focus mainly on poorly controlled emotions, and the criteria for ODD are more evenly distributed between behavioral and emotional symptoms.[3] The challenges in behavioral and emotional regulation present in all 3 of these conditions warrant inclusion when discussing disruptive behavior disorders.

This chapter focuses on ODD, CD, and intermittent explosive disorder, as they are more common in children and adolescents, compared to pyromania (which describes multiple episodes of deliberate and purposeful fire setting) and kleptomania (which describes recurrent failure to resist impulses to steal items even though the items are not needed for personal use or for their monetary value).[3] Although attention-deficit/hyperactivity disorder (ADHD) may be considered a disruptive behavior disorder, it is discussed in detail in Chapter 18, ADHD.

Oppositional Defiant Disorder

The *DSM-5* states that a child who meets criteria for a diagnosis of ODD must have "a pattern of angry/irritable mood, argumentative/defiant behavior, or vindictiveness lasting at least 6 months."[3] In addition, the child must display 4 or more irritable, defiant, and/or vindictive behaviors. The child's age and developmental level must be taken into consideration, and the disturbance in behavior must cause clinically significant impairment in academic, social, or occupational functioning. A child is precluded from being diagnosed with ODD if the behaviors occur exclusively during the course of substance use, a mood or psychotic disorder, or if the child also meets criteria for disruptive mood dysregulation disorder.[3]

Conduct Disorder

The *DSM-5* describes the diagnosis of CD as "a repetitive and persistent pattern of behavior in which the basic rights of others or major age-appropriate societal norms or rules are violated."[3] Children with CD must have met at least 3 criteria in the past 12 months, with at least one criterion present in the past 6 months, from any of the following categories: aggression to people and animals, destruction of property, deceitfulness or theft, and serious violations of rules. The behaviors must result in clinically significant impairment in academic, social, or occupational functioning, and criteria cannot be met for antisocial personality disorder.[3]

In the *DSM-5,* the diagnosis of CD is coded based on age at onset. An individual with "CD, childhood-onset type" is described as having the presence of at least one criterion characteristic of CD prior to 10 years of age. An individual with "CD, adolescent-onset type" is described as having the absence of any criterion of CD prior to 10 years of age. An individual with "CD, unspecified onset" has an unknown age of onset.[3]

Intermittent Explosive Disorder

The *DSM-5* describes intermittent explosive disorder as "recurrent behavioral outbursts representing a failure to control aggressive impulses."[3] This can manifest as either verbal aggression or physical aggression occurring twice weekly, on average, for a period of 3 months. To meet criteria for the diagnosis, there must be 3 behavioral outbursts involving damage, destruction of property, and/or physical assault within a 12-month period. An individual with intermittent explosive disorder must have a chronological age (or equivalent developmental level) of at least 6 years. The recurrent outbursts are not premeditated, are grossly out of proportion to any trigger, are associated with significant impairment in functioning, and are not better explained by another mental health or medical disorder.[3]

Other Specified Disruptive, Impulse-Control, and Conduct Disorder and Unspecified Disruptive, Impulse-Control, and Conduct Disorder

The diagnosis of other specified disruptive, impulse-control, and conduct disorder applies to presentations in which symptoms characteristic of disruptive, impulse-control, and conduct disorder cause significant impairment but do not meet full criteria for any of the diagnoses in this category, and the clinician chooses to indicate the specific reason the diagnostic criteria are met.[3] The diagnosis of unspecified disruptive, impulse- control, and conduct disorder also applies to presentations in which criteria are not fully met, but in this case the clinician chooses not to indicate the reason for which the diagnostic criteria were met.[3] Much of the information applicable for ODD, intermittent explosive disorder, or CD can be useful in caring for a child who is diagnosed with either the other specified or unspecified categorizations. Therefore, this chapter primarily focuses on disruptive behavior disorders categorized by ODD, CD, and intermittent explosive disorder.

Epidemiology of Disruptive Behavior Disorders

It may not be possible to determine the prevalence of disruptive behaviors because many do not cause sufficient impairment to warrant a medical diagnosis. However, noncompliant and oppositional behaviors comprise some of the most common concerns among parents and are the most frequently reported behavior problems seen by primary care pediatricians.[5] Overall, about 5% of children between the ages of 6 and 18 years meet *DSM-IV* criteria for either ODD or CD at any given time, while the combined prevalence of these disorders is approximately 7% according to *DSM-5*.[3,6] The lifetime prevalence rates of each are slightly higher, ranging from 9% to 13% for ODD and 3% to 16% for CD.[7,8] In a US population survey of adolescents, the lifetime prevalence rate of *DSM-IV* intermittent explosive disorder was reported to be 7.8%.[9] The diagnosis of ODD, intermittent explosive disorder, or CD is more common in boys, although oppositional behavior per se may be equally common between both genders.[10]

Assessment of Children With Disruptive Behaviors

Primary pediatric health care professionals care for children with varying levels of disruptive behaviors. Therefore, it is important for clinicians to evaluate the child's behaviors and the parents' responses to determine if the parent-child interaction may be inadvertently perpetuating the child's negative behaviors. Parents often place demands on their children, such as cleaning up their toys, and some of these demands may seem aversive to the child. The child may respond to this aversive event by displaying a coercive response, such as yelling or having a tantrum. Parents may respond to the coercive response by removing the original aversive demand, and this negatively reinforces the child's noncompliant behavior. The child is likely to continue to yell or have a tantrum when future demands are placed because the child has learned that he will get his own way by doing so. Another response the parent could make to the yelling or tantrum is to try to comfort the child and explain the reason for the request. This parental attention positively reinforces the child's noncompliant behavior, and thus the child may continue to manifest these coercive responses because he has learned that he will get attention for them. Alternatively, the parent may respond to the child's coercive response by presenting another aversive event, such as yelling or loudly repeating the request. The child may ultimately respond to the parent's demand, but the child learns to respond only to the parent's more aversive demands, such as yelling or stating commands loudly. If any of these maladaptive parent-child interactions continue over time, a persistent and worsening pattern of noncompliance and defiance may develop.[11] When the primary pediatric health care professional recognizes that the parent-child interaction is heading in a negative direction, he or she can play a crucial role in providing guidance and offering effective techniques that the parent can use. A more effective parent response to a child's protests may include a simple and single repetition of the request, followed by verbal acknowledgment that complying with the request may be difficult from the child's perspective, and firm limit setting on worsening behavior (see Chapter 7, Basics of Child Behavior and Primary Care Pediatric Management of Common Behavioral Problems).

In addition to intervening when problem behaviors are described, the primary pediatric health care professional should evaluate the disruptive behaviors to determine if a medical diagnosis such as ODD, CD, or intermittent explosive disorder should be made. While specific antisocial acts occur in up to 80% of youths,[12] children who meet criteria for a diagnosis of ODD, CD, or intermittent explosive disorder display a persistent history of multiple problem behaviors.

Important Points to Consider When Taking the History

Although children may present to the primary pediatric health care professional with any number of disruptive behaviors, the most common referral symptoms for disruptive behavior disorders are fighting, stealing, lying, cruelty, fire-setting, substance abuse, and sexual misconduct.[1] When taking the history, it is important to obtain information from several sources, including the child, parents, and teachers. The primary pediatric health care professional should learn as much as possible about the parenting style, parent-child interactions, and the child's strengths, as this information can be valuable for treatment planning and implementation of interventions.[6] The child's age and gender must be taken into account. At different ages, children display different types of disruptive behaviors, with property and status offenses more prevalent at older ages.[10] Males are more likely to use physical attacks and females are more likely to use indirect, verbal, and relational violence.[13]

Important Questions to Ask in the History

In assessing a child with disruptive behaviors, it is helpful to use the criteria described in the *DSM*-5 for the diagnoses of ODD, CD, and intermittent explosive disorder to guide the history. For example, in a child who displays aggression, it is important to determine what type of aggression the child shows, such as verbal, physical, etc, and to whom the aggression is directed, such as parents, other children, animals, etc. The clinician should ask how long these behaviors have occurred and if there were any significant changes in the child's life prior to the onset of the disruptive behaviors. It is also important to ask parents, teachers, and other adult caregivers how disruptive these behaviors are. Individuals with CD are often unable to appreciate other's welfare and have little or no remorse about harming others.[14] Therefore, they may not be able to understand and report how their behaviors are negatively impacting others.

Primary pediatric health care professionals may find the following brief questions helpful in determining whether criteria for the diagnosis of ODD are likely to be met. Research has shown that a positive response for all 3 is 91% specific for meeting *DSM-IV* criteria on full interview, and a negative response is 94% sensitive for ruling out ODD.[15,16]

1. Has your child, in the past 3 months, been spiteful or vindictive, or blamed others for his or her own mistakes? (Any "yes" is a positive response.)

2. How often is your child touchy or easily annoyed, and how often has your child lost his or her temper, argued with adults, or defied or refused adults' requests? (Greater than or equal to 2 times weekly is a positive response.)

3. How often has your child been angry and resentful or deliberately annoying to others? (Greater than or equal to 4 times weekly is a positive response.)

It is important for primary pediatric health care professionals to be sure to perform a thorough assessment of the child's psychosocial functioning to assess for comorbidities or alternative diagnoses. Areas to assess include attention, level of activity and impulsiveness, social interactions, and communication skills. Other factors to consider when evaluating a child with disruptive behaviors include anxiety, mood disorders, cognitive and/or learning problems, substance abuse, and history of physical or sexual abuse.

Supplements to Clinical Interview

Standardized questionnaires can aid the primary pediatric health care professional in evaluating disruptive behavior. Two commonly used rating scales for ADHD are the Conners Rating Scales–Revised and the Vanderbilt ADHD Diagnostic Parent and Teacher Rating Scales. These include information about oppositional and disruptive behaviors, and thus can be useful.[17] In addition, more broadly based behavioral rating scales, such as the Eyberg Child Behavior Inventory[18] (a parent rating scale), and the Child Behavior Checklist[19] (a child rating scale), can serve as an adjunct to taking a clinical history. Finally, the Modified Overt Aggression Scale[20] is another useful supplement to the clinical interview in evaluating disruptive behavior.

The diagnoses of ODD, CD, and intermittent explosive disorder are made clinically. Outside of research purposes or a medical history and physical examination indicating abnormal neurological status, neuroimaging is not recommended. No laboratory work is routinely performed. If active substance abuse is suspected, a urine drug screen should be considered. In addition, if sexual abuse or unprotected sexual activity is present, testing for sexually transmitted infections may be warranted.[6]

Risk Factors for the Development of Disruptive Behavior Disorders

The many known risk factors for the development of disruptive behavior disorders can be classified into the following categories: biological, individual, family, and social/school (Box 21.1).[6] Rather than 1 risk factor acting in isolation, it seems that the accumulation of risk factors may be critical to the development of disruptive behavior disorders.[21] Disruptive behavior disorders most likely have a multifactorial etiology, including some degree of genetic vulnerability and environmental and/or social contributors.[22] Overall, some of the most commonly cited risk factors include low socioeconomic status, history of rejection or abuse, and parental challenges, including antisocial behaviors, substance abuse, and dysfunctional parenting.

Box 21.1. Risk Factors for the Development of Disruptive Behavior Disorders

Biological
- Genetic
- Antenatal and perinatal complications
- Brain injury, brain disease
- Male sex
- Environmental toxins, such as lead

Family
- Single-parent household or family divorce
- Domestic violence
- Lack of permanent family
- Parental substance abuse or antisocial behavior
- Child maltreatment or neglect
- Parent-child conflict
- Excessive parental control
- Lack of parental supervision
- Maternal depression or anxiety

Individual
- Cognitive impairment
- Difficult temperament
- Aggressiveness
- Hyperactivity, impulsivity
- Attention problems
- Language impairment
- Reading problems

Social/School
- Low socioeconomic status
- Rejection by peers
- Association with deviant peers
- History of being bullied
- Neighborhood violence
- Disorganized or dysfunctional school
- Intense exposure to violence via media

One interesting study evaluated the effect of poverty on the prevalence of oppositional and conduct disorders. In this study, 9- to 13-year-old rural children, of whom one-quarter were Native American and the remaining were predominantly white, were given annual psychiatric examinations for 8 years. Halfway through the study, a casino opened up on the reservation, which gave every Native American family an income supplement, moving 14% of study families out of poverty. The non–Native American families were unaffected. Reducing poverty among Native American families resulted in a reduction of oppositional and conduct problems in their children. The mechanisms by which this occurred seemed to be related to fewer demands on parents' time, fewer single parents, and better parental supervision, rather than purely related to increased income.[23]

While many risk factors are well known, the anatomical basis for disruptive behavior disorders is less well established. However, neuroimaging studies have found the frontal lobe to be associated with violence and aggression.[21] In addition, atypical frontal lobe functioning, as detected via electroencephalogram, has been suggested as the basis for the negative affective style displayed in children with ODD.[24] A meta-analysis of functional magnetic resonance imaging (fMRI) studies found that the most consistent dysfunction in youths with disruptive behavior disorders is in the rostro-dorsomedial, fronto-cingulate, and ventral-striatal regions that mediate reward-based decision-making.[25] Neurotransmitters have also been investigated to ascertain what role they play in relation to disruptive behaviors. Serotonin has been linked to aggression, though research remains ongoing to further elucidate its precise relationship to ODD and CD.[21]

Comorbidities of Disruptive Behavior Disorders

Disruptive behavior disorders are often comorbid with other conditions. The most frequently reported comorbid conditions are ADHD, major depression, and substance disorders. Attention-deficit/hyperactivity disorder occurs 10 times more frequently in children with disruptive behavior disorders, and major depression occurs 7 times more frequently, compared with children who do not have a diagnosis of a disruptive behavior disorder.[15] A child between the ages of 11 to 14 years with a diagnosis of CD is 4 times more likely to have substance disorders by age 18 years.[26] Many other psychiatric and developmental disorders are more prevalent in children with disruptive behavior disorders compared with the general population. These include mood disorders and anxiety disorders,[8] as well as learning and cognitive disorders.[27] Given the high number of comorbid conditions associated with disruptive behavior disorders, it is important for primary pediatric health care professionals to routinely assess attention, mood, substance use, and school functioning in children and adolescents presenting with disruptive behaviors.

Treatment

Children who meet criteria for the diagnoses of ODD, CD, or intermittent explosive disorder generally require the care of a psychiatrist, developmental-behavioral pediatrician, or psychologist who can work in conjunction with the primary pediatric health care professional.[1] Disruptive behavior disorders tend to be chronic conditions, and this should be taken into account when planning treatment. Treatments are more effective if initiated early. A structured psychosocial intervention should be the first line of treatment for ODD and CD. Treatments should involve the parents; in most cases, core goals of treatment include improving parenting skills and parent-child interactions.[6]

Psychosocial Treatments

Psychosocial treatments have the best evidence for treating disruptive behaviors. Evidence-based psychosocial treatments include parent management training, multimodal interventions (eg, multisystemic therapy), and individual interventions (eg, cognitive behavioral therapy), each of which will be described in this chapter.

Parent management training is an effective and well-studied intervention.[28] The theory behind this intervention is that the disruptive behavior, at least in part, is due to a maladaptive parent-child interaction. Thus, a parent is taught a new set of skills to use with the child, including ways to reward prosocial behaviors and ways to address noncompliant behaviors.[27] A challenge with parent management training is that it requires a committed parent, and it may not be successful with more dysfunctional families.[6]

Multimodal interventions include a more comprehensive system for change. While parent management training does not necessarily enhance the child's ability to make friends or perform well in school, multimodal interventions may include enabling the child to improve his or her problem-solving skills and working with the child's teacher to improve the child's educational functioning.[6] Some types of multimodal programs and therapies are multisystemic therapy, which targets adolescents with severe CD, and Families and Schools Together, which targets children with CD who are starting school.[6] While programs such as wilderness camps and boot camps may sometimes be considered to provide multimodal interventions, there is no solid evidence for their effectiveness. The main concern with these programs is that the skills children develop in these isolated settings will not generalize, and these settings enable antisocial peers to congregate together.[6]

Individual interventions provide children with problem-solving skills training. Through teaching, children are taught to find adaptive solutions to their problems in areas such as coping with anger and social skills. Techniques such as role playing, structured activities, modeling the behavior, stories, and the use of games facilitate teaching. In some cases, modified cognitive-behavioral therapy and day treatment may be part of the intervention.[7] Individual interventions are most effective when used in conjunction with a broader treatment program that also addresses parenting, social, and school interventions.[21]

Pharmacotherapy

Pharmacotherapy should never be the primary treatment for disruptive behavior disorders, although medication might be considered in children with comorbid conditions, such as ADHD, anxiety, or depression.[6,21] When using stimulants in children with ADHD and disruptive behavior disorders, careful monitoring and supervision should be implemented, given the high prevalence of substance use and abuse in this population.[29]

Prognosis

Although ODD and CD seem to be closely related, their relationship is complex. Some children presenting with a diagnosis of ODD in childhood ultimately evolve into a diagnosis of CD, often after puberty. Other children may exhibit disruptive behaviors for a short time and/or will continue to carry a diagnosis of ODD, though it will not evolve into CD. Boys with ODD are more likely to be diagnosed with CD later than girls.[30]

Some children with CD will go on to develop a profile consistent with the diagnosis of antisocial personality disorder. In fact, the *DSM-5* criteria for antisocial personality disorder require evidence of CD prior to the age of 15 years.[3] However, most children diagnosed with CD will not develop antisocial personality disorder in adulthood.[6] Individuals with either ODD or CD are at greater risk for comorbid intermittent explosive disorder.[3]

Predictors of Outcome

In general, studies have shown that the higher the number of disruptive behaviors a child exhibits, the worse the long-term outcome.[6] Aggressive, antisocial symptoms, fire setting, family dysfunction, and substance abuse are associated with a poor prognosis.[1] Among children who have ODD, those with temperamental traits of oppositionality have a poorer prognosis compared with children in whom the oppositional behavior occurred as an outcome of an acute event.[1] Adolescents with severe externalizing behaviors are more likely to leave school early and report global adversity throughout life compared with those with few or no externalizing behaviors.[31] It is hard to determine if their experiences in adolescence (eg, getting into trouble, turbulent family relationships) lead to more difficulties in life, or if the adult difficulties are primarily due to the underlying disruptive behaviors.

Conclusion

Disruptive behaviors and their associated diagnoses of ODD, CD, and intermittent explosive disorders are a common reason that parents seek medical care from a primary pediatric health care professional. Therefore, it is helpful to understand the risk factors, assessment, and treatment for children with disruptive behaviors. While disruptive behavior disorders are often chronic, early identification and intervention of problem behaviors can often improve the functioning of affected children and families.

References

1. Harris J. Disruptive behavior disorders. In: McMillan J, RFeigin R, DeAngelis C, Jones M, eds. *Oski's Pediatrics: Principles and Practice*. 4th ed. Philadelphia, PA: Lippincott Williams & Wilkins; 2006:629–634
2. Hoffenaar PJ, Hoeksma JB. The structure of oppositionality: response dispositions and situational aspects. *J Child Psychol Psychiatry*. 2002;43(3):375–385
3. American Psychiatric Association. *Diagnostic and Statistical Manual of Mental Disorders*. 5th ed. Arlington, VA: American Psychiatric Publishing; 2013
4. American Psychiatric Association. *Diagnostic and Statistical Manual of Mental Disorders*. 4th ed. Text rev. Washington, DC: American Psychiatric Publishing; 2000
5. MacDonald EK. Principles of behavioral assessment and management. *Pediatr Clin North Am*. 2003;50(4):801–816
6. Rey J, Walter G, Soutullo C. Oppositional defiant and conduct disorders. In: Martin A, Volkmar F, eds. *Lewis's Child and Adolescent Psychiatry: A Comprehensive Textbook*. 4th ed. Philadelphia, PA: Lippincott Williams & Wilkins; 2007:454–466
7. Farmer EM, Compton SN, Burns BJ, Robertson E. Review of the evidence base for treatment of childhood psychopathology: externalizing disorders. *J Consult Clin Psychol*. 2002;70(6):1267–1302
8. Nock MK, Kazdin AE, Hiripi E, Kessler RC. Prevalence, subtypes, and correlates of DSM-IV conduct disorder in the National Comorbidity Survey Replication. *Psychol Med*. 2006;36(5):699–710

9. McLaughlin KA, Green JG, Hwang I, Sampson NA, Zaslavsky AM, Kessler RC. Intermittent explosive disorder in the National Comorbidity Survey Replication Adolescent Supplement. *Arch Gen Psychiatry.* 2012;69(11):1131–1139

10. Lahey BB, Schwab-Stone M, Goodman SH, et al. Age and gender differences in oppositional behavior and conduct problems: a cross-sectional household study of middle childhood and adolescence. *J Abnorm Psychol.* 2000;109(3):488–503

11. Forehand R, McMahon R. *Helping the Noncompliant Child: A Clinician's Guide to Parent Training.* New York, NY: The Guilford Press; 1981

12. Greydanus DE, Pratt HD, Patel DR, Sloane MA. The rebellious adolescent. Evaluation and management of oppositional and conduct disorders. *Pediatr Clin North Am.* 1997;44(6):1457–1485

13. Crick NR, Grotpeter JK. Relational aggression, gender, and social-psychological adjustment. *Child Dev.* 1995;66(3):710–722

14. Searight HR, Rottnek F, Abby SL. Conduct disorder: diagnosis and treatment in primary care. *Am Fam Physician.* 2001;63(8):1579–1588

15. Angold A, Costello EJ. Toward establishing an empirical basis for the diagnosis of oppositional defiant disorder. *J Am Acad Child Adolesc Psychiatry.* 1996;35(9):1205–1212

16. Hamilton SS, Armando J. Oppositional defiant disorder. *Am Fam Physician.* 2008;78(7):861–866

17. Collett BR, Ohan JL, Myers KM. Ten-year review of rating scales. V: scales assessing attention-deficit/hyperactivity disorder. *J Am Acad Child Adolesc Psychiatry.* 2003;42(9):1015–1037

18. Burns GL, Patterson DR. Factor structure of the Eyberg Child Behavior Inventory: a parent rating scale of oppositional defiant behavior toward adults, inattentive behavior, and conduct problem behavior. *J Clin Child Psychol.* 2000;29(4):569–577

19. Lengua LJ, Sadowski CA, Friedrich WN, Fisher J. Rationally and empirically derived dimensions of children's symptomatology: expert ratings and confirmatory factor analyses of the CBCL. *J Consult Clin Psychol.* 2001;69(4):683–698

20. Ratey JJ, Gutheil CM. The measurement of aggressive behavior: reflections on the use of the Overt Aggression Scale and the Modified Overt Aggression Scale. *J Neuropsychiatry Clin Neurosci.* 1991;3(2):S57–S60

21. Burke JD, Loeber R, Birmaher B. Oppositional defiant disorder and conduct disorder: a review of the past 10 years, part II. *J Am Acad Child Adolesc Psychiatry.* 2002;41(11):1275–1293

22. Jaffee SR, Caspi A, Moffitt TE, et al. Nature × nurture: genetic vulnerabilities interact with physical maltreatment to promote conduct problems. *Dev Psychopathol.* 2005;17(1):67–84

23. Costello EJ, Compton SN, Keeler G, Angold A. Relationships between poverty and psychopathology: a natural experiment. *JAMA.* 2003;290(15):2023–2029

24. Baving L, Laucht M, Schmidt MH. Oppositional children differ from healthy children in frontal brain activation. *J Abnorm Child Psychol.* 2000;28(3):267–275

25. Alegria AA, Radua J, Rubia K. Meta-analysis of fMRI studies of disruptive behavior disorders. *Am J Psychiatry.* 2016;173(11):1119–1130

26. Elkins IJ, McGue M, Iacono WG. Prospective effects of attention-deficit/hyperactivity disorder, conduct disorder, and sex on adolescent substance use and abuse. *Arch Gen Psychiatry.* 2007;64(10):1145–1152

27. Gottlieb SE, Friedman SB. Conduct disorders in children and adolescents. *Pediatr Rev.* 1991;12(7):218–223

28. Woolfenden SR, Williams K, Peat JK. Family and parenting interventions for conduct disorder and delinquency: a meta-analysis of randomised controlled trials. *Arch Dis Child.* 2002;86(4):251–256

29. Pappadopulos E, Macintyre Ii JC, Crismon ML, et al. Treatment recommendations for the use of antipsychotics for aggressive youth (TRAAY). Part II. *J Am Acad Child Adolesc Psychiatry.* 2003;42(2):145–161

30. Rowe R, Maughan B, Pickles A, Costello EJ, Angold A. The relationship between DSM-IV oppositional defiant disorder and conduct disorder: findings from the Great Smoky Mountains Study. *J Child Psychol Psychiatry.* 2002;43(3):365–373

31. Colman I, Murray J, Abbott RA, et al. Outcomes of conduct problems in adolescence: 40 year follow-up of national cohort. *BMJ.* 2009;338:a2981

CHAPTER 22

Anxiety and Mood Disorders

Viola Cheung, DO, FAAP

Michele L. Ledesma, MD, FAAP

Carol C. Weitzman, MD, FAAP

Introduction

Anxiety disorders are a group of disorders categorized by excessive fear that results in behavioral disturbances and impairment in activities of daily living. Mood disorders are diagnoses of which a disturbance in mood, either depression or mania, is the underlying disorder that causes functional impairment as well as cognitive and somatic changes. Among youth aged 13 to 17 years, there is an estimated lifetime prevalence of 31.9% for anxiety disorders and 14.3% for mood disorders,[1] as defined in the *Diagnostic and Statistical Manual of Mental Disorders,* Fifth Edition (*DSM-5*).[2] In total, approximately 11% to 20% of children in the United States will have a behavioral or emotional disorder at any given time.[3] These statistics indicate that behavior and emotional problems are common throughout childhood and begin early in life. Among all children meeting criteria for a behavioral or emotional disorder, anxiety and mood disorders are some of the most prevalent psychiatric conditions seen in children and adolescents.[4] Anxiety and depressive symptoms at low levels, however, have been shown to have an evolutionary benefit.[5] The absence of anxiety may lead to injury or death, as anxiety symptoms increase alertness and reduce the probability of missing potential threats. Withdrawing motivation and decreasing activity may allow a person to conserve his or her efforts in situations in which that energy would be wasted or worsen the situation.[5] The challenge for busy primary pediatric health care professionals is to know when symptoms are transient, developmentally appropriate, or suggestive of a more significant anxiety and mood problem that is maladaptive and causing impairment in functioning across settings.

Primary pediatric health care professionals play an important role in promoting the social-emotional health of children (see Chapter 12, Social and Emotional Development), and they often serve as an entry point to behavioral health services and treatment. Because of frequent contact with families and the opportunity to see children and adolescents before symptoms have become frank disorders, primary pediatric health care professionals are well-positioned to assess the severity of a child's problem, offer brief intervention and treatment, and assess the need for more intensive services. Ideally, primary care clinicians should feel competent to identify, manage, and advocate for children with anxiety and mood disorders and to know when to refer to developmental-behavioral pediatrics, child psychiatry, or other behavioral health professionals; however, this is not always the case. The reasons are multifactorial and include time limitations, reimbursement constraints, and lack of behavioral health professionals to whom patients can be referred to once identified.[6] In a study survey of 832 pediatric primary care providers, 77% felt that the greatest barrier to treating mental/behavioral health problems was the lack of time.[7] Nearly half of surveyed pediatricians reported lack of confidence in their ability to treat child mental/behavioral health problems due to lack of training in identifying such problems.[6] To address this, there are increasing numbers of resources available to promote mental/behavioral health competencies.[8,9]

The American Academy of Pediatrics (AAP) Task Force on Mental Health and the Bright Futures Periodicity Schedule recommends that mental/behavioral health surveillance questions be asked at all health care visits, including topics such as school performance and sleep hygiene.[10] Standardized behavior rating scales can aid clinical judgment and often can be incorporated into pediatric primary care settings. These scales are not designed to make a diagnosis but to help the primary care clinician determine whether there is a problem requiring further exploration.

History and key questions are often the most useful way to begin to assess the severity of a behavioral problem. Although caregivers may be able to report accurately on behaviors that are observed, children should be directly interviewed, as they are most qualified to describe mood and/or anxiety symptoms, and sometimes these feelings have not been previously disclosed. In addition, input from people actively involved in the child's life outside of the home environment, such as teachers, is extremely useful in allowing the primary pediatric health care professional to have a better understanding of the impact of these symptoms on a child's daily functioning.

Parents and children may be reluctant to bring their anxiety and depressive symptoms to the attention of a medical professional due to concerns of being "labeled" with a mental health disorder or fear of being treated with medication; however, adolescents report an increased willingness to disclose mental health information if their confidentiality is assured.[11] Low emotional competence in the adolescent or child, which is defined as the ability to manage and express emotions and negative attitudes related to seeking professional help, is also another barrier to a person's willingness to disclose information about mental health problems.[12] Additionally, parents have decreased recognition of the significance of the child's distress and the impact it is having on the child, especially as these are internalizing symptoms.[13] Family dysfunction and parental psychopathology, such as maternal depression, may also influence the presentation of the child's symptoms more negatively. Therefore, primary pediatric health care professionals must convey an interested and nonjudgmental attitude toward their families in order to encourage the child or adolescent and parent to share their concerns.[14]

Anxiety Disorders

Introduction

Anxiety disorders are a group of disorders categorized by excessive fear resulting in behavioral disturbances and impairment in activities of daily living. *Fear* is defined as an emotional response to a real or perceived imminent threat. *Anxiety* is the anticipation of a future threat.[2] While it is common for children to experience fear or anxiety transiently, children with anxiety disorders overestimate and misperceive the danger of situations they fear, and these fears persist in an excessive way beyond developmentally appropriate periods.[15] Age-typical anxiety and fear in childhood tends to follow a developmental sequence. Young children develop attachment to their caregivers early in life and experience normative fears at separation, such as at bedtime or when being dropped off at child care or preschool. As children begin to explore the environment around them, fear of animals or objects in their environment develops as a protective response.[16] When children enter school and engage in more complex peer interactions, performance and social fears emerge. While children with age-typical fears will try to avoid or escape triggers that provoke their anxiety, children with anxiety disorders often go to extreme lengths.

The presentation of anxiety disorders can vary, and children may present in less expected ways. For example, they may present with somatic complaints, such as stomachaches, headaches, and nausea, or they may present with irritability, oppositionality, or anger, particularly when they are confronted with their fear trigger. Children, particularly younger children, do not always recognize that their fear and worry are excessive, which can make detection of an anxiety problem more difficult.[17]

Epidemiology

Anxiety disorders are the most common psychiatric disorders presenting in children and adolescents, with prevalence rates as high as 20%,[17,18] and they are often the earliest mental health problems to emerge in children.[19] Although preschoolers with anxiety disorders are often not recognized and may not be as clearly differentiated as in older children, overall prevalence rates have been reported to be similar to those in older children, with reported rates of 19.4%.[20] Anxiety disorders are often undertreated, with only 18% of adolescents with an anxiety disorder receiving treatment.[21] Obsessive-compulsive disorder (OCD) affects approximately 1% of children, and this increases to up to 4% in late adolescence.[22] The prevalence rates for posttraumatic stress disorder (PTSD) vary but have been estimated to be between 3% and 6% in an unreferred population.[23] In children with a history of sexual abuse, nearly 50% may develop PTSD,[24] and approximately 5% of children develop PTSD after exposure to natural disasters.[25]

There are a number of different types of anxiety disorders. Obsessive-compulsive disorder, which had been included within anxiety disorders in prior iterations of the *Diagnostic and Statistical Manual,* is now in a new section in the *DSM-5*[2] ("Obsessive-Compulsive and Related Disorders"), and PTSD is now described in *DSM-5* under the section of "Trauma and Stressor-related Disorders."[2] Despite their inclusion outside of "Anxiety Disorders" in the *DSM-5*, they are included within this chapter, as many treatments are similar for both.

Anxiety disorders may be differentiated from each other by situations that trigger the anxiety or fear. Separation and specific phobias emerge first, with performance anxiety and social phobia/social anxiety emerging later in childhood; these are followed by panic disorder and OCD in adolescence. Generalized anxiety disorder is the most common type of anxiety disorder, and panic disorder and agoraphobia are the least common.[18] The gender profiles of the different anxiety disorders vary over childhood. Overall, anxiety disorders and PTSD are more prevalent in girls compared to boys, with prevalence ratios reaching 2:1 to 3:1 by adolescence.[2,23]

Anxiety disorders tend to be enduring, and more than three-quarters of young adults with psychiatric disorders report first having a diagnosis between the ages of 11 and 18 years.[3] A specific anxiety disorder may persist or change to another anxiety disorder later, or there may be a syndrome shift to multiple anxiety disorders, depression, and/or substance use disorders. Preventing this "cascade of psychopathology" is one key reason for early recognition and treatment.[26]

Comorbidity within anxiety disorders and between other psychiatric disorders is common. In a recent population-based study of preschoolers, approximately 23% of children met criteria for 2 anxiety disorders, and 8% met criteria for 3. Preschoolers with generalized anxiety disorder were most likely to have a co-occurring anxiety or nonanxiety disorder.[20] The literature often refers to the "pediatrics anxiety disorder triad," which consists of generalized anxiety disorder, social phobia/social anxiety disorder, and separation anxiety disorder, as these tend to co-occur, have similar trajectories, and respond similarly to pharmacological and behavioral treatment. In a study that examined the comorbidity of 1,035 adolescents between 12 and 17 years old, the comorbidity rate within anxiety disorders was 14.1%, and it was 51% for other psychiatric disorders, such as depression, somatoform disorders, and substance use disorders, with depression being the most common.[27]

There are many risk factors for developing an anxiety disorder. There is significant heritability, and some studies have indicated that children of parents with an anxiety disorder are 7 times more likely to develop an anxiety disorder than children whose parents have no mental health disorder.[28] Recent studies suggest that genes account for as much as 30% of the variance in childhood anxiety. Temperamental factors, such as shyness or behavioral inhibition, which also have a genetic component, also play a role. Additional factors associated with developing an anxiety disorder include insecure attachment, parental characteristics that include overprotection, lack of warmth, significant criticism, parental negative beliefs about a child's coping ability leading to low expectations and high accommodation, and environmental factors, such as living in poverty or high psychosocial stress.[28]

Risk factors for the development of PTSD include childhood characteristics, including IQ and temperament, early environmental conditions, such as loss of a parent before 1 year of age, self-perception of the severity and impact of the traumatic exposure, and genetic predisposition.[29,30]

Etiology and Pathophysiology

The etiology of anxiety disorders is almost always multifactorial. Although there are clear genetic underpinnings, developmental and psychosocial vulnerabilities, as well as acute and chronic stressors, contribute to their genesis and presentation.

Many studies have investigated the heritability of anxiety disorders in familial and twin studies, and there is evidence that the brain-derived neurotrophic factor (BDNF) protein may play a role. The BDNF protein regulates neuronal survival, and lower levels of this protein have been associated with anxiety disorders.[31] On neuroimaging studies, anxiety disorders are related to atypical activity of the prefrontal cortex–amygdala circuitry. Functional imaging studies have shown decreased activity in the right orbitofrontal cortex and anterior cingulate cortex and increased activity in the amygdala, which is linked to fear responses. In studies where subjects were shown pictures of faces with angry, disgusted, or fearful expressions, people with generalized anxiety disorder showed increased activation of the amygdala and decreased activation of the ventrolateral prefrontal cortex (VLPFC).[32] Activity of the VLPFC has been shown to be inversely related to the severity of anxiety symptoms, and both cognitive behavioral therapy (CBT) and fluoxetine have been shown to increase activity in the VLPFC. Biological abnormalities in the levels of neurotransmitters in the central nervous system, such as serotonin, gamma-aminobutyric acid (GABA), dopamine, and glutamate, have been associated with anxiety disorders.[33] The exact mechanism in which brain neurotransmitter levels modulate anxiety symptoms has been unclear, and there have been many theories postulated. Although medications that prevent the reuptake of serotonin, thereby increasing serotonin levels, have been correlated with a reduction in anxiety symptoms, the exact mechanism of this is unclear.[33] Levels of GABA, the major inhibitory neurotransmitter, have been postulated to be lower in people with anxiety disorders.[34] Dopamine may increase amygdala activation, heightening anxiety symptoms; however, increases in dopamine have also been shown to reduce anxiety and result in positive feelings of self-efficacy and confidence.[35,36] Neurochemical studies have correlated glutamate and glutamatergic tone, the major excitatory neurotransmitter in the brain, in the anterior cingulate with symptom severity in generalized anxiety disorder.[16,36]

Obsessive-compulsive disorder has been found to be familial in origin, with higher lifetime prevalence in people with first-degree relatives.[37] Neurobiological studies have revealed dysfunction in the orbitofrontal cortex, temporolimbic cortices, caudate nuclei, and thalamus, and recent evidence has suggested a larger network of cerebral dysfunction than previously appreciated.[38] Similar to non-OCD anxiety disorders, how neurotransmitters modulate OCD symptoms in the brain is not entirely clear.

However, increased levels of glutamate, a predominant excitatory neurotransmitter, have been found in the cerebrospinal fluid (CSF) of patients with OCD.[39]

Exposure to traumatic events in early childhood may have a lifelong effect on the functioning of the cortisol system and stress regulation that may increase the risk of PTSD later in life (see Chapter 3, Environmental Influences on Child Development and Behavior).

Changes from *DSM-IV-TR* to *DSM-5*

There have been several changes to the section on "Anxiety Disorders" in the *DSM-5*[2] from the *DSM-IV-TR*. In the *DSM-5*, OCD, PTSD, and acute stress disorder are no longer categorized under "Anxiety Disorders." Separation anxiety disorder is now included in "Anxiety Disorders" and can now have an onset after age 18 years. There have also been changes to the diagnostic criteria for agoraphobia, specific phobia, and social anxiety disorder, along with changes in symptom duration requirements. In the *DSM-5*, anxiety symptoms need to be present for at least 6 months for everyone, not only for people under 18 years of age. In addition, in the *DSM-5*, what was previously known as social phobia is now called social anxiety disorder. Lastly, a new developmental subtype of PTSD, Posttraumatic Stress Disorder in Children 6 Years and Younger, is described and makes use of developmentally appropriate criteria for young children.

DSM-5 Categories and Definitions
– Separation Anxiety Disorder (F93.0)

Separation anxiety disorder is defined by excessive fear or anxiety when experiencing or anticipating separation from a caregiver (or someone the individual is attached to) that lasts at least 4 weeks in children and adolescents and 6 months or more in adults and causes significant impairment. The child may become socially withdrawn, exhibit sadness, or have difficulty concentrating on work or play. Children with separation anxiety disorder tend to restrict social experiences away from home or attachment figures, and there is often excessive worry of potential harm, such as illness, injury, disasters, or death, to the attachment figure. The child may also experience excessive worry about getting lost or being kidnapped, if separated from his or her attachment figure. Additional problems triggered by separation or fear of separation may include sleep disturbances (eg, refusal to sleep alone), repeated nightmares, and somatic symptoms (which may include headaches, stomachaches, nausea, and/or vomiting).

– Selective Mutism (F94.0)

Selective mutism is the persistent failure to speak in certain social situations, while speaking in other ones. The symptoms last longer than 1 month, and their onset is generally before 5 years of age. The child may speak at home or with immediate family members but may not verbally respond to others when spoken to. The failure to speak is not due to any underlying expressive language deficit, and the child does not have any speech disturbances. Selective mutism results in impairment of social communication, occupational, and academic achievement.

– Specific Phobia (F40.2XX)

In specific phobias, the child experiences excessive circumscribed fear or anxiety about a specific object or situation and actively avoids the phobic object or situation. The fear or anxiety is out of proportion to the actual risk. Children may have more than one specific phobia. Exposure to the phobic object or situation consistently results in immediate fear or anxiety, which may be manifested in crying, tantrums, freezing, or clinging behaviors. For a diagnosis, a specific phobia must last for at least 6 months and result in functional impairment in home, work, school, or social interactions. There are *International Classification of Diseases, Tenth Revision* codes for specific phobias.

– Social Anxiety Disorder (F40.10)

Social anxiety disorder is categorized by excessive fear or anxiety in one or more social situations in which the child or adolescent perceives or worries about being judged negatively by both peers and adults. The child or adolescent avoids social situations due to fears that he or she may be negatively evaluated or may be embarrassed. These symptoms must persist for at least 6 months.

– Panic Disorder (F41.0)

A panic disorder is diagnosed when a child or adolescent has recurrent panic attacks. A panic attack is a sudden intense fear or discomfort that reaches a peak within minutes. The panic attacks appear to occur without an obvious trigger, although most people identify a stressor several months before their first panic attack. The child or adolescent may go from a calm state to an anxious state and experience heightened autonomic nervous system symptoms, such as accelerated heart rate, sweating, shaking, shortness of breath, chest pain or discomfort, abdominal distress, numbness or tingling, and/or have a fear of dying or losing control. Other symptoms may include feelings of unreality or being detached from oneself. To meet criteria for panic disorder, a child or adolescent must have persistent concern or worry about additional panic attacks, and this worry must last greater than 1 month in duration. Many children who present with panic attacks will undergo lengthy and costly medical investigations.

– Agoraphobia (F40.00)

This is defined by fear or intense anxiety involving 2 or more situations, including using public transportation, being in open or enclosed spaces, standing in line or being in a crowd, or being outside of the home alone. Children or adolescents with agoraphobia often have thoughts that something terrible might happen in the above situations. They may avoid situations or insist on the presence of a companion due to perceived difficulty escaping or being unable to find help in the event of incapacitating or embarrassing symptoms. Symptoms must be present 6 months or longer.

– Generalized Anxiety Disorder (F41.1)

A child or adolescent with a generalized anxiety disorder worries excessively about routine life circumstances, multiple events, and/or activities for at least 6 months. These children or adolescents usually find it difficult to control their worries and have concerns related to their competence or quality of their performance, and whether or not others are evaluating them. They exhibit at least 3 symptoms that include feeling on edge, fatigue, difficulty concentrating, irritability, muscle tension, and sleep disturbance. Functional impairment is often secondary to the associated symptoms and the considerable time spent worrying.[2]

– Obsessive-Compulsive Disorder (F42)

A child or adolescent with obsessive-compulsive disorder has uncontrollable obsessions, which are defined as recurrent thoughts that are intrusive and unwanted, and compulsions, which are defined as repetitive behaviors or mental acts that he or she feels to the urge to repeat over and over. Obsessions and compulsions may be related to themes of contamination, symmetry, and fear of harm to oneself and others.

– Posttraumatic Stress Disorder (F43.10)

This occurs after exposure to one or more traumatic events—actual or threatened death, serious injury, or sexual violence—either by directly experiencing or witnessing the traumatic event, having the traumatic event occur to a close family member or friend, or having repeated exposure to the consequences of the traumatic event more than through electronic media alone. Children aged 6 years or younger may not experience the traumatic event themselves but may witness it. Symptoms include: (1) *intrusion symptoms,* such as re-experiencing recurrent and distressing memories and dreams, dissociative reactions, intense psychological distress, and/or marked physiological reactions; (2) *persistent avoidance* of associated stimuli; (3) *negative alterations in cognition and mood* associated with the traumatic event or feelings of detachment; and (4) marked alterations in arousal and reactivity associated with the traumatic event.

Anxiety Screening Tools

Structured and semistructured diagnostic interviews, self-report rating scales, and clinician-rated instruments are the most common methods for identifying and measuring anxiety in the pediatric population.[40] Screening questions should use developmentally appropriate language, have adequate psychometric properties, and be based on criteria as highlighted in the *DSM*. Ideally, information should be obtained from multiple informants, including parents and teachers.[17,41] For children 8 years or older, self-reported measures for anxiety may include the Multidimensional Anxiety Scale for Children (MASC) or the Screen for Child Anxiety Related Emotional Disorders (SCARED). Younger children should be screened with parent report measures or interviewed with the use of visual aids, such as a feeling or mood thermometer. Measures such as the Children's Yale Brown Obsessive Compulsive scale,[42] which is not particularly amenable to use in pediatric primary care, or the Obsessive-Compulsive Inventory–Child Version[43] can be used to assess for obsessive or compulsive symptoms.

It is often necessary for the clinician to ask questions specifically about trauma and symptoms of PTSD because children and adolescents are unlikely to volunteer information.[44] Repeated evaluation over time may be necessary, as symptoms may present months or years after a traumatic incident.[44] School-based screening should be considered after community-level traumatic events.[45] There are several well-validated tools available that can be used by primary pediatric health care professionals for screening both trauma exposure and symptoms of PTSD, including the Child PTSD Symptom Scale, Traumatic Events Screening Inventory, and UCLA Child/Adolescent PTSD Reaction Index.

If the screening measures are positive for anxiety symptoms, the primary pediatric health care professional should determine which anxiety disorder might be present, the severity, and the degree of functional impairment. Instruments available to screen for anxiety disorders, OCD, and PTSD are detailed in Tables 22.1–22.3.

Differential Diagnosis

The differential diagnoses of anxiety disorders include hyperthyroidism, pheochromocytoma, migraines, medication side effects, excessive caffeine intake, attention-deficit/hyperactivity disorder (ADHD), other mental health problems, and/or learning disabilities.[4,17]

Although the defining characteristic of PTSD is that it is triggered by a traumatic event, other mental health disorders may be preceded by trauma as well. An acute stress reaction refers to the development of fear behaviors lasting from 3 days to 1 month after a traumatic event and may be a precursor to PTSD. Depression and anxiety are often comorbid with PTSD. Specific phobias and dissociative disorders have also been known to occur in response to a traumatic event. Finally, any neurological damage that may have occurred due to the traumatic event should be assessed.

Treatment

Due to the shortage of mental/behavioral health professionals in almost all communities, primary pediatric health care professionals often need to become involved with the treatment and ongoing symptom reassessment of children with anxiety disorders. In follow-up studies of children who received treatment for their anxiety disorders, there was a decreased risk of developing another mental health disorder after 3 to 4 years.[46] Pharmacological and nonpharmacological options are available to treat anxiety disorders. In children with mild to moderate anxiety or OCD symptoms, CBT is the first recommended line of treatment,[17] although evidence supporting CBT for children under 7 years old is lacking.[47,48] In children and adolescents with moderate to severe anxiety disorders or OCD, a partial response to psychotherapy alone, or complex comorbid conditions, a multimodal treatment approach is often needed. This approach includes pharmacotherapy, CBT, and family therapy.[17,22,49] Clinical trials in the Child/Adolescent Anxiety Multimodal Study (CAMS), which was a 6-year randomized controlled trial involving 488 children and adolescents between the ages of 7 and 17 years who had diagnoses of separation anxiety disorder, generalized anxiety disorder, and social phobia,

Table 22.1. Screening Tools for the Identification of Anxiety Disorders

Measure	Description	No. of Items	Format	Approximate time to complete	Age	Availability
The Revised Children's Manifest Anxiety Scale, Second Edition (RCMAS-2)	Yes/No checklist Measures physiological symptoms, worry, and inattentiveness associated with anxiety problems. Measures overall anxiety levels and academic stress, test anxiety, peer and family conflicts, and drug problems.	49 items Short Form (10 items) available	Child self-report	5–10 minutes	6–19 years	Western Psychological Services www.wpspublish.com
The Screen for Childhood Anxiety Disorders, Revised (SCARED-R)	3-point scale Assesses for 5 domains of anxiety including: panic/somatic, generalized anxiety, separation anxiety, social phobia, and school phobia.	66 items	Parent completed Child self-report	10 minutes	8–18 years	In the public domain University of Pittsburgh Child and Adolescent Bipolar Spectrum Services http://pediatricbipolar.pitt.edu/resources/instruments
Multidimensional Anxiety Scale for Children, 2nd Edition (MASC2)	Assesses for the presence of anxiety symptoms Measures symptoms in the following scales: separation anxiety/phobias, GAD index, social anxiety, obsessions and compulsions, physical symptoms, harm avoidance	50 items	Parent completed Child self-report	15 minutes	8–19 years	Pearson Clinical www.pearsonclinical.com
The Spence Children's Anxiety Scale (SCAS)	4-point frequency scale Assesses for 6 domains of anxiety including: generalized anxiety, panic/agoraphobia, social phobia, separation anxiety, OCD, and physical injury fears	38 items, parent form 44 items, child form Preschool scale: 28 items, parent completed 22 items, teacher completed	Parent completed Child self-report Teacher completed	10 minutes	8–15 years Preschool scale: 3–6 years	In the public domain www.scaswebsite.com

Abbreviations: GAD, generalized anxiety disorder; OCD, obsessive-compulsive disorder.

Table 22.2. Screening Tools for the Identification of Obsessive-Compulsive Disorder

Measure	Description	No. of Items	Format	Approximate Time to Complete	Age Range	Availability
Children's Yale Brown Obsessive Compulsive Scale	5-part interview and checklists that assess OCD symptoms and severity Contains 5 sections that include: instructions, obsessions checklist, severity ratings for obsessions, compulsions checklist, and severity rating for compulsions.	40-item obsessions checklist 40-item compulsions checklist 10-item severity rating	Clinician interview followed by severity rating checklist	May take up to 120 minutes to administer and score.	6–17 years	In the public domain www.cappcny.org/home/media/CYBOCS.pdf
Obsessive-Compulsive Inventory–Child Version	3-point frequency scale Assesses the frequency of OCD symptoms and the amount of distress caused by the symptoms.	21 items	Child self-report	10–15 minutes	7–17 years	Edna Foa, PhD Department of Psychiatry University of Pennsylvania 3535 Market Street, 6th Floor Philadelphia, PA 19104 Phone: (215) 746–3327 Email: foa@mail.med.upenn.edu

Abbreviation: OCD, obsessive-compulsive disorder.

Table 22.3. Screening Tools for the Identification of Traumatic Experiences and Symptoms of Posttraumatic Stress Disorder

Tool	Description	No. of Items	Format	Approximate Time to Complete	Age Range	Availability
Child Post-Traumatic Stress Reaction Index	5-point frequency scale Assesses for some of the symptoms for PTSD as well as guilt, impulse control, somatic symptoms, and regressive behaviors.	20 items	Clinician interview	10–20 minutes	6–17 years	Email: drned@earthlink.net
Child PTSD Symptom Scale	4-point frequency scale Assesses PTSD diagnostic criteria and symptom severity.	26 items	Child self-report	10–15 minutes	8–18 years	Edna Foa, PhD Department of Psychiatry University of Pennsylvania 3535 Market Street, 6th Floor Philadelphia, PA 19104 Phone: (215) 746–3327 Email: foa@mail.med.upenn.edu
Traumatic Events Screening Inventory for Children (TESI-C)	Yes/No checklist Assesses a child's experience of a variety of potential traumatic events including current and previous injuries, hospitalizations, domestic violence, community violence, disasters, accidents, physical abuse, and sexual abuse.	16 items	Semi-structured interview	10–30 minutes	4+ years	In the public domain www.ptsd.va.gov
UCLA PTSD Reaction Index	5-point frequency scale Assesses a child's trauma history and the full range of DSM-5 PTSD diagnostic criteria	48 items	Semi-structured interview	15–20 minutes	7–12 years (Child) 13+ years (Adolescent)	www.reactionindex.com

Abbreviations: DSM-5, Diagnostic and Statistical Manual of Mental Disorders, 5th Edition; PTSD, posttraumatic stress disorder; UCLA, University of California, Los Angeles.

compared the efficacy of pharmacotherapy (sertraline) alone, behavioral intervention (CBT) alone, or a combination of pharmacotherapy and behavioral intervention together. The results showed that combination treatment was more effective than monotherapy with pharmacotherapy or CBT alone.[4,49] The Pediatric Obsessive Compulsive Disorder Treatment Study (POTS), a multicenter, randomized clinical trial of 112 children and adolescents with OCD who were 7 to 17 years old, was designed to compare the efficacy of sertraline treatment only, CBT only, and a combination of sertraline and CBT, or placebo. The results showed that monotherapy with either sertraline or CBT alone or combination therapy was more effective than placebo. As in the CAMS, combined treatment of sertraline and CBT was the most effective treatment.[50] There were comparable rates of improvements in patients who received either sertraline or CBT alone. For PTSD, trauma-focused cognitive behavioral therapy (TF-CBT) has the largest evidence base and is proven to be the most effective treatment for PTSD among all psychological therapies.[51]

– Behavioral Intervention

Nonpharmacological treatment includes cognitive behavioral interventions, psychodynamic psychotherapy, and family therapy.[15] Children with anxiety actively seek escape from and avoidance of their anxiety triggers in order to prevent distress. Cognitive behavioral therapy works by examining the relationship between cognitions, behaviors, and feelings.[21,52] Components of CBT include: (1) psychoeducation; (2) teaching children adaptive coping skills, such as relaxation techniques like deep breathing; (3) changing negative self-talk and distorted negative expectations; (4) exposing children through gradual desensitization to feared stimuli, so that they can tolerate and modify negative emotions; and (5) relapse prevention plans.[17] The goal of CBT is to teach children to experience their symptoms and deal more effectively with them rather than to avoid or escape them.[15] Cognitive behavior therapy performed individually or in a group setting is comparable and has been effective in treating anxiety disorders in children. Individual programs, such as Coping Cat, have been shown to be effective in treating children with anxiety disorders by reducing symptoms and functional impairment,[53] and these improvements have been shown to be sustained up to 1 year later.[54] Group cognitive behavior therapy, such as Social Effectiveness Training for Children, may offer opportunities for peer modeling and social interactions and has been beneficial for children with all anxiety disorders, especially social phobia.[21,48]

Parents and families play an important role in the development and maintenance of child anxiety. The quality of the parent-child relationship and parenting behaviors have been associated with anxiety symptoms in children.[28] Nearly all parents of anxious children report accommodating their child's avoidant and escape behaviors. Accommodation predicts symptom severity, degree of child impairment, family dysfunction and distress, and poor treatment outcomes.[55] Therefore, in treating childhood anxiety disorders, parental anxiety, parenting styles, and parent-child interactions need to be addressed. Both excessive accommodation or being overly demanding, which denies the child's fear and delegitimizes the anxiety, need to be replaced with support, which acknowledges the child's distress but also affirms confidence in the coping abilities of the child.

The first step of any treatment for PTSD is ensuring the child's safety, as ongoing trauma can undermine any effective treatment.[44] Treatment planning for PTSD should also incorporate appropriate interventions for comorbid mental health disorders, such as anxiety, depression, and substance abuse.[45] Psychotherapy remains the first-line treatment for children and adolescents with PTSD.[45] Trauma-focused cognitive-behavioral therapy has been shown to be effective in treating the core symptoms of PTSD, as well as trauma-related depression and anxiety.[51] Trauma-focused cognitive-behavioral therapy utilizes exposure therapy and adds skill-building modules following the PRACTICE acronym: *p*sychoeducation and parenting skills, *r*elaxation skills, *a*ffect regulation skills, *c*ognitive coping, *t*rauma narrative, *i*n vivo mastery, *c*hild-parent sessions, and *e*nhancing future safety and development. There is evidence for the use of TF-CBT across a wide range of traumatic experiences, including sexual abuse, domestic violence, traumatic loss, and acts of terrorism.[44]

For children who have experienced large-scale disasters or community violence, group CBT protocols, such as Cognitive-Behavioral Intervention for Trauma in Schools (CBITS), have been shown to be effective and provide a component of psychoeducation for teachers addressing the potential impact of trauma on classroom behavior and learning.[45]

Involving parents in PTSD treatment is more effective than treating the child or adolescent alone. Parents and other family members need psychoeducation, as they may themselves have PTSD, feel guilty for not protecting the child, or may be inadvertently triggering a child's symptoms with reminders of the trauma.[44] Child-parent psychotherapy is a dyadic therapy intended for children 3 to 5 years of age that combines elements of TF-CBT with attachment theory and is a relationship-based model for children who have experienced family trauma such as domestic violence.[45]

– Pharmacotherapy

Due to the lack of research in the use of medications to treat childhood anxiety disorders, many medications used to treat children with anxiety disorders are considered off-label.[49] In 2014, duloxetine became the only medication approved by the US Food and Drug Administration (FDA) for the treatment of generalized anxiety disorder in children. However, multiple randomized trials of children and adolescents with anxiety disorders have shown reduction in anxiety symptoms with the use of selective serotonin reuptake inhibitors (SSRIs), including sertraline,[56] fluvoxamine,[57] paroxetine,[58] and fluoxetine[59] over placebo in children with generalized anxiety disorder, social phobia, and separation anxiety disorder[21,49] In addition, clinical trials of escitalopram,[60] citalopram,[61] and duloxetine[62] have been shown to be effective in decreasing anxiety symptoms in children versus placebo.[21] In deciding which SSRI to use, it may be helpful for the primary pediatric health care professional to inquire about positive responses with SSRIs in first-degree relatives, as enzymes that metabolize the SSRIs may have a genetic disposition. The greatest safety evidence otherwise is for fluvoxamine, which had the highest rate of clinical response and tolerance in a comparison meta-analysis of 16 clinical trials. The results of this comparison study showed that the probability of efficacy in ascending order was placebo, venlafaxine (a selective serotonin-norepinephrine reuptake inhibitor [SNRI]), sertraline, paroxetine, fluoxetine, and fluvoxamine, with fluvoxamine being the most efficacious. In addition, fluoxetine, fluvoxamine, and paroxetine were better tolerated than sertraline and venlafaxine.[63]

The effects of SSRI medications may not be seen for 4 to 8 weeks, but early effects of SSRI medication have been reported in the first 1 to 2 weeks. If a child experiences absent or partial response with the maximum dosage for at least 6 to 8 weeks on the first SSRI, a second SSRI should be trialed.[21] If a child fails a second SSRI at the maximum tolerated or recommended dose, a referral to a child psychiatrist or developmental-behavioral pediatrician should be considered. When remission is achieved, treatment should be continued for at least 6 to 12 months before consideration of discontinuing the medication. SSRI medications need to be tapered over a minimum of 1 to 2 months in order to avoid flulike symptoms, including agitation, dizziness, nausea, headache, and fatigue. These side effects are often reversed by resuming the preceding SSRI dose and decreasing the dose at a more gradual rate. SSRIs are typically well-tolerated, with the most common side effects being gastrointestinal (GI) symptoms, sleep difficulties, and sexual dysfunction. Gastrointestinal symptoms tend to be self-limited and are rarely severe enough to warrant discontinuation. More significant adverse reactions may include disinhibition, agitation, mania, or psychosis. Up to 2% of children taking SSRIs experience the emergence of suicidal thoughts and behaviors. There is an increased risk during the first 9 days of treatment or if the starting doses are higher than usual, confirming the need for close follow-up during the titration period.[17] Clinicians should watch for the development of serotonin syndrome, a potentially severe adverse effect of SSRIs and SNRIs. Serotonin syndrome is a triad of mental status changes, autonomic hyperreactivity, and neuromuscular abnormalities and symptoms that can range from mild to life-threatening.[64] Most cases will present within 24 hours of the initiation or change in dosage. Guidelines for prescribing SSRIs are detailed in Table 22.4.

Selective serotonin-norepinephrine reuptake inhibitors, such as venlafaxine ER, have also been shown efficacious in the treatment of anxiety disorders; however, an increase in suicidal ideation has been noted.[4,65] Tricyclic antidepressants (TCAs) and benzodiazepines have also been used to treat childhood anxiety disorders, although the safety and efficacy of these medications in children have not been established. Tricyclic antidepressants are not commonly used due to side effects, including QTc prolongation and the need for close monitoring of a child's vital signs, electrocardiogram parameters, and blood levels. Emergency treatment of anxiety symptoms with benzodiazepines has been effective for adults due to their rapid onset, although randomized controlled trials using alprazolam were not found to be any more effective than placebo in reducing anxiety symptoms in children.[21] In general, benzodiazepines are not appropriate for long-term treatment because they cause sedation and induce tolerance and withdrawal symptoms, as well as having the potential for abuse,[32] but there may be a limited role in the acute phase of treatment.[66]

Table 22.4. Medications for the Treatment of Anxiety Disorders and Depression

Medication	FDA Approval for Children	Starting Dose	Effective Dose Range	Recommended Administration	Half-Life	Cytochrome Metabolic Pathway	Common Side Effects
Selective Serotonin Reuptake Inhibitors (SSRIs)							Sedation, insomnia, confusion, headache, fatigue, dry mouth, sweating, tremor, orthostatic hypotension, GI distress, sexual dysfunction
Fluoxetine	For Depression: ages 8–17 For OCD: ages 7–17	5–10 mg daily	20–80 mg daily	AM	48–72 hrs Half-life of active metabolite (norfluoxetine) is 2 weeks	Major: 2D6 Minor: 2C19 Enzyme Inhibition: 2D6, 2C19, 3A4	Bruising and rare bleeding
Escitalopram	For Depression: ages 12–17	5–10 mg daily	10 mg daily Maximum: 20 mg daily	AM	27–32 hrs	2C19 No significant actions on CYP450 isoenzymes	
Citalopram	Safety and efficacy has not been established for less than 18 years of age.	10–20 mg daily	20 mg daily Maximum: 60 mg daily	AM	23–45 hrs	Major: 2C19, 3A4 Minor: 2D6 Enzyme Inhibition: 2D6	
Sertraline	For OCD: ages 6–17	25–50 mg daily	50–100 mg daily Maximum: 150–200 mg daily	AM	22–36 hrs Half-life of metabolite is 62–104 hrs	2C9 Enzyme Inhibition: 2D6, 3A4, 2C9	

Table 22.4. Medications for the Treatment of Anxiety Disorders and Depression (*continued*)

Medication	FDA Approval for Children	Starting Dose	Effective Dose Range	Recommended Administration	Half-Life	Cytochrome Metabolic Pathway	Common Side Effects
Selective Serotonin Reuptake Inhibitors (SSRIs)							**Sedation, insomnia, confusion, headache, fatigue, dry mouth, sweating, tremor, orthostatic hypotension, GI distress, sexual dysfunction**
Paroxetine	Safety and efficacy has not been established for less than 18 years of age.	Panic disorder: 5–10 mg daily; increase by 10 mg every 2–4 weeks Social anxiety disorder: 20 mg daily; increase by 10–20 mg every 4–6 weeks	Panic disorder: 10–40 mg daily Social Anxiety Disorder: 20–60mg Maximum: 40–60 mg daily	PM	24 hrs Inactive metabolites	2D6 Enzyme Inhibition: 2D6, 2C9	Significant withdrawal symptoms Suicidal ideation
Fluvoxamine	For OCD: ages 8–17	25 mg daily; increase by 25 mg daily every 4–7 days	50–200 mg daily Maximum: 200–300 mg daily	HS	9–28 hrs	1A2, 2D6 Enzyme Inhibition: Major:1A2 Minor: 2C9, 2C19, 3A4	

Table 22.4. Medications for the Treatment of Anxiety Disorders and Depression (*continued*)

Medication	FDA Approval for Children	Starting Dose	Effective Dose Range	Recommended Administration	Half-Life	Cytochrome Metabolic Pathway	Common Side Effects
Serotonin–Norepinephrine Reuptake Inhibitors (SNRIs)							
Venlafaxine	Safety and efficacy has not been established for less than 18 years of age.	37.5–75 mg daily	75–150 mg daily Maximum: 150 mg daily	BID QD (XR formulation)	3–7 hrs Half-life of active metabolite is 9–13 hrs	2D6 Enzyme Inhibition: 2D6, 3A4	SIADH, hyponatremia, nausea and dizziness
Duloxetine	FDA approved for GAD in children	30 mg daily	30–60 mg daily Maximum: 60 mg daily	QD	12 hrs	1A2, 2D6 Enzyme Inhibition: 2D6	Urinary retention
Benzodiazepines							Fatigue, drowsiness, impaired mental speed, impaired visuospatial and visuomotor abilities, decreased concentration, paradoxical hyperactivity
Lorazepam	Safety and efficacy has not been established in children less than 12 years of age.	0.5 mg daily	Maximum: 6 mg daily	BID-TID	10–20 hrs	No active metabolites	
Diazepam	Yes, for children 6 months and up for sedation	2 mg divided BID-TID	Maximum: 40 mg daily divided BID-TID	BID-TID	20–50 hrs	2C19, 3A4 Accumulates on chronic dosing	

Table 22.4. Medications for the Treatment of Anxiety Disorders and Depression (*continued*)

Medication	FDA Approval for Children	Starting Dose	Effective Dose Range	Recommended Administration	Half-Life	Cytochrome Metabolic Pathway	Common Side Effects
Tricyclic Antidepressants							
Clomip-ramine	Yes, for children with OCD above the age of 10	25 mg daily	3 mg/kg or 100 mg daily Maximum: 3 mg/kg or 200 mg daily	HS	17–28 hrs	1A2, 2D6 Enzyme Inhibition: 2D6	Insomnia, blurred vision, constipation, sweating, hypotension, EKG changes, GI distress

Abbreviations: AM, morning; BID, twice a day; EKG, electrocardiogram; GAD, generalized anxiety disorder; GI, gastrointestinal; HS, at bedtime; OCD, obsessive-compulsive disorder; PM, evening; QD, once a day; TID, 3 times a day;

In contrast to non-OCD-related anxiety disorders, there are FDA-approved medications to treat children with OCD. These include clomipramine and fluvoxamine in children 10 years of age or older, fluoxetine, and sertraline.[67] Pharmacological treatment with citalopram and paroxetine has also been effective in treatment of OCD symptoms, although there is no current FDA approval for their use.[68] A meta-analysis of 12 randomized, controlled medication trials conducted to compare the treatment efficacy of pediatric OCD medications—such as paroxetine, fluoxetine, fluvoxamine, sertraline, and clomipramine—showed that clomipramine had greater effect in reducing OCD symptoms in comparison to the SSRIs.[69] As clomipramine is a tricyclic antidepressant, guidelines for medication monitoring include EKG and blood levels as mentioned previously. Therefore, due to their more favorable side-effect profiles, SSRI medications are still the first-line pharmacological treatment for OCD in the pediatric population.

Selective serotonin reuptake inhibitors are the first-line treatment for adults with PTSD, but there is limited evidence of their efficacy in children and adolescents. In randomized, controlled trials for adolescent PTSD, sertraline,[70] and fluoxetine[71] were found to be no more effective than placebo, but they may be effective in patients who present with significant symptoms of depression.[72] Citalopram has shown promise in open-label trials. Sympatholytic drugs, such as clonidine, guanfacine, prazosin, and propranolol, are used to decrease hyperarousal and symptoms of increased heart rate, anxiety, and impulsivity in children with PTSD.[45,73] Benzodiazepines are generally not recommended for treating symptoms of panic and anxiety.[44] Atypical antipsychotics are frequently prescribed to treat emotional dysregulation, aggression, and psychotic symptoms as well as anxiety, but large-scale studies are lacking. In smaller trials, mood stabilizers, such as carbamazepine, oxcarbazepine, and divalproex appear to decrease PTSD symptoms, anger, and irritability.[73]

Tips for Primary Pediatric Health Care Professionals

Primary pediatric health care professionals can offer education about anxiety symptoms and brief supportive counseling to children and families. Quick attempts to alleviate a child's anxiety by inadvertently encouraging escape, avoidance, and parental accommodation are rarely helpful and send a powerful, negative message that an anxious child cannot develop coping skills and needs excess protection rather than support. It is also important not to convey a sense of blame to parents for accommodations they are providing but instead empower them by explaining how a change in their behavior can help their child. It is critical not to "take sides" with one or the other parent but encourage them to support each other in changing practices. A few well-placed questions about how much a child's anxiety symptoms are "taking over," how much parents feel they are participating in their child's anxiety routines, and how much they need to modify their daily lives as a result can be revealing.

When to Refer

Children who should be referred to a mental health/behavioral specialist include those who have failed 2 courses of an SSRI, SNRI, or have had significant adverse effects; those with severe symptomatology; and those with PTSD, OCD, and substance-induced anxiety.

Mood Disorders

Introduction

Mood disorders in children and adolescents comprise both ends of the affective spectrum from depression to mania. They are associated with negative academic, social, and health outcomes, including mood disorders in adulthood, substance abuse, early pregnancy and parenthood, and increased suicide risk.[74] They often coexist with other disorders, including ADHD, anxiety, conduct disorders, and substance abuse; mood disorders and their associated comorbidities contribute significantly to morbidity and mortality throughout the lifespan.

Although the diagnosis of mood disorders in the pediatric population is based primarily on adult criteria,[2] symptoms of mood disorders in children and adolescents may differ from those of adults. Importantly, irritability may be a more pronounced symptom than depressed mood or mania; also, what may appear to be boredom can instead be lack of motivation or fatigue.[75] Bipolar disorder in children has been known to present with more rapid mood cycling as opposed to discrete mood cycles.[76] Mood disorders may also present with somatic symptoms, as children may interpret symptoms of depression or mania as symptoms of physical illness.

Epidemiology

Data released by the Centers for Disease Control and Prevention (CDC) on Mental Health Surveillance Among Children from 2005–2011 based on several nationally representative survey systems, including the National Center for Health Statistics, the National Health Interview Survey, the National Health and Nutrition Examination Survey, the National Survey on Drug Use and Health, and the Youth Risk Behavior and Surveillance System (YRBS), estimated that 3.9% of children from 3 to 17 years of age had ever received a diagnosis of depression, and the prevalence of depression among children in the same age group was estimated at 2.1% (current) to 3.0% (in the past 12 months) based on parental report.[77] Among adolescents surveyed, rates were considerably higher, with the self-reported rate of depression in the past 2 weeks at 6.7% and the lifetime prevalence by age 17 years reported to be 12.0%.[77] This is somewhat lower than the findings of the National Comorbidity Survey Replication Adolescent Supplement (NCS-A), which reported a prevalence rate of 14.3% for mood disorders, with a median age of onset of 13 years.[1] In the Great Smoky Mountains Study of youth aged 9 to 21 years, there was an imputed cumulative prevalence rate of 11.2% for any mood disorder.[78] There are notable gender differences in the prevalence of depression in adolescence, with females reporting higher rates (17.5% to 18.2%) compared to males (7.7% to 12.8%).[77,78] Among prepubertal children, however, boys are more likely to meet criteria for depression.

For bipolar disorders, the NCS-A found a prevalence rate of 2.9% for bipolar I and II disorders combined, with a lifetime prevalence of 4.3% for adolescents aged 17 to 18 years.[79] A meta-analysis of 12 studies from 6 countries, including the United States, found a mean prevalence rate of 1.8% for pediatric bipolar disorders.[80] There was no gender difference found, which is consistent with the literature from adult studies.[81]

Psychosocial risk factors associated with depression include a family history of depression and/or anxiety, dysfunctional family relationships, poor social supports,[82] a history of early trauma or abuse,[83] stressors such as academic difficulties and bullying,[84] substance abuse, and early sexual activity. Having a negative or maladaptive coping style,[85] a sense of hopelessness,[86] and low self-esteem are considered personality risk factors. Medical risk factors include low birth weight, a history of concussion[87] or traumatic brain injury,[88] chronic medical illness, and prior diagnoses of anxiety and conduct disorders.[89] Gender identity is an important factor, and children and adolescents who identify as gay, bisexual, lesbian, and/or transgender are reported to have higher rates of depression and suicidal ideation.[79] Protective factors include family connectedness and social supports, the presence of caring adults,[20] positive coping strategies, and having a strong belief system.[86]

The strongest risk factor for pediatric bipolar disorder is a family history of bipolar disorder.[90] Other risk factors include a history of severe childhood trauma and intrauterine exposure to drugs.

Comorbidity is common in mood disorders, and studies have shown that 50% to 90% of youth with depression will have a comorbid diagnosis. In the NCS-A, anxiety disorders and disruptive behavior disorders (ODD and CD) were most strongly associated with depression, with about a 4-fold increased risk for major depressive disorder. There was about a 3-fold increased risk of major depressive disorder (MDD) for ADHD and for substance use disorders.[91] In bipolar disorder, ADHD (52% to 84%), ODD (72% to 88%), severe MDD (85% to 89%), and anxiety (51% to 56%) were the most common comorbid conditions.[92] Mood disorders are also associated with medical complications later in life, including accelerated atherosclerosis and early cardiovascular disease.[93]

Based on the CDC's most recent data from 2014, suicidal risk is the most worrisome concern related to depression, and suicide is the second leading cause of death among youth in the United States. The overall suicide rate for children aged 10 to 19 years was 4.5 per 100,000 in 2010 (higher for boys [6.9 per 100,000] than for girls [2.0 per 100,000]) and has increased to 5.36 per 100,000 in 2014.[94] Alarmingly, the suicide rate among children aged 10 to 14 years more than doubled from 0.9% in 2009 to 2.1% in 2014.[95] The rate of suicidal ideation reported in the YRBS was 15.8% nationwide and was higher among girls (19.3%) than for boys (12.5%).[77] Up to 32% of patients with depression will make a suicide attempt at some time during adolescence or young adulthood, and up to 7% will commit suicide. In autopsy studies, 50% to 60% of adolescent suicide victims had a depressive disorder at the time of death.[96]

Given these statistics, any assessment of mood disorders must include assessment of safety concerns and safety planning for worsening suicidal or homicidal behavior.[79] Children who present with more severe depression, a poorer functional status, and insomnia are at increased risk for suicidal behaviors.[96] Feelings of worthlessness and hopelessness are more likely to be associated with thoughts of death, suicidal ideation, suicidal plans, and attempted suicides.[75] Parent-child conflict has been found to be a significant factor in prepubertal victims.[97]

Etiology and Pathophysiology

Genetic and epigenetic causes, developmental and psychosocial vulnerabilities, and acute and chronic stressors comprise the myriad factors that can contribute to the emergence and endurance of a mood disorder.

Many studies have investigated the heritability of mood disorders in familial and twin studies, and there is evidence that genes on several chromosomes, including the *RORA*, *RORB*, and *GRM8* genes, may be implicated.[32] However, the pathogenesis of depression appears to involve epigenetic mechanisms in several genes rather than specific depression genes.

Psychosocial stressors contribute to gene-environment interactions. There is evidence that stress induces modifications in the hypothalamic-pituitary-adrenal axis, and the overproduction of stress hormones has been found to cause reduced neurogenesis in the hippocampus, which has been associated with adolescent and adult depression.[98] It is important to note that stress-related pathology causing epigenetic changes can be transmitted transgenerationally.[98]

On neuroimaging studies, adolescent depression has been found to be associated with hyperactivation of the amygdala and the subgenual anterior cingulate cortex (ACC).[98] The successful treatment of symptoms of depression by a variety of methods, including deep brain stimulation and medication, decreases the activation in the subgenual ACC.[32]

Neurotransmitters, particularly norepinephrine, serotonin, dopamine, and acetylcholine, are implicated in the course of depression.[32] The "monoaminergic hypothesis" of depression was one of the first neurobiological theories to be elucidated by neuroanatomical studies, and it proposed that deficiencies of norepinephrine, serotonin, and dopamine occurred in depression. Subsequent research has shown that while these neurotransmitters are somehow involved, studies of metabolites in the CSF, blood, and urine have yet to definitively show this deficiency, which suggests that other pathogenic factors are involved.[99] Immune mechanisms have also been implicated in the pathogenesis of depression. Inflammatory cytokines have been found in increased levels in blood and CSF, and it has been proposed that cytokines may influence the metabolism and neuroendocrine functions of neurotransmitters.[99]

Familial, twin, and adoption studies indicate that bipolar disease is highly heritable, with rates up to 80% in some studies. However, no specific gene has been identified, and bipolar disease is considered genetically complex.[100] Children with bipolar disorder often have neurocognitive impairments involving verbal memory and visual-spatial memory, processing speed, working memory, and social cognition.[101] Neuroimaging studies have shown reduced ACC and amygdala volumes[100] as well as corpus callosum volumes and more white matter abnormalities. Inflammatory cytokines have likewise been implicated.

Changes from *DSM-IV-TR* to *DSM-5*

Under the *DSM-IV-TR*, there was a single mood disorder category; in the *DSM-5*, mood disorders are grouped into two categories: depressive disorders, including disorders that involve primarily depressed mood, and bipolar disorders, covering disorders that involve an element of mania or hypomania. Diagnostic changes include the addition of new diagnoses: disruptive mood dysregulation disorder and persistent depressive disorder (which replaces dysthymia and chronic major depressive disorder). Additional changes include the addition of the specifier "with mixed features" (ie, features of both mania and depression) to both depressive and bipolar disorders, and the removal of bereavement as an exclusion for depression. Also, Bipolar I and II disorders emphasize changes in energy and activity in addition to mood. Finally, the designation "Other Specified" disorders was created, and the "NOS" diagnoses were eliminated.[2]

DSM-5 Categories and Definitions
– Depressive Disorders

The depressive disorders include major depressive disorder, persistent depressive disorder, disruptive mood dysregulation disorder, and premenstrual dysphoric disorder, as well as depressive disorders due to substance abuse, medication, or another medical condition. The common feature of all these disorders is the presence of sad, empty, or irritable mood accompanied by functional impairment.[2]

Major Depressive Disorder (F32.0–9, F33.0–9)

Major depressive disorder is characterized by discrete episodes (although diagnosis is possible based on one episode) of either persistent depressed mood (or irritable mood in children or adolescents) or anhedonia lasting at least 2 weeks, along with the presence of 4 additional symptoms, including significant weight loss or poor weight gain in children, insomnia or hypersomnia, psychomotor agitation or retardation, fatigue, feelings of worthlessness or guilt, inability to concentrate or indecisiveness, or recurrent thoughts of death, suicidal ideation, or a suicide attempt.

Persistent Depressive Disorder (formerly dysthymia, F34.1)

Persistent depressive disorder is a more chronic form of depression that can be diagnosed when depressed or irritable mood persists for at least 1 year in children (at least 2 years in adults), along with at least 2 additional symptoms, including decreased or increased appetite, insomnia or hypersomnia, low energy or fatigue, low self-esteem, poor concentration or difficulty making decisions, or feelings of hopelessness.

It is important to keep in mind that *DSM* symptom criteria are not adapted for age or gender. In children, depression may present differently depending on the development of the child. *DSM* criteria have been found to have lower diagnostic validity in children, as they present with more diverse symptomatology, including vegetative symptoms, anxiety, conduct problems, body dysmorphic symptoms, and deliberate vomiting, in addition to suicidal ideation.

Sleep disturbances are important symptoms of mood disorders, and altered circadian rhythms are often seen in mood disorders.[102] Persistent insomnia in a person with a history of depressive episodes is a risk factor for relapse.[32]

– Bipolar and Related Disorders

Classically, bipolar disorder and mania were considered uncommon in children. However, retrospective analyses of adult patients with bipolar disorder suggested that symptoms began much earlier than previously believed, and analyses of several longitudinal research samples suggested that children can present with symptoms of mania.[79]

Although the same criteria are used for diagnosis in children and adults, there is often more rapid cycling and mixed states described in children,[103] and pediatric bipolar disorder tends to have a more chronic course.[104] High rates of comorbid disruptive behavior disorders, including ADHD and ODD, are commonly found.[103]

Although primary pediatric health care professionals are not expected to be the primary behavioral health care clinicians for a child with bipolar disorder, they play a critical role in screening, diagnosis, care coordination, and monitoring for medical complications of treatment.[79] They should also be aware that suicide risk is particularly high in bipolar disorder, with about one-third of patients attempting suicide in their lifetimes.[2]

Bipolar I Disorder (F31.0–9)

Bipolar I is diagnosed in individuals who meet criteria for a manic episode, defined as a distinct period of abnormally elevated and persistently elevated, expansive, or irritable mood lasting at least 1 week and present most of the day, nearly every day. Mania manifests as at least 3 of the following (4 if mood is only irritable): inflated self-esteem or grandiosity, decreased need for sleep (getting by with little or no need for sleep, as opposed to insomnia, which is difficulty falling or staying asleep), increased talking or pressured speech, flight of ideas, racing thoughts, distractibility, an increase in goal-directed activity or psychomotor agitation, and excessive involvement in activities with a potential for significant consequences. These manic episodes may have been preceded by and may be followed by periods of hypomania or major depression, although it is not necessary for diagnosis. Juvenile mania often presents as labile and erratic changes in mood and energy levels with irritability and belligerence being more common than euphoria. In young children, excessive silliness, hypersexuality, decreased need for sleep, and daredevil and reckless acts are also seen.

Bipolar II Disorder (F31.81)

In contrast, Bipolar II disorder is characterized by the occurrence of a current or past hypomanic episode and at least one current or past episode of major depression. Hypomania is defined as a distinct period of abnormally and persistently increased activity or energy, lasting at least 4 consecutive days and persisting most of the day, nearly every day. Bipolar II is differentiated from Bipolar I based on the presence of milder symptoms of mania (hence the term hypomania) alternating with symptoms of depression.

Cyclothymic Disorder (F34.0–9)

Cyclothymic disorder is characterized by chronic, fluctuating mood, including numerous distinct periods of hypomanic symptoms and periods of depressive symptoms that do not meet criteria for a diagnosis of either Bipolar II disorder or MDD.

Screening Tools

The US Preventive Services Task Force (USPSTF), the National Institute for Health and Clinical Excellence, the American Academy of Child and Adolescent Psychiatry (AACAP), and the AAP recommend annual, routine screening for depression for children aged 11 to 21 years, as well as assessing for suicide risk factors at each well-child visit.[74] However, the USPSTF cautions that there is limited evidence of a direct link between screening for depression in children and adolescents in primary care settings and depression outcomes.[105] Standardized screening measures are important in predicting risk, but clinicians should not rely solely on them to make a diagnosis.[3] History and presentation are key components of an evaluation. Several screening instruments are available for depression (as detailed in Table 22.5) that can be administered and scored within the setting of a primary care practice. Among these, the Beck Depression Inventory and the Patient Health Questionnaire for Adolescents reported the highest sensitivities (approximately 89%) and specificities (approximately 75%).[105–107] Providers should also assess suicide risk in children and adolescents with depression using structured screening and interview tools, if feasible.[74] Currently, there is no consensus or well-validated screening tool available for the assessment of bipolar disorders in children, although there is some data on the use of scales such as the Child Mania Rating Scale and Young Mania Rating Scale.

Differential Diagnoses

The main differential diagnoses of mood disorders are other mood disorders, as depression is often the first symptom of pediatric bipolar disorder, and youth with depressive disorders often experience manic episodes.[104]

Disruptive behavior disorders, such as ADHD, ODD, and conduct disorder, are frequently comorbid with mood disorders.[91,92] The primary distinguishing features of mood disorders are their episodic nature, and particularly in bipolar disorders, distinct symptoms of mania. As such, it is important to determine that the mood episode symptoms and behavior represent a significant departure from baseline functioning. Also, although youth with disruptive behavior disorders may defy bedtime rules, they do not typically have a decreased need for sleep. Grandiosity, hypersexuality, racing thoughts, and flight of ideas are also distinct characteristics of bipolar disorders.[104]

There is also some symptom overlap between anxiety disorders and mood disorders; specifically, children and adolescents may present with symptoms such as irritability and sleep disturbance. Children with generalized anxiety typically have more chronic symptoms, such as chronic irritability, restlessness, and impaired concentration.[104]

Table 22.5. Screening Tools for the Identification of Depressive Disorders

Scale	Description	No. of Items	Format	Approximate Time to Complete	Age Range	Availability
Children's Depression Inventory, 2nd Edition (CDI-2)	3-point scale Assesses cognitive, affective, and behavioral signs of depression. Scale and subscale scores report on emotional problems, functional problems, negative mood, physical symptoms, negative self-esteem, interpersonal problems, and ineffectiveness.	28 items (full version) 12 items (short version)	Parent completed Child self-report (full and short versions) Teacher completed	5 minutes (short version) 15 minutes (full version)	6–17 years	Pearson Clinical www.pearsonclinical.com
Beck Depression Inventory, 2nd Edition (BDI-II)	4-point frequency scale with a total cutoff score of 20 for moderate depression Assesses the severity of depressive symptoms.	21 items	Child self-report or clinician interview	5–10 minutes	13–80 years	Pearson Clinical www.pearsonclinical.com
Mood and Feelings Questionnaire (MFQ)	3-point scale Designed to measure depressive symptoms.	11 items (short form) 32 items (long form)	Parent completed Child self-report	5–10 minutes (short version)	8–16 years	In the public domain Duke Developmental Epidemiology Program http://devepi.mc.duke.edu
Children's Depression Rating Scale, Revised (CDRS-R)	7-point scale Interview format is intended to engage children who are withdrawn and isolated.	17 items	Clinician interview	15–20 minutes	6–12 years	Western Psychological Services www.wpspublish.com
Patient Health Questionnaire (PHQ-2, PHQ-9)	4-point frequency scale Based on the depression module of the PHQ. The first two items are used to screen for depression, and if positive, the entire scale can then be used to assess symptom severity; question 9 screens for suicidal ideation.	9 items	Child self-report	5 minutes	13–17 years Adult	In the public domain www.phqscreeners.com
Pediatric Symptom Checklist	3-point frequency scale Screens for general psychosocial functioning. Attention, internalizing, and externalizing subscales can be obtained.	35 items	Parent completed Child self-report	5 minutes	3–16 years PSC-Y: 11+ years	In the public domain AAP Bright Futures https://brightfutures.aap.org/

Abbreviation: PHQ, Patient Health Questionnaire.

Adjustment disorder with depressed mood is an important differential. Although depressive symptoms often occur in the context of psychosocial stressors, an adjustment disorder occurs in response to a specific stressor, the symptoms are out of proportion in severity and intensity to the stressor, and it resolves once the stressor is eliminated.[2]

It can be difficult to differentiate pediatric schizophrenia from mood disorders, particularly when psychotic symptoms are present. Typically, the cognitive deficits are milder in mood disorders, while hallucinations, loosening of associations, and disordered thinking are more prominent in schizophrenia.[104]

An important differential is a comorbid substance use disorder, and a thorough history and assessment of substance use is critical, as either intoxication or withdrawal may precipitate manic or depressive symptoms. Judicious use of laboratory tests, such as drug panels, may be indicated and can also improve diagnostic accuracy.[104]

As with all mental/behavioral health disorders, mood symptoms due to a general medical condition must be carefully assessed.

Treatment

Because of the chronicity and potentially dangerous outcomes of untreated depression, primary pediatric health care professionals need to be able to screen for and diagnose mood disorders, as well as assess the risk for suicide in children and adolescents. Additionally, because of the shortage of mental health professionals, primary pediatric health care professionals may provide treatment and ongoing symptom reassessment. Both pharmacological and nonpharmacological options are supported by evidence.

– Depressive Disorders

The main treatment modalities for mood disorders are psychotherapy and medication. Psychotherapy, such as CBT and interpersonal therapy (IPT), is the first-line treatment for mild to moderate depression and should be combined with medication for moderate to severe depression.[108] There is evidence for both psychotherapy and medications based on large, randomized clinical trials that show reduction of symptoms based on both standardized measures and neuroimaging.[79]

When a clinician diagnoses a child or adolescent with depression, the patient should receive a minimum of 8 weeks of treatment, either psychotherapy or medication at an appropriate dose. Depression should be assessed regularly during treatment using structured tools in order to track progress and inform ongoing treatment, and treatment should continue until symptom remission is sustained and there is no longer any functional impairment. Both primary care and specialty providers should consider treatment adjustments for adolescents whose symptoms do not remit.[74]

Nonpharmacological Treatment

For mild to moderate depression, nonpharmacological treatment, including counseling and psychotherapy, is the first-line treatment. Providers should offer brief, supportive counseling and psychoeducation about depression to the child and family, as well as to the school. Supportive management, including advice on nutrition, exercise, and sleep, and problem-solving should be offered.[108] For mild depression, this may be adequate treatment.[74]

A meta-analysis of different psychotherapy modalities, which included CBT, IPT, behavioral problem-solving, relaxation, and attachment-based therapy, found these treatments to be equally efficacious.[108] Of these, CBT is widely considered the treatment of choice for depression in adolescents and adults. CBT for depression seeks to restructure distorted negative thinking; address helplessness, hopelessness, and hostility; encourage active behaviors; teach mood monitoring; and help with goal-setting and problem-solving.[79] Many studies have shown the effectiveness of CBT in individual and group settings. Although there is inconclusive evidence of its efficacy in prepubertal children,[109] there is increasing data that combined parent and child treatment may be more effective than treatment directed at the child alone.[110]

IPT, in contrast to CBT, focuses on a patient's relationships with family and peers, coping with stressors with others, and problem-solving ways to make relationships more positive.[79] IPT has been shown to be at least as efficacious as CBT for adolescent depression.[108] For both CBT and IPT, evidence shows small, positive benefits in terms of depression prevention and symptom reduction both immediately following treatment and for up to 12 months, but there is limited evidence of its durability beyond 1 year.[108,111] Mindfulness-based CBT has been shown to be effective in preventing relapse of depression in adults, and there is preliminary evidence of its efficacy in adolescents.[112]

Other therapeutic modalities include family therapy, individual psychodynamic therapy, and school- and community-based interventions, although evidence supporting these is more limited.[109] There is also growing evidence that exercise is an effective adjunct to pharmacological treatment.[113] Additionally, clinicians are urged to promote resilience in children and families who have endured a stressful event, such as by building on a social support network, encouraging community involvement, and working with teachers and other professionals involved in a child's life.

Pharmacological Treatment

Medications are indicated for moderate to severe depression, as well as mild to moderate depression that has not responded to psychotherapy after 6–8 weeks.[74,108]

Large clinical trials have concluded that the combination of medication and psychotherapy is superior to either alone. In fact, a meta-analysis has shown that on their own, SSRIs are less effective in pediatric than in adult MDD, and only about 60% of adolescents will respond to an adequate medication trial after 6 to 8 weeks.[114] In the Treatment for Adolescents with Depression Study (TADS), treatment with fluoxetine was compared to CBT and combination treatment, and it was found that the combination of fluoxetine and CBT was superior to monotherapy with either.[72] For initial nonresponders, the Treatment of Resistant Depression in Adolescents (TORDIA) trial found that adding CBT to a medication switch (ie, to an alternate SSRI) was more effective than a medication switch alone to either an alternate SSRI or to venlafaxine. Among the participants in the TADS study who elected to enroll in a 3.5-year naturalistic follow-up (patients who were given placebo were given the option of receiving active treatment), nearly half (47%) experienced a recurrent major depressive episode, but overall, global functioning was sustained and continued to improve gradually.[115]

The primary classes of medication to treat pediatric depression are SSRIs, SNRIs, and TCAs. FDA-approved SSRIs for treatment of depression are fluoxetine and escitalopram.[79] Fluoxetine has long been established to be superior to placebo both for symptom reduction and preventing relapse;[116] however, it is important to keep in mind that there have been high response rates to placebo as well.[108] In comparison to other antidepressants, fluoxetine has been found to be significantly more effective than other SSRIs, as well as more effective than nortriptyline, and it has been found to be more tolerable than imipramine and duloxetine.[117]

Like treatment for anxiety disorders, the effect of SSRIs may be seen after 1 to 2 weeks, but patients should be advised that full efficacy may take 4 to 8 weeks. Failure to respond to a second SSRI warrants referral to a developmental-behavioral pediatrician or child and adolescent psychiatrist.[47,108]

SSRIs have been linked to suicidal ideation and carry a black-box warning as a result of a meta-analysis that found that the average risk of suicidal ideation to be increased (4% compared to 2% in placebo) in patients taking SSRIs, although no completed suicides occurred.[108] As a result of this black-box warning, SSRI prescriptions for children and adolescents decreased, and this decrease was associated with an increase in suicide rates.[118] Subsequent analyses found mixed data, with other studies reporting a decrease in suicidal thoughts and behaviors mediated through a decrease in depression symptoms. Overall, the risk of suicidal thoughts and behaviors is estimated to be at 1% to 2% for children and adolescents.[47] Nevertheless, parents and adolescents must be informed of this risk and involved in the decision to weigh the risks of treatment and nontreatment. Patients should be monitored closely at the initiation of treatment, and both parents and children should have an action plan if suicidal thoughts emerge. Another uncommon but serious adverse effect is manic activation, that is, switching to symptoms of mania, including elevated arousal, affect, and energy level, which can occur in 2% to 10% of patients, although it has been estimated that less than 2% actually become manic. Patients with symptoms of mania and a family history of bipolar disorder may be at higher risk.[79] The FDA recommends that depressed youths be seen weekly for the first 4 weeks and every 2 weeks afterwards, and if face-to-face appointments are not possible, evaluations should be carried out by telephone.[108]

SNRIs and TCAs are also used in adults but have not been approved for use in children. There is evidence to support the efficacy of venlafaxine, but safety profiles have not been established and suicidality is a strong concern.[119] TCAs have not been shown to be more effective than placebo in pooled studies, and cardiac side effects and the need for close monitoring are important considerations.[120]

Once remission is achieved, patients should continue to be followed every 3 months, and medication should be continued for at least 6 to 12 months of stability.[74,121]

– Bipolar and Related Disorders

A multimodal treatment approach combining psychopharmacology and adjunctive psychosocial therapies is the mainstay of treatment for bipolar disorders in children and adolescents.[103] Although primary pediatric health care professionals will not solely manage bipolar disorder, familiarity with evidence-based treatments is helpful.

Nonpharmacological Treatment

Psychotherapy for bipolar disorders includes both individual and family therapies. Commonly used modalities include family psychoeducation, family-focused treatment for adolescents (FFT-A), dialectical behavior therapy (DBT), and child and family-focused cognitive behavioral therapy (CFF-CBT).[122]

In both family psychoeducation and FFT-A, treatment strategies include increasing knowledge and understanding of bipolar disorder and its treatment, improving communication skills, and cultivating problem-solving and coping skills. Family psycho-education additionally is aimed at increasing the child's and family's sense of support.[123] DBT is a modified form of cognitive behavioral therapy (CBT) and targets emotional dysregulation by teaching coping skills to both individuals and families.[124] CFF-CBT integrates principles of FFT with CBT and is based on specific problems of children and families, biological theories of excessive reactivity, and the role of environmental stressors in the outcome.[125]

Pharmacological Treatment

Mood stabilizers used for bipolar disorders include the second-generation antipsychot-ics (SGAs), such as risperidone, aripiprazole, and lithium, and antiepileptic drugs (AEDs), such as carbamazepine and divalproex.[122]

SGAs approved for the treatment of bipolar disorders in pediatrics are risperidone, aripiprazole, olanzapine, and quetiapine. Risperidone has been shown to have response rates of 59% to 63%,[126] while studies of aripiprazole demonstrate response rates of 63%.[127] Lithium is commonly used in adults, and although pediatric studies are lacking, the Collaborative Lithium Trial (CoLT) showed that lithium was effective for treating symp-toms of mania in about half the participants.[128] Antiepileptic drugs have also been used in adults, and there is some evidence of their efficacy in children.[79] Open label studies of carbamazepine[129] and divalproex[130] have demonstrated symptomatic improvement. When compared against each other in the Treatment of Early Age Mania (TEAM) study, however, risperidone was found to be superior to lithium and divalproex, and response rates to lithium and divalproex did not differ.[126]

The most common side effects of the SGAs are nausea, vomiting, constipation, sedation, and headache, which in most cases improve over time. Of greater concern are the meta-bolic adverse effects, including weight gain, hypertension, dyslipidemia, and insulin sensitivity. Primary pediatric health care professionals may need to manage these side effects by offering nutritional counseling and anticipatory guidance, as well as referral to endocrinology if necessary. Weight, blood pressure, and laboratory studies, including cholesterol, glucose, and insulin levels, should be monitored periodically.[131] Rare but serious adverse effects associated with the SGAs include extrapyramidal movement disorders, such as dystonias and tardive dyskinesia.

In the CoLT trial, lithium was generally well-tolerated and was not associated with weight gain;[128] however, it is known to cause thyroid dysfunction. Adverse effects of AEDs vary but include sedation, dizziness, GI symptoms, weight gain, and rash. As in all cases, primary pediatric health care professionals must also be wary of drug-drug interactions when prescribing medication for other conditions.[79]

Suicide Risk and Safety Planning

Suicide is a risk in both depression and bipolar disorders. Both the AAP and the AACAP recommend that all management must include screening for suicidality and the establishment of a safety plan, which includes restricting legal means, engaging a concerned third party, and developing a plan for communication should the patient become acutely suicidal or homicidal.[108,132] Of note, a review of suicide prevention contracts found detrimental outcomes, including an increased association with suicidal attempts and completed suicides, and are not recommended.[133] Screening tools, such as the Suicide Assessment Five-step Evaluation and Triage (SAFE-T) and the Columbia Suicide Severity Rating Scale (CSSRS), are freely available. When a suicidal patient is identified, the clinician should determine whether the patient warrants hospitalization.[121] Further, access to firearms is a major risk factor for completed suicide, and there is a strong association between having a gun in the home and increased risk of suicide among adolescents.[134] The AAP recommends counseling parents to remove guns from the home or restrict access to them, and this should be stressed for patients with mood disorders, other significant mental health problems, substance abuse problems, or a history of suicide attempts.[134]

Tips for Primary Pediatric Health Care Professionals

The most important role of a primary pediatric health care professional is to develop a therapeutic alliance with the child or adolescent and the family, and to remain a safe, nonjudgmental, and concerned party. Pediatric primary care clinicians should be prepared to offer psychoeducation and brief supportive counseling, including advice on sleep, exercise, nutrition, and coping strategies, along with initial medical management for children and adolescents presenting with milder symptoms. Because adolescents tend not to come to primary care practices frequently, opportunistic interventions integrated into routine primary care consultations may be beneficial. Lastly, primary pediatric health care professionals will benefit from identifying local resources and fostering collaboration with mental/behavioral health providers in order to provide quality mental/behavioral health care.

When to Refer

Children and adolescents who should be referred to mental/behavioral health specialists include those who have failed 2 courses of an SSRI or SNRI or have had significant adverse effects; those with moderate to severe symptoms; those with known or suspected bipolar disorder; and those who express suicidal ideation or have made a suicide attempt.

Resources

Journal Articles

Weitzman C, Wegner L, American Academy of Pediatrics Section on Developmental and Behavioral Pediatrics, et al. Promoting optimal development: screening for behavioral and emotional problems. *Pediatrics.* 2015;135(2):384–395

Zuckerbrot, RA, Cheung AH, Jensen PS, et al. Guidelines for adolescent depression in primary care (GLAD-PC): I. Identification, assessment, and initial management. *Pediatrics.* 2007;120(5):e1299–e1312

Lewandowski RE, Acri MC, Hoagwood KE, et al. Evidence for the management of adolescent depression. *Pediatrics.* 2013;132(4):e996–e1009

Birmaher B, Brent D; AACAP Work Group on Quality Issues, et al. Practice parameter for the assessment and treatment of children and adolescents with depressive disorders. *J Am Acad Child Adolesc Psychiatry.* 2007;46(11):1503–1526

Connolly SD, Bernstein GA; Work Group on Quality Issues. Practice parameter for the assessment and treatment of children and adolescents with anxiety disorders. *J Am Acad Child Adolesc Psychiatry.* 2007;46(2):267–283

Cohen JA, Bukstein O, Walter H, et al. Practice parameter for the assessment and treatment of children and adolescents with posttraumatic stress disorder. *J Am Acad Child Adolesc Psychiatry.* 2010;49(4):414–430

Geller DA, March J. Practice parameter for the assessment and treatment of children and adolescents with obsessive-compulsive disorder. *J Am Acad Child Adolesc Psychiatry.* 2012;51(1):98–113

McClellan J, Kowatch R, Findling RL; Workgroup on Quality Issues. Practice parameter for the assessment and treatment of children and adolescents with bipolar disorder. *J Am Acad Child Adolesc Psychiatry.* 2007;46(1):107–125

Web Sites

AAP Mental Health Screening and Assessment Tools for Primary Care
www.aap.org/en-us/advocacy-and-policy/aap-health-initiatives/
Mental-Health/Documents/ MH_ScreeningChart.pdf

AAP Bright Futures Mental Health Toolkit
www.brightfutures.org/mentalhealth/pdf/tools.html

AAP Anxiety Module
This module provides information on initial management and recognition of children with mild to moderate anxiety in the primary care setting.
www.aap.org/en-us/advocacy-and-policy/aap-health-initiatives/
Mental-Health/Pages/Module-2-Anxiety.aspx

AAP Trauma Toolbox for Primary Care
www.aap.org/en-us/advocacy-and-policy/aap-health-initiatives/
healthy-foster-care-america/Pages/Trauma-Guide.aspx

AACAP Depression Resource Center
www.aacap.org/aacap/families_and_youth/resource_centers/depression_
resource_center/Home.aspx

Anxiety BC
This Web site provides practical techniques for families and clinicians to use to help manage anxious feelings their children may experience.
http://www.anxietybc.com

The Developmental-Behavioral Pediatrics Online Community Web Site
This Web site provides information on developmental, behavioral, and emotional problems.
www.dbpeds.org/

International OCD Foundation Web Site
https://iocdf.org/

National Center for PTSD
www.ptsd.va.gov

National Child Traumatic Stress Network
www.nctsn.org

National Institutes of Mental Health
www.nimh.nih.gov

The Reach Institute
Guidelines for Adolescent Depression in Primary Care (GLAD-PC) Toolkit
www.glad-pc.org

SAFE-T Suicide Assessment Five-step Evaluation and Triage
http://stopasuicide.org/assets/docs/Safe_T_Card_Mental_Health_
Professionals.pdf

Stop a Suicide Today
A suicide prevention resource.
www.stopasuicide.org

References

1. Merikangas KR, He JP, Burstein M, et al. Lifetime prevalence of mental disorders in U.S. adolescents: results from the National Comorbidity Survey Replication—Adolescent Supplement (NCS-A). *J Am Acad Child Adolesc Psychiatry.* 2010;49(10):980–989
2. American Psychiatric Association. *Diagnostic and Statistical Manual of Mental Disorders.* 5th ed. Arlington, VA: American Psychiatric Association; 2013
3. Weitzman C, Wegner L; American Academy of Pediatrics Section on Developmental and Behavioral Pediatrics, et al. Promoting optimal development: screening for behavioral and emotional problems. *Pediatrics.* 2015;135(2):384–395
4. Wehry AM, Beesdo-Baum K, Hennelly MM, Connolly SD, Strawn JR. Assessment and treatment of anxiety disorders in children and adolescents. *Curr Psychiatry Rep.* 2015;17(7):52
5. Nesse RM. Proximate and evolutionary studies of anxiety, stress and depression: synergy at the interface. *Neurosci Biobehav Rev.* 1999;23(7):895–903
6. Heneghan A, Garner AS, Storfer-Isser A, Kortepeter K, Stein RE, Horwitz SM. Pediatricians' role in providing mental health care for children and adolescents: do pediatricians and child and adolescent psychiatrists agree? *J Dev Behav Pediatr.* 2008;29(4):262–269
7. Horwitz SM, Kelleher KJ, Stein RE, et al. Barriers to the identification and management of psychosocial issues in children and maternal depression. *Pediatrics.* 2007;119(1):e208–e218
8. American Academy of Pediatrics Committee on Psychosocial Aspects of Child and Family Health, Task Force on Mental Health. Policy statement—The future of pediatrics: mental health competencies for pediatric primary care. *Pediatrics.* 2009;124(1):410–421
9. American Academy of Pediatrics. *Addressing Mental Health Concerns in Primary Care: A Clinician's Toolkit.* Elk Grove Village, IL: American Academy of Pediatrics; 2010
10. Foy JM; American Academy of Pediatrics Task Force on Mental Health. Enhancing pediatric mental health care: report from the American Academy of Pediatrics Task Force on Mental Health. Introduction. *Pediatrics.* 2010;125(suppl 3):S69–S74
11. Ford CA, Millstein SG, Halpern-Felsher BL, Irwin CE, Jr. Influence of physician confidentiality assurances on adolescents' willingness to disclose information and seek future health care. A randomized controlled trial. *JAMA.* 1997;278(12):1029–1034
12. Rickwood D, Deane FP, Wilson CJ, Ciarrochi J. Young people's help-seeking for mental health problems. *AeJAMH.* 2005;4(3):218–251
13. Varni JW, Thissen D, Stucky BD, et al. Item-level informant discrepancies between children and their parents on the PROMIS(*) pediatric scales. *Qual Life Res..* 2015;24(8):1921–1937
14. Wissow LS, Roter DL, Wilson ME. Pediatrician interview style and mothers' disclosure of psychosocial issues. *Pediatrics.* 1994;93(2):289–295
15. Kendall PC. Treating anxiety disorders in children: results of a randomized clinical trial. *J Consult Clin Psychol.* 1994;62(1):100–110
16. Blackford JU, Pine DS. Neural substrates of childhood anxiety disorders: a review of neuroimaging findings. *Child Adolesc Psychiatr Clin N Am.* 2012;21(3):501–525
17. Connolly S, Bernstein G, Work Group on Quality Issues. Practice parameter for the assessment and treatment of children and adolescents with anxiety disorders. *J Am Acad Child Adolesc Psychiatry.* 2007;46(2):267–283
18. Costello EJ, Egger HL, Angold A. The developmental epidemiology of anxiety disorders: phenomenology, prevalence, and comorbidity. *Child Adolesc Psychiatr Clin N Am.* 2005;14(4):631–648
19. Beesdo K, Knappe S, Pine DS. Anxiety and anxiety disorders in children and adolescents: developmental issues and implications for DSM-V. *Psychiatr Clin North Am.* 2009;32(3):483–524
20. Franz L, Angold A, Copeland W, Costello EJ, Towe-Goodman N, Egger H. Preschool anxiety disorders in pediatric primary care: prevalence and comorbidity. *J Am Acad Child Adolesc Psychiatry.* 2013;52(12):1294–1303

21. Siegel RS, Dickstein DP. Anxiety in adolescents: update on its diagnosis and treatment for primary care providers. *Adolesc Health Med Ther.* 2012;3:1–16

22. Geller DA, March J. Practice parameter for the assessment and treatment of children and adolescents with obsessive-compulsive disorder. *J Am Acad Child Adolesc Psychiatry.* 2012;51(1):98–113

23. Kilpatrick DG, Ruggiero KJ, Acierno R, Saunders BE, Resnick HS, Best CL. Violence and risk of PTSD, major depression, substance abuse/dependence, and comorbidity: results from the National Survey of Adolescents. *J Consult Clin Psychol.* 2003;71(4):692–700

24. Wolfe DA, Sas L, Wekerle C. Factors associated with the development of posttraumatic stress disorder among child victims of sexual abuse. *Child Abuse Negl.* 1994;18(1):37–50

25. Shannon MP, Lonigan CJ, Finch AJ, Jr., Taylor CM. Children exposed to disaster: I. Epidemiology of post-traumatic symptoms and symptom profiles. *J Am Acad Child Adolesc Psychiatry.* 1994;33(1):80–93

26. Copeland WE, Shanahan L, Costello EJ, Angold A. Childhood and adolescent psychiatric disorders as predictors of young adult disorders. *Arch Gen Psychiatry.* 2009;66(7):764–772

27. Essau CA. Comorbidity of anxiety disorders in adolescents. *Depress Anxiety.* 2003;18(1):1–6

28. Drake KL, Ginsburg GS. Family factors in the development, treatment, and prevention of childhood anxiety disorders. *Clin Child Fam Psychol Rev.* 2012;15(2):144–162

29. Koenen KC, Moffitt TE, Poulton R, Martin J, Caspi A. Early childhood factors associated with the development of post-traumatic stress disorder: results from a longitudinal birth cohort. *Psychol Med.* 2007;37(2):181–192

30. Cornelis MC, Nugent NR, Amstadter AB, Koenen KC. Genetics of post-traumatic stress disorder: review and recommendations for genome-wide association studies. *Curr Psychiatry Rep.* 2010;12(4):313–326

31. Suliman S, Hemmings SM, Seedat S. Brain-Derived Neurotrophic Factor (BDNF) protein levels in anxiety disorders: systematic review and meta-regression analysis. *Front Integr Neurosci.* 2013;7:55

32. Carlson NR, Birkett MA. Schizophrenia and the affective disorders. *Physiology of Behavior.* 12th ed. Boston, MA: Pearson; 2016:519–551

33. Bystritsky A, Khalsa SS, Cameron ME, Schiffman J. Current diagnosis and treatment of anxiety disorders. *P T.* 2013;38(1):30–57

34. Lydiard RB. The role of GABA in anxiety disorders. *J Clin Psychiatry.* 2003;64(suppl 3):21–27

35. Schneier FR, Abi-Dargham A, Martinez D, et al. Dopamine transporters, D2 receptors, and dopamine release in generalized social anxiety disorder. *Depress Anxiety.* 2009;26(5):411–418

36. Strawn JR, Dominick KC, Patino LR, Doyle CD, Picard LS, Phan KL. Neurobiology of pediatric anxiety disorders. *Curr Behav Neurosci Rep.* 2014;1(3):154–160

37. Hanna GL, Himle JA, Curtis GC, Gillespie BW. A family study of obsessive-compulsive disorder with pediatric probands. *Am J Med Genet B Neuropsychiatr Genet.* 2005;134b(1):13–19

38. Whiteside SP, Port JD, Abramowitz JS. A meta-analysis of functional neuroimaging in obsessive-compulsive disorder. *Psychiatry Res.* 2004;132(1):69–79

39. Chakrabarty K, Bhattacharyya S, Christopher R, Khanna S. Glutamatergic dysfunction in OCD. *Neuropsychopharmacology.* 2005;30(9):1735–1740

40. The Research Units on Pediatric Psychopharmacology Anxiety Study Group. The Pediatric Anxiety Rating Scale (PARS): development and psychometric properties. *J Am Acad Child Adolesc Psychiatry.* 2002;41(9):1061–1069

41. Muris P, Dreessen L, Bogels S, Weckx M, Melick Mv. A questionnaire for screening a broad range of DSM-defined anxiety disorder symptoms in clinically referred children and adolescents. *J Child Psychol Psychiatry.* 2004;45(4):813–820

42. Scahill L, Riddle MA, McSwiggin-Hardin M, et al. Children's Yale-Brown Obsessive Compulsive Scale: reliability and validity. *J Am Acad Child Adolesc Psychiatry.* 1997;36(6):844–852

43. Foa EB, Coles M, Huppert JD, Pasupuleti RV, Franklin ME, March J. Development and validation of a child version of the obsessive compulsive inventory. *Behav Ther.* 2010;41(1):121–132

44. Gerson R, Rappaport N. Traumatic stress and posttraumatic stress disorder in youth: recent research findings on clinical impact, assessment, and treatment. *J Adolesc Health.* 2013;52(2):137–143

45. Cohen JA. Practice parameter for the assessment and treatment of children and adolescents with posttraumatic stress disorder. *J Am Acad Child Adolesc Psychiatry.* 2010;49(4):414–430

46. Last CG, Perrin S, Hersen M, Kazdin AE. A prospective study of childhood anxiety disorders. *J Am Acad Child Adolesc Psychiatry.* 1996;35(11):1502–1510

47. Southammakosane C, Schmitz K. Pediatric psychopharmacology for treatment of ADHD, depression, and anxiety. *Pediatrics.* 2015;136(2):351–359

48. Mohatt J, Bennett S, Walkup J. Treatment of separation, generalized, and social anxiety disorders in youths. *Am J Psychiatry.* 2014;171(7):741–748

49. Strawn JR, McReynolds DJ. An evidence-based approach to treating pediatric anxiety disorders. *Curr Psychiatr.* 2012;11(9):16–21

50. Pediatric OCD Treatment Study (POTS) Team. Cognitive-behavior therapy, sertraline, and their combination for children and adolescents with obsessive-compulsive disorder: the Pediatric OCD Treatment Study (POTS) randomized controlled trial. *JAMA.* 2004;292(16):1969–1976

51. Gillies D, Maiocchi L, Bhandari AP, Taylor F, Gray C, O'Brien L. Psychological therapies for children and adolescents exposed to trauma. *Cochrane Database Syst Rev.* 2016;10:Cd012371

52. Cartwright-Hatton S, Roberts C, Chitsabesan P, Fothergill C, Harrington R. Systematic review of the efficacy of cognitive behaviour therapies for childhood and adolescent anxiety disorders. *Br J Clin Psychol.* 2004;43(Pt 4):421–436

53. Podell JL, Mychailyszyn M, Edmunds J, Puleo CM, Kendall PC. The Coping Cat program for anxious youth: the FEAR plan comes to life. *Cogn Behav Pract.* 2010;17(2):132–141

54. Kendall PC, Flannery-Schroeder E, Panichelli-Mindel SM, Southam-Gerow M, Henin A, Warman M. Therapy for youths with anxiety disorders: a second randomized clinical trial. *J Consult Clin Psychol.* 1997;65(3):366–380

55. Lebowitz ER, Panza KE, Bloch MH. Family accommodation in obsessive-compulsive and anxiety disorders: a five-year update. *Expert Rev Neurother.* 2016;16(1):45–53

56. Rynn MA, Siqueland L, Rickels K. Placebo-controlled trial of sertraline in the treatment of children with generalized anxiety disorder. *Am J Psychiatry.* 2001;158(12):2008–2014

57. Walkup JT, Labellarte MJ, Riddle MA, et al. Fluvoxamine for the treatment of anxiety disorders in children and adolescents. *N Engl J Med.* 2001;344(17):1279–1285

58. Wagner KD, Berard R, Stein MB, et al. A multicenter, randomized, double-blind, placebo-controlled trial of paroxetine in children and adolescents with social anxiety disorder. *Arch Gen Psychiatry.* 2004;61(11):1153–1162

59. Birmaher B, Waterman GS, Ryan N, et al. Fluoxetine for childhood anxiety disorders. *J Am Acad Child Adolesc Psychiatry.* 1994;33(7):993–999

60. Isolan L, Pheula G, Salum GA, Jr., Oswald S, Rohde LA, Manfro GG. An open-label trial of escitalopram in children and adolescents with social anxiety disorder. *J Child Adolesc Psychopharmacol.* 2007;17(6):751–760

61. Chavira DA, Stein MB. Combined psychoeducation and treatment with selective serotonin reuptake inhibitors for youth with generalized social anxiety disorder. *J Child Adolesc Psychopharmacol.* 2002;12(1):47–54

62. Strawn JR, Prakash A, Zhang Q, et al. A randomized, placebo-controlled study of duloxetine for the treatment of children and adolescents with generalized anxiety disorder. *J Am Acad Child Adolesc Psychiatry.* 2015;54(4):283–293

63. Uthman OA, Abdulmalik J. Comparative efficacy and acceptability of pharmacotherapeutic agents for anxiety disorders in children and adolescents: a mixed treatment comparison meta-analysis. *Curr Med Res Opin.* 2010;26(1):53–59

64. Boyer EW, Shannon M. The serotonin syndrome. *N Engl J Med.* 2005;352(11):1112–1120

65. Silverstone P. Qualitative review of SNRIs in anxiety. *J Clin Psychiatry.* 2004;65(suppl 17):19–28

66. Strawn JR, Sakolsky DJ, Rynn MA. Psychopharmacologic treatment of children and adolescents with anxiety disorders. *Child Adolesc Psychiatr Clin N Am.* 2012;21(3):527–539

67. McClellan JM, Werry JS. Evidence-based treatments in child and adolescent psychiatry: an inventory. *J Am Acad Child Adolesc Psychiatry.* 2003;42(12):1388–1400

68. Geller DA, Wagner KD, Emslie G, et al. Paroxetine treatment in children and adolescents with obsessive-compulsive disorder: a randomized, multicenter, double-blind, placebo-controlled trial. *J Am Acad Child Adolesc Psychiatry.* 2004;43(11):1387–1396

69. Geller DA, Biederman J, Stewart SE, et al. Which SSRI? A meta-analysis of pharmacotherapy trials in pediatric obsessive-compulsive disorder. *Am J Psychiatry.* 2003;160(11):1919–1928

70. Robb AS, Cueva JE, Sporn J, Yang R, Vanderburg DG. Sertraline treatment of children and adolescents with posttraumatic stress disorder: a double-blind, placebo-controlled trial. *J Child Adolesc Psychopharmacol.* 2010;20(6):463–471

71. Robert R, Tcheung WJ, Rosenberg L, et al. Treating thermally injured children suffering symptoms of acute stress with imipramine and fluoxetine: a randomized, double-blind study. *Burns.* 2008;34(7):919–928

72. March JS, Silva S, Petrycki S, et al. The Treatment for Adolescents with Depression Study (TADS): long-term effectiveness and safety outcomes. *Arch Gen Psychiatry.* 2007;64(10):1132–1143

73. Strawn JR, Keeshin BR, DelBello MP, Geracioti TD, Jr., Putnam FW. Psychopharmacologic treatment of posttraumatic stress disorder in children and adolescents: a review. *J Clin Psychiatry.* 2010;71(7):932–941

74. Lewandowski RE, Acri MC, Hoagwood KE, et al. Evidence for the management of adolescent depression. *Pediatrics.* 2013;132(132):e996–e1009

75. Liu X, Gentzler AL, Tepper P, et al. Clinical features of depressed children and adolescents with various forms of suicidality. *J Clin Psychiatry.* 2006;67(9):1442–1450

76. Baweja R, Mayes SD, Hameed U, Waxmonsky JG. Disruptive mood dysregulation disorder: current insights. *Neuropsychiatr Dis Treat.* 2016;12:2115–2124

77. Perou R, Bitsko RH, Blumberg SJ, et al. Mental health surveillance among children—United States, 2005–2011. *MMWR Suppl.* 2013;62(2):1–35

78. Copeland W, Shanahan L, Costello J, Angold A. Cumulative prevalence of psychiatric disorders by young adulthood: a prospective cohort analysis from the Great Smoky Mountains Study. *J Am Acad Child Adolesc Psychiatry.* 2011;50(3):252–261

79. Tang MH, Pinsky EG. Mood and Affect Disorders. *Pediatr Rev.* 2015;36(2):52–61

80. Van Meter AR, Moreira ALR, Youngstrom EA. Meta-analysis of epidemiologic studies of pediatric bipolar disorder. *J Clin Psychiatry.* 2011;72(9):1250–1256

81. Duax JM, Youngstrom EA, Calabrese JR, Robert L. Findling MD. Sex differences in pediatric bipolar disorder. *J Clin Psychiatry.* 2007;68:1565–1573

82. Stice E, Ragan J, Randall P. Prospective relations between social support and depression: differential direction of effects for parent and peer support? *J Abnorm Psychol.* 2004;113(1):155–159

83. Heim C, Nemeroff CB. The role of childhood trauma in the neurobiology of mood and anxiety disorders: preclinical and clinical studies. *Biol Psychiatry.* 2001;49(12):1023–1039

84. Saluja G, Iachan R, Scheidt PC, Overpeck MD, Sun W, Giedd JN. Prevalence of and risk factors for depressive symptoms among young adolescents. *Arch Pediatr Adolesc Med.* 2014;158(8):760–765

85. Thompson RJ, Mata J, Jaeggi SM, Buschkuehl M, Jonides J, Gotlib IH. Maladaptive coping, adaptive coping, and depressive symptoms: variations across age and depressive state. *Behav Res Ther.* 2010;48(6):459–466

86. Breton JJ, Labelle R, Berthiaume C, et al. Protective factors against depression and suicidal behaviour in adolescence. *Can J Psychiatry.* 2015;60(2 Suppl 1):S5-S15

87. Chrisman SP, Richardson LP. Prevalence of diagnosed depression in adolescents with history of concussion. *J Adolesc Health.* 2014;54(5):582–586

88. Tsai MC, Tsai KJ, Wang HK, et al. Mood disorders after traumatic brain injury in adolescents and young adults: a nationwide population-based cohort study. *J Pediatr.* 2014;164(1):136–141, e131

89. Stringaris A, Lewis G, Maughan B. Developmental pathways from childhood conduct problems to early adult depression: findings from the ALSPAC cohort. *Br J Psychiatry.* 2014;205(1):17–23

90. Miklowitz DJ, Chang KD. Prevention of bipolar disorder in at-risk children: theoretical assumptions and empirical foundations. *Dev Psychopathol.* 2008;20(3):881–897

91. Avenevoli S, Swendsen J, He J-P, Burstein M, Merikangas KR. Major depression in the national comorbidity survey–adolescent supplement: prevalence, correlates, and treatment. *J Am Acad Child Adolesc Psychiatry.* 2015;54(1):37–44.e2

92. Joshi G, Wilens T. Comorbidity in pediatric bipolar disorder. *Child Adolesc Psychiatr Clin N Am.* 2009;18(2):291–319, vii-viii

93. Goldstein BI, Carnethon MR, Matthews KA, et al. Major depressive disorder and bipolar disorder predispose youth to accelerated atherosclerosis and early cardiovascular disease. *Circulation.* 2015;132:965–986

94. Centers for Disease Control and Prevention. *Fatal Injury Reports 1999-2015.* 2016; https://webappa.cdc.gov/sasweb/ncipc/mortrate.html. Accessed November 27, 2017

95. Curtin SC, Hedegaard H, Minino AM, Warner M. Quickstats: death rates for motor vehicle traffic injury, suicide, and homicide among children and adolescents aged 10–14 years—United States, 1999–2014. *MMWR Morb Mortal Wkly Rep.* 2016;65(43):1203

96. Barbe RP, Williamson DE, Bridge JA, et al. Clinical differences between suicidal and nonsuicidal depressed children and adolescents. *J Clin Psychiatry.* 2005;66(4):492–498

97. Soole R, Kõlves K, De Leo D. Suicide in children: a systematic review. *Arch Suicide Res.* 2015;19(3):285–304

98. Blom EH, Ho TC, Connolly CG, et al. The neuroscience and context of adolescent depression. *Acta Pediatrica.* 2015;105:358–365

99. Ferrari F, Villa RF. The neurobiology of depression: an integrated overview from biological theories to clinical evidence. *Mol Neurobiol.* 2017;54(7):4847–4865

100. Roybal DJ, Singh MK, Cosgrove VE, et al. Biological evidence for a neurodevelopmental model of pediatric bipolar disorder. *Isr J Psychiatry Relat Sci.* 2012;49(1):28–43

101. Frias A, Palma C, Furriols N. Neurocognitive impairments among youth with pediatric bipolar disorder: a systematic review of neuropsychological research. *J Affect Disord.* 2014;166:297–306

102. Bechtel W. Circadian rhythms and mood disorders: are the phenomena and mechanisms causally related? *Front Psychiatry.* 2015;6:118

103. McClellan J, Kowatch R, Findling RL, Work Group on Quality Issues. Practice parameter for the assessment and treatment of children and adolescents with bipolar disorder. *J Am Acad Child Adolesc Psychiatry.* 2007;46(1):107–125

104. Singh MK, Ketter T, Chang KD. Distinguishing bipolar disorder from other psychiatric disorders in children. *Curr Psychiatry Rep.* 2014;16:516

105. Forman-Hoffman V, McClure E, McKeeman J, et al. Screening for major depressive disorder in children and adolescents: a systematic review for the U.S. Preventive Services Task Force. *Ann Intern Med.* 2016;164(5):342–349

106. Dolle K, Schulte-Korne G, O'Leary AM, von Hofacker N, Izat Y, Allgaier AK. The Beck depression inventory—II in adolescent mental health patients: cut-off scores for detecting depression and rating severity. *Psychiatry Res.* 2012;200(2–3):843–848

107. Richardson LP, McCauley E, Grossman DC, et al. Evaluation of the patient health questionnaire (PHQ-9) for detecting major depression among adolescents. *Pediatrics.* 2010;126(6):1117–1123

108. Birmaher B, Brent D, Bernet W, et al. Practice parameter for the assessment and treatment of children and adolescents with depressive disorders. *J Am Acad Child Adolesc Psychiatry.* 2007;46(11):1503–1526

109. Forti-Buratti MA, Saikia R, Wilkinson EL, Ramchandani PG. Psychological treatments for depression in pre-adolescent children (12 years and younger): systematic review and meta-analysis of randomised controlled trials. *Eur Child Adolesc Psychiatry.* 2016;25:1045–1054

110. Compton SN, March JS, Brent D, Albano AMt, Weersing R, Curry J. Cognitive-behavioral psychotherapy for anxiety and depressive disorders in children and adolescents: an evidence-based medicine review. *J Am Acad Child Adolesc Psychiatry.* 2004;43(8):930–959

111. Hetrick SE, Cox GR, Witt KG, Bir JJ, Merry SN. Cognitive behavioural therapy (CBT), third-wave CBT and interpersonal therapy (IPT) based interventions for preventing depression in children and adolescents. *Cochrane Database Syst Rev.* 2016;(8):CD003380

112. Ames CS, Richardson J, Payne S, Smith P, Leigh E. Mindfulness-based cognitive therapy for depression in adolescents. *Child Adolesc Ment Health.* 2014;19(1):74–78

113. Kvam S, Kleppe CL, Nordhus IH, Hovland A. Exercise as a treatment for depression: a meta-analysis. *J Affect Disord.* 2016;202:67–86

114. Varigonda AL, Jakubovski E, Taylor MJ, Freemantle N, Coughlin C, Bloch MH. Systematic review and meta-analysis: early treatment responses of selective serotonin reuptake inhibitors in pediatric major depressive disorder. *J Am Acad Child Adolesc Psychiatry.* 2015;54(7):557–564

115. Peters AT, Jacobs RH, Feldhaus C, et al. Trajectories of functioning into emerging adulthood following treatment for adolescent depression. *J Adolesc Health.* 2016;58(3):253–259

116. Graham J. Emslie MD, Beth D. Kennard PD, Taryn L. Mayes MS, et al. Fluoxetine versus placebo in preventing relapse of major depression in children and adolescents. *Am J Psychiatry.* 2008;165(4):459–467

117. Cipriani A, Zhou X, Del Giovane C, et al. Comparative efficacy and tolerability of antidepressants for major depressive disorder in children and adolescents: a network meta-analysis. *Lancet.* 2016;388(10047):881–890

118. Gibbons RD, Brown CH, Hur K, et al. Early evidence on the effects of regulators' suicidality warnings on SSRI prescriptions and suicide in children and adolescents. *Am J Psychiatry.* 2007;164(9):1356–1363

119. Emslie GJ, Findling RL, Yeung PP, Kunz NR, Li Y. Venlafaxine ER for the treatment of pediatric subjects with depression: results of two placebo-controlled trials. *J Am Acad Child Adolesc Psychiatry.* 2007;46(4):479–488

120. Geller B, Reising D, Leonard HL, Riddle MA, Walsh BT. Critical review of tricyclic antidepressant use in children and adolescents. *J Am Acad Child Adolesc Psychiatry.* 1999;38(5):513–516

121. Cheung AH, Kozloff N, Sacks D. Pediatric depression: an evidence-based update on treatment interventions. *Curr Psychiatry Rep.* 2013;15(8):381

122. Washburn JJ, West AE, Heil JA. Treatment of pediatric bipolar disorder: a review. *Minerva Psichiatr.* 2011;52(1):21–35

123. Fristad MA, MacPherson HA. Evidence-based psychosocial treatments for child and adolescent bipolar spectrum disorders. *J Clin Child Adolesc Psychol.* 2014;43(3):339–355

124. Goldstein TR, Axelson DA, Birmaher B, Brent DA. Dialectical behavior therapy for adolescents with bipolar disorder: a 1-year open trial. *J Am Acad Child Adolesc Psychiatry.* 2007;46(7):820–830

125. Pavuluri MN, Graczyk PA, Henry DB, Carbray JA, Heidenreich J, Miklowitz DJ. Child- and family-focused cognitive-behavioral therapy for pediatric bipolar disorder: development and preliminary results. *J Am Acad Child Adolesc Psychiatry.* 2004;43(5):528–537

126. Geller B, Luby JL, Joshi P, et al. A randomized controlled trial of risperidone, lithium, or divalproex sodium for initial treatment of bipolar I disorder, manic or mixed phase, in children and adolescents. *Arch Gen Psychiatry.* 2012;69(5):515–528

127. Findling RL, Nyilas M, Forbes RA, et al. Acute treatment of pediatric bipolar I disorder, manic or mixed episode, with aripiprazole: a randomized, double-blind, placebo-controlled study. *J Clin Psychiatry.* 2009;70(10):1441–1451

128. Findling RL, Robb A, McNamara NK, et al. Lithium in the acute treatment of bipolar I disorder: a double-blind, placebo-controlled study. *Pediatrics.* 2015;136(5):885–894

129. Joshi G, Wozniak J, Mick E, et al. A prospective open-label trial of extended-release carbamazepine monotherapy in children with bipolar disorder. *J Child Adolesc Psychopharmacol.* 2010;20(1):7–14

130. Findling RL, Frazier TW, Youngstrom EA, et al. Double-blind, placebo-controlled trial of divalproex monotherapy in the treatment of symptomatic youth at high risk for developing bipolar disorder. *J Clin Psychiatry.* 2007;68:781–788

131. Pringsheim T, Panagiotopoulos C, Davidson J, Ho J, Canadian Alliance for Monitoring Effectiveness and Safety of Antipsychotics in Children (CAMESA) guideline group. Evidence-based recommendations for monitoring safety of second-generation antipsychotics in children and youth. *Paediatr Child Health.* 2011;16(9):581–589

132. Zuckerbrot RA, Cheung AH, Jensen PS, Stein RE, Laraque D, GLAD-PC Steering Group. Guidelines for adolescent depression in primary care (GLAD-PC): I. Identification, assessment, and initial management. *Pediatrics.* 2007;120(5):e1299–e1312

133. Edwards SJ, Sachmann MD. No-suicide contracts, no-suicide agreements, and no-suicide assurances: a study of their nature, utilization, perceived effectiveness, and potential to cause harm. *Crisis.* 2010;31(6):290–302

134. Dowd MD, Sege RD, Gardner HG, et al. Firearm-related injuries affecting the pediatric population. *Pediatrics.* 2012;130(5):e1416–e1423

CHAPTER 23

Basics of Psychopharmacological Management

Eugenia Chan, MD, MPH, FAAP

Katherine A. Trier, MD, FAAP

Peter J. Chung, MD, FAAP

According to recent estimates from the National Health Interview Survey, up to 7.5% of children from 6 to 17 years of age are prescribed medication to treat a behavioral or emotional difficulty.[1] Due to the limited availability of specialty providers, such as developmental-behavioral pediatricians and child and adolescent psychiatrists, the burden of first-line diagnosis and treatment often falls upon the patient's primary pediatric health care professional, within the context of a medical home. Further, the American Academy of Pediatrics (AAP) states, "Pediatric primary care providers have unique opportunities and a growing sense of responsibility to prevent and address mental health and substance abuse problems in the medical home."[2]

Despite this AAP statement, nearly 50% of children with mental/behavioral health needs are unable to access appropriate treatment.[3] Many primary pediatric health care professionals feel responsible for the identification, but not necessarily the ongoing medical management, of many mental/behavioral health disorders.[4] Although mandatory rotations in developmental-behavioral pediatrics during pediatric residency training have increased pediatricians' familiarity with the treatment of common childhood mental/behavioral health conditions, relatively few pediatric residency graduates rate their mental/behavioral health treatment skills as "very good" or "excellent."[5] Further, many family physicians, pediatric nurse practitioners, and physician assistants who provide primary care to children and adolescents receive no formal training in developmental-behavioral pediatrics.

This chapter will review general principles for using psychotropic medications in children and adolescents with developmental-behavioral disorders, and it will provide additional information regarding the evidence base and clinical use of these agents to treat hyperactive and disruptive behaviors, aggression and self-injury, anxiety and mood disorders, rigid and compulsive behaviors, and sleep problems. Where available, the authors will reference clinical practice guidelines and evidence-based practices, although off-label uses will also be discussed. Information regarding epidemiology, diagnosis, and non-pharmaceutical treatment options for the disorders discussed is provided elsewhere in this volume (see Chapter 8, Development and Disorders of Feeding, Sleep, and Elimination; Chapter 18, Attention-Deficit/Hyperactivity Disorder; Chapter 19, Autism Spectrum Disorder; Chapter 21, Disruptive Behavior Disorders; and Chapter 22, Anxiety and Mood Disorders).

General Principles for Using Psychotropic Medications in Children and Adolescents

Identify the primary underlying developmental-behavioral disorder rather than treat the symptoms. A thorough diagnostic evaluation to accurately identify the underlying developmental-behavioral disorder is necessary before developing a treatment plan. Behavioral and mood problems can be complex in their presentation and etiology. Is the child appearing inattentive primarily because of a short attention span or pervasive anxiety, or secondary to demands and expectations at school that exceed his or her underlying developmental abilities? Does the child act aggressively because of mood dysregulation, impulsivity, or a lack of appropriate social regard? Inappropriate medication use can mask, exacerbate, and delay identification of the underlying problem(s). A variety of screening instruments and assessment tools, as discussed elsewhere in this manual, along with careful interview of the child and his or her caregivers, can help the primary pediatric health care professional arrive at a likely diagnosis (see Chapter 9, Developmental and Behavioral Surveillance and Screening Within the Medical Home; Chapter 10, Developmental Evaluation; Chapter 11, Making Developmental-Behavioral Diagnoses; Chapter 15, Cognitive Development and Disorders; Chapter 17, Learning Disabilities; Chapter 18, Attention-Deficit/Hyperactivity Disorder; Chapter 19, Autism Spectrum Disorder; Chapter 21, Disruptive Behavior Disorders; and Chapter 22, Anxiety and Mood Disorders).

Consider medication as a component of a multimodal approach to treatment. For most developmental-behavioral disorders, a multimodal approach of medication and evidence-based psychosocial treatments yields the best outcomes. These may be employed sequentially (eg, parent behavioral training, then stimulant medication, if needed, to treat attention-deficit/hyperactivity disorder [ADHD] in preschool-aged children) or concurrently (eg, cognitive behavioral therapy [CBT] and antidepressant medication for depression in adolescents). Psychotropic medications generally do not "fix" the problem, but they can enable the child to participate in and benefit from the psychosocial treatments.

Carefully review any previous trials of medication treatment. Clinicians should review previous medication trials. Important details, such as the child's age at the time the medication was tried, the target behaviors or symptoms, dosing and titration schedule, experience of side effects, and the reasons for treatment failure or discontinuation, provide guidance as to the next steps of treatment. Medications that have failed in the past may be relatively contraindicated; however, if the clinician determines that the medication had been used inappropriately or inadequately (eg, wrong dose, wrong target, or not titrated sufficiently), another trial may be warranted.

Ensure that the patient's caregivers understand the targets of treatment, the timing of effects, and the potential for side effects. Educating patients and caregivers regarding the medication's expected effects on symptoms and potential adverse effects is a critical component of medication management. Caregivers should have a clear understanding of the reasons for prescribing medication, the potential risks and benefits of the medication, and realistic expectations for how well and how quickly a medication will address the target symptoms. Discussing potential adverse effects and how they might be addressed (eg, change dose, change timing, or change medication) can increase the likelihood of adherence to medication treatment. The importance of routine monitoring should also be emphasized.

Make thoughtful medication choices based on available evidence and personal experience. Available clinical practice guidelines can provide recommendations for appropriate first- and second-line medication classes to treat a given developmental-behavioral disorder (eg, methylphenidate- and amphetamine-based preparations for ADHD), but primary pediatric health care professionals may often feel overwhelmed by the rapidly increasing array of medication choices within a medication class. While promising, pharmacogenetic testing to guide medication selection has not yet become part of routine clinical practice. In the absence of head-to-head trials comparing the relative efficacy of one specific medication to another, clinicians should use a common-sense approach for developing their own expertise with psychotropic medications:

* Understand which medications are FDA approved for treatment in children and adolescents.
* Become familiar with at least 1 to 2 medications within a given medication class or subclass, taking into account options for children who may not be able to swallow pills.
* Develop a standard practice for choosing and starting a first-line medication and switching to a second-line medication, if needed.

Start low, go slow, and titrate for best effect. In general, most psychoactive medications should be started at the lowest doses and gradually increased to reach optimal effect. Patients should be monitored for effectiveness as well as side effects with each dose change. The "best" dose is the one that offers the most acceptable balance between the optimal effect on target symptoms while minimizing side effects.

Keep it simple. Adherence to medication is more likely when the medication regimen is as simple as possible. For example, an extended-release stimulant administered once daily is usually easier for families than an immediate-release stimulant administered 2 or 3 times a day. When possible, using a single medication rather than a combination of medications is recommended. Avoid adding a new medication to treat the side effects of an existing medication.

Monitor regularly for effectiveness and side effects. Once the patient is on an effective medication dose and regimen, the patient should be routinely monitored for side effects and continuing effectiveness by way of parent, teacher, or self-report. Monitoring can be conducted informally or via the use of standardized checklists and questionnaires. As an individual's brain develops, body habitus increases and academic and social-emotional demands evolve, so the medication dose and/or type may need to be adjusted.

Consider discontinuing treatment at least on an annual basis. Although many children prescribed psychotropic medication will likely require long-term treatment, the prescribing clinician should periodically evaluate whether medication continues to be necessary. For patients who have achieved target goals, or whose symptoms and behaviors appear to have resolved, a trial off the medication can identify those who no longer require it.

Treatment of Hyperactivity, Impulsivity, and Inattention

The AAP has published clinical recommendations for the treatment of ADHD (see Chapter 18, Attention-Deficit/Hyperactivity Disorder), as summarized below.[6,7]

- Preschool-aged children (4 to 5 years): Parent- or teacher-based behavior therapy is recommended as first-line treatment; methylphenidate is recommended only if behavioral therapy does "not demonstrate significant improvement and there is moderate-to-severe continuing disturbance in the child's function."
- Elementary school–aged (6 to 11 years of age): Stimulant therapy is recommended as the first line of therapy along with behavioral therapy, parent training, and/or school intervention; nonstimulant therapy is the second line.
- Adolescents (12 to 18 years of age): Medication treatment is recommended with consideration for the addition of behavior therapy.

Stimulants

Psychostimulant medications have been used in practice since the 1960s for the treatment of hyperactivity and inattention, and these medications have a substantial evidence base demonstrating their efficacy in children (including preschoolers), adolescents, and adults. All stimulant medications have FDA approval for the treatment of ADHD in children ≥6 years of age. Only immediate-release dextroamphetamine and its derivatives are approved for use in children from 3 to 5 years of age. (See Table 23.1.)

Stimulants appear to exert their effect by increasing the available amount of dopamine and norepinephrine for neurotransmission in the synapses of the prefrontal cortex and especially in the striatum. Methylphenidate inhibits reuptake of dopamine, while amphetamine both stimulates release of dopamine and norepinephrine, as well as inhibits their uptake. Stimulants are easily absorbed and readily cross the blood-brain barrier; they bind poorly to plasma proteins and are rapidly excreted in the urine (on average, in 4 hours). The maximum drug effects occur while the medication is increasing in serum levels, not when a steady state has been achieved.[8] Due to this pharmacokinetic profile, when stimulants were first used for ADHD, immediate-release stimulants would have to be administered multiple times per day, usually with at least one dose administered at school. This treatment regimen was associated with difficulties coordinating with school personnel, interruptions in the child's academic schedule, risk of stigma for the student, variability in the time of medication administration (resulting in gaps of medication coverage), and a higher potential for abuse or diversion.

Table 23.1. Stimulant Medications Used for Treatment of ADHD

	Drug (generic)	Brand Name	Duration	Formulation and Administration	Pediatric Dosing
Long-acting medications	Methylphenidate	Concerta	10 to 12 hours	• 18, 27, 36, 54 mg extended-release capsules • Swallow whole	**Initial** (≥6 years old): 18 mg/day **Max:** 54 mg/day (72 mg/day adolescents)
		Daytrana	10 to 12 hours	• 10, 15, 20, 30 mg extended-release patch • Apply 2 hours before desired effect • Remove 2 hours before desired end point	**Initial** (≥6 years old): 10 mg/day **Max:** 30 mg/day
		Quillivant XR	12 hours	• 5 mg/mL suspension	**Initial** (≥6 years old): 10–20 mg/day **Max:** 60 mg/day
		QuilliChew ER	10 to 12 hours	• 20 (scored), 30 (scored), 40 (not scored) mg extended-release chewable tablets	**Initial** (≥6 years old): 20 mg/day **Max:** 60 mg/day
		Aptensio XR	12 hours	• 10, 15, 20, 30, 40, 50, 60 mg	**Initial** (≥6 years old): 10 mg/day **Max:** 60 mg/day
	Dexmethylphenidate	Focalin XR	10 to 12 hours	• 5, 10, 15, 20, 25, 30, 35, 40 mg extended-release capsules • Swallow whole; sprinkle on applesauce	**Initial** (≥6 years old): 5 mg/day **Max:** 30 mg/day
	Amphetamine	Adderall XR (mixed amphetamine salts)	10 to 12 hours	• 5, 10, 15, 20, 25, 30 mg extended-release capsules • Swallow whole; sprinkle on applesauce	**Initial** (≥6 years old): 10 mg/day **Max:** 30 mg/day
		Dyanavel XR (amphetamine)	10 to 12 hours	• 2.5 mg/mL suspension • Bubblegum flavor	**Initial** (≥6 years old): 2.5–5 mg/day **Max:** 20 mg/day
		Adzenys XR-ODT (amphetamine)	10 to 12 hours	• 3.1, 6.3, 9.4, 12.5, 15.7, 18.8 mg oral disintegrating tablet • Orange flavor	**Initial** (≥6 years old): 6.3 mg/day **Max:** 12.5 mg/day (6 to 12 years); 18.8 mg/day (13 to 17 years)
	Lisdexamfetamine	Vyvanse	10 to 12 hours	• 20, 30, 40, 50, 60, 70 mg extended-release capsules • Swallow whole; dissolve in water	**Initial** (≥6 years old): 30 mg/day **Max:** 70 mg/day

Table 23.1. Stimulant Medications Used for Treatment of ADHD (*continued*)

	Drug (generic)	Brand Name	Duration	Formulation and Administration	Pediatric Dosing
Intermediate-acting medications	Dextroamphetamine sulfate	Dexedrine Spansule	6 to 8 hours	• 5, 10, 15 mg time-release capsules • Swallow whole; sprinkle on applesauce	**Initial** (≥6 years old): 5 mg, once or twice daily **Max:** 40 mg/day
	Methylphenidate	Metadate ER	6 to 8 hours	• 20 mg extended-release tablets • Swallow whole	**Initial** (≥6 years old): 20 mg/day (after use of short-acting meds) **Max:** 60 mg/day
		Ritalin SR	6 to 8 hours	• 20 mg extended-release tablets • Swallow whole	**Initial** (≥6 years old): 20 mg/day (after use of short-acting meds) **Max:** 60 mg/day
		Metadate CD	8 hours	• 10, 20, 30, 40, 50, 60 mg extended-release capsules • Swallow whole; sprinkle on applesauce	**Initial** (≥6 years old): 20 mg/day **Max:** 60 mg/day
		Methylin ER	6 to 8 hours	• 10, 20 mg extended-release tablets • Swallow whole	**Initial** (≥6 years old): 10 mg/day **Max:** 60 mg/day
		Ritalin LA	8 hours	• 10, 20, 30, 40 mg extended-release capsules • Swallow whole; sprinkle on applesauce	**Initial** (≥6 years old): 20 mg/day **Max:** 60 mg/day

Table 23.1. Stimulant Medications Used for Treatment of ADHD (*continued*)

	Drug (generic)	Brand Name	Duration	Formulation and Administration	Pediatric Dosing
Short-acting medications	Amphetamine mixed salts	Adderall	4 to 6 hours	• 5, 7.5, 10, 12.5, 15, 20, 30 mg tablets • Swallow whole	**Initial** 3 to 5 years old: 2.5 mg/day; ≥6 years old: 5 mg, once or twice daily **Max:** 40 mg/day
	Dexmethylpheni-date	Focalin	3 to 5 hours	• 2.5, 5, 10 mg scored tablets • Swallow whole	**Initial** (≥6 years old): 2.5 mg twice daily **Max:** 20 mg/day
	Dextroamphet-amine sulfate	Dexedrine	4 to 6 hours	• 5, 10 mg scored tablets, 5 mg/5 mL solution • Swallow tablets whole	**Initial** 3 to 5 years old: 2.5 mg daily; ≥6 years old: 5 mg, once or twice daily **Max:** 40 mg/day
	Methylphenidate	Methylin	3 to 5 hours	• 5 mg/5 mL, 10 mg/5 mL solution; 2.5, 5, 10 mg chewable tablets	**Initial** (≥6 years old): 5 mg, twice daily **Max:** 60 mg/day
		Ritalin	3 to 5 hours	• 5, 10, 20 mg tablets • Swallow whole	**Initial** (≥6 years old): 5 mg, twice daily **Max:** 60 mg/day
	Methamphetamine	Desoxyn	3 to 5 hours	• 5 mg tablets • Swallow whole	**Initial** (≥6 years old): 5 mg, once or twice daily **Max:** 25 mg/day

Abbreviations: ADHD, attention-deficit/hyperactivity disorder; CD, controlled delivery; ER, extended release; LA, long acting; ODT, orally disintegrating tablet; SR, sustained release; XR, extended release.

Advances in drug development have resulted in a greater variety of extended-release stimulant formulations that allow for less frequent dosing as well as new extended-release formulations for children who are unable to swallow pills. Examples include the following:

- Wax matrix medications (eg, Ritalin SR [methylphenidate hydrochloride]) were designed to disperse the drug slowly over time; however, this formulation has been shown to result in decreased efficacy with delay to effect, limiting its clinical use.
- Beaded capsules (eg, Ritalin LA [methylphenidate hydrochloride], Metadate CD [methylphenidate hydrochloride], Focalin XR [dexmethylphenidate], Adderall XR [mixed amphetamine salts]) utilize a combination of enteric coated beads with different rates of dissolution (ie, immediate and delayed) to mimic BID (twice per day) dosing. These capsules can be opened and the contents mixed into a spoonful of foods with a pureed consistency (eg applesauce, pudding, whipped cream, and ice cream), so long as the individual ingests the spoonful without chewing the beads. Because the beads may adhere to the side of a cup, parents should be discouraged from administering the medication in liquid.
- The osmotic-controlled release oral delivery system (OROS) of Concerta (methylphenidate hydrochloride) uses osmotic pressure in the gut to propel drug contents out of the capsule via a small port. The capsule must be swallowed whole and is passed in the stool.
- The prodrug Vyvanse (lisdexamfetamine) consists of dextroamphetamine bound to lysine, and it is inert until the lysine is cleaved by red blood cells. The sustained effect of the medication is related to the rate of first-pass hepatic or intestinal metabolism. The capsule can be dissolved in water.
- Transdermal applications such as Daytrana (methylphenidate hydrochloride) allow for sustained release of methylphenidate across the skin for an extended period of time. Patches can be easily administered on the hip and then removed 3 hours prior to the desired stop time. Skin irritation may occur with regular administration, so patients should be counseled to alternate sides of administration from day to day. Patches that fall off due to sweat or moisture must be replaced. Permanent skin lightening may also occur.
- New extended-release suspensions include Quillivant XR (methylphenidate hydro-chloride) and Dyanavel XR (mixed amphetamine-dextroamphetamine); these allow for more precise dose titration, which can be useful for children who have difficulty tolerating standard doses of other extended-release stimulants.
- New chewable (eg, QuilliChew ER [methylphenidate hydrochloride]) and oral disinte-grating tablets (eg, Adzenys XR-ODT [amphetamine]) extended-release formulations offer additional options for children who are unable to swallow pills.

– Initiation and Titration

In general, randomized controlled trials (RCTs) have not consistently demonstrated the superiority of one stimulant formulation over another; clinicians are encouraged to initiate a trial with stimulant medications that have a well-established evidence base. The ADHD Medication Guide (**http://www.adhdmedicationguide.com/**), made available online by Cohen Children's Center, is updated frequently with new developments and includes pictures of pills for easy identification.

Common clinical practice is to initiate a methylphenidate or amphetamine preparation at the lowest dose and then titrate on a per-visit rate (eg, monthly to every few months) based on parent, teacher, and/or self report of the patient's response and experience of side effects. Parents who are somewhat ambivalent about medication, however, may be too quickly satisfied with suboptimal improvements on a low dose, even if there is on-going impairment due to ADHD symptoms. In contrast to community-based "care as usual," stimulant titration protocols using parent and teacher rating scales at regular, scheduled (weekly to monthly) intervals often result in more rapid attainment of optimal dosing and efficacy in the research setting.[9]

Clinicians may choose to utilize a more aggressive (eg, "forced-dose") titration schedule when starting a stimulant. One approach is to dispense 30 capsules of a medication and have the patient try 3 different doses, each for 5 days at a time, with follow-up in 2 weeks. For example, 30 capsules of dexmethylphenidate extended release 5 mg can be distributed with instructions to take 1 capsule (5 mg) for 5 days, 2 capsules (10 mg) for 5 days, and 3 capsules (15 mg) for 5 days. Titration can be halted if there are significant side effects lasting more than a few days. At the 2-week follow-up visit, the clinician and caregiver can decide which dose is the most appropriate. If the initial stimulant choice does not demonstrate a favorable risk-benefit balance, a trial of another stimulant is recommended. Studies have demonstrated that approximately 75% to 80% of individuals with ADHD will respond to either methylphenidate or amphetamine.

– Side Effects

All stimulant medications share a similar adverse effect profile, although the experience of individual patients can vary depending on the medication, formulation, and dose. The presence of significant adverse effects with a particular preparation in one stimulant class (eg, methylphenidate) does not necessarily preclude a trial with a different preparation in the same class.

Common side effects include headaches, stomachaches, mild increases in heart rate or blood pressure, appetite suppression, and difficulty with sleep onset. Headaches and stomachaches may spontaneously resolve as the individual adjusts to the medication and may also improve when the stimulant is administered with food. Sleep onset difficulty generally does not resolve over time and is typically related to the length of drug duration or to "rebound" effects after the medication has worn off. Both irritability and mood dysregulation can occur, most often in the mid to late afternoon or early evening as the medication effect wears off. These adverse drug events may limit tolerance of the medication, if they outweigh the benefit to the child. Alternatively, clinicians may adjust the medication regimen to minimize side effects.

Uncommon side effects of stimulant medication treatment include stimulant-induced psychosis (visual, auditory, or tactile hallucinations or psychotic thoughts), aggression, or behavioral disinhibition and/or mania. These may occur with high doses or in individuals predisposed toward schizophrenia or bipolar disorder.[10] The oft-cited "zombie" effect is also usually associated with too high a dose.

The relationship between chronic administration of stimulants and growth is complex. While the primary concern has been poor weight gain and likelihood of attaining adult height due to decreased caloric intake from appetite suppression, other mechanisms, such as stimulant effects on central nervous system growth regulation, changes induced in hepatic metabolism, and alterations in cartilage, have also been proposed. Emerging evidence suggests that any deleterious effects on growth may be primarily on growth rate (ie, children will eventually reach their true adult height) or may be quite modest, dose-dependent, and reversible with discontinuation of the drug.[11,12] Common clinical practices to diminish negative effects on weight and height include increasing caloric intake, administering appetite stimulants (eg, cyproheptadine), and taking "drug holidays" on weekends or vacations; however, these have not been supported by research. When deciding to decrease, interrupt, or discontinue medication treatment due to effects on weight, the clinician should take into account the potential benefits to the individual in academic, social, and behavioral functioning. There is no indication to cease stimulant therapy over the summer, for example, simply to "give the brain a break."

The relationship between tics and stimulant use is controversial. Although there has historically been concern that stimulants may worsen tic behaviors, tics wax and wane over time; increased frequency of tics may be due to the natural history of the disorder rather than to stimulant use. The presence of a tic disorder concurrent with ADHD is no longer considered a contraindication for stimulant use;[13] however, if transient tics develop or tics clearly worsen while on medication, an alternative therapy may be indicated. Clinicians may opt to try an "ABAB" withdrawal trial in which the medication is withdrawn and reintroduced in a scheduled fashion to monitor for effects on tic frequency.

Finally, much concern has been raised regarding the possible cardiac side effects of stimulant use. Stimulants have been associated with minor increases in systolic blood pressure (SBP, ≤7 mmHg) and heart rate (≤10 bpm); 5% to 15% of treated individuals may have more significant changes in these parameters (defined as SBP ≥ 120 mmHg, increases in SBP ≥20 mmHg, or increase in heart rate ≥20 bpm), but these are typically transient.[14] However, in the early 2000s, cases of sudden death among individuals taking stimulant medication were reported, raising concern about the possible arrhythmogenic effects of stimulants. In 2005, the FDA added a warning to mixed amphetamine salts that "sudden death has been reported in association with amphetamine treatment at usual doses in children with structural cardiac abnormalities." In May 2008, the American Heart Association (AHA) released recommendations that all individuals with ADHD who are being considered for stimulant therapy should be carefully evaluated for potential cardiac abnormalities. Evaluations should include a thorough family history, investigation of potential subtle cardiac signs and symptoms in the individual (eg, palpitations, syncope, or chest pain with exercise), a detailed cardiac exam, and a consideration for a screening electrocardiogram (ECG), preferably read by a pediatric cardiologist. In August 2008, the AAP and AHA released a joint statement clarifying that screening ECGs were reasonable to consider, but not mandatory to obtain, and that "treatment of a patient with ADHD should not be withheld because an ECG is not done."[15] In current clinical practice, it is generally held that cardiology clearance for stimulant treatment is indicated only if concerning elements arise in the individual's history, family history, or physical exam. Clinicians are urged to document pertinent negative findings in the medical record prior to beginning treatment with a stimulant.

Alpha-2 Agonists

Alpha-2 agonists, available as clonidine and guanfacine, have also demonstrated efficacy in the treatment of hyperactivity and inattention. Clonidine was initially developed in the 1960s as a treatment for hypertension and acts on the alpha-2 receptors 2A, 2B, and 2C in the prefrontal cortex. Guanfacine was developed in the late 20th century and more specifically binds to alpha-2A receptors (therefore exerting less effect on blood pressure). Alpha-2 receptors in the prefrontal cortex have been implicated in the maintenance of attention and focus. The exact mechanism of action for these medications is not well understood. It is theorized that these medications enhance the transmission of dopamine and norepinephrine in this region, albeit through different mechanisms than with stimulants. Alpha-2 agonists were used off-label in the treatment of ADHD until the FDA approved their use in the early 21st century (2009 and 2010) for children 6 years and older. Only the extended-release forms of clonidine and guanfacine have FDA approval as monotherapy for ADHD as well as adjuncts to stimulants. In clinical practice, however, off-label use of immediate-release clonidine and guanfacine is common. Although alpha-2 agonists are not approved for other psychiatric disorders, they are sometimes used for the treatment of oppositional behavior, aggression, and delayed sleep onset.

Extended-release alpha-2 agonists have demonstrated efficacy in decreasing ADHD symptoms.[16] The effect size of these medications (0.7) is moderate but smaller than the large stimulant effect size of 1.0. Effects are not immediate and may take 2 to 4 weeks to become apparent. Therefore, practice parameters by the AAP and the American Academy of Child and Adolescent Psychiatry (AACAP) classify alpha-2 agonists as second-line therapies. They may be used as monotherapy in individuals who have not been able to tolerate any stimulant. Clinicians may also choose to utilize an alpha-2 agonist as first-line therapy in children with comorbid diagnoses of ADHD and autism spectrum disorder (ASD), given the possibility of higher rates of stimulant side effects experienced in this population. Finally, alpha-2 agonists may function well to target defiant behavior in children with ADHD (although a stimulant remains the first-line treatment).[17]

Alpha-2 agonists also have a role in combination therapy. They can be particularly useful as adjunctive therapies if a patient is not able to tolerate a higher dose of stimulant but continues to show impairment due to ADHD symptoms. Unlike stimulants, alpha-2 agonists demonstrate coverage throughout the day and can be helpful particularly for individuals who struggle with attention problems in the afternoon or evening (after a stimulant has worn off). Individuals with ADHD and co-occurring tics may benefit from the use of an alpha-2 agonist, although, as stated previously, stimulants are still recommended as a first-line therapy even if tics are present. Those individuals with ADHD and sleep difficulties may also benefit from the addition of an alpha-2 agonist.

For short-acting alpha-2 agonists (typically given twice daily), clinicians should start with an evening dose (0.05–0.1 mg of clonidine or 0.5–1 mg of guanfacine) for 3 to 7 days to allow the body to acclimate to the medication and then increase the frequency to twice daily. The medication dose can be increased in a stepwise fashion every 3 to 7 days to the maximum tolerated dose. Short-acting formulations typically come in tablets and can be divided in half for finer dose manipulation. Long-acting medications should be similarly titrated in a stepwise fashion. Clinicians should start an initial evening dose (guanfacine extended-release 1 mg or clonidine extended-release 0.1 mg) and increase as tolerated every 1 to 4 weeks. Long-acting formulations must be swallowed whole. Alpha-2 agonists are typically excreted in the urine.

As with stimulants, dosing of alpha-2 agonists is generally limited by the side effects rather than directed by weight-based targets (although average and maximum doses can be seen in Table 23.2). The most common adverse effects of alpha-2 agonists include fatigue, sedation, and somnolence, with higher rates being reported with clonidine than with guanfacine. These effects are dose dependent and may decrease over time as an individual becomes accustomed to the medication; however, if these side effects do not improve within the first week, they are unlikely to resolve. For those taking a short-acting formulation, sedation may decrease if patients are changed to a long-acting medication (especially if it can be given in the evening). Anticholinergic effects, such as dry eyes, dry mouth, and constipation, can also be seen. Some concerns have been raised about possible QT prolongation, particularly for guanfacine, but a meta-analysis of available data did not demonstrate clinically significant events; screening ECGs are not indicated.[18] Alpha-2 agonists may result in mild decreases of systolic and diastolic blood pressure, but the changes are usually trivial in the pediatric population. However, sudden cessation of alpha-2 agonists, especially when individuals are taking higher doses, can precipitate a withdrawal syndrome, which includes increased blood pressure, headache, tremor, restlessness, and nausea. It is recommended that when stopping the medication, clinicians gradually taper the dose, with adjustments made every 3 to 7 days.

Table 23.2. Nonstimulant Medications Used for Treatment of ADHD					
	Drug (generic)	**Brand**	**Duration**	**Forms and Administration**	**Pediatric Dose**
Nonstimulant (approved for treatment of ADHD by the FDA)	Atomoxetine	Strattera	10 to 12 hours	• 10, 18, 25, 40, 60, 80, 100 mg capsules • Swallow whole.	**Initial <70 kg:** 0.5 mg/kg/day **≥70 kg:** 40 mg/day **Max:** 1.4 mg/kg/day or 100 mg/day
	Guanfacine ER	Intuniv	12 hours	• 1, 2, 3, 4 mg extended-release tablets • Swallow whole.	**Initial (≥6 years old):** 1 mg/day **Max:** 4 mg/day
	Clonidine ER	Kapvay	12 hours	• 0.1 mg extended-release tablets • Swallow whole.	**Initial (≥6 years old):** 0.1 mg/day **Max:** 0.4 mg/day
Nonstimulant (not approved by the FDA for treatment of ADHD)	Clonidine	Catapres	See package insert.	• 0.1, 0.2, 0.3 mg tablets or transdermal system • Swallow tablets whole; when titrated to optimal, stable oral dose, may switch to equivalent transdermal dose.	**Initial <45 kg:** 0.05 mg/day **≥45 kg:** 0.1 mg/day **Max:** 0.4 mg/day, in divided doses
	Guanfacine	Tenex	See package insert.	• 1, 2 mg tablets • Swallow tablets whole; if switching from immediate release (IR), discontinue IR and titrate dose of extended release (ER) starting with 1 mg daily.	**Initial <45 kg:** 0.5 mg/day **≥45 kg:** 1 mg/day **Max:** 4 mg/day

Abbreviations: ADHD, attention-deficit/hyperactivity disorder; FDA, US Food and Drug Administration.

Atomoxetine

Atomoxetine (Strattera) is a selective norepinephrine reuptake inhibitor that is generally used as second-line therapy for the treatment of ADHD. It is FDA approved as monotherapy for children ≥6 years of age. As with many psychiatric medications, the exact mechanism of action is unclear. It is theorized that atomoxetine may selectively inhibit mechanisms of norepinephrine reuptake in the synaptic clefts of the prefrontal cortex, resulting in similar neurochemical changes seen in stimulant use. Atomoxetine is metabolized by the liver (CYP2D6) and should be used with caution in individuals who have hepatic problems or those who are taking CYP2D6 inhibitors, such as fluoxetine.

Atomoxetine appears to have efficacy for individuals with ADHD and other comorbid disorders, especially anxiety.[19] It does not appear to exacerbate tics and may actually decrease tic severity. As with to alpha-2 agonists, medication efficacy is consistent over the course of the day without the waxing and waning effects seen in stimulant therapy. Finally, unlike stimulants, atomoxetine has a low potential for abuse or misuse, making it an attractive option for clinicians or individuals who are uncomfortable with using controlled substances. However, the effect size of atomoxetine is estimated to be around 0.7, which is less than the effect size of stimulants. In addition, it may take 2 to 4 weeks for atomoxetine to develop its therapeutic effect.

Atomoxetine can be given in a single dose or divided into twice-daily doses. Clinicians should start atomoxetine at the initial dose of 0.5 mg/kg/day and gradually increase every 3 to 7 days to the target dose, generally 1.2 mg/kg. The medication can be discontinued without weaning the dose. However, restarting the medication requires a retitration to the target dose, and the effects may take 2 to 4 weeks to be seen; medication "holidays" are discouraged.

Common side effects of atomoxetine include difficulty with sleep, decreased appetite, somnolence, irritability, gastrointestinal symptoms, and sexual dysfunction. Dividing the dose twice daily often helps ameliorate side effects.[20] Pediatric patients may also demonstrate mild increases in hemodynamic markers, such as heart rate and blood pressure, but these changes typically resolve on follow-up evaluation. There may be mild deleterious effects on adult height, although these changes appear to be reversible.

In 2005, based on 12 different RCTs, the FDA issued a black box warning for atomoxetine regarding the increased risk of suicidal thinking. Meta-analyses regarding atomoxetine's adverse drug events have largely demonstrated that this increased risk is likely clinically insignificant, but clinicians should still caution caregivers and individuals to monitor for the development of any such symptoms.[21] Similarly, although severe hepatitis has been reported during drug development, this is rarely seen in clinical practice and is reversible upon drug discontinuation. There is no indication for obtaining serial liver function enzymes for monitoring purposes. Parents and individuals should be cautioned about the signs and symptoms of acute hepatitis and instructed to seek appropriate medical care if necessary.

Clinical Monitoring for Medication Treatment of ADHD

Regardless of the treatment regimen, individuals receiving psychotropic medication for symptoms of ADHD should be periodically evaluated for medication effectiveness and side effects. Vital signs, especially heart rate and blood pressure, as well as growth parameters, should be measured at each visit. Rating scales, such as the Swanson, Nolan, and Pelham Questionnaire or the National Institute for Children's Health Quality (NICHQ) Vanderbilt Assessment Scales, can be provided to the teacher(s) and parents(s) and tracked for changes over time. Informal teacher reports or comments written on progress reports and report cards can also be valuable sources of information. Individuals may also provide self-reported symptom severity, although research suggests that teenagers and young adults may underreport impairments when compared with teacher and parent feedback.[22] Checklists such as the Adult ADHD Self-Report Scale (ASRS) are available for use and have emerging evidence of reliability in the adult population.[23]

Teenagers and young adults often express the desire to stop treatment for ADHD as they transition into adulthood.[24] Decisions to discontinue treatment for ADHD must involve carefully weighing the costs of treatment versus the potential harm of untreated ADHD symptomatology. Some children may appear to "grow out" of their ADHD as neuromaturation of the prefrontal lobe results in improved attention and executive functioning. However, although ADHD has been historically considered a disorder of childhood, research has demonstrated as many as one-third of adolescents and adults with childhood ADHD report ongoing functional impairment due to ADHD symptoms, with additional risks for other psychiatric disorders or adverse psychosocial outcomes.[25, 26] Reflecting this change, the *Diagnostic and Statistical Manual of Mental Disorders,* Fifth Edition,[27] categorizes ADHD as a neurodevelopmental disorder rather than a disruptive behavior disorder, has included symptoms seen in adults, and has lowered the diagnostic threshold in individuals 17 years of age and older. Adults diagnosed with ADHD in childhood have been shown to be at higher risk for a number of negative psychosocial outcomes, including: (1) problems with occupational, financial, and social functioning; (2) psychiatric disorders, such as conduct disorder, oppositional defiant disorder, antisocial personality disorder, and substance use disorders; (3) criminal activity; and (4) mortality (often from accidents).[26,28] Discontinuation of treatment for ADHD in adulthood is common, which is concerning given the potential benefits of stimulants on decreasing comorbid disorders such as substance abuse.[29,30] Young adults going to college should be counseled and monitored for concurrent substance abuse and misuse, as well as abuse and diversion of ADHD medication. This should include a careful evaluation of the psychosocial history, including a history of substance use.[31] Treatments may need to be adjusted around the individual's class or work schedule, although a lack of consistent symptom coverage may leave the patient vulnerable to deficits of executive function, potentially resulting in increased rates of high-risk sexual activity, unplanned pregnancy, driving accidents, and criminal activity.

Treatment of Aggression, Irritability, and Self-Injury

Antipsychotics were first developed in the 1950s and historically have been the first-line treatment of psychosis in adults and children. Initial diagnostic indications for use included schizophrenia and bipolar disorder. However, as the FDA began approving the use of antipsychotics for other disorders, including ASD, rates of prescribing antipsychotic medications increased tenfold between 1993 and 2010. Currently, aggression is the more common target of antipsychotic therapy in the pediatric population. Of more concern is the increasing frequency of off-label use; in a recent national study, only 34% of antipsychotic prescriptions were for FDA-approved indications, while 24% of prescriptions were for ADHD, 14% were for psychoses, and 15% were for "no mental disorder diagnosis."[32]

"Typical" antipsychotics (ie, "first-generation" antipsychotics [FGAs]) exert their effects by binding to dopamine D_2 receptors in the tuberoinfundibular, mesolimbic, and pre-frontal limbic pathways. By comparison, "atypical" antipsychotics (ie, "second-generation" antipsychotics [SGAs]) have relatively weaker affinity for the D_2 receptors and also bind to serotonin 5-hydroxytryptophan-2A ($5HT_{2A}$) receptors. SGAs are thought to have fewer neurological side effects than FGAs, making them more attractive for long-term use. However, some have suggested that the safety profile of SGAs has been falsely promoted through the use of inappropriate comparisons (eg, comparing high-dose FGAs to low-dose SGAs), publication bias, and spurious marketing practices. Meta-analyses suggest that the classification of antipsychotics into "first" and "second" generation is a meaningless distinction, as each antipsychotic has an individual efficacy and rate of adverse events.[33]

For primary pediatric health care professionals, the 2 antipsychotics most likely to be used are risperidone (Risperdal) and aripiprazole (Abilify). Risperidone is FDA approved for the treatment of irritability in children with ASD from 5 to 16 years of age; aripiprazole is approved for the same symptoms in children with ASD from 6 to 17 years of age. Studies of antipsychotic medication treatment of children with ASD have not demonstrated improvements in social communication or social interaction.[34] Although several RCTs have demonstrated the benefit of antipsychotics in children with disruptive behavior disorders, including conduct disorder and oppositional defiant disorder,[35] there is currently no FDA indication for antipsychotics in these conditions. Aripiprazole has been shown in several studies to be beneficial for nonsuicidal self-injury; however, most of this research concerns adolescents and adults with borderline personality disorder or anxiety disorders who engage in practices such as cutting, carving, and burning.[36] Risperidone and aripiprazole are also approved for use in the pediatric population for the treatment of schizophrenia and bipolar disorder, but these conditions are relatively rare and are best deferred to subspecialty care.

Antipsychotics should be started at low doses and gradually titrated every 2 to 4 weeks. The AACAP recommends that the lowest effective dose should be utilized for the shortest amount of time (given the significant side effects outlined in the next section), and the adult maximum dose should not be exceeded (Table 23.3). Benefits may not be apparent until 4 weeks of treatment is complete. In general, antipsychotics are metabolized by the liver and excreted in the urine; many SGAs are processed by cytochrome P450 (CYP) enzymes, and active levels may be affected when a patient is cotreated with a CYP inhibitor or inducer.[37] Antipsychotics should be gradually tapered, with doses decreased by 25% every 7 days. Sudden discontinuation of medication can result in symptoms of withdrawal, including agitation, activation, insomnia, psychosis, and dyskinesia.

Table 23.3. Second-generation Antipsychotics That Are FDA Approved for Use in Children					
Drug (generic)	Brand	Forms and Administration	Starting Dose	Effective Dose	Maximum Dose
Risperidone	Risperdal	**Tablet:** 0.25 mg, 0.5 mg, 1 mg, 2 mg, 3 mg, 4 mg **Liquid:** 1 mg/mL **Dissolving tablet:** 0.5 mg, 1 mg, 2 mg, 3 mg, 4 mg	0.25–0.5 mg/day	0.5–1 mg/day for autism; 2.5 mg/day for bipolar disorder; 3 mg/day for schizophrenia	3 mg/day for children; 6 mg/day for adolescents
Aripiprazole	Abilify	**Tablet:** 2 mg, 5 mg, 10 mg, 15 mg, 20 mg, 30 mg **Liquid:** 1 mg/mL **Dissolving tablet:** 10 mg, 15 mg	2 mg/day	5–10 mg/day	30 mg/day

Abbreviation: FDA, US Food and Drug Administration.

Both FGAs and SGAs are associated with several concerning side effects that have garnered additional attention as national prescribing rates have increased. Although rates of individual side effects may differ from drug to drug, patients taking any antipsychotic should be closely monitored for the following potential adverse effects.

– Metabolic Effects

All antipsychotics carry a risk for increased appetite and subsequent weight gain, with the mean weight increase being greater for risperidone than for aripiprazole.[38,39] Pediatric patients gain more weight per month than adults do when treated with an SGA.[40] Elevations in blood glucose and dyslipidemia can occur, depending on the antipsychotic; risperidone appears to have an intermediate effect and aripiprazole a minimal effect on blood glucose and lipids.[41] Individuals who take an SGA have an increased risk of developing diabetes mellitus,[42] which may be mediated by weight gain and/or direct effects of antipsychotics on insulin resistance.[43,44] There is insufficient literature regarding the effects of chronic dyslipidemia induced by SGA therapy in the pediatric population.

Although effects on insulin resistance and dyslipidemia are more likely to occur in patients with increased weight gain, they have also been reported independent of weight effects. Therefore, all patients prescribed antipsychotics should have blood glucose and lipid profiles monitored closely. In a joint statement issued by the American Diabetes Association, the American Psychiatric Association, and the American Association of Clinical Endocrinologists, an expert panel recommended the following:[45]

1. If possible, baseline screening prior to starting a medication (and referrals as appropriate), including
   a. A personal and family history of diabetes, dyslipidemia, hypertension, and cardiovascular disease
   b. Body mass index (BMI)
   c. Waist circumference
   d. Blood pressure
   e. Fasting blood glucose
   f. Fasting lipid profile
2. BMI at 4 weeks, 8 weeks, 12 weeks, and quarterly thereafter
3. Blood pressure, fasting blood glucose, and fasting lipid profile at 12 weeks
4. Personal and family history, waist circumference, blood pressure, and fasting blood glucose annually
5. Fasting lipid profile every 5 years
6. More frequent screening if clinically indicated

– Extrapyramidal Symptoms

Extrapyramidal symptoms (EPS) result from dopamine antagonism in the basal ganglia and manifest as neuromotor abnormalities. EPS include akathisia (restlessness), parkinsonism (cogwheel rigidity and tremor), dystonia (muscle spasms), bradykinesia (slow movement), tremor, and tardive dyskinesia (jerky and repetitive movements of the facial muscles). EPS are most commonly associated with FGA but may still occur with SGA use, especially in the pediatric population.[46] Tardive dyskinesia is often the most concerning EPS because it may be permanent, even after discontinuation of the drug. Rates of tardive dyskinesia following short-term treatment with SGAs are low in the pediatric population, but there is insufficient literature regarding chronic use.[47] The AACAP recommends using structured tools like the Abnormal Involuntary Movement Scale or Neurological Rating Scale at baseline and at regular intervals during treatment with an antipsychotic.[48,49] Acute management of EPS includes the administration of anticholinergic agents, such as diphenhydramine or benztropine. Should EPS develop, the clinician may choose to reduce the dose of the antipsychotic or attempt another formulation.

– Cardiovascular Effects

Antipsychotic use has been associated with short-term cardiovascular changes, including tachycardia, hypotension, pericarditis, and QTc interval alterations. Risperidone has been shown to increase the QTc, while aripiprazole may decrease the QTc. Most research on possible long-term effects of SGA use has not demonstrated any clinically significant and sustained impacts on the cardiovascular system.[50,51] Nevertheless, the AACAP refers to guidelines from the AHA,[52] which recommend obtaining family history for sudden or unexplained deaths, the patient's history for syncope or palpitations, and performing additional cardiac evaluations if the sustained resting heartbeat is >130 bpm, the PR interval is >200 milliseconds, the QRS is >120 milliseconds, or the QTc is >460 milliseconds.

– Prolactin Levels

Prolactin is a hormone produced by the anterior pituitary and is normally inhibited by dopamine. The D_2 binding of antipsychotics can result in increased prolactin levels within 1 to 9 days. Hyperprolactinemia, defined as >20 ng/mL for adult men and >25 ng/mL for adult women, can result in issues such as sexual problems and gynecomastia.[53] Hyperprolactinemia is described more often with FGAs than with SGAs, although risperidone does appear to result in sustained increases in prolactin levels. Adverse drug events such as gynecomastia have gained attention due to the increased frequency of lawsuits in which claimants allege the drug manufacturers did not provide sufficient warning about gynecomastia. In the absence of symptoms of hyperprolactinemia, however, the AACAP does not recommend baseline or routine monitoring of prolactin levels. Should symptoms of hyperprolactinemia develop, the clinician may choose to decrease or discontinue the antipsychotic or try a different antipsychotic. Clinicians should be careful to document discussions regarding the potential risk of hyperprolactinemia (as well as other adverse effects) when considering antipsychotic treatment.

– Neuroleptic Malignant Syndrome

Neuroleptic malignant syndrome (NMS) is a rare but serious adverse effect of antipsychotic use. Symptoms include muscle rigidity, fever, altered consciousness, and autonomic dysfunction; these symptoms typically occur within 2 weeks of initiation of therapy or dose adjustments. NMS requires immediate medical attention, which often includes treatment in the intensive care setting, including aggressive fever control and administration of muscle relaxants. Clinicians may choose to restart a lower-potency antipsychotic following an occurrence of NMS, but it is recommended to start with a lower dose and titrate slowly. A history of NMS also predisposes individuals to negative reactions to anesthesia, so patients and families should be encouraged to share this information prior to any prospective surgical procedures.

Treatment of Anxiety and Mood Disorders

Recent epidemiological studies suggest that the prevalence of pediatric anxiety disorders may be as high as 25% to 32%, and the prevalence of mood disorders is approximately 11%.[54-57] In general, for most mild to moderate anxiety and mood disorders, first-line treatment should be CBT without medication; for more severe disorders, a combination of CBT with an antidepressant in the selective serotonin reuptake inhibitor (SSRI) or serotonin-norepinephrine reuptake inhibitor (SNRI) classes is recommended (see Chapter 22, Anxiety and Mood Disorders). Many SSRIs and SNRIs are FDA approved to treat certain anxiety and mood disorders in the pediatric population (Table 23.4). Response to psychological or medication treatment should be monitored over time through the use of symptom rating scales administered on a periodic basis. Useful screeners are brief and address symptom severity. Validated and reliable screeners for pediatric anxiety and depressive disorders include the Screen for Child Anxiety Related Emotional Disorders (SCARED),[58] the Spence Children's Anxiety Scale (SCAS),[59] and the Childhood Depression Screener (ChilD-S).[60]

Anxiety Disorders

The SSRIs fluoxetine, fluvoxamine, and sertraline have FDA indications for treatment of pediatric obsessive-compulsive disorder (OCD), and the SNRI duloxetine is FDA approved for treatment of generalized anxiety disorder. Use of SSRIs and SNRIs for treatment of other pediatric anxiety disorders, therefore, is off label. Nevertheless, they have been shown to be effective in reducing anxiety symptoms in children and adolescents, and SSRIs and SNRIs are considered to be the first- and second-line medication choice, respectively, for treating anxiety disorders in childhood.[61-63]

Tricyclic antidepressants, such as clomipramine and imipramine, have also been used to treat pediatric anxiety disorders, but these are considered third-line after the SSRIs and SNRIs due to limited support for efficacy and greater adverse effects, including anticholinergic symptoms and potential for cardiotoxicity.

Benzodiazepines, such as clonazepam, lorazepam, and alprazolam, have not been extensively studied in children, and thus have a limited role for medication treatment of pediatric anxiety. A benefit of benzodiazepines is their short onset of action (minutes to hours). Thus, benzodiazepines may be used to relieve impairing anxiety in certain acute situations (eg, flying) or when initiating an SSRI in order to provide immediate symptom relief while waiting for the SSRI to reach therapeutic levels in children with severe symptoms. Common adverse effects include agitation, disinhibition, and impaired memory and learning. Clinicians should consider the risk of abuse, addiction, and diversion when prescribing a benzodiazepine. Suggested starting doses for clonazepam and alprazolam are 0.25 mg once or twice daily.

Depressive and Mood Disorders

Medication treatment is indicated for children and adolescents with moderate to severe major depression, dysthymia, or depressive symptoms with functional impairment, ideally in combination with CBT for greater efficacy.[64] Children and adolescents with milder forms of major depression who have not responded to CBT are also candidates for antidepressant medication.

As with anxiety disorders, the medication of choice for treating pediatric depressive disorders is an SSRI. Both fluoxetine and escitalopram are FDA approved for treatment of major depression in children older than 7 years of age. Fluoxetine is recommended as first-line treatment based on more evidence of efficacy relative to other SSRIs to treat pediatric depression. Approximately 60% of adolescents experience symptomatic improvement after initiation of SSRI treatment.[65,66] For those who do not respond to the initial SSRI, a second-line agent, such as sertraline, citalopram, escitalopram, or venlafaxine should be considered.[67,68]

There is insufficient evidence to support the use of other antidepressants, such as tricyclic antidepressants or bupropion, for treating depressive disorders in children.

Clinical Use of SSRIs and SNRIs

SSRIs and SNRIs should be initiated at the lowest available dose for 7 days, then increased incrementally to an initial therapeutic dose while monitoring for side effects. If symptomatic improvement is not evident after 6 to 8 weeks, then the dose should be increased again for another trial until either the maximum dose is reached or side effects become intolerable. Children may require doses similar to adults due to more rapid metabolism.

While SSRIs and SNRIs are generally well tolerated, clinicians should monitor children for the following adverse effects:

- Physical effects include nausea, headache, diarrhea, insomnia, sweating, or vivid dreams. These are usually transient but can be mitigated by reducing the dose or slowing the rate of upward titration.
- Psychiatric effects include disinhibition, agitation, mania or hypomania, and worsened anxiety. These are relatively uncommon and usually improve by reducing the medication dose.
- In 2004, the FDA issued a black box warning indicating an increased risk for suicidal thinking or behavior (suicidality) among individuals taking antidepressant medication.[69] However, this increased risk was among individuals treated with SSRIs for depression, not anxiety or OCD.[66] The risk of untreated depression should be weighed against the likely benefit of these medications for children and adolescents with depression.
- Effects of serotonin syndrome are anxiety, agitation, delirium, diaphoresis, tachycardia, hypertension, hyperthermia, gastrointestinal distress, muscle rigidity, tremor, and hyperreflexia. This can occur when multiple medications (eg, SSRI, SNRI, bupropion, and trazodone, among others) interact to increase serotonergic neurotransmission.

The FDA recommends the following monitoring schedule for patients prescribed antidepressants:[70]

- Weekly for the first 4 weeks
- Biweekly during the second month
- Monthly beginning in the third month, unless there are changes in medication, symptoms, or functioning, or if there is concurrent substance use

Once an effective treatment has been established, children should remain on that medication for at least 12 months. When a trial off medication is desired, SSRIs must be tapered by decreasing the dose by 25% to 50% weekly in order to avoid discontinuation symptoms such as dizziness, fatigue, chills, myalgia, dysphoria, and gastrointestinal distress. Medication should be resumed if the patient's symptoms recur.

Primary pediatric health care professionals should consider consultation or referral to a subspecialist for patients with severe mood or anxiety disorders, suicidal thinking, co-occurring anxiety and depression, concurrent substance use, or those who have not responded to treatment.

Table 23.4. Selective Serotonin Reuptake Inhibitor (SSRI) and Serotonin-Norepinephrine Reuptake Inhibitor (SNRI) Medications in Children and Adolescents

Medication	FDA Indication	Dosing	Maintenance Dose Range	Elimination Half-Life
SSRIs				
Fluoxetine	**Major depression:** ≥8 years **OCD:** ≥7 years	**Start:** 5 mg (child); 10 mg (adolescent) Increase by 20 mg increments.	10–80 mg	2 to 6 days
Fluvoxamine	**OCD:** ≥8 years	**Start:** 25 mg (child); 50 mg (adolescent) Increase by 25 to 50 mg increments.	50–300 mg (divide dose to minimize side effects)	16 hours
Paroxetine	—	**Start:** 5–10 mg; Increase by 5 mg (child) to 10 mg (adolescent) increments.	10–60 mg	20 hours
Sertraline	**OCD:** ≥6 years	**Start:** 12.5–25 mg; Increase by 12.5 mg (child) to 25 mg (adolescent).	50–200 mg	26 hours
Citalopram	—	**Start:** 10–20 mg; Increase by 10 mg.	60 mg	35 hours
Escitalopram	**Major depression:** ≥12 years	**Start:** 5–10 mg; Increase by 5 mg.	20 mg	30 hours
SNRIs				
Duloxetine	**GAD:** ≥7 years	**Start:** 30 mg; Increase by 30 mg.	120 mg	12 hours
Venlafaxine	—	**Start:** 37.5 mg; Increase by 37.5 mg (child) to 75 mg (adolescent).	150–225 mg	11 hours

Abbreviations: GAD, generalized anxiety disorder; FDA, US Food and Drug Administration; OCD, obsessive-compulsive disorder; SNRI, serotonin-norepinephrine reuptake inhibitor; SSRI, selective serotonin reuptake inhibitor.

Treatment of Compulsive, Rigid, and Repetitive Behaviors

Obsessive-Compulsive Disorder

Obsessive-compulsive disorder is characterized by recurrent intrusive thoughts, images or urges (obsessions) that typically cause anxiety or distress and by repetitive mental or behavioral acts (compulsions) that the child feels driven to perform.[27]

Selective serotonin reuptake inhibitors are first-line medications for OCD because of their demonstrated efficacy and safety in this age group. FDA-approved SSRIs for the treatment of OCD in children include sertraline, fluoxetine, and fluvoxamine. SSRIs should be initiated at low doses and titrated gradually to a therapeutic dose. Depending on clinical response, additional dose adjustments should be given a 6- to 12-week trial until the maximum effective dose with the minimum side effects is achieved. Effective treatment of OCD symptoms typically requires higher doses than those used to treat depression or anxiety disorders.

The tricyclic antidepressant clomipramine is also effective for treating OCD in children. However, its use is limited by potentially significant side effects, including delayed cardiac conduction and, rarely, sudden cardiac death. Prior to initiating clomipramine, clinicians should screen for underlying cardiovascular illnesses and obtain a baseline blood pressure, pulse, and ECG. Blood pressure, pulse, and repeat ECG should be obtained with any increase in dose.

Rigid and Repetitive Behaviors

Rigid and repetitive behaviors are often problematic in children with ASD. First-line treatments should involve behavioral interventions such as the techniques utilized by applied behavior analysis (ABA) therapy. To date, little evidence supports the use of medications to treat repetitive behaviors.

Based on their efficacy for treating compulsive behavior in children with OCD, SSRIs have been used to treat repetitive behaviors in children with ASD; however, there is currently an insufficient strength of evidence to support the use of SSRIs for repetitive behaviors in ASD.[71] Medications that have been effective in reducing rigid and repetitive behaviors in children with ASD include atypical antipsychotics (eg, risperidone), antiepileptic drugs (eg, valproate), and anxiolytics (eg, buspirone).[72-74] However, these medications have significant side effect profiles, and children should be monitored closely while undergoing treatment.

Treatment of Sleep Disorders

Sleep plays a critical role in early brain development, problem-solving, and memory consolidation.[75] However, as many as 30% of children and adolescents experience sleep problems that their parents deem as "significant."[76] Sleep disorders are even more prevalent in children with comorbid neurobehavioral conditions, including ADHD, ASD, depression, anxiety, and psychosis. Sleep difficulties in children should be addressed and treated in a timely manner, as lack of sleep can contribute to behavioral and academic impairments as well as difficulties with emotional regulation. In addition, when children sleep fewer hours than needed or sleep less regularly, parents also experience disrupted sleep, leading to implications for the entire family.

Sleep disorders can result from conditioning factors (environmental), the absence of consistent sleep schedules or routines, psychological factors, and medical factors. Clinicians should first obtain a thorough sleep history. Most pediatric sleep disorders are related to poor sleep hygiene, so the clinician's initial step in management should be to improve the sleeping environment.

Clinicians should also evaluate for medical conditions that may impede sleep, including obstructive sleep apnea, sleep-related asthma, gastroesophageal reflux, obesity, thyroid disorders, and restless leg syndrome. In addition, medications used to treat other medical conditions may interfere with sleep. For instance, albuterol used to treat asthma, certain liquid antibiotics, and certain tricyclic antidepressants all have been demonstrated to have a potentially negative impact on sleep.[77,78] Clinicians should interview adolescents separately to ascertain the use of caffeine, energy drinks, alcohol, nicotine, and other recreational drugs.

Only after behavioral and environmental contributors to poor sleep have been addressed should the clinician consider initiating a medication for sleep. No medications have specific FDA indications for sleep disorders in children. Given the limited evidence regarding long-term use of sleep medications in children, prescribers should aim to treat children with the lowest effective dose of medication for a limited period of time. Medication to help with sleep should be used only as an *adjunct* to nonpharmacological strategies. In a national study of sleep medication prescribing practices by pediatricians, antihistamines were the most commonly prescribed medication, followed closely by clonidine.[75] However, clinicians should consider the specific sleep complaint, potential medication interactions, and side effect profile in selecting a medication to assist with sleep.

For children with transient disruptions in their sleep schedules, such as when a child is traveling, commonly prescribed, short-term medications include antihistamines, such as diphenhydramine and hydroxyzine, or hormone analogs, such as melatonin. These tend to have a quick onset and short duration of action. Antihistamines, such as diphenhydramine, are the most commonly prescribed medications used to assist with sleep in children. While antihistamines are well tolerated and can be helpful in inducing sleep in older children, tolerance quickly develops, and children can become dependent upon these medications for sleep. Other common antihistamine side effects include residual sedative effects during the daylight hours or paradoxical hyperactivity. Melatonin has been shown to improve initiation and maintenance of sleep in children with a range of neurodevelopmental disorders. Melatonin should be taken on an empty stomach, 90 minutes prior to bedtime.[79,80] Liquid preparations of melatonin contain ethanol, so these should be avoided. Instead, parents should crush melatonin pills and mix with food or drink when administering to children who do not yet swallow pills.

The FDA does not regulate dietary supplements, and thus the concentration of the active ingredients can vary among different brands of melatonin.

Although frequently prescribed for sleep disturbances, clonidine is a powerful rapid eye movement suppressant that can affect blood pressure. Therefore, its use should be reserved for those children who continue to experience significant sleep disruptions leading to impairments in daily functioning, despite first-line medication treatment. Similarly, benzodiazepines should only be used as a brief, second-line therapy, as tolerance and dependency can rapidly develop with prolonged use. Chloral hydrate has historically been used for sleep induction in children with neurological impairments. However, as high doses are frequently required and daytime sedation is a common side effect, the use of this drug is more limited.

Children with neurobehavioral disorders often have comorbid sleep disorders, such as difficulty initiating sleep, difficulty staying asleep, disordered sleep/wake schedules, and circadian rhythm disorders. These can be further exacerbated by medications used to treat the underlying condition. For example, stimulants used to treat ADHD commonly lead to prolonged sleep onset. It is often helpful to choose a medication for a co-occurring sleep disorder that can be synergistic in treating their primary neurobehavioral condition. Psychiatric medications often chosen for their beneficial sleep-inducing effects are included in Table 23.5.

| Table 23.5. Medications With Sleep-Inducing Effects Used to Treat Various Neurobehavioral Disorders ||
Neurobehavioral diagnosis	First-line medication(s) for sleep
Attention-deficit/hyperactivity disorder (ADHD)	Clonidine, imipramine, melatonin
Depression	Imipramine, amitriptyline, trazodone
Bipolar disorder	Risperidone, olanzapine, quetiapine
Anxiety disorder	Lorazepam, clonazepam, imipramine, melatonin, diphenhydramine
Posttraumatic stress disorder (PTSD)	Clonidine, imipramine
Psychotic disorders	Risperidone, olanzapine, quetiapine
Autism spectrum disorder (ASD)	Risperidone, melatonin

As with any disorder, it is important for the primary pediatric health care professional to know when a patient should be referred for more specialized care. Should significant sleep disruptions persist despite behavioral measures and appropriately dosed medications, a referral is likely warranted. Children receiving multiple medications are at risk for medication interactions and should also be referred. Suggested doses for sleep medications are listed in Table 23.6.

Table 23.6. Suggested Dosing for Pediatric Sleep Medications				
Medication	**Category**	**Indication**	**Recommended Dose**	**Side Effects/ Warnings**
Diphenhydramine	Antihistamine	Sleep induction	10–100 mg	Paradoxical hyperactivity, daytime drowsiness, tolerance
Hydroxyzine	Antihistamine	Sleep induction	10–100 mg	Paradoxical hyperactivity, daytime drowsiness, tolerance
Melatonin	Hormone analog	Sleep induction, regulating circadian rhythms	1–10 mg	FDA does not regulate the manufacture of this drug; concentration of active ingredient may vary
Chloral hydrate	Sedative–hypnotic	Historical use for children with neurodevelopmental disorders	25–50 mg/kg 30 minutes before bed	High doses needed, daytime sedation
Lorazepam	Benzodiazepine	Arousal disorders	0.5–1 mg	Treat for <2 weeks to decrease risk of tolerance
Diazepam	Benzodiazepine	Arousal disorders	2.5–5 mg	Treat for <2 weeks to decrease risk of tolerance
Clonazepam	Benzodiazepine	Arousal disorders	0.25–0.5 mg	Treat for <2 weeks to decrease risk of tolerance; significant residual daytime sleepiness
Imipramine	Tricyclic antidepressant	Arousal disorders	10–100mg	Increased risk of suicidal thoughts, potential drug interactions, anticholinergic symptoms, potential cardiotoxicity
Trazodone	Atypical antidepressant	Sleep induction	25–100mg	Dizziness, dry mouth, nausea, priapism
Gabapentin	Anticonvulsant	Arousal disorders	50–300 mg (max 150 mg in younger children)	Leukopenia, skin rash, vertigo, hyperglycemia
Clonidine	Alpha-agonist	Sleep induction	0.05–0.2 mg	Abrupt discontinuation can lead to rebound hypertension and nightmares
Risperidone	Atypical antipsychotic	Sleep induction/maintenance	0.25–2 mg	Tardive dyskinesia, weight gain, galactorrhea, cardiac effects, blood count abnormalities
Olanzapine	Atypical antipsychotic	Sleep induction/maintenance	2.5–10 mg	Tardive dyskinesia, weight gain, galactorrhea, cardiac effects, blood count abnormalities
Quetiapine	Atypical antipsychotic	Sleep induction/maintenance	50–100 mg	Tardive dyskinesia, weight gain, galactorrhea, cardiac effects, blood count abnormalities

Abbreviations: ADHD, attention-deficit/hyperactivity disorder; FDA, US Food and Drug Administration; SNR , serotonin-norepinephrine reuptake inhibitor.

Conclusion

Pharmacological management of behavioral health and developmental conditions in pediatrics is often complex. Children frequently present with more than one diagnosis and may benefit from a combination of medications targeting each diagnosis. It is important for primary pediatric health care professionals to recognize when to refer to a more specialized level of care. Treatment algorithms driven by evidence can empower the general practitioner to serve as the first responder to mental or behavioral challenges and to initiate therapy with a standard medication, particularly if there is a wait for the patient to be seen by a specialist. However, primary pediatric health care professionals should consider referral to a developmental-behavioral pediatrician or child and adolescent psychiatrist when a child does not respond to standard treatment regimens, including several medication treatment trials, or when a child presents with multiple comorbid behavioral or mental health conditions.

References

1. Howie LD, Pastor PN, Lukacs SL. Use of medication prescribed for emotional or behavioral difficulties among children aged 6-17 years in the United States, 2011-2012. NCHS data brief, no 148. Hyattsville, MD: National Center for Health Statistics. 2014. https://www.cdc.gov/nchs/data/databriefs/db148.pdf. Accessed January 16, 2018
2. American Academy of Pediatrics Committee on Psychosocial Aspects of Child and Family Health and Task Force on Mental Health. Policy statement—The future of pediatrics: mental health competencies for pediatric primary care. *Pediatrics*. 2009;124(1):410–421
3. Simon AE, Pastor PN, Reuben CA, Huang LN, Goldstrom ID. Use of mental health services by children ages six to 11 with emotional or behavioral difficulties. *Psychiatr Serv*. 2015;66(9):930–937
4. Stein REK, Horwitz SM, Storfer-Isser A, Heneghan A, Olson L, Hoagwood KE. Do pediatricians think they are responsible for identification and management of child mental health problems? Results of the AAP periodic survey. *Ambul Pediatr*. 2008;8(1):11–17
5. Horwitz SM, Caspary G, Storfer-Isser A, et al. Is developmental and behavioral pediatrics training related to perceived responsibility for treating mental health problems? *Acad Pediatr*. 2010;10(4):252–259
6. American Academy of Pediatrics Subcommittee on Attention-Deficit/Hyperactivity Disorder; Steering Committee on Quality Improvement and Management, Wolraich M, et al. ADHD: clinical practice guideline for the diagnosis, evaluation, and treatment of attention-deficit/hyperactivity disorder in children and adolescents. *Pediatrics*. 2011;128(5):1007–1022
7. American Academy of Pediatrics. Implementing the key action statements: an algorithm and explanation for process of care for the evaluation, diagnosis, treatment, and monitoring of ADHD in children and adolescents. *Pediatrics*. 2011:128(5)SI1–SI21
8. Wolraich ML, Doffing MA. Pharmacokinetic considerations in the treatment of attention-deficit hyperactivity disorder with methylphenidate. *CNS Drugs*. 2004;18(4):243–250
9. Vitiello B, Severe JB, Greenhill LL, et al. Methylphenidate dosage for children with ADHD over time under controlled conditions: lessons from the MTA. *J Am Acad Child Adolesc Psychiatry*. 2001;40(2):188–196
10. Berman SM, Kuczenski R, McCracken JT, London ED. Potential adverse effects of amphetamine treatment on brain and behavior: a review. *Mol Psychiatry*. 2009;14(2):123–142
11. Faraone SV, Biederman J, Morley CP, Spencer TJ. Effect of stimulants on height and weight: a review of the literature. *J Am Acad Child Adolesc Psychiatry*. 2008;47(9):994–1009
12. Harstad EB, Weaver AL, Katusic SK, et al. ADHD, stimulant treatment, and growth: a longitudinal study. *Pediatrics*. 2014;134(4):e935–e944
13. Pidsosny IC, Virani A. Pediatric psychopharmacology update: psychostimulants and tics—past, present and future. *J Can Acad Child Adolesc Psychiatry*. 2006;15(2):84–86
14. Hammerness PG, Karampahtsis C, Babalola R, Alexander ME. Attention-deficit/hyperactivity disorder treatment: what are the long-term cardiovascular risks? *Expert Opin Drug Saf*. 2015;14(4):543–551
15. American Academy of Pediatrics/American Heart Association clarification of statement on cardiovascular evaluation and monitoring of children and adolescents with heart disease receiving medications for ADHD: May 16, 2008. *J Dev Behav Pediatr*. 2008;29(4):335

16. Hirota T, Schwartz S, Correll CU. Alpha-2 agonists for attention-deficit/hyperactivity disorder in youth: a systematic review and meta-analysis of monotherapy and add-on trials to stimulant therapy. *J Am Acad Child Adolesc Psychiatry*. 2014;53(2):153–173

17. Connor DF, Findling RL, Kollins SH, et al. Effects of guanfacine extended release on oppositional symptoms in children aged 6–12 years with attention-deficit hyperactivity disorder and oppositional symptoms: a randomized, double-blind, placebo-controlled trial. *CNS Drugs*. 2010;24(9):755–768

18. Martinez-Raga J, Knecht C, de Alvaro R. Profile of guanfacine extended release and its potential in the treatment of attention-deficit hyperactivity disorder. *Neuropsychiatr Dis Treat*. 2015;11:1359–1370

19. Dell'Agnello G, Zuddas A, Masi G, Curatolo P, Besana D, Rossi A. Use of atomoxetine in patients with attention-deficit hyperactivity disorder and comorbid conditions. *CNS Drugs*. 2009;23(9):739–753

20. Greenhill LL, Newcorn JH, Gao H, Feldman PD. Effect of two different methods of initiating atomoxetine on the adverse event profile of atomoxetine. *J Am Acad Child Adolesc Psychiatry*. 2007;46(5):566–572

21. Reed VA, Buitelaar JK, Anand E, et al. The safety of atomoxetine for the treatment of children and adolescents with attention-deficit/hyperactivity disorder: a comprehensive review of over a decade of research. *CNS Drugs*. 2016;30(7):603–628

22. Barkley RA, Fischer M, Smallish L, Fletcher K. The persistence of attention-deficit/hyperactivity disorder into young adulthood as a function of reporting source and definition of disorder. *J Abnorm Psychol*. 2002;111(2):279–289

23. Adler LA, Spencer T, Faraone SV, et al. Validity of pilot Adult ADHD Self-Report Scale (ASRS) to rate adult ADHD symptoms. *Ann Clin Psychiatry*. 2006 Jul-Sep;18(3):145–148

24. Turgay A, Goodman DW, Asherson P, et al. Lifespan persistence of ADHD: the life transition model and its application. *J Clin Psychiatry*. 2012;73(2):192–201

25. Yoshimasu K, Barbaresi WJ, Colligan RC, et al. Childhood ADHD is strongly associated with a broad range of psychiatric disorders during adolescence: a population-based birth cohort study. *J Child Psychol Psychiatry*. 2012;53(10):1036–1043

26. Barbaresi WJ, Colligan RC, Weaver AL, Voigt RG, Killian JM, Katusic SK. Mortality, ADHD, and psychosocial adversity in adults with childhood ADHD: a prospective study. *Pediatrics*. 2013;131(4):637–644

27. American Psychiatric Association. *Diagnostic and Statistical Manual of Mental Disorders*. 5th ed. Arlington, VA: American Psychiatric Association; 2013

28. Brook JS, Brook DW, Zhang C, Seltzer N, Finch SJ. Adolescent ADHD and adult physical and mental health, work performance, and financial stress. *Pediatrics*. 2015;131(1):5–13

29. Humphreys KL, Eng T, Lee SS. Stimulant medication and substance use outcomes: a meta-analysis. *JAMA Psychiatry*. 2013;70(7):740–749

30. Groenman AP, Oosterlaan J, Rommelse NNJ, et al. Stimulant treatment for attention-deficit hyperactivity disorder and risk of developing substance use disorder. *Br J Psychiatry*. 2013;203(2):112–119

31. Harstad E, Levy S; American Academy of Pediatrics Committee on Substance Abuse. Attention-deficit/hyperactivity disorder and substance abuse. *Pediatrics*. 2014;134(1):e293–e301

32. Sohn M, Moga DC, Blumenschein K, Talbert J. National trends in off-label use of atypical antipsychotics in children and adolescents in the United States. *Medicine (Baltimore)*. 2016;95(23):e3784

33. Leucht S, Corves C, Arbter D, Engel R, Li C, Davis JM. Second-generation versus first-generation antipsychotic for schizophrenia: a meta-analysis. *Lancet*. 2009;373(9657):31–41

34. Ji NY, Findling RL. An update on pharmacotherapy for autism spectrum disorder in children and adolescents. *Curr Opin Psychiatry*. 2015;28(2):91–101

35. Pandina GJ, Aman MG, Findling RL. Risperidone in the management of disruptive behavior disorders. *J Child Adolesc Psychopharmacol*. 2006;16(4):379–392

36. Turner BJ, Austin SB, Chapman AL. Treating nonsuicidal self-injury: a systematic review of psychological and pharmacological interventions. *Can J Psychiatry*. 2014;59(11):576–585

37. Urichuk L, Prior TI, Dursun S, Baker G. Metabolism of atypical antipsychotics: involvement of cytochrome P450 enzymes and relevance for drug-drug interactions. *Curr Drug Metab*. 2008;9(5):410–418

38. Almandil NB, Liu Y, Murray ML, Besag FMC, Aitchison KJ, Wong ICK. Weight gain and other metabolic adverse effects associated with atypical antipsychotic treatment of children and adolescents: a systematic review and meta-analysis. *Paediatr Drugs*. 2013;15(2):139–150

39. Maayan L, Correll CU. Weight gain and metabolic risks associated with antipsychotic medications in children and adolescents. *J Child Adolesc Psychopharmacol*. 2011;21(6):517–535

40. Safer DJ. A comparison of risperidone-induced weight gain across the age span. *J Clin Psychopharmacol*. 2004;24(4):429–436

41. Cohen D, Bonnot O, Bodeau N, Consoli A, Laurent C. Adverse effects of second-generation antipsychotics in children and adolescents: a Bayesian meta-analysis. *J Clin Psychopharmacol*. 2012;32(3):309–316

42. Andrade SE, Lo JC, Roblin D, et al. Antipsychotic medication use among children and risk of diabetes mellitus. *Pediatrics*. 2011;128(6):1135–1141

43. Newcomer JW. Second-generation (atypical) antipsychotics and metabolic effects: a comprehensive literature review. *CNS Drugs*. 2005;19(suppl 1):1–93

44. Deng C. Effects of antipsychotic medications on appetite, weight, and insulin resistance. *Endocrinol Metab Clin North Am*. 2013;42(3):545–563

45. Consensus development conference on antipsychotic drugs and obesity and diabetes. *Diabetes Care*. 2004;27(2):596–601

46. Correll CU, Sheridan EM, DelBello MP. Antipsychotic and mood stabilizer efficacy and tolerability in pediatric and adult patients with bipolar I mania: a comparative analysis of acute, randomized, placebo-controlled trials. *Bipolar Disord*. 2010;12(2):116–141

47. Correll CU, Kane JM. One-year incidence rates of tardive dyskinesia in children and adolescents treated with second-generation antipsychotics: a systematic review. *J Child Adolesc Psychopharmacol*. 2007;17(5):647–656

48. Menzies V, Farrell SP. Schizophrenia, tardive dyskinesia, and the Abnormal Involuntary Movement Scale (AIMS). *J Am Psychiatr Nurses Assoc*. 2002;8(2):51–56

49. Sipe JC, Knobler RL, Braheny SL, Rice GPA, Panitch HS, Oldstone MBA. A neurological rating scale (NRS) for use in multiple sclerosis. *Neurology*. 1984;34(10):1368–1368

50. Alda JA, Muñoz-Samons D, Tor J, et al. Absence of change in corrected QT interval in children and adolescents receiving antipsychotic treatment: a 12 month study. *J Child Adolesc Psychopharmacol*. 2016;26(5):449–457

51. Jensen KG, Juul K, Fink-Jensen A, Correll CU, Pagsberg AK. Corrected QT changes during antipsychotic treatment of children and adolescents: a systematic review and meta-analysis of clinical trials. *J Am Acad Child Adolesc Psychiatry*. 2015;54(1):25–36

52. Gutgesell H, Atkins D, Barst R, et al. AHA Scientific Statement: cardiovascular monitoring of children and adolescents receiving psychotropic drugs. *J Am Acad Child Adolesc Psychiatry*. 1999;38(8):1047–1050

53. Aboraya A, Fullen JE, Ponieman BL, Makela EH, Latocha M. Hyperprolactinemia associated with risperidone: a case report and review of literature. *Psychiatry (Edgmont)*. 2004;1(3):29–31

54. Achenbach TM, Howell CT, McConaughy SH, Stanger C. Six-year predictors of problems in a national sample of children and youth: I. Cross-informant syndromes. *J Am Acad Child Adolesc Psychiatry*. 1995;34(3):336–347

55. Kessler RC, Avenevoli S, Costello EJ, et al. Prevalence, persistence, and sociodemographic correlates of DSM-IV disorders in the National Comorbidity Survey Replication Adolescent Supplement. *Arch Gen Psychiatry*. 2012;69(4):372–380

56. Merikangas KR, He J-P, Burstein M, et al. Lifetime prevalence of mental disorders in U.S. adolescents: results from the National Comorbidity Survey Replication—Adolescent Supplement (NCS-A). *J Am Acad Child Adolesc Psychiatry*. 2010;49(10):980–989

57. Avenevoli S, Swendsen J, He J-P, Burstein M, Merikangas KR. Major depression in the national comorbidity survey-adolescent supplement: prevalence, correlates, and treatment. *J Am Acad Child Adolesc Psychiatry*. 2015;54(1):37–44.e2

58. Birmaher B, Brent DA, Chiappetta L, et al. Psychometric properties of the Screen for Child Anxiety Related Emotional Disorders (SCARED): a replication study. *J Am Acad Child Adolesc Psychiatry*. 1999;38(10):1230–1236

59. Brown-Jacobsen, AM, Wallace, DP, and SP Whiteside. Multimethod, multi-informant agreement, and positive predictive value in the identification of child anxiety disorders using the SCAS and ADIS-C. *Assessment*. 2011 Sep;18(3):382–392

60. Allgaier AK, Krick K, Opitz A, Saravo B, Romanos M, Schulte-Körne G. Improving early detection of childhood depression in mental health care: the Children's Depression Screener (ChilD-S). *Psychiatry Res*. 2014;217(3):248–252

61. POTS Team. Cognitive-behavior therapy, sertraline, and their combination for children and adolescents with obsessive-compulsive disorder: the Pediatric OCD Treatment Study (POTS) randomized controlled trial. *JAMA*. 2004;292(16):1969–1976

62. Rynn MA, Walkup JT, Compton SN, et al. Child/adolescent anxiety multimodal study: evaluating safety. *J Am Acad Child Adolesc Psychiatry*. 2015;54(3):180–190

63. Uthman OA, Abdulmalik J. Comparative efficacy and acceptability of pharmacotherapeutic agents for anxiety disorders in children and adolescents: a mixed treatment comparison meta-analysis. *Curr Med Res Opin*. 2010;26(1):53–59

64. March J, Silva S, Petrycki S, et al. Fluoxetine, cognitive-behavioral therapy, and their combination for adolescents with depression: Treatment for Adolescents With Depression Study (TADS) randomized controlled trial. *JAMA*. 2004;292(7):807–820

65. Hetrick SE, McKenzie JE, Cox GR, Simmons MB, Merry SN. Newer generation antidepressants for depressive disorders in children and adolescents. *Cochrane Database Syst Rev.* 2012;11:CD004851

66. Correll CU, Kratochvil CJ, March JS. Developments in pediatric psychopharmacology: focus on stimulants, antidepressants, and antipsychotics. *J Clin Psychiatry.* 2011;72(5):655–670

67. Gibbons RD, Hur K, Brown CH, Davis JM, Mann JJ. Benefits from antidepressants: synthesis of 6-week patient-level outcomes from double-blind placebo-controlled randomized trials of fluoxetine and venlafaxine. *Arch Gen Psychiatry.* 2012;69(6):572–579

68. Brent D, Emslie G, Clarke G, et al. Switching to another SSRI or to venlafaxine with or without cognitive behavioral therapy for adolescents with SSRI-resistant depression: the TORDIA randomized controlled trial. *JAMA.* 2008;299(8):901–913

69. Friedman RA. Antidepressants' black-box warning—10 years later. *N Engl J Med* 2014 Oct 30;371(18):1666–1668

70. Rynn M, Puliafico A, Heleniak C, Rikhi P, Ghalib K, Vidair H. Advances in pharmacotherapy for pediatric anxiety disorders. *Depress Anxiety.* 2011;28(1):76–87

71. McPheeters ML, Warren Z, Sathe N, et al. A systematic review of medical treatments for children with autism spectrum disorders. *Pediatrics.* 2011;127(5):e1312–e1321

72. McDougle CJ, Scahill L, Aman MG, et al. Risperidone for the core symptom domains of autism: results from the study by the Autism Network of the of the Research Units on Pediatric Psychopharmacology. *Am J Psychiatry.* 2005;162(6):1142–1148

73. Hollander E, Soorya L, Wasserman S, et al. Divalproex sodium vs. placebo in the treatment of repetitive behaviours in autism spectrum disorder. *Int J Neuropsychopharmacol.* 2006;9(2):209–213

74. Chugani DC, Chugani HT, Wiznitzer M, et al. Efficacy of low-dose buspirone for restricted and repetitive behavior in young children with autism spectrum disorder: a randomized trial. *J Pediatr.* 2016;(Mar):45–53

75. Schnoes CJ, Kuhn BR, Workman EF, Ellis CR. Pediatric prescribing practices for clonidine and other pharmacologic agents for children with sleep disturbance. *Clin Pediatr (Phila).* 2006;45(3):229–238

76. Connor DF, Meltzer BM. Sleep disorders. In: *Pediatric Psychopharmacology Fast Facts,* New York, NY: W. W. Norton & Company, Inc.; 2006:493

77. Ferber R. The sleepless child. In: Guilleminault C, ed. *Sleep and Its Disorders in Children.* New York: Raven Press; 1987:141

78. Roux FJ, Kryger MH. Medication effects on sleep. *Clin Chest Med.* 2010; 31(2):397–405

79. Wasdell MB, Jan JE, Bomben MM, et al. A randomized, placebo-controlled trial of controlled release melatonin treatment of delayed sleep phase syndrome and impaired sleep maintenance in children with neurodevelopmental disabilities. *J Pineal Res.* 2008;44(1):57–64

80. Gringras P, Gamble C, Jones AP, et al. Melatonin for sleep problems in children with neurodevelopmental disorders: randomised double masked placebo controlled trial. *BMJ.* 2012; 345:e6664

CHAPTER 24

Complementary Health Approaches in Developmental and Behavioral Pediatrics

Thomas D. Challman, MD, FAAP

Scott M. Myers, MD, FAAP

Justin is a 4-year-old boy who was diagnosed with autism spectrum disorder (ASD) at the age of 2 years, when he presented with severe communication impairments, joint attention deficits, and repetitive behaviors. His parents come to your office with information they found on the Internet regarding a special diet that other parents have reported to be helpful for children with ASD. They also have some questions about the value of certain vitamins and other supplements. Justin is in a well-designed preschool program and is receiving intensive applied behavior analysis services. How should you address their concerns?

Primary pediatric health care professionals and caregivers should consider several important questions when evaluating the merits of a particular treatment that is being promoted for children with developmental-behavioral disorders. What is the scientific rationale and evidence regarding the use of these therapies individually or in combination for children with developmental-behavioral concerns? What are the potential risks of these therapies? Is it plausible that these approaches should be expected to have efficacy in improving the symptoms of a developmental-behavioral disorder based on what we already know about neuroscience and how the body works? How does one balance the desire of a parent to pursue a particular treatment with the right of a child not to be subjected to unsubstantiated therapies that may be ineffective or even harmful? And importantly, how do we help caregivers learn the skills they need to critically evaluate the large number of remedies popularized on the Internet and social media?

Complementary Health Approaches: Definition and Background

One of the challenges of assessing therapies that fall outside mainstream or standard medical care is the ill-defined and shifting boundary that differentiates these treatments from accepted medical practices. Many definitions for this group of therapies have been used over the years. Complementary and alternative medicine has been defined as "a broad domain of healing resources that encompasses all health systems, modalities, and practices and their accompanying theories and beliefs, other than those intrinsic to the politically dominant health systems of a particular society or culture in a given historical period,"[1] and as practices "not presently considered an integral part of conventional medicine."[2] The term *complementary medicine* has been used to describe nonstandard approaches that are used with conventional medicine, and the term *alternative medicine* has been used to refer to therapies that are a replacement for mainstream medical practices. The National Center for Complementary and Integrative Health (NCCIH), an NIH center, currently uses the term *complementary health approaches* (CHAs) when referring to treatments that fall outside the mainstream of standard medical care, and *integrative health* to convey the idea of using standard and nonstandard therapies in a coordinated manner.[3]

NCCIH categorizes CHAs into 2 main domains: natural products and mind-body practices. Natural products include botanical agents, vitamins, minerals, and special diets, whereas mind-body practices include such approaches as massage therapy, yoga, chiropractic, and acupuncture. The diversity and varied scientific plausibility of practices included under the umbrella of CHAs highlights the importance of evaluating the specific merits of individual therapies and methods (some of which, eg, vitamin supplements, may be considered either CHAs or conventional depending on the context in which they are being used).

The use of CHAs is common among adults,[4-6] and population-based data indicate that the use of these therapies is as high as 12% in the general pediatric population.[7-9] CHAs are used more commonly in children of parents who use these therapies themselves and are associated with higher levels of parental education.[10-13] Significant variability has been reported among selected outpatient and inpatient pediatric groups.[11,12,14-20] The use of CHAs does appear to be widespread among children with chronic medical conditions.[21-27] High rates of use have also been reported among children with developmental and behavioral disorders, including ASD, attention-deficit/hyperactivity disorder (ADHD), and other developmental-behavioral disorders.[13,28-40]

There has been increased interest in research into CHAs over the past 20 years. The National Center for Complementary and Alternative Medicine (renamed NCCIH) was created in 1998 for the purpose of investigating complementary and alternative practices using the methods of rigorous scientific study and disseminating authoritative information regarding CHAs to the public and professionals. Unfortunately, few NIH-funded projects related to CHAs have been directed at issues relevant to pediatrics, and limited information has been developed proving or disproving the value of specific complementary health approaches.

How to Evaluate Therapies

Families of children with developmental and behavioral disorders, and the clinicians caring for these children, should ask certain questions to help them identify therapies that have an insufficient evidence base or are scientifically implausible. These questions can be grouped into 3 main categories that pertain to the theoretical basis of the therapy, the evidence base of the therapy, and the tactics used to promote the therapy (Table 24.1[41,42]).

Table 24.1. Twelve Questions to Ask About a Complementary or Alternative Therapies[41,42]
Questions related to the underlying theoretical basis for the therapy
1. Is the treatment based on a theory that is overly simplistic?
2. Is the treatment based on proposed forces or principles that are inconsistent with accumulated knowledge from other scientific disciplines?
3. Has the treatment changed little over a very long period of time?
Questions related to the scientific evaluation of the therapy
4. Is it possible to test the treatment claim?
5. Have well-designed studies of the treatment been published in the peer-reviewed medical literature?
6. Do proponents of the treatment cherry-pick data that support the value of the treatment, while ignoring contradictory evidence?
7. Do proponents of the treatment assume a treatment is effective until there is sufficient evidence to the contrary?
8. Do proponents claim that a particular treatment cannot be studied in isolation but only in combination with a package of other interventions or practices?
Questions related to the promotion and marketing of the therapy
9. Is the treatment promoted as being free of adverse effects?
10. Is the treatment promoted primarily through the use of anecdotes?
11. Do proponents of the treatment use scientific-sounding but nonsensical terminology to describe the treatment?
12. Is the treatment promoted for a wide range of physiologically diverse conditions?

Evaluating the Theoretical Basis of a Therapy

Therapies considered complementary and alternative have diverse origins and arise from a variety of theoretical frameworks. The following questions can help identify therapies that have a weak theoretical foundation:

1. Is the treatment based on a theory that is overly simplistic?
2. Is the treatment based on proposed forces or principles that are inconsistent with accumulated knowledge from other scientific disciplines?
3. Has the treatment changed little over a very long period of time?

Many of the nonstandard therapies used in children with developmental-behavioral disorders are based on hypotheses that do not account for much of what we already know about the neurobiology of these disorders. For example, the belief that ASD is caused by a discrete toxic environmental insult has gained traction, facilitated by the rapid spread of misinformation on the Internet. While environmental factors that modify disease expression certainly should be explored even in disorders that have a strong genetic basis, therapies (eg, chelation therapy) based in a belief about the role of some environmental trigger are unjustified in the absence of good evidence that the particular environmental factor is actually etiologically related to the disorder. There should also not be a blind leap to link associated medical issues to the etiology of a particular developmental-behavioral disorder. For example, even if medical issues, such as gastrointestinal dysfunction, occur more commonly in children with ASD, it does not necessarily follow that these issues are causally related to the core neurobehavioral features—to contend otherwise necessitates that a body of evidence about the neurobiology of ASD be disregarded. While treating a GI problem, or any other associated medical problem, is certainly important for the overall health and comfort of a child with a developmental-behavioral disorder, the claim that treatment of these associated medical issues should ameliorate core neurobehavioral features is currently not supported by available evidence. One should look no further than trisomy 21 to find a disorder in which various gastrointestinal and immune abnormalities are common but not related in a cause-effect manner to the fundamental neurodevelopmental issues.

Certain complementary health approaches also appear to be quite disconnected from what we already understand about how the natural world works. Therapeutic touch, for example, is based on the belief that an energy "biofield" exists in proximity to the human body and that imbalances in this energy field are responsible for human disease (including developmental disturbances). Practitioners of therapeutic touch believe that this energy field can be manipulated manually and can result in objective improvements in some aspect of physical functioning. This theory is fundamentally inconsistent with much of the accumulated knowledge in biology and physics. While people may certainly experience subjective improvement in some symptom after undergoing therapeutic touch, the mechanism for this improvement is likely based in placebo effects and not in the adjustment of "energy" imbalances. Another energy-based practice, acupuncture, also illustrates the principle that therapies remaining unchanged for many years (or centuries) may not be undergoing the error correction that is a necessary element of scientific practices.

While the scientific investigation of novel therapies is an important pursuit and is a primary mission of NCCIH, some therapies do not merit any further study given that their underlying theoretical basis is so implausible or at odds with an accumulation of reliable, reproducible knowledge from other scientific disciplines. The appropriateness of considering plausibility in determining which novel therapies are worthy of formal investigation is especially relevant when research resources are limited.

Evaluating the Evidence Base for a Therapy

The question of whether a particular treatment can actually do what it claims to do is a fundamental issue that should concern clinicians who care for children with developmental-behavioral disorders. Several questions can shed light on whether there is an adequate evidence base to support the use of a specific therapy. Is it possible to test the treatment claim? Have well-designed studies of the treatment been published in the peer-reviewed medical literature? Do proponents of the treatment cherry-pick data that support the value of the treatment while ignoring contradictory evidence? Do proponents of the treatment assume a treatment is effective until there is sufficient evidence to the contrary? Do proponents claim that a particular treatment cannot be studied in isolation but only in combination with a package of other interventions or practices?

The evidence base for CHAs in developmental-behavioral disorders remains quite limited, and some of the most widely used therapies are not supported by any published studies. Summary recommendations for the use of various complementary health approaches in developmental-behavioral disorders are outlined in Table 24.2. There is insufficient evidence to indicate any broad value for the various alternative medical systems (traditional Chinese medicine, Ayurvedic medicine, naturopathy, and homeopathy) in the treatment of developmental-behavioral disorders. There have been efforts to test traditional Chinese medicine methods in developmental-behavioral disorders including ADHD, cerebral palsy, and intellectual disabilities, although significant methodological deficiencies limit any conclusions that can be drawn from these studies. Homeopathy, which has a highly questionable scientific basis, has not been shown to be beneficial in the treatment of ADHD.[43]

Mind-body practices, including sensory integration therapy, massage, auditory integration training, and chiropractic manipulation, have a similar lack of supporting evidence. Although sensory integration therapies enjoy widespread use among children with developmental-behavioral disorders, there is limited evidence supporting the therapeutic value of these methods,[44] and further rigorous research is needed. A number of studies of massage in infants have been published, but there is not convincing evidence of measurable developmental benefits in preterm or low birth weight infants or in children with ASD.[45,46] Similarly, there have been several trials of auditory integration training (which is based on the hypothesis that abnormal auditory perception contributes to various developmental and behavioral symptoms) in children with ASD, but there is not sufficient evidence to support its use.[47] Other manipulative or body-based practices, including optometric visual training, craniosacral therapy, and chiropractic manipulation, lack scientific plausibility and do not have any current role in the treatment of children with developmental-behavioral disorders. Children with trisomy 21 and atlantoaxial instability may be particularly susceptible to injury from chiropractic manipulation.

Table 24.2. Summary Recommendations for the Use of Selected Complementary and Alternative Therapies in Developmental-Behavioral Disorders Based on Available Evidence

Not recommended: insufficient or absent empiric support (or strong evidence of inefficacy), low plausibility

- Homeopathy
- Chiropractic
- Auditory integration therapy
- Vestibular stimulation
- Vision therapy, visual perceptual training
- Reflexology
- Craniosacral therapy
- Patterning, Doman-Delacato method
- Acupuncture
- Therapeutic touch
- Magnet therapy
- Reiki, Qi gong
- Hypnosis
- Pharmacological doses of vitamins (except in known metabolic disorders)
- Herbal remedies
- Chelation therapy
- Secretin in ASD
- Hyperbaric oxygen
- Antifungal agents
- Antiviral agents
- Antioxidants
- Immunoglobulins
- Stem cell therapy
- Gluten-free, casein-free diet in ASD

More research needed: limited empiric support, limited plausibility

- Biofeedback, EEG/EMG biofeedback
- Meditation, relaxation techniques
- Music therapy
- Massage
- Sensory integration therapy
- Omega-3 fatty acids
- Oxytocin
- Transcranial magnetic stimulation

Adequate empiric evidence to support current use

- Melatonin for prolonged sleep latency

Abbreviations: ASD, autism spectrum disorder; EEG, electroencephalogram; EMG, electromyogram.

Electroencephalographic biofeedback has been promoted for the treatment of children with ADHD and remains under investigation. However, it is not yet a well-validated treatment approach in this population. Meditation and relaxation training have been investigated in children with ADHD, cerebral palsy, and intellectual disabilities, and short-term improvements in certain behavioral measures have been observed in some studies.

Energy therapies, including therapeutic touch and acupuncture, are based in the belief that energy fields are present around all living organisms and that a disturbance in these fields is a cause of disease. There is no convincing evidence that acupuncture is beneficial in the treatment of any developmental-behavioral disorder, and most published studies have been uncontrolled or had unreliable outcome measures. There are no published studies of therapeutic touch in children with developmental-behavioral disorders, and the theoretical basis of this particular therapy remains highly questionable.

"Natural products" (as defined by NCCIH) include special diets, vitamins, supplements, and similar interventions. While these approaches can potentially have greater biological plausibility than many other complementary therapies, many also have weak or non-existent evidence of efficacy in the treatment of developmental-behavioral disorders. Dietary manipulations have long been used in attempts to effect a positive change in the behavior or developmental functioning of children with various disorders. The Feingold diet (based on the hypothesis that various food additives are the cause of hyperactive behavior) gained popularity in the 1970s, and early trials did not show any consistently positive effect.[48] Subsequent data have suggested the possibility that certain food additives may exert negative behavioral effects in subgroups of young children.[49] Oligoantigenic diets arose from the belief that food allergies may play a role in the etiology of hyperactive behavior. There are 6 controlled trials of oligoantigenic diets in children with ADHD between 1985 and 1997 listed in the Cochrane Central Register of Controlled Trials that have been reviewed both positively and negatively.[50,51] Effect sizes in these studies were not large. A more recent study indicated a beneficial effect of a carefully monitored elimination diet in a group of children with ADHD,[52] although a clear role for such an intervention in ADHD management remains undetermined.

The gluten- and casein-free (GF-CF) diet has gained widespread popularity in children with ASD. There have been several trials of this diet, which is based on the unproved hypothesis that peptides derived from gluten and casein cross into the bloodstream from the GI tract and subsequently exert a central nervous system effect that leads to behavioral abnormalities. Despite its widespread use, the scientific literature does not support the GF-CF diet as a treatment for children with ASD.[53–55]

Various vitamins, minerals, and other supplements are commonly used in ASD and other developmental-behavioral disorders.[32,34] Vitamin B_6 and magnesium are among the most widely studied supplements. While some investigations have shown apparent benefits, many of these studies had methodological shortcomings, and the best data currently do not support the combined use of these supplements in the treatment of ASD.[56] There has also been considerable interest in omega-3 fatty acids as a potential therapy for various developmental-behavioral disorders. At the present time, evidence remains inadequate to either support or refute the value of polyunsaturated fatty acid treatment in children with ADHD, specific learning disorders, or ASD.[57-59] Sleep disturbances are extremely common in children with developmental-behavioral disorders, and melatonin has been used as a treatment to shorten prolonged sleep latency and increase total sleep time. There is growing evidence that supports the use of melatonin for this purpose.[60]

More invasive nonstandard biomedical interventions in developmental-behavioral disorders include heavy metal chelation and hyperbaric oxygen therapy (HBOT). Chelation therapy has potentially serious adverse effects, including death.[61] In 2008, an NIH-funded study of chelation in ASD was suspended over safety concerns. Current evidence does not support a therapeutic role for chelation in the treatment of ASD.[62] HBOT remains popular in some regions for children with cerebral palsy and other developmental-behavioral disorders despite a lack of replicated experimental evidence showing any value in these conditions. A review in 2003 concluded that there is insufficient evidence to determine whether hyperbaric oxygen treatment improves functional outcome in children with cerebral palsy.[63] HBOT has also been promoted for the treatment of ASD. A recent systematic review identified one randomized controlled trial of hyperbaric oxygen in children with ASD.[64] In this single trial, there was no evidence of improvement in the core communication or behavioral features, and there was an increased risk of barotrauma in the treatment group.

Instead of following a logical, forward-moving process in which credible therapies are studied and either verified or discarded, the scientific community has commonly been forced to disprove the value of untenable therapies already in wide use. The use of secretin in ASD is one such example. A small case series published in 1998 reported improvement in language and social features in 3 children with ASD who had undergone diagnostic endoscopy.[65] The gastrointestinal hormone secretin, which had been used during these endoscopy procedures, subsequently was widely touted (on the Internet and in the media) as a therapy for ASD, and thousands of children were treated. However, numerous subsequent controlled trials indicated that secretin is no more effective than placebo.[66]

Certain complementary health approaches are framed in such a way that objective analysis of efficacy is discouraged. For example, some therapies (eg, therapeutic touch) have been described as being highly dependent on the skill of individual practitioners. This creates an environment in which studies that do not show benefit for the therapy can be more easily dismissed by believers. Another common ploy used to obscure evidence of inefficacy is for a claim to be made that a specific therapy cannot be studied in isolation; rather, a large package of interventions, or entire systems of care, must be evaluated. This makes the creation of an appropriately controlled study difficult and may serve to hide the fact that a particular therapy has no measurable benefit.

While it is appropriate to recognize that there are different levels of scientific evidence, not all evidence should be viewed as carrying equal weight. The evidence at the top of this hierarchy should most strongly inform clinical decision-making. Much of the evidence (for instance, individual anecdotes) that supports the value of CHAs in developmental-behavioral disorders does not even reach Level 5 in the Oxford Centre for Evidence-based Medicine classification of levels of evidence (Table 24.3)[67] and is woefully inadequate to support any positive recommendation for the use of these therapies. Unfortunately, even the peer-reviewed medical literature contains studies in which the conclusion of a positive effect of a particular treatment for children with a developmental-behavioral disorder is undercut by analytical flaws. It is crucial for primary pediatric health care professionals attempting to practice evidence-based medicine to read the peer-reviewed literature with an appropriately critical eye. Clinicians and researchers should continue to advocate for rigorous, well-designed clinical studies to prove or disprove the efficacy of specific complementary health approaches for children with developmental-behavioral disorders.[68]

Level	Evidence
Table 24.3. Oxford Centre for Evidence-based Medicine Levels of Evidence[67] (For definitions of terms used, see glossary at http://www.cebm.net/glossary/)	
1a	Systematic review (with homogeneity) of randomized controlled trials (RCT)
1b	Individual RCT (with narrow confidence interval)
1c	All or none*
2a	Systematic review (with homogeneity) of cohort studies
2b	Individual cohort study (including low-quality RCT; eg, <80% follow-up)
2c	"Outcomes" research; ecological studies
3a	Systematic review (with homogeneity) of case-control studies
3b	Individual case-control study
4	Case-series (and poor quality cohort and case-control studies)
5	Expert opinion without explicit critical appraisal, or based on physiology, bench research, or "first principles"

*Met when all patients died before the therapy became available, but some now survive on it, or when some patients died before the therapy became available, but none now die on it.

Adapted from Oxford Centre for Evidence-Based Medicine - Levels of Evidence 2009.

Evaluating the Strategies Used to Promote a Therapy

Additional useful information about a therapy can be gleaned from an analysis of the methods by which the therapy is promoted and marketed. Is the treatment promoted as being free of adverse effects? Is the treatment promoted primarily through the use of anecdotes? Does advertising for a therapy use scientific-sounding, but nonsensical, terminology? Is it promoted for a wide range of physiologically diverse conditions?

Certain treatments, particularly herbal remedies, may be advertised as natural, with the unspoken implication being that the therapy is safer than conventional medicines. This, of course, is not necessarily the case, and there are a variety of potential health risks associated with herbs and supplements.[69] Advocates for a particular CHA, when challenged about the safety of their therapy, may respond with the *tu quoque* logical error of pointing out the risks of conventional medical approaches. The safety of a therapy cannot be viewed in a strictly dichotomous fashion because treatments are never either safe or unsafe. Rather, the risks of a particular treatment need to be balanced against the anticipated benefits. Even a small risk of harm (physical or nonphysical) should not be accepted in a therapy that presents no prospect of benefit.

Complementary therapies are often promoted through the use of anecdotes and testimonials. The Internet has been a major driving force in the popularization of many of these therapies. Because of the various biases that inevitably color our perceptions of what we observe, however, anecdotes can never take the place of more objective methods of analysis (eg, controlled trials) that serve to minimize these biases. Any treatment promoted exclusively through testimonials should be viewed with great caution.

Therapies that are advertised as being effective for a wide range of diverse conditions also warrant increased scrutiny. It is often possible to construct a convoluted narrative that links multiple different health problems back to a single purported cause. Such narratives may appear to have a scientific veneer, but upon closer inspection have serious fundamental flaws. We should rightfully question whether disorders with quite different underlying physiological bases should be treatable with a single one-size-fits-all biomedical intervention. Any benefit observed from such a treatment is very likely nonspecific (ie, a placebo response) and not related to the proposed mechanism of action of the therapy.

Counseling Families of Children With Developmental-Behavioral Disorders About CHAs

Virtually every article written about the use of CHAs in children with chronic medical conditions concludes with the recommendation that medical professionals need to discuss the use of these therapies with the caregivers of these children. What, then, should be said? The American Academy of Pediatrics has suggested that providers increase their knowledge about nonstandard practices, be able to critically analyze the merits of specific therapies, identify potential safety risks, provide families with information about all therapeutic options, and emphasize the importance of investigating nonstandard practices using rigorous scientific methodology.[70] However, it is challenging to put such recommendations into practice when there is little or no reliable evidence of safety or efficacy to draw upon.

Even for complementary health approaches that have been tested in an appropriately rigorous manner, an all too common occurrence is that proponents develop such a strong belief in the therapy itself that they are blinded to the reality that all available evidence indicates the therapy has no greater benefit than a placebo. When this occurs, believers in the therapy often propose further investigation (to study an ever-smaller component of an herb, a different patient population, etc.) in an effort to continue the search for evidence that the therapy has value. Caregivers of children with developmental-behavioral disorders may also consider evidence of inefficacy in an idiosyncratic manner. One of the first controlled trials of secretin in children with ASD showed that secretin was no more effective than placebo in improving behavioral and communication features.[71] Despite these findings, when parents of the participants in this study were informed of the negative results, a large percentage expressed interest in continuing the treatments. This suggests that caregivers of children with developmental-behavioral disorders may be considerably influenced by factors other than what the scientific community considers acceptable evidence regarding their decisions about which treatments to pursue for their children. One potential explanation is that when anxiety is high as a consequence of having a child with a condition that has unclear etiology and uncertain outcome, a caregiver may have a greater likelihood of adopting a belief that might be viewed as unscientific. Such beliefs can be powerfully reinforced by the social milieu (eg, support groups or social media) in which parents may find themselves immersed. A major challenge for the scientific community is to find new ways to actively influence these networks to accept and disseminate accurate, scientifically supported information. It remains to be seen whether the most vocal proponents of CHAs are willing to change their practices in response to scientific evidence; unfortunately, the fact that some therapies with solid evidence of inefficacy are still commonly used in children with developmental-behavioral disorders suggests otherwise.

The need for primary pediatric health care professionals to be accepting of diverse healing traditions is commonly invoked as a reason why CHAs should not be marginalized by the medical community.[72] However, only a small minority of caregivers of children with ASD cite cultural reasons as important in their decision to pursue a particular complementary health approach.[32] Analysis of other surveys of CHAs in children with ASD illustrates that most of the therapies that are being commonly used have their origins in scientifically implausible beliefs about the etiology of the disorder, as opposed to being associated with any particular cultural or religious tradition.[31,33,34]

Primary pediatric health care professionals need to use several different approaches when discussing CHAs with families. Families should be strongly advised to avoid those therapies that are clearly risky and have insufficient evidence of efficacy (for example, chelation therapy in ASD). Therapies for which there is adequate evidence of safety and efficacy in children with developmental-behavioral disorders should be recommended; however, few complementary health approaches currently fall into this category. A larger group of therapies may have some degree of potential plausibility but have not been adequately tested. These therapies should not yet be promoted but should undergo more rigorous clinical investigation. Finally, the small number of practices that are clearly part of cultural or religious traditions can usually be supported, assuming there are no major anticipated safety concerns. Primary pediatric health care professionals should not be afraid to use reasoned arguments to dissuade families from pursuing inappropriate therapies because no one else may be willing or able to confront the health fads that have the potential to create risks for children with developmental-behavioral disorders and their families.

Ethical Considerations

The story of Justin at the beginning of this chapter highlights some of complexities inherent in evaluating the ethics of complementary health approaches in children with developmental-behavioral disorders. Principles that need to be considered within an ethical framework include beneficence, nonmaleficence, autonomy, justice, and truthfulness. In the case of the use of CHAs in children, these principles may come into direct conflict with one another, and clinicians must give careful attention to each when rendering advice about nonstandard medical practices.

A primary pediatric health care professional has the responsibility to administer therapies that are beneficial to the patient and society. The importance of basing treatment decisions on the best available evidence is paramount—as is the need for the scientific community to continue to develop reliable and valid evidence. It is challenging to know, however, whether the principle of beneficence is truly being upheld in situations where there is no reliable data supporting the value of a therapy, or if all we have are indirect or weak surrogate outcome measures (eg, parental perceptions of the effectiveness of the therapy). An equally difficult situation arises when the safety of a nonstandard therapy is considered. Again, safety data for many commonly used CHAs are lacking. In a child who is receiving multiple therapies with unproven efficacy but that are broadly safe, how should we consider the aggregate burden on the child and family? At some point, this approach could be viewed as primarily fulfilling a need to do something as opposed to actually contributing to the well-being of the child. Primary pediatric health care professionals need to continue to carefully balance the principles of beneficence, nonmaleficence, and autonomy in deciding whether it is justifiable to recommend (or tacitly support) a treatment that is ineffective, lacks a sufficient evidence base, or is based on an implausible, underlying theoretical framework.

The ethical principle of justice often relates to the fair allocation of medical resources and treatments. This principle has been invoked in discussions regarding the lack of access to CHAs.[73] Consideration should also be given, however, to the flip side of this argument. In situations in which CHA proponents promote attitudes that decrease the use of medical practices (eg, immunizations[74]) that have clear individual and public health value, the unjust distribution of health services may be a collateral result of nonstandard therapies. Time spent in an ineffective therapy may also detract from the pursuit of other interventions known to be effective (particularly if the cost of the ineffective therapy creates undue financial burdens for the family).

Placebo and other expectancy effects may account for a significant proportion of the benefit perceived by users of CHAs. Some proponents would argue that the mechanism of efficacy is less important than the fact that benefit occurs. In fact, the use of *de facto* placebos may be quite common in conventional medical practice as well.[75] The deception that occurs, however, when a provider prescribes an innocuous but ineffective therapy purely to achieve some degree of placebo effect runs counter to the ethical principle of truthfulness. Although a potential role for the clinical use of placebos in developmental-behavioral pediatrics has been suggested,[76] a consensus has not been reached on the appropriateness of this notion.

Conclusion

Although the use of CHAs is widespread among children with developmental-behavioral disorders, there is a paucity of reliable data supporting the value of most of these approaches. Some treatments that have their origin as a complementary or alternative therapy may ultimately develop a sufficient evidence base that supports their widespread use. Until this occurs, medical professionals should remain appropriately skeptical, and the rational scientific community needs to remain on guard against therapies, whether viewed as complementary or conventional, whose use is not justified by the available evidence.[77] Pediatricians in the medical home benefit from a continuous, longitudinal relationship with patients and their families. When a primary pediatric health care professional builds a therapeutic relationship with a family through a trusting, open relationship, the family is likely to be more willing to disclose CHA use and to consider clinician advice regarding these therapies. Truly family-centered care should include efforts to teach families of children with developmental-behavioral disorders to evaluate therapeutic claims critically and to clearly understand the potential hazards (physical, emotional, and financial) that can accompany the use of unproved therapies.

References

1. Zollman C, Vickers A. What is complementary medicine? *BMJ*. 1999;319(7211):693–696
2. National Center for Complementary and Alternative Medicine, ed. *Expanding Horizons of Healthcare: Five Year Strategic Plan 2001–2005*. Washington, DC: US Department of Health and Human Services; 2000
3. National Center for Complementary and Integrative Health. Complementary, alternative, or integrative health: what's in a name? https://nccih.nih.gov/health/integrative-health. Updated June 2016. Accessed December 26, 2017
4. Barnes PM, Powell-Griner E, McFann K, Nahin RL. Complementary and alternative medicine use among adults: United States, 2002. *Adv Data*. 2004;343:1–19
5. Stussman BJ, Black LI, Barnes PM, Clarke TC, Nahin RL. Wellness-related use of common complementary health approaches among adults: United States, 2012. *Natl Health Stat Report*. 2015(85):1–12
6. Posadzki P, Watson LK, Alotaibi A, Ernst E. Prevalence of use of complementary and alternative medicine (CAM) by patients/consumers in the UK: systematic review of survey. *Clin Med*. 2013;13(2):126–131
7. Yussman SM, Ryan SA, Auinger P, Weitzman M. Visits to complementary and alternative medicine providers by children and adolescents in the United States. *Ambul Pediatr*. 2004;4(5):429–435
8. Davis MP, Darden PM. Use of complementary and alternative medicine by children in the United States. *Arch Pediatr Adolesc Med*. 2003;157(4):393–396
9. Black LI, Clarke TC, Barnes PM, Stussman BJ, Nahin RL. Use of complementary health approaches among children aged 4–17 years in the United States: National Health Interview Survey, 2007–2012. *Natl Health Stat Report*. 2015(78):1–19
10. Davis MF, Meaney FJ, Duncan B. Factors influencing the use of complementary and alternative medicine in children. *J Altern Complement Med*. 2004;10(5):740–742
11. Sawni-Sikand A, Schubiner H, Thomas RL. Use of complementary/alternative therapies among children in primary care pediatrics. *Ambul Pediatr*. 2002;2(2):99–103
12. Spigelblatt L, Laine-Ammara G, Pless IB, Guyver A. The use of alternative medicine by children. *Pediatrics*. 1994;94(6 Pt 1):811–814
13. Akins RS, Krakowiak P, Angkustsiri K, Hertz-Picciotto I, Hansen RL. Utilization patterns of conventional and complementary/alternative treatments in children with autism spectrum disorders and developmental disabilities in a population-based study. *J Dev Behav Pediatr*. 2014;35(1):1–10

14. Ottolini MC, Hamburger EK, Loprieato JO, et al. Complementary and alternative medicine use among children in the Washington, DC area. *Ambul Pediatr.* 2001;1(2):122–125

15. Simpson N, Roman K. Complementary medicine use in children: extent and reasons. A population-based study. *Br J Gen Pract.* 2001;51(472):914–916

16. Wilson KM, Klein JD. Adolescents' use of complementary and alternative medicine. *Ambul Pediatr.* 2002;2(2):104–110

17. Madsen H, Andersen S, Nielsen RG, et al. Use of complementary/alternative medicine among paediatric patients. *Eur J Pediatr.* 2003;162(5):334–341

18. Sibinga EM, Ottolini MC, Duggan AK, Wilson MH. Parent-pediatrician communication about complementary and alternative medicine use for children. *Clin Pediatr (Phila).* 2004;43(4):367–373

19. Jean D, Cyr C. Use of complementary and alternative medicine in a general pediatric clinic. *Pediatrics.* 2007;120(1):e138–e141

20. Robinson N, Blair M, Lorenc A, et al. Complementary medicine use in multi-ethnic paediatric outpatients. *Complement Ther Clin Pract.* 2008;14(1):17–24

21. Feldman DE, Duffy C, De Civita M, et al. Factors associated with the use of complementary and alternative medicine in juvenile idiopathic arthritis. *Arthritis Rheum.* 2004;51(4):527–532

22. Junker J, Oberwittler C, Jackson D, Berger K. Utilization and perceived effectiveness of complementary and alternative medicine in patients with dystonia. *Mov Disord.* 2004;19(2):158–161

23. Magi T, Kuehni CE, Torchetti L, et al. Use of complementary and alternative medicine in children with cancer: a study at a Swiss university hospital. *PLoS One.* 2015;10(12):e0145787

24. Markowitz JE, Mamula P, delRosario JF, et al. Patterns of complementary and alternative medicine use in a population of pediatric patients with inflammatory bowel disease. *Inflamm Bowel Dis.* 2004;10(5):599–605

25. Sidora-Arcoleo K, Yoos HL, McMullen A, Kitzman H. Complementary and alternative medicine use in children with asthma: prevalence and sociodemographic profile of users. *J Asthma.* 2007;44(3):169–175

26. Vlieger AM, Blink M, Tromp E, Benninga MA. Use of complementary and alternative medicine by pediatric patients with functional and organic gastrointestinal diseases: results from a multicenter survey. *Pediatrics.* 2008;122(2):e446–e451

27. Adams D, Dagenais S, Clifford T, et al. Complementary and alternative medicine use by pediatric specialty outpatients. *Pediatrics.* 2013;131(2):225–232

28. Höfer J, Hoffmann F, Bachmann C. Use of complementary and alternative medicine in children and adolescents with autism spectrum disorder: a systematic review. *Autism.* 2017;21(4):387–402

29. Kaale A, Roge B, Bonnet-Brilhaut F, et al. Prevalence and correlates of use of complementary and alternative medicine in children with autism spectrum disorder in Europe. *Eur J Pediatr.* 2015;174(10):1277–1285

30. Perrin JM, Coury DL, Hyman SL, et al. Complementary and alternative medicine use in a large pediatric autism sample. *Pediatrics.* 2012;130(suppl 2):S77–S82

31. Levy SE, Mandell DS, Merhar S, Ittenbach RF, Pinto-Martin JA. Use of complementary and alternative medicine among children recently diagnosed with autistic spectrum disorder. *J Dev Behav Pediatr.* 2003;24(6):418–423

32. Hanson E, Kalish LA, Bunce E, et al. Use of complementary and alternative medicine among children diagnosed with autism spectrum disorder. *J Autism Dev Disord.* 2007;37(4):628–636

33. Harrington JW, Rosen L, Garnecho A, Patrick PA. Parental perceptions and use of complementary and alternative medicine practices for children with autistic spectrum disorders in private practice. *J Dev Behav Pediatr.* 2006;27(suppl 2):S156–S61

34. Wong HH, Smith RG. Patterns of complementary and alternative medical therapy use in children diagnosed with autism spectrum disorders. *J Autism Dev Disord.* 2006;36(7):901–909

35. Bussing R, Zima BT, Gary FA, Garvan CW. Use of complementary and alternative medicine for symptoms of attention-deficit hyperactivity disorder. *Psychiatr Serv.* 2002;53(9):1096–1102

36. Gross-Tsur V, Lahad A, Shalev RS. Use of complementary medicine in children with attention deficit hyperactivity disorder and epilepsy. *Pediatr Neurol.* 2003;29(1):53–55

37. Sinha D, Efron D. Complementary and alternative medicine use in children with attention deficit hyperactivity disorder. *J Paediatr Child Health.* 2005;41(1–2):23–26

38. Hurvitz EA, Leonard C, Ayyangar R, Nelson VS. Complementary and alternative medicine use in families of children with cerebral palsy. *Dev Med Child Neurol.* 2003;45(6):364–370

39. Prussing E, Sobo EJ, Walker E, Dennis K, Kurtin PS. Communicating with pediatricians about complementary/alternative medicine: perspectives from parents of children with Down syndrome. *Ambul Pediatr.* 2004;4(6):488–494

40. Sanders H, Davis MF, Duncan B, et al. Use of complementary and alternative medical therapies among children with special health care needs in southern Arizona. *Pediatrics.* 2003;111(3):584–587

41. Lilienfeld SO, Lynn SJ, Lohr JM, eds. *Science and Pseudoscience in Clinical Psychology.* New York, NY: Guilford Press; 2003

42. Nickel R. Controversial therapies for young children with developmental disabilities. *Infants Young Child.* 1996;8:29–40

43. Coulter MK, Dean ME. Homeopathy for attention deficit/hyperactivity disorder or hyperkinetic disorder. *Cochrane Database Syst Rev.* 2007(4):005648

44. Weitlauf AS, Sathe NA, McPheeters ML, Warren Z; Agency for Healthcare Research and Quality. Interventions targeting sensory challenges in children with autism spectrum disorder—an update. *Comparative Effectiveness Review No. 186.* AHRQ publication 17-EHC004-EF. https://effectivehealthcare.ahrq.gov/topics/asd-interventions/research-2017/. Published May 2017. Accessed November 16, 2017

45. Vickers A, Ohlsson A, Lacy JB, Horsley A. Massage for promoting growth and development of preterm and/or low birth-weight infants. *Cochrane Database Syst Rev.* 2004;(2):000390

46. Lee MS, Kim JI, Ernst E. Massage therapy for children with autism spectrum disorders: a systematic review. *J Clin Psychiatry.* 2011;72(3):406–411

47. Sinha Y, Silove N, Hayen A, Williams K. Auditory integration training and other sound therapies for autism spectrum disorders (ASD). *Cochrane Database Syst Rev.* 2011;(12):CD003681

48. Wender, EH. The food additive-free diet in the treatment of behavior disorders: a review. *J Dev Behav Pediatr.* 1986(7):35–42

49. Bateman B, Warner JO, Hutchinson E, et al. The effects of a double blind, placebo controlled, artificial food colourings and benzoate preservative challenge on hyperactivity in a general population sample of preschool children. *Arch Dis Child.* 2004(89):506–511

50. Arnold LE. Alternative/complementary treatments for attention deficit hyperactivity disorder. In: Rogers BT, Montgomery TR, Lock TM, Accardo PJ, eds. *Attention Deficit Hyperactivity Disorder: The Clinical Spectrum.* Baltimore, MD: York Press; 2001:197–207

51. Accardo PJ. Other therapies. In: Accardo PJ, Blondis TA, Whitman BY, Stein MA, eds. *Attention Deficits and Hyperactivity in Children and Adults.* 2nd ed. New York, NY: Marcel Dekker; 2000:633–651

52. Pelsser LM, Frankena K, Toorman J, et al. A randomised controlled trial into the effects of food on ADHD. *Eur Child Adolesc Psychiatry.* 2009(18):12–9

53. Millward C, Ferriter M, Calver S, Connell-Jones G. Gluten- and casein-free diets for autistic spectrum disorder. *Cochrane Database Syst Rev.* 2008;(2):003498

54. Hyman SL, Stewart PA, Foley J, et al. The gluten-free/casein-free diet: a double-blind challenge trial in children with autism. *J Autism Dev Disord.* 2016;46(1):205–220

55. Sathe N, Andrews JC, McPheeters ML, Warren ZE. Nutritional and dietary interventions for autism spectrum disorder: a systematic review. *Pediatrics.* 2017;139(6):pii: e20170346

56. Nye C, Brice A. Combined vitamin B_6-magnesium treatment in autism spectrum disorder. *Cochrane Database Syst Rev.* 2005;(4):CD003497

57. Gillies D, Sinn JKH, Lad SS, Leach MJ, Ross MJ. Polyunsaturated fatty acids (PUFA) for attention deficit hyperactivity disorder (ADHD) in children and adolescents. *Cochrane Database Syst Rev.* 2012;(7):CD007986

58. Tan M, Ho JJ, Teh K. Polyunsaturated fatty acids (PUFAs) for children with specific learning disorders. *Cochrane Database Syst Rev.* 2016;(9):CD009398

59. Voigt RG, Mellon MW, Katusic SK, et al. Dietary docosahexaenoic acid supplementation in children with autism. *J Pediatr Gastroenterol Nutr.* 2014 Jun;58(6):715–722

60. Schwichtenberg AJ; Malow BA. Melatonin treatment in children with developmental disabilities. *Sleep Med Clin.* 10(2):181–187

61. Brown MJ, Willis T, Omalu B, Leiker R. Deaths resulting from hypocalcemia after administration of edetate disodium: 2003–2005. *Pediatrics.* 2006;118(2):e534–e536

62. James S, Stevenson SW, Silove N, Williams K. Chelation for autism spectrum disorder (ASD). *Cochrane Database Syst Rev.* 2015;(5):CD010766

63. McDonagh M, Carson S, Ash J. *Hyperbaric Oxygen Therapy for Brain Injury, Cerebral Palsy, and Stroke.* Rockville, MD: Agency for Healthcare Research and Quality, US Department of Health and Human Services; 2003. AHRQ publication 03-E050. https://archive.ahrq.gov/downloads/pub/evidence/pdf/hypox/hyperox.pdf. Published September 2003. Accessed December 26, 2017

64. Xiong T, Chen H, Luo R, Mu D. Hyperbaric oxygen therapy for people with autism spectrum disorder (ASD). *Cochrane Database Syst Rev.* 2016;(10):CD010922

65. Horvath K, Stefanatos G, Sokolski KN, et al. Improved social and language skills after secretin administration in patients with autistic spectrum disorders. *J Assoc Acad Minor Phys.* 1998;9(1):9–15

66. Williams K, Wray JA, Wheeler DM. Intravenous secretin for autism spectrum disorders (ASD). *Cochrane Database Syst Rev.* 2012;(4):CD003495

67. Oxford Centre for Evidence-Based Medicine Web site. http://www.cebm.net/oxford-centre-evidence-based-medicine-levels-evidence-march-2009/. Accessed December 26, 2017

68. Dawson G. Questions remain regarding the effectiveness of many commonly used autism treatments. *Pediatrics.* 2017;139(6):e20170730

69. Lee JY, Jun SA, Hong SS, et al. Systematic review of adverse effects from herbal drugs reported in randomized controlled trials. *Phytotherapy Research.* 2016;30(9):1412–1419

70. American Academy of Pediatrics Committee on Children With Disabilities. Counseling families who choose complementary and alternative medicine for their child with chronic illness or disability. *Pediatrics.* 2001;107(3):598–601

71. Sandler AD, Sutton KA, DeWeese J, et al. Lack of benefit of a single dose of synthetic human secretin in the treatment of autism and pervasive developmental disorder. *N Engl J Med.* 1999;341(24):1801–1806

72. Kaptchuk TJ, Eisenberg DM. Varieties of healing. 1: medical pluralism in the United States. *Ann Intern Med.* 2001;135(3):189–195

73. Vohra S, Cohen MH. Ethics of complementary and alternative medicine use in children. *Pediatr Clin North Am.* 2007;54(6):875–884

74. Busse JW, Kulkarni AV, Campbell JB, Injeyan HS. Attitudes toward vaccination: a survey of Canadian chiropractic students. *CMAJ.* 2002;166(12):1531–1534

75. Tilburt JC, Emanuel EJ, Kaptchuk TJ, Curlin FA, Miller FG. Prescribing "placebo treatments": results of national survey of US internists and rheumatologists. *BMJ.* 2008;337:a1938

76. Sandler A. Placebo effects in developmental disabilities: implications for research and practice. *Ment Retard Dev Disabil Res Rev.* 2005;11(2):164–170

77. Singer A; Ravi R. Complementary and alternative treatments for autism part 2: identifying and avoiding non-evidence-based treatments. *AMA J Ethics.* 2015;17(4):375–380

CHAPTER 25

Social and Community Services for Children With Developmental Disabilities and/or Behavioral Disorders and Their Families

Dinah L. Godwin, MSW, LCSW

Sherry Sellers Vinson, MD, MEd, FAAP

Introduction

Developmental disabilities and many behavioral disorders are lifelong chronic conditions with no medical cures. Even acute behavioral disorders that seem to resolve are often rooted in a child's neurobiology, from which other behavior problems may arise over a lifetime (see Chapter 11, Making Developmental-Behavioral Diagnoses). While modern medicine provides pharmacological treatments to decrease symptoms of these conditions, patients and their families continue to present to their primary pediatric health care professionals with problems that are not amenable to medication alone. While not always easy to find, there are both governmental and nonprofit programs available to support children with chronic developmental-behavioral disorders and their families. The American Academy of Pediatrics (AAP) emphasizes that primary pediatric health care professionals should provide a medical home for these patients— linking them and their families to appropriate services and resources, including community-based resources—in a coordinated effort to achieve optimal outcomes.[1] Research has indicated that families of children with developmental-behavioral disorders want their primary pediatric health care professionals to help coordinate their children's care in the manner advised by the AAP, including putting them in touch with parents of children with similar disorders.[2] For these reasons, primary pediatric health care professionals need to be familiar with social and community services available to children with developmental disabilities and behavioral disorders and their families.

Care Coordination and Case Management

From the time of the initial diagnosis of a developmental disability or behavioral disorder, primary pediatric health care professionals make multiple recommendations for their patients that involve accessing services provided by a third party not under the clinician's or parent's control. For example, primary care clinicians often write orders or make recommendations for therapies (eg, speech, occupational, physical, or behavioral therapies), school services (eg, remedial special educational instruction or accommodations and modifications), and evaluations in other clinics (eg, audiology, ophthalmology, or medical genetics); some of these may require the patient's parent to be reliant on a third party with regard to scheduling and payment. The need for additional third parties to address new situations continues for life, given the chronic nature of many developmental-behavioral disorders. This can cause patients, their caregivers, and their health care professionals ongoing stress due to lack of control. Both primary care clinicians and parents of individuals with developmental-behavioral disorders report confusion over the exact services needed from each of the third parties, frustration over wait times for appointments, and inconsistency regarding insurance or Medicaid coverage for the services.[3,4]

Primary pediatric health care professionals' designation of a care coordinator and provision of care coordination services within their practices help clinicians navigate the health care system and access needed services for all of their patients, including those with developmental-behavioral disorders. Building such care coordination services within a pediatric practice is one of the emphasized cornerstones of the AAP family-centered medical home model, so much so that the AAP provides the tools for such coordination through a Web site (**https://medicalhomeinfo.aap.org**; click on the "Tools and Resources" link on the home page). This Web site also has information regarding Title V Maternal and Child Health Bureau's children with special health care needs programs and other resources and services available in individual states under "National and State Initiatives" located at the top of the home page.

Various agencies, insurance plans, and most state Medicaid programs offer case managers who can serve as care coordinators for eligible patients. This care coordination is limited to patients meeting inclusion criteria for having a case manager. In the cases of patients eligible for such a service through a managed care organization, the role of the case manager may be limited to seeking only the services aimed at disease management, with no coordination for educational, social support, or secondary behavioral health needs. In light of these possible limitations with use of outside sources, care coordination within the primary care pediatric practice is preferred, since these services would be available to all patients, addressing all condition-related needs and not simply those considered a medical treatment.[5] At times, however, the use of an outside case manager might be needed. The Henry J. Kaiser Family Foundation Web site provides helpful information about each state's Medicaid case management services (**kff.org/medicaid/state-indicator/targeted-case-management**).

Effective care coordination links families to individuals who can (1) help caregivers understand the health care needs of their child and maintain their child's health history; (2) provide information regarding their child's medical condition; (3) identify the medical, social, educational, and mental health services their child may need; (4) assist in applying for services for which the child is eligible; (5) develop a written comprehensive plan of care; (6) arrange for services to be provided and monitor the provision of services; (7) follow up on referrals; (8) arrange for transportation; and (9) coordinate

593

Chapter 25: Social and Community Services for Children With Developmental Disabilities
and/or Behavioral Disorders and Their Families

among service providers.[6] The staff member chosen to be the care coordinator can vary, although there are some indications that the most effective choice with regard to cost and family satisfaction would be a nurse.[7]

Addressing specific nonmedical needs of individuals with developmental-behavioral disorders and their families has various benefits. One study showed that care coordination in the context of a patient-centered medical home helped alleviate the economic burden on families of children with attention-deficit/hyperactivity disorder (ADHD).[8] Another study showed that having an individual provide case management and counseling for grandparents raising grandchildren with developmental disabilities increased the grandparents' sense of empowerment and caregiving mastery while decreasing their depressive symptoms.[9] Case managers also seem to be the key to successful vocational programs for children with developmental disabilities transitioning to adulthood, and they offer hope for reducing the maltreatment of children with disabilities, estimated to be around 3 to 4 times higher than the maltreatment of children without disabilities.[10,11] Care coordination seems to improve continuity of care, decreases delayed or missed services, and improves caregiver satisfaction with medical care.[12,13] Such coordination also seems to reduce fragmented or duplicative care, length and cost of hospital stays, and caregiver stress.[14] Unfortunately, despite the evidence base for care coordination, many families continue to report difficulty accessing these services. In a study involving parents of children with autism spectrum disorder, only 14% of parents who needed care coordination felt that they received the services they needed. The more highly resourced parents in this study (ie, white, English-speaking parents with higher educational levels and private insurance coverage) reported the greatest gaps between their perceived need and receipt of adequate care coordination support.[15] In general, parents of children with autism report significantly more difficulty accessing services than parents of children with other developmental disabilities or behavioral disorders,indicating the critical importance of implementing care coordination systems for these families.[16]

Children's Mental Health Services

The 2009–2010 National Survey of Children with Special Health Care Needs showed that of the approximately 12,042 children in the survey with a chronic emotional, behavioral, or developmental problem, 27.6% of those children required counseling or other mental health services.[17] However, 5.6% of children with special health care needs were not able to receive these services. Mental health services were the most common unmet need reported, particularly for low-income and uninsured children.[17] These data are consistent with findings over the past 30 years.[18] Among children receiving special education services, emotional and behavioral problems are now the most frequently reported reason for limitations in the children's daily activities.[19] Even among young children (from birth to 3 years of age) with developmental disabilities, a significant number have behavior problems consistent with a psychiatric disorder, including tantrums, aggression, oppositional behaviors, hyperactivity, and self-injury.[20] Intervention from behavioral health providers, including behavior therapists and/or psychiatrists, is essential in helping to ameliorate the impact of these behaviors on the child and family. Caring for a child with mental health care needs affects the financial well-being and family caregiving burden more than caring for a child with other special health care needs.[21]

Undoubtedly, primary pediatric health care professionals and their office staff who are aware of and can access children's mental health services, while counseling families to alleviate some of the stigma of referral to a mental health provider, can offer hope to the numbers of families projected to have such needs in their practices. Primary pediatric health care professionals can obtain information about state and local mental health services through the National Alliance on Mental Illness (**www.nami.org**) and Mental Health America (**www.mentalhealthamerica.net**). Another Web site, **www.psychologytoday.com**, provides links to psychiatrists, psychotherapists, and other behavioral health providers by city, state, or zip code.

Supplemental Medical Insurance and Other Financial Assistance Programs

The cost of raising a child with a developmental-behavioral disorder can be staggering for families. A recent study found that the lifetime cost of raising a child with autism, for example, was $1.4 million, and the cost of raising a child with both autism and an intellectual disability was $2.4 million. The most significant financial factors involved the expenses associated with lost parental productivity as well as the cost of special education services.[22] The Medical Expenditure Panel Surveys of 1999 and 2000 targeting families of youth with disabilities younger than 18 years revealed that these families paid approximately 11% of health care bills out of pocket, with the financial burden worse on families having the most severely affected children, the lowest incomes, and/or the least health insurance.[23] The 2009–2010 National Survey of Children with Special Health Care Needs reported that 21.6% of families of the youth with chronic physical, developmental, behavioral, or emotional conditions on the survey list reported that their child's health care caused financial problems, and 25% of these surveyed families had to cut back or quit work because of their child's condition. In addition, 23.6% of the surveyed families reported their children experienced unmet health care needs.[17] Despite the availability of Medicaid and the State Children's Health Insurance Program (SCHIP) to low-income parents with uninsured children with developmental-behavioral disorders, many parents who qualify for these programs report not using them due to the belief that they are not eligible for the programs or because they feel that the application process is too difficult.[24] Expansion of insurance coverage options available through the health care marketplace as part of the Patient Protection and Affordable Care Act (ACA) has reduced the number of uninsured individuals; however, children, including those with special health care needs, were not a priority in the development of the ACA, as adults comprised the majority of the uninsured population.[25] Given these factors, it is critical for primary pediatric health care professionals or their office

595

Chapter 25: Social and Community Services for Children With Developmental Disabilities
and/or Behavioral Disorders and Their Families

staff to know how to guide families in accessing and applying for supplemental medical insurance and other financial assistance programs that may be available to children with developmental-behavioral disorders and their families.

A key financial assistance program for children with disabilities is Supplemental Security Income (SSI), which provides a monthly financial benefit to families of children with disabilities who meet financial eligibility criteria. Primary pediatric health care professionals can assist families by providing a clear, concise summary of medical records that document the child's disability to the Social Security Administration. In addition, health care professionals who work with children with disabilities should become familiar with the Medicaid waiver programs in their state, as these provide funding and supplemental services to individuals with disabilities with the goal of helping families with their caregiving needs. Some states have long waiting lists for these Medicaid waiver services, so primary pediatric health care professionals should refer families to these programs as early as possible. Helpful Web sites for clinicians to learn more about financial assistance programs for children and families are included in Table 25.1.

Table 25.1. Financial Assistance Web Sites		
Web Address	**Agency Name**	**Information Available**
www.ssa.gov	Social Security Administration	Supplemental Security Income (SSI), Social Security Disability Insurance (SSDI), and other Social Security benefits
www.healthcare.gov	Federal Web site administered by the Centers for Medicare and Medicaid Services	Public and private insurance options, including those available through the health care marketplace
www.hhs.gov	US Department of Health and Human Services	Temporary Assistance for Needy Families (TANF), Supplemental Nutrition Assistance Program (SNAP), and other social service programs
www.benefits.gov	Official benefits Web site of the US government	State-specific information on governmental programs, including public insurance benefits, TANF, SNAP, and other social service programs

Educational and Advocacy Services

Because primary pediatric health care professionals are often the first individuals to express a concern regarding a child's development or behavior or the first with whom parents share a concern, they are in a unique position to be able to access appropriate early childhood and special education services for their patients. Children with developmental-behavioral disorders may need special education and related services to be successful in school. Strock-Lynskey and Keller[26] detail the history of special education laws beginning with Section 504 of the Rehabilitation Act of 1973. This Act was the impetus for subsequent laws that provide civil rights protections to individuals with special needs, require rehabilitation services in schools, and prohibit discrimination by institutions receiving federal funds. The first law governing the provision of special education services was passed in 1975 with the Education of All Handicapped Children Act (EHA, PL 94–142), which established the right to a *free and appropriate education* for all children with disabilities from 5 to 21 years of age in the *least restrictive environment,* regardless of the functioning level of the child's abilities. In 1986, an amendment to the EHA extended the provision of special educational services to include early childhood intervention for children from birth to 3 years of age and special education to children from 3 to 5 years of age. In 1990, PL 94–142 was reauthorized and renamed the Individuals with Disabilities Education Act (IDEA, PL 101–476). IDEA has been amended twice, in 1997 and 2004, with one of the 2004 provisions emphasizing a family-centered approach by "strengthening the role and responsibility of parents and ensuring that families of such children have meaningful opportunities to participate in the education of their children at school and at home."[27] These laws have also been expanded over the years to include more children with special health care needs living in their local communities, including children in residential settings, in hospitals, or those who are homebound. Partnerships, family choice, and the provision of information needed for parents to become advocates are supported by these laws. In addition, advocates for children with developmental-behavioral disorders can also depend on the Americans with Disabilities Act of 1990, which "prohibits the denial of education services, programs or activities to students with disabilities and prohibits discrimination against all such students," and Section 504 of the Rehabilitation Act (details at **https://www2.ed.gov/about/offices/list/ocr/504faq.html**).[28] The 2015 Every Student Succeeds Act (ESSA), which replaced the 2002 No Child Left Behind (NCLB) law, continued the NCLB requirement that public schools be held accountable for the educational achievement of students with disabilities.

Infants and young children under 3 years of age with a suspected developmental delay or behavior disorder, as well as children with a medically diagnosed physical or mental condition having a high probability of resulting in delays, are eligible for early childhood intervention referral under Part C of IDEA (see Chapter 6, Early Intervention). Children from 3 to 21 years of age may qualify for special education services through their local public school district under one or more of the following eligibility categories: autism, intellectual disability, specific learning disability, orthopedic impairment, other health impairment (OHI), auditory impairment, deafness, visual impairment, deaf-blindness, emotional disturbance, speech impairment, traumatic brain injury, and multiple disabilities (see Chapter 20, Interpreting Psychoeducational Testing Reports, Individualized Family Service Plans [IFSP], and Individualized Education Program Plans [IEP]).

Primary pediatric health care professionals can assist families whose children have a developmental-behavioral disorder with a timely referral for early childhood intervention, and they can support a parent's request for a school district special education and related services (such as occupational therapy, physical therapy, and speech/language therapy) evaluation. Physicians are the only individuals who can identify children whose health conditions affect their strength, vitality, or alertness and allow them to access special education services and modifications through the OHI eligibility category,

597

Chapter 25: Social and Community Services for Children With Developmental Disabilities
and/or Behavioral Disorders and Their Families

which requires a licensed physician's documentation. OHI eligibility includes ADHD, developmental coordination disorders, and other medical conditions that negatively impact the child's education. While not within the realm of special education, Section 504 of the Rehabilitation Act also allows for special accommodations, such as preferential seating and extra testing time, which the clinician can advise parents to seek as needed for their children.

Many families of children with developmental-behavioral disorders have become increasingly knowledgeable about the laws governing their child's educational rights and have developed advocacy skills to ensure provision of services. Educational advocacy has become a recognized need and service of many disability groups. Across the country, there are seminars, trainings, and conferences for parents and professionals devoted to ensuring the educational rights of children with disabilities. Nonetheless, there are many children who are not yet receiving the services they need in order to maximize their potential. The 2009–2010 National Survey of Children with Special Health Care Needs found that nearly half of school-aged children with developmental problems had difficulty accessing services, and 16.9% did not have an Individualized Education Program (IEP).[30]

The AAP clinical report on the IDEA for children with special educational needs emphasizes the importance of developing a thorough understanding of the early intervention and special education processes and the critical role of pediatric health care professionals in supporting the child's receipt of appropriate services.[31] A primary pediatric health care professional does a great service for the child and parents by listening to parents' concerns in a time-limited clinic visit and guiding them to the appropriate early intervention or school district evaluations, even when the clinician does not observe the stated behavior or delay. While primary pediatric health care professionals do not have a direct role in remediation, they are able to initiate interventions aimed at helping the child meet his or her full potential. They can monitor the child's progress, help parents identify their child's strengths, and advocate for needed educational and therapeutic programs from year to year. They can also help families understand their child's developmental levels and abilities and accept realistic goals for their child. Community agencies, such as local chapters of The Arc (**www.thearc.org**), provide training for parents on special education and advocacy skills and may also provide educational advocates to accompany parents to their children's IEP meetings at school to assist them in accessing the most appropriate special educational and therapeutic services for their children. State contact information and other resources related to IDEA may be found at **https://www2.ed.gov/about/contacts/state/index.html** and **http:// idea.ed.gov.**

Functional Behavioral Analysis/Behavior Management Counseling Services

Both mothers and fathers of children with disabilities exhibit high rates of depressive symptoms associated with child behavior problems, parental stress, coping style, and support.[32,33] Interventions that provide parents with behavioral training while also addressing their well-being reduce parental distress.[34,35] Parents can better implement child behavioral management with specific behavioral counseling.

A practical and evidence-based method for helping parents manage their child's behavior problems is to align them with individuals who can provide a home-based functional behavioral assessment (FBA) and then provide in-home behavior management counseling services to the parents. Providing services in the setting where the problem behavior occurs helps the parents understand what triggers the child's behavior as well as what strategies are most effective in modifying the behavior. In-home behavior management counseling is most commonly available through board certified behavior analysts (BCBAs) for families of children with autism, although it is effective for children with all types of developmental-behavioral disorders. When in-home services are not available, parents can consult with a therapist, counselor, or psychologist in a clinical setting to work on behavior management. Evidence-based group parent management training programs, such as Triple P (Positive Parenting Program) and 1–2-3 Magic, are also available to help parents learn positive behavior management strategies and effective ways to respond to challenging behaviors.

Similarly, schools also use FBAs and behavioral plans to help teachers and other staff members optimally work with a child with behavioral problems in their setting. The behavior therapist performing the FBA observes and precisely describes the specific maladaptive behaviors, including when they happen and when they stop. The behavior analyst uses the information from the observation to understand the factors influencing the behaviors and the triggers and consequences of the behaviors to determine the driving forces behind each behavior. The behavior analyst then provides school personnel and parents with training and guidance on ways to bring about appropriate changes in the child's behavior. Resources for FBA can be found at The Center for Effective Collaboration and Practice (**www.air.org/resource/functional-assessment-and-behavioral-intervention-plans**) or on the Wrightslaw Web site (**www.wrightslaw.com/info/discipl.fba.jordan.pdf**).

Support Groups

Parent-to-parent support is a resource of great value that clinicians can offer to parents as they adjust and cope with their child's diagnosis of a developmental-behavioral disorder. Having adequate support helps decrease the feelings of stress and social isolation that often follow the initial diagnosis. When a child is diagnosed with a developmental-behavioral disorder, the impact can be overwhelming and can affect family relationships. The time immediately following the diagnosis, often described as "a critical period" for families, is a particularly apt time for referral to parent support resources.[36] During this critical period, parents can be confused about where to obtain appropriate early educational and therapeutic services, which services are most effective and most evidence-based, and how to pay for them. It can greatly help for a parent to speak to another

599

Chapter 25: Social and Community Services for Children With Developmental Disabilities
and/or Behavioral Disorders and Their Families

parent whose child has the same or similar diagnosis, who has been through the same process of adjustment, and with whom they can share their feelings and gain answers in how to navigate the systems of care.

As time passes, parents of children with developmental-behavioral disorders run the gamut of emotions, from joy to despair, as they navigate the systems of care—therapeutic, educational, and psychological—to help their child and family. Primary pediatric health care professionals may feel unprepared in how to advise and advocate for these primarily nonmedical interventions. Parent support groups and parent-to-parent networks offer information, advice, and often an experienced hand to help with finding educational, social service, and other needed community resources. As children age, or as families move to other cities, these networks provide needed information regarding local schools, therapists, and extracurricular activities.

There are many options for support, both for specific disabilities and behavioral disorders and for disabilities of unknown etiology. Formal group meetings with special topics, online support through Facebook groups and other social media, gatherings at houses of worship, and many times an informal network of parents all provide opportunities to those who want to band together to energize their spirits, decrease their sense of isolation, and enhance their abilities to meet their children's needs. There are groups available for both parents, as well as separate mothers' and fathers' groups, as parents often differ in adaptation to their child's diagnosis.[37] There are also sibling groups for brothers and sisters of children with developmental-behavioral disorders, where they can develop friendships and gain support from those in similar circumstances.[38] Grandparent and other kin caregiver support groups allow for information sharing as well. In our mobile society, support groups help those whose extended families live elsewhere. The Internet has extended the ability of parents to bridge miles and even countries to network with each other, especially in cases involving children with rare disorders.[39] Family Voices is a national advocacy and support group of families of children with special health care needs and has affiliates in each state and territory of the United States (**www.familyvoices.org**).

Research demonstrates the benefits of parent-to-parent support, showing that parents are "uniquely qualified to help each other."[40] Primary pediatric health care professionals can help by keeping a close eye on parental well-being, supporting and encouraging parents' efforts to seek out other parents of children with developmental-behavioral disorders. They and their staff should provide support organization information at the onset of diagnosis and thereafter as needed. Primary pediatric health care professionals can access parent group listings by state at **www.yellowpagesforkids.com**.

Respite Care

Raising a child with a developmental-behavioral disorder presents many challenges, affecting all family relationships. Respite care is short-term temporary care that provides parents and caregivers with important time off from the constancy of their child care responsibilities. This family support service is often critical for the long-term stability of the family and child at home. Caregivers take pride in their ability to provide good care for their child; however, one result of this devoted caregiving is often a lack of time and energy for personal, marital, and family activities, which results in social isolation. Many hours are spent on therapy appointments, obtaining medical supplies and equipment, modifying the home to ensure safety, and advocating for school and community services. The physical, emotional, and financial demands may be overwhelming, adversely affecting the health and well-being of all family members.[41-43] Because the family is the child's best resource, families need respite services to avoid the burnout that often accompanies the provision of 24-hour care. Respite care helps to maintain family stability and to enable children with developmental-behavioral disorders to remain in a nurturing home. In-home and out-of-home respite options are based on the parent's needs, funding, and availability. A few hours, a few days, or weeks at a time helps to replenish a parent's or caregiver's energy. It has been reported that respite care is the most requested family support service for children with developmental-behavioral disorders.[44] This report is not surprising, because a respite allows parents and caregivers a chance to spend time with a spouse, friends, or their children without disabilities, who may often be overshadowed by their sibling's needs. Respite care helps to increase positive family interactions and enables families and caregivers to cope with chronic and potentially stressful situations. By decreasing parent and caregiver stress, respite care reduces the possibility of maltreatment, known to be increased among children with developmental-behavioral disorders compared to children without such disorders in the general population. The US Department of Health and Human Services estimated that the rate of maltreatment for children with disabilities was 31%.[45] A 2007 AAP clinical report noted that children with behavioral disorders are at highest risk of maltreatment and that neglect is the most common type of maltreatment across all disability types.[46] A respite also provides opportunities for children with developmental-behavioral disorders to meet new people and friends and to enjoy new experiences outside the home. Their siblings may be included as well. These activities can increase the child's self-esteem while improving parent and caregiver relationships.

Respite options may include in-home respite care providers; daytime, overnight, or weekend respite programs; "parents' night out" events at local faith communities or community organizations; or day or overnight summer camps for children with disabilities. Funding for these services varies greatly from state to state but may be available through Medicaid waiver programs or other community agencies. A corollary benefit to participating in parent support groups and networks is that parents may be able to arrange an informal respite by trading child care responsibilities with other parents of children with disabilities.

Primary pediatric health care professionals can help by asking parents about their needs for supportive care and by monitoring for burnout. Such inquiries acknowledge the extra care that these parents provide, a recognition parents complain is often missing.[47] They can encourage and support families in this endeavor by having information regarding community respite services available in their offices and by completing required medical documentation for respite care services. Because they know firsthand the impact of care,

601

Chapter 25: Social and Community Services for Children With Developmental Disabilities
and/or Behavioral Disorders and Their Families

they can also be advocates in the community for more available and diverse respite options to meet the needs of these parents and caregivers. A state-by-state listing of respite care services can be found at **www.archrespite.org**.

Personal Care Attendant Services

Caring for a child with a developmental-behavioral disorder who also has self-care limitations can require additional assistance at home. Primary pediatric health care professionals should be aware that personal care attendant services are a health care benefit provided under the Medicaid plan of each state as an optional, not required, service that states may select, so that children with developmental-behavioral disorders can receive services to assist in day-to-day living in their community. Children with severe physical and medical disabilities can receive assistance to help with mobility and self-care skills, allowing these children to enjoy and participate in their home and community life. Children with severe behavioral disorders can have supervision to help perform daily tasks, communicate, and learn new skills. Personal care attendants can assist with activities of daily living, such as eating, bathing, brushing teeth, toileting, and dressing, as well as with positioning, lifting, transferring, exercising, and adaptive skill building.[48]

Personal care attendant services allow children with developmental-behavioral disorders to live at home in a nurturing environment with parents, siblings, or other extended family members or caregivers. Families are often able to choose, hire, and supervise service providers for their children through Medicaid self-direction, known in many states as Consumer Directed Services, a potentially more effective, less costly approach to care.[49] Regardless of the severity of their disability or behavioral difficulties, with personal care services, children are able to function as a member of a family, attend school, and participate more fully in social and recreational activities in their communities, with an improved quality of life for the child, family, and community.

Primary pediatric health care professionals can assist families in accessing personal care attendant services by completing required forms that document the severity of the disability and define the services and supports that are needed. This is a time-consuming task, not often reimbursable, but well appreciated by families and service providers. Primary care clinicians can also help by advocating for these services with the appropriate state officials and groups.

Counseling Regarding Long-term Legal and Financial Planning Issues

Just as parents of children with typical development need advice about designing a will that addresses care of their minor children in case of parental demise, the parents of children with developmental-behavioral disorders need to do the same, although often in a more detailed fashion to specifically address disability, behavior, financial, and guardianship issues. In addition, parents of children with developmental-behavioral disorders need guidance and legal help to plan for their children's adulthood and to write specific instructions for their adult children's care, if they as parents are no longer able to give care or to be available to make decisions regarding this care.

Even parents of children with milder disabilities, such as dyslexia or ADHD, may need to consider special adult provisions for their children, if the parents anticipate that the income of their adult children with milder disabilities may be less than that of their unaffected adult children. Parents of children with certain behavioral disorders may also need to address ways to protect against these children unwisely spending inherited money as adults. Parents of children with developmental-behavioral disorders limiting their independence, as well as parents of children whose conditions require long-term medical treatment and/or prevent adult decision-making, need to deal with the financial and legal aspects of these situations well before their children reach 18 years of age.

Finding appropriate counseling regarding long-term legal and financial planning issues is of paramount importance to families of children with developmental-behavioral disorders. Regulations limiting the amount of assets or income an individual can have and still receive benefits, such as Supplemental Security Income (SSI) and Medicaid, are confusing and change often. Therefore, parents need professionals who listen to them and who understand the issues of families like theirs. Special needs attorneys and special needs planners have knowledge of and experience with relevant legal and financial issues, including tax laws and regulations governing Medicaid, SSI, other governmental benefits, other available programs (eg, the tax-advantaged ABLE savings accounts), health insurance options, estate planning, special needs trusts, and legal options (eg, guardianship, power of attorney, or other alternatives to guardianship). Fortunately, well-respected national, state, and local organizations serving individuals with specific disabilities or disorders offer help to families with regard to knowing what the families need to do and where to find appropriate professionals to help them.

Primary pediatric health care professionals and their office staff are in a unique position to advise parents of their patients with developmental-behavioral disorders regarding long-term planning for their children and finding appropriate financial and/or legal counseling for this planning to take place. Because the primary care clinician is usually one of the first professionals to talk with the parents regarding their children's diagnoses and usually follows the children on a longitudinal basis, the primary pediatric health care professional and his or her staff can advise parents to begin planning for their children's future as soon as possible, as in some states, long-term care lists like those for Medicaid waivers may take from 8 to 14 years before services become available. Primary pediatric health care professionals should advise all parents, including those with limited financial resources, to begin estate planning and establish special needs trusts. While this information is difficult for parents to hear, it should be given in a sensitive manner soon after a diagnosis is given to avoid potential loss of eligibility for certain government programs, while still seeing to the child's supplemental needs. At each clinic visit, primary pediatric health care professionals can update anticipatory guidance for what the children are likely to need as adults and remind parents that at 22 years of age, even individuals with severe disabilities will transition out of previously guaranteed

603

Chapter 25: Social and Community Services for Children With Developmental Disabilities
and/or Behavioral Disorders and Their Families

services, such as public school/special education and certain governmental programs. Primary pediatric health care professionals can also guide parents toward reputable Web sites and organizations offering appropriate financial and legal counseling to address their children's needs. While the benefit of helping families with appropriate long-term planning for their children with developmental-behavioral disorders is intuitive, there are some studies that document this benefit.[50,51] Resources to assist families in obtaining information about long-term legal and financial planning can be found at **http://kidshealth.org/en/parents/needs-planning.html**.

Extracurricular Activities and Summer Camps

Extracurricular activities, such as clubs, sports, scouting, art, dance, theatre, and music, are an important part of the educational experience of all students, including children with developmental-behavioral disorders. Children with developmental-behavioral disorders may experience low self-esteem related to their inability to keep up academically and socially with peers. Their need for special education and related services often sets them apart from the general student population, and often peers and siblings reinforce their feelings of being different and less capable than other children.[52]

Participation in athletic and creative activities provides children with developmental-behavioral disorders with opportunities to develop self-confidence and experience success in fun and nonstressful ways. Participation in these activities may also help the child and his or her family to identify a child's special talent that can be a huge boost to that child's self-esteem.

Federal laws governing special education services recognize the importance of extracurricular activities. The IDEA amendments of 1997 included a "statement of program modifications or supports for school personnel that will be provided for students with disabilities to participate in extracurricular and other nonacademic activities. School districts shall take steps to provide nonacademic and extracurricular services in such manner as necessary to afford children with disabilities an equal opportunity for participation in those services and activities."[53]

Nonschool-sponsored extracurricular activities are available through the Special Olympics, special needs scouting, YMCA programs, disability groups (eg, The Arc or United Cerebral Palsy [UCP]), as well as through city parks and recreation departments. Specialty programs, such as hippotherapy or adaptive aquatics, offer recreational activities specifically for children with disabilities.

Summer camps are an additional extracurricular activity. Not only do they provide children with developmental-behavioral disorders with the opportunity to experience success outside the classroom; they also allow these children to be like their siblings and same-age peers who go to camp. Both day and overnight camps support the development of independence and self-esteem. Specialty camps help children to understand and cope with a specific disability or chronic illness, while also enjoying horseback riding, swimming, and other fun activities. Children with even the most severe disabilities can enjoy the opportunity to be away from home, while their parents may enjoy the temporary respite from child care duties.[54]

Primary pediatric health care professionals can help parents with selecting extracurricular activities, summer programs, and camps appropriate for their child's developmental level. As clinicians, their letters of support and medical input regarding the level of participation and care needs will aid activity and camp directors in planning and programming for children with developmental-behavioral disorders. In addition, they can address their medical treatment of these children toward maximizing their ability to participate in these activities.[55] The primary pediatric health care professional's support for extracurricular activities and summer camps emphasizes their value for children with developmental-behavioral disorders. Information about extracurricular activities and summer camps for children with special health care needs can be found in Table 25.2.

Table 25.2. Extracurricular Program Web Sites		
Web Address	**Program Name**	**Purpose/Mission**
www.specialolympics.org	Special Olympics	Adaptive sports programs for children and youth with intellectual and developmental disabilities
www.bestbuddies.org	Best Buddies International	Global volunteer movement that creates opportunities for one-to-one friendships, integrated employment, and leadership development for people with intellectual and developmental disabilities
www.scouting.org/disabilitiesawareness.aspx	Boy Scouts of America	Information on special needs scouting and inclusion of children and youth with disabilities
www.acacamps.org	American Camp Association	Information on accredited day and overnight camp programs, including a search tool to find special needs camps
www.kidscamps.com	Private Web site	Private Web site that includes a search tool to find day and overnight camps, including those for children and youth with special needs

Assistive Technology

Assistive technology resources now provide children with developmental-behavioral disorders with an extensive array of tools to communicate their needs and to demonstrate their abilities to learn. Access to these resources in the educational setting is mandated by IDEA. Assistive technology can help children with disabilities to more fully participate with typical peers in both school and extracurricular settings. These resources can also help children better connect and communicate with family, friends, and the world outside. Children with even the most severe conditions may benefit from

605

Chapter 25: Social and Community Services for Children With Developmental Disabilities
and/or Behavioral Disorders and Their Families

assistive technology. For instance, communication devices operated by eye movement hold much promise for children whose motor impairment prevents speaking and hand or foot movement.[56] Primary pediatric health care professionals should request an assistive technology evaluation for even their youngest patients with developmental disabilities.[57] Such evaluations can be requested through early childhood intervention programs for children from birth to 3 years of age, through special education programs for children and adolescents from 3 to 21 years of age, and through agencies such as United Cerebral Palsy (UCP). Additional resource information may be found on the Web site for the Accessible Technology Coalition (**http://atcoalition.org/**).

Conclusion

Laws and resources will change over time. However, when primary pediatric health care professionals partner with parents to identify and access all community and social services available to children with developmental-behavioral disorders and their families, they can develop the most comprehensive plans for ensuring that these children reach their full potential.

Resources

Due to each state and local government having their own services for individuals with developmental-behavioral disorders, primary pediatric health care professionals and caregivers should also use Internet search engines to look for specific services in their state and local area. In addition, primary care clinicians and caregivers should use Internet search engines to look for specific diagnosis-related national, state, and local organizations, as Web sites for such organizations often aid in finding needed services.

Case Management
www.kff.org/medicaid/state-indicator/targeted-case-management

Children's Mental Health Services
www.nami.org
www.mentalhealthamerica.net
www.psychologytoday.com

Supplemental Medical Insurance and Other Financial Assistance Programs
Medicaid, CHIP, Health Care Marketplace:
www.healthcare.gov

SSI:
www.ssa.gov

Other financial assistance and benefits:
www.hhs.gov or www.benefits.gov

Educational Advocacy Services

http://idea.ed.gov

State education agency contact information:

www2.ed.gov/about/contacts/state/index.html

www.thearc.org

Support Groups

www.yellowpagesforkids.com

www.familyvoices.org

Functional Behavioral Analysis/In-Home Behavior Management
Counseling Services

www.air.org/resource/functional-assessment-and-behavioral-intervention-plans

www.wrightslaw.com/info/discipl.fba.jordan.pdf

Respite Care

www.archrespite.org

Personal Attendant Care

Use Internet browser to search for "personal care services" and the name of your state to yield information.

Counseling Regarding Long-term Legal and Financial Planning Issues

http://kidshealth.org/en/parents/needs-planning.html

http://www.ablenrc.org/about/what-are-able-accounts

Extracurricular Activities/Summer Camps

www.specialolympics.org

www.bestbuddies.org

http://www.scouting.org/disabilitiesawareness.aspx

www.acacamps.org

www.kidscamps.com

The last two Web sites include camp search tools that enable searches for camps that serve individuals with disabilities and other special populations.

Assistive Technology

http://atcoalition.org/

The Accessible Technology Coalition provides information and resources on assistive technology options for individuals with developmental disabilities.

http://ucp.org/resources/assistive-technology/

The Web site for the national organization, United Cerebral Palsy, includes information on assistive technology as well as links to state-specific assistive technology programs.

607

Chapter 25: Social and Community Services for Children With Developmental Disabilities and/or Behavioral Disorders and Their Families

General

www.thearc.org

The Arc is the world's largest community-based organization for people with intellectual and developmental disabilities. The Arc is devoted to promoting and improving support and services for all people with intellectual and developmental disabilities and their families.

www.autism-society.org

Official site of Autism Society of America with contact information for state and local affiliates.

www.autismspeaks.org

Information for families and providers on autism and related services; includes helpful toolkits for families and information on research and advocacy efforts.

https://brightfutures.aap.org

The Bright Futures section of the American Academy of Pediatrics Web site has extensive information for professionals and families of children with disabilities.

www.cdc.gov

Centers for Disease Control and Prevention.

www.disAbilitiesbookspress.com

Books of interest for parents of children with disabilities, family members, and professionals who serve children and families.

www.easterseals.com

Services to ensure that people living with disabilities have equal opportunities to live, learn, work, and play; includes listing of state and local affiliates.

www.epilepsy.com

Information on services for individuals with epilepsy.

www.familyconnect.org/parentsitehome.aspx

Information on resources and services for individuals who are blind or visually impaired.

www.familyvoices.org

Family-to-family health and education information, including state and local affiliates.

http://fragilex.org/

National Fragile X Foundation.

www.gallaudet.edu/clerc-center.html

Information on resources and services for deaf and hard of hearing individuals.

http://www.gottransition.org/index.cfm

Information and resources on health care transition for providers, patients and families.

https://medicalhomeinfo.aap.org

National center of medical home initiatives for children with special health care needs (tools for coordinating care, state resources and more).

www.nacdd.org

National Association of Councils on Developmental Disabilities.

www.ndss.org

National Down Syndrome Society.

http://www.pacer.org

Parent training and information center for families of children with disabilities; Web site also links to the National Bullying Prevention Center.

www.parentcenterhub.org

Center for Parent Information and Resources. Information in English and Spanish for parents of children with disabilities.

www.rarediseases.org

National Organization for Rare Disorders; information and networking site for families affected by rare genetic and medical conditions.

www.spinabifidaassociation.org

Spina Bifida Association.

www.ucp.org

A "one-stop resource guide" for cerebral palsy for every US state and territory.

www.wrightslaw.com

Information about special education law, education law, and advocacy.

References

1. American Academy of Pediatrics Council on Children With Disabilities. Care coordination in the medical home: integrating health and related systems of care for children with special health care needs. *Pediatrics.* 2005;116(5):1238–1244
2. Zajicek-Farber ML, Lotrecchiano GR, Long TM, Farber JM. Parental perceptions of family centered care in medical homes of children with neurodevelopmental disabilities. *Matern Child Health J.* 2015;19(8):1744–1755
3. Boudreau AA, Perrin JM, Goodman E, Kurowski D, Cooley WC, Kuhlthau K. Care coordination and unmet specialty care among children with special health care needs. *Pediatrics.* 2014;133(6):1046–1053
4. Litt JS, McCormick MC. Care coordination, the family-centered medical home, and functional disability among children with special health care needs. *Acad Pediatr.* 2015;15(2):185–190.
5. Antonelli RC, McAllister JW, Popp J. *Making Care Coordination a Critical Component of the Pediatric Health System: A Multidisciplinary Framework.* New York, NY: The Commonwealth Fund. 2009;10(21):1–26

609

Chapter 25: Social and Community Services for Children With Developmental Disabilities and/or Behavioral Disorders and Their Families

6. Council on Children with Disabilities and Medical Home Implementation Project Advisory Committee. Patient- and family-centered care coordination: a framework for integrating care for children and youth across multiple systems. *Pediatrics*. 2014;133(5):e1451–e1460

7. Antonelli RC, Stille CJ, Antonelli D. Care coordination for children and youth with special health care needs: a descriptive, multisite study of activities, personnel costs, and outcomes. *Pediatrics*. 2008;122(1):e209–e216

8. Ronis SD, Baldwin CD, Blumkin A, Kuhlthau K, Szilagyi PG. Patient-centered medical home and family burden in attention-deficit hyperactivity disorder. *J Dev Behav Pediatr*. 2015;36(6):417–25

9. McCallion P, Janicki M, Kolomer S. Controlled evaluation of support groups for grandparent caregivers of children with developmental disabilities and delays. *Am J Ment Retard*. 2004;109(5):352–361

10. Gilson SF. Case management and supported employment: a good fit. *J Case Manag*. 1998;7(1):10–17

11. Lightfoot E, LaLiberte T. Approaches to child protection management for cases involving people with disabilities. *Child Abuse Negl*. 2006;30(4):381–391

12. Miller K. Care coordination impacts on access to care for children with special health care needs enrolled in Medicaid and CHIP. *Matern Child Health J*. 2014;18(4):864–872

13. Hamilton LJ, Lerner CF, Presson AP, Klitzer TS. Effects of a medical home program for children with special health care needs on parental perceptions of care in an ethnically diverse patient population. *Matern Child Health J*. 2013;17(3):463–469

14. Lin SC, Margolis B, Yu SM, Adirim TA. The role of medical home in emergency department use for children with developmental disabilities in the United States. *Pediatr Emerg Care*. 2014;30(8):534–539

15. Sobotka SA, Francis A, Vander Ploeg Booth K. Associations of family characteristics with perceptions of care among parents of children with autism. *Child Care Health Dev*. 2016;42(1):135–140

16. Vohra R, Madhavan S, Sambamoorthi U, St Peter C. Access to services, quality of care, and family impact for children with autism, other developmental disabilities, and other mental health conditions. *Autism*. 2014;18(7):815–826

17. US Department of Health and Human Services Health Resources Services Administration. *The National Survey of Children with Special Health Care Needs: Chartbook 2009–2010*. http://mchb.hrsa.gov/cshcn0910/more/pdf/nscshcn0910.pdf. Accessed November 27, 2017

18. Witt W, Riley A, Coiro MJ. Childhood functional status, family stressors, and psychosocial adjustment among school-aged children with disabilities in the United States. *Arch Pediatr Adolesc Med*. 2003;157(7):687–695

19. Pastor PN, Reuben CA. Trends in parent-reported emotional and behavioral problems among children using special education services. *Psychiatr Serv*. 2015;66(6):656–659

20. Fox RA, Keller KM, Grede PL, Bartosz AM. A mental health clinic for toddlers with developmental delays and behavior problems. *Res Dev Disabil*. 2007;28(2):119–129

21. Busch SH, Barry CL. Mental health disorders in childhood: assessing the burden on families. *Health Aff (Millwood)*. 2007;26(4):1088–1095

22. Buescher AV, Cidav Z, Knapp M, Mandell DS. Costs of autism spectrum disorders in the United Kingdom and the United States. *JAMA Pediatr*. 2014;168(8):721–728

23. Newacheck PW, Inkelas M, Kim SE. Health services use and health care expenditures for children with disabilities. *Pediatrics*. 2004; 114(1):79–85

24. Haley J, Kenney G. Low-income uninsured children with special health care needs: why aren't they enrolled in public health insurance programs? *Pediatrics*. 2007;119(1):60–68

25. Feldman HM, Buysse CA, Hubner LM, Huffman LC, Loe IM. Patient Protection and Affordable Care Act of 2010 and children and youth with special health care needs. *J Dev Behav Pediatr*. 2015;36(3):207–217

26. Strock-Lynskey D, Keller D. Integrating a family-centered approach into social work practice with families of children and adolescents with disabilities. *J Soc Work Disabil Rehabil*. 2006;6(1–2):111–1134

27. 108th Congress. Public Law 108–446. http://idea.ed.gov/. Accessed November 27, 2017

28. US Department of Education. Protecting students with disabilities: frequently asked questions about Section 504 and the education of children with disabilities. http://www2.ed.gov/about/offices/list/ocr/504faq.html. Accessed November 27, 2017

29. US Department of Education. No Child Left Behind provision gives schools new flexibility and ensures accountability for students with disabilities. http://www2.ed.gov/nclb/freedom/local/specedfactsheet.html. Accessed November 27, 2017

30. Lindly OJ, Sinche BK, Zuckerman KE. Variation in educational services receipt among US children with developmental conditions. *Acad Pediatr*. 2015;15(5):534–543

31. Lipkin PH, Okamoto J; Council on Children with Disabilities and Council on School Health. The Individuals with Disabilities Education Act (IDEA) for children with special educational needs. *Pediatrics*. 2015;136:(6):e1650–e1662

32. Lee J. Maternal stress, well-being, and impaired sleep in mothers of children with developmental disabilities: a literature review. *Res Dev Disabil*. 2013;34(11):4255–4273

33. Rosenthal DG, Learned N, Liu YH, Weitzman M. Characteristics of fathers with depressive symptoms. *Matern Child Health J.* 2013;17(1):119–128

34. Colalillo S, Johnston C. Parenting cognition and affective outcomes following parent management training: a systematic review. *Clin Child Fam Psychol Rev.* 2016;19(3):216–235

35. Child Welfare Information Gateway. Parent education to strengthen families and reduce the risk of maltreatment. Washington, DC: US Department of Health and Human Services, Children's Bureau; 2013 https://www.childwelfare.gov/pubPDFs/parented.pdf. Accessed November 27, 2017

36. Rahi JS, Manaras I, Tuomainen H, Hundt GL. Meeting the needs of parents around the time of diagnosis of disability among their children: evaluation of a novel program for information, support, and liaison by key workers. *Pediatrics.* 2004;114(4):e477–e482

37. Keller D, Honig AS. Maternal and paternal stress in families with school-aged children with disabilities. *Am J Orthopsychiatry.* 2004;74(3):337–348

38. Roberts RM, Ejova A, Giallo R, Strohm K, Lillie M, Fuss B. A controlled trial of the SibworkS group program for siblings of children with special needs. *Res Dev Disabil.* 2015;43–44:21–31

39. Baum LS. Internet parent support groups for primary caregivers of a child with special health care needs. *Pediatr Nurs.* 2004;30(5):381–381, 401

40. Kerr SM, McIntosh JB. Coping when a child has a disability: exploring the impact of parent-to-parent support. *Child Care Health Dev.* 2000;26(4):309–321

41. Cowen PS, Reed DA. Effects of respite care for children with developmental disabilities: evaluation of an intervention for at risk families. *Public Health Nurs.* 2004;19(4):272–283

42. Strunk JA. Respite care for families of special needs children: a systematic review. *J Dev Phys Disabil.* 2010;22(6):615–630

43. Harper A, Taylor Dyches T, Harper J, Olsen Roper S, South M. Respite care, marital quality, and stress in parents of children with autism spectrum disorder. *J Autism Dev Disord.* 2013;43(11):2604–2616

44. Johnson CP, Kastner TA, American Academy of Pediatrics Committee/Section on Children With Disabilities. Helping families raise children with special health care needs at home. *Pediatrics.* 2005;115(2):507–511

45. Child Welfare Information Gateway. The risk and prevention of maltreatment of children with disabilities. Washington, DC: US Department of Health and Human Services, Administration for Children and Families, Children's Bureau; 2012 https://www.childwelfare.gov/pubs/prevenres/focus/. Accessed November 27, 2017

46. Hibbard RA, Desch LW; American Academy of Pediatrics Committee on Child Abuse and Neglect, Council on Children With Disabilities. Maltreatment of children with disabilities. *Pediatrics.* 2007;119(5):1018–1025

47. Roberts I, Lawton D. Acknowledging the extra care parents give their disabled children. *Child Care Health Dev.* 2001;27(4):307–319

48. The Henry J. Kaiser Family Foundation. Medicaid benefits: personal care services. https://www.kff.org/medicaid/state-indicator/personal-care-services. Accessed November 27, 2017

49. Caldwell J, Heller T. Longitudinal outcomes of a consumer-directed program supporting adults with developmental disabilities and their families. *Intellect Dev Disabil.* 2007;45(3):161–173

50. Heller T, Caldwell J. Supporting aging caregivers and adults with developmental disabilities in future planning. *Ment Retard.* 2006;44(3):189–202

51. Botsford AL, Rule D. Evaluation of a group intervention to assist aging parents with permanency planning for an adult offspring with special needs. *Soc Work.* 2004;49(3):423–431

52. Blanchard LT, Gurka MJ, Blackman JA. Emotional, developmental, and behavioral health of American children and their families: a report from the 2003 National Survey of Children's Health. *Pediatrics.* 2006;117 (6):e1202–e1212

53. Individuals with Disabilities Education Act Amendments of 1997, Section 614(d)(1)(A)(iii)

54. Briery B, Rabian B. Psychosocial changes associated with participation in a pediatric summer camp. *J Pediatr Psychol.* 1999;24(2):183–190

55. Accardo J, Shapiro BK. Neurodevelopmental disabilities: beyond the diagnosis. *Semin Pediatr Neurol.* 2005;12(4):242–249

56. Borgestig M, Sandqvist J, Parsons R, Falkmer T, Hemmingsson H. Eye gaze performance for children with severe physical impairments using gaze-based assistive technology—a longitudinal study. *Assist Technol.* 2016;28(2):93–102

57. Desch LW, Gaebler-Spira D; American Academy of Pediatrics Council on Children With Disabilities. Prescribing assistive-technology systems: focus on children with impaired communication. *Pediatrics.* 2008;121(6):1271–1280

CHAPTER 26

Transition to Adult Medical Care

Peter J. Smith, MD, MA, FAAP

Kruti R. Acharya, MD, FAAP

Stephen H. Contompasis, MD, FAAP

Introduction

This chapter provides an overview of the many challenges to achieving transition in health care for young adults with developmental-behavioral disorders. It provides an overview of the complexity of the issues across systems, policies, practices, and beliefs, from the personal level to the population level. The resource section at the end of this chapter provides primary pediatric health care professionals with some current assets that may enable them to better achieve transition for their patients with developmental-behavioral disorders or special health care needs, leading to improved outcomes for all involved.

> "*For in every adult there dwells the child that was, and in every child there lies the adult that will be.*"
>
> John Connolly, *The Book of Lost Things*

What Is Known?

As a result of improvements in living conditions and medical advances over the last few decades, individuals with developmental-behavioral disorders have experienced an increase in life expectancy. Prior to these improvements, children with developmental-behavioral disorders were primarily cared for by pediatric health care professionals in pediatric systems of health care. For the purposes of this chapter, we will consider children with developmental-behavioral disorders as those children with functional impairments in cognitive (including learning and intellectual disabilities), neurobehavioral (including attention-deficit/hyperactivity disorder [ADHD], autism spectrum disorder [ASD], and other neuropsychiatric disorders [eg, anxiety disorders, mood disorders, thought disorders, and posttraumatic disorders]) and motor (including cerebral palsy, muscular dystrophies, and spina bifida) development.

The transition to adult health care is complicated in part by a bifurcated pediatric and adult health care system. Health care benefits may also change because of age-out limits for public insurance programs; loss of access to comprehensive, medically necessary services guaranteed by early and periodic screening, diagnostic, and treatment service regulations; and changes for individuals receiving Supplemental Security Income (SSI). Across the United States, pediatric and adult health care systems vary tremendously with differences related to geography (eg, urban versus rural), affiliations with academic health systems and publicly funded systems, availability of care coordination supports, and access to insurance. Furthermore, the adult health care system differs from the pediatric system in structure (eg, availability of social work support) and processes (eg, shared decision making, roles of primary and specialty providers) as well as in experience and capacity to accept younger adults with certain childhood-onset conditions.

All adolescents and young adults, regardless of disability status, who grow out of pediatric care transition to adult medical care; however, many may not have the knowledge and skills to navigate new adult care systems. In order to successfully transition to adult health care, adolescents and young adults need support and guidance from their families, referring pediatric providers, and accepting adult providers. However, only 40% of Youth With Special Health Care Needs (YSHCN), which includes youth with developmental-behavioral disorders, receive the necessary supports and services to successfully transition to adult health care, work, and independence, with this rate being even lower for minority and low-income YSHCN.[1] Moreover, youth with developmental-behavioral disorders experience disparities in transition services, and youth with autism spectrum disorder (ASD) are significantly less likely to receive health care transition services than youth with other special health care needs.[2] Youth with ASD and a comorbid developmental disability are even less likely to receive health care transition services.[2]

Without support, youth with developmental-behavioral disorders are especially at risk of serious consequences of a poorly coordinated transition. They are at risk for lapses in primary and subspecialty care, increased emergency department utilization, poorer health outcomes, and worse quality of life.[3,4]

When planning transition for young adults with developmental disabilities, common concerns are issues related to self-determination and supported decision-making. Guardianship is one example of a legal process to appoint a guardian for an individual deemed to have incapacitated decision-making capacity. All persons are deemed capable before the law until it can be demonstrated before a court that the person requires some supervision.[5] In addition to assessing competency to make medical decisions, other skill areas that are reviewed include general supervision and safety, finding housing, employment, education, buying and selling property, making contracts, and controlling one's finances. Alternatives to full guardianship (eg, limited guardianship, representative payee, or power of attorney) exist and should be explored to guarantee that individuals with developmental disabilities retain as much autonomy as they are able. Primary pediatric health care professionals serving youth with developmental disabilities should be keenly aware of the need for guardianship determination by 18 years of age and should advise patients and families according to current state policy, practices, and procedures. Avoiding doing so could create a situation where a child without the ability to make medical decisions is in a vulnerable position, and his or her parents are blocked from participating until a court determination of guardianship is established.[6]

During the process of health care transition, there are 4 main stakeholders: patients, families, referring health care providers, and receiving health care providers. Each of these groups has specific roles and responsibilities to promote a successful transition process.

What Are the Goals?

Across groups, there is a shared goal to promote the individual patient's effective navigation of the complicated health care system, or, more simply stated, to promote that the individual patient does not fall through the cracks. However, each group also has unique concerns and apprehensions.

As adolescents with developmental-behavioral disorders transition to adult care, it is especially important for them to feel that clinicians maintain respect for their personal autonomy. Even though this goal is universal across different patient populations, it is especially important for young adults with known cognitive disabilities that their health care professionals presume that they possess decision-making capacity. Health care professionals can help this process by becoming more knowledgeable about these issues and achieving better practice though specific training in interviewing and examination to both assess decision-making capacity and support the autonomy of patients with developmental-behavioral disorders.[7] Providers may use a transition readiness tool to assess self-management skills and track mastery of important health competencies.

Even though transition-age youth and their families both share the same goals, there is a tension for parents within their relationships with their children: They must balance their competing goals of wanting to empower their children to achieve maximal independence while simultaneously wanting to promote their children's safety. Of course, this is a universal tension in all parenting. However, because individuals with developmental-behavioral disorders experience unique risks during their time as adolescents and into adulthood, their parents have unique tensions to resolve.[8]

Different types of health care providers have different goals for the process of transition. Primary pediatric health care professionals want to find knowledgeable and compatible adult health care professionals who are willing to accept patients with developmental-behavioral disorders. Adult health care professionals who accept these patients want to provide quality care for a patient population with whom they are likely less familiar. These issues are described in more detail in the American Academy of Pediatrics (AAP) policy statement, "A Consensus Statement on Health Care Transitions for Young Adults With Special Health Care Needs."[9]

> "*The best laid schemes o' Mice an' Men,*
> *Gang aft agley.*"

Robert Burns, *To a Mouse*

What Are the Barriers?

There are at least 2 major types of barriers for individuals with developmental-behavioral disorders that stand in the way to successful transitions. The first category of barrier is institutional and administrative, and the second is attitudinal. Both types of barriers are important, and they also frequently interact dynamically.

The institutional and administrative health transition barriers identified for youth with developmental-behavioral disorders and their families are as follows: (1) lack of information about the transition process and available adult health care providers; (2) lack of explicit and continuous attention to youth's needs for decision-making supports; (3) reticence among caregivers about relinquishing care and decision-making responsibilities; (4) difficulties in letting go of long-standing pediatric relationships; (5) difficulties finding adult providers available to care for young adults with developmental-behavioral disorders; (6) low utilization of medical and behavioral health care, changes in program eligibility for adult services, insurance, and disability assistance; (7) lack of coordination and communication between pediatric and adult providers to facilitate a smooth transition; and (8) inadequate care coordination support and funding for activities to manage the transfer and integration to adult care.

Lack of adequate reimbursement for the often time-consuming and difficult tasks of care management leads either to health care teams that are struggling to stay financially viable if they try to offer this important portion of care or to health care teams that limit or entirely avoid accepting patients with significant developmental-behavioral disorders into their practices. Furthermore, there are significant challenges related to payment structures. For example, the chapter structure of the *International Classification of Diseases, Tenth Revision, Clinical Modification* (*ICD-10-CM*) groups developmental conditions with mental health disorders as Chapter 5, Mental, Behavioral and Neurodevelopmental Conditions (F01–F99). If an adult payer (ie, insurance company) carves out all Chapter 5 codes, it may be extremely difficult for patients with developmental conditions to have their medical care covered. Primary care providers increasingly refer these patients to subspecialists because they cannot offer this care within the business constraints that are part of the current fee-for-service model. It is hoped that a transition to value-based models will result in a meaningful increase in the payments for health care management, but this is far from certain and still in the future.

The second set of barriers to successful transition is attitudes that can be divided into 3 groups: those of families, those of the individuals themselves, and those of health care professionals. First, parents of individuals with developmental-behavioral disorders may find it difficult to let go of their trusted pediatric providers and institutions with whom they often have longstanding relationships. Building new trusting relationships with new adult providers and systems is difficult. Families may also be reluctant to let go of their children. As mentioned earlier, all parents and caregivers experience tension between balancing their desire to keep their children safe and their desire to promote their children's independence. However, this tension is particularly acute for parents of children with developmental-behavioral disorders. Their children have to navigate an inherently more complex transition, their children are frequently less personally able to make the transition without significant supports, and parents have usually been the ones to supply the majority of that support. Especially for children with cognitive impairments, behavioral and mental health concerns, or significantly life-threatening medical conditions, families are reasonably reluctant to trust systems that they have too often experienced as broken, unreliable, and not up to the task of supporting their loved ones.

The second group of attitude barriers can be found in individuals with developmental-behavioral disorders who are in the state of not knowing what is possible. Simply put, they don't know what they don't know and may have low expectations. One common example of this occurs when adult individuals with developmental-behavioral disorders are not aware that they have a right to privacy and are specifically not aware that their parents do not have to continue to accompany them into the exam room at medical clinic visits.[9] Conflict may also occur between young adults and their parents when seeking social and employment opportunities.

Finally, like families, pediatric health care professionals who have served children with developmental-behavioral disorders have worries about their patients, and these worries (again, like those of families) are often based in lived experiences, especially related to the care of children with cognitive impairments, behavioral/mental health concerns, or significantly life-threatening medical conditions. Pediatric health care professionals are well aware of the lack of support for these children, their families, and themselves. They are also aware that there may be no clear protocols or systems to help identify adult health care professionals who accept transitioning patients.

The majority of referring and receiving health care providers have limited knowledge about the adult life outcomes of individuals with developmental-behavioral disorders, which impacts how they care for patients. For example, many are unaware or lack confidence in explaining the tremendous improvements in the function and life expectancy of individuals with Down syndrome and may therefore not explore the issues of sexuality, dating, marriage, driving, employment, mental health, or other topics that they routinely discuss with other adolescents and young adults.

Additional System-Level Challenges

As currently structured, funding sources create systematic barriers. Frequently, there are changes in sources and eligibility criteria for health care funding that can occur when a person ages out of some programs and into others. For example, until 21 years of age, the federal government mandates what is covered as Medicaid supported services; after

21 years of age, states determine what services they will offer. Similarly, SSI eligibility is based on parental income for those younger than 18 years; however, for those 18 years of age and over, it is determined by one's employment potential and income. Because of the age limits and different eligibility criteria, individuals must reapply for SSI when they turn 18 years of age, as if they are brand new to the system. Even if an individual with a developmental-behavioral disorder received SSI benefits until 18 years of age, he or she may not quality for SSI as an adult. In addition, state waiver services may change for those older than 21 years, or access may be dependent on early application owing to long wait lists. Waivers are state programs that provide supports for individuals who meet an institutional level of care through Medicaid home and community-based services and are also referred to as *1915(c) programs.*

Although developmental-behavioral disorders are the most prevalent chronic medical disorders encountered in pediatric medicine (see Chapter 1, Child Development: The Basic Science of Pediatrics), subspecialty-level pediatric providers are scarce, and equivalent subspecialty-level adult health care providers are nonexistent. Of the 118,292 pediatricians currently certified by the American Board of Pediatrics, only 775 are subspecialty board–certified in Developmental-Behavioral Pediatrics, and only 255 are subspecialty board–certified in Neurodevelopmental Disabilities.[10] This does not represent 1,030 different subspecialists, as some individuals possess both certifications. These few pediatric physicians are trained specifically in the many varied areas related to the long-term care of children with developmental-behavioral disorders, including developmental outcomes, educational policy, coordination of care, family systems dynamics, and governmental services and supports.

Training and board certification in internal medicine does not have a single learning objective specifically directed toward developmental behavioral disorders, so internal medicine physicians have reason to wonder whether they have the appropriate training to care for this important and growing population of adults.[11,12] Many unfortunately feel compelled to refuse to accept patients in this population because they feel ill prepared to do so.[13] Adult health care professionals who work in underserved areas (including rural areas and inner cities where there are workforce shortages of therapists, case managers, and subspecialty referral networks) often struggle to supply the needed resources for their patients of all ages, and the transitional period is 1 epoch that highlights these struggles.

Not only does the lack of an equivalent adult subspecialty have significant clinical effects; it also affects at least 3 pernicious structural problems: (1) The shape and content of medical school curricula are usually entirely lacking in any competencies specifically related to developmental-behavioral disorders across the lifespan, (2) the shape and direction of research programs rarely are driven by questions about the medical and social problems of developmental-behavioral disorders, and (3) the shape and advocacy initiatives directed toward addressing population health and public policy programs rarely address the unique needs of developmental-behavioral disorders. For instance, although educational programs often take into account language and cultural barriers, they almost never take into account barriers due to intellectual disability, autism, or other developmental-behavioral disorders. Another example is found in the lack of appropriate equipment designed for examination rooms or radiology suites to accommodate an individual who uses a wheelchair for mobility. All of these problems stem from the simple fact that on most medical school committees, research review committees, agency boards, and public health councils, there is no one present with any "skin in the game" relative to developmental-behavioral disorders. While many health systems have developed transition programs for cystic fibrosis, congenital heart disease, sickle cell disease, and inflammatory bowel disease, these same health systems have not given the same institutional support for transitional programs for individuals with developmental-behavioral disorders. This disparity may be attributable in large part to the availability of adult pulmonologists, cardiologists, hematologists, and gastroenterologists versus the lack of adult specialists in developmental-behavioral disorders.

What Can Be Done?

There are several areas of possible intervention that have great potential for improving the number of individuals with developmental-behavioral disorders who successfully transition from pediatric to adult health care systems. These areas of advancing high-quality medical home practice include care coordination activities, medical and post-graduate education reforms, health care financing changes, public health education initiatives, and innovative research funding programs.[14]

In the area of medical education, it will be important to institute clear, formal learning objectives related to the needs of individuals with developmental-behavioral disorders, including objectives related to transitions. There have been successful initiatives to increase the formal training and general awareness of previously underrepresented issues within medical school curricula (eg, efforts to improve knowledge, skills, and attitudes related to lesbian, gay, bisexual, transgender, and questioning individuals and potential medical issues), and these prior experiences point to the potential for a similar initiative for individuals with developmental-behavioral disorders, especially including transition as a specific issue to be addressed.[15] Likewise, residency training programs, fellowship training programs, and continuing medical education (CME) programs could all be updated to include general competencies in transition and specific competencies related to the transition of individuals with developmental-behavioral disorders. Deliberate placement of medical students and residents into clinical settings where quality medical homes provide care coordination should be encouraged. Further, there will need to be an exploration of the creation of an adult medicine subspecialty that is dedicated to the care of individuals with developmental-behavioral disorders. Approaches that address the needs of doctors-in-training (from medical school through fellowship) and the needs of currently practicing providers (CME) will be important. These educational initiatives have the potential to transform the attitudes of clinicians in a way that moves transitions from being an afterthought to a central organizing principle in their care of these patients. These initiatives will, of course, require the infusion of new financial and administrative resources.

In clinical practice, the potential evolution toward value-based financing systems offers tremendous potential regarding an increase in the payments to support the time and administrative efforts of primary care medical homes and other health care teams who are coordinating care, including coordinating efforts within supportive transitions.[16] However, these processes are slow and uneven, and there is tremendous regional variation in the pace and direction of change. Without clear and effective changes to the current payment systems, which undervalue the time and work of care coordination (including that needed for successful transitions), no amount of educational programs will be generally effective—if clinical teams are not reimbursed at least enough to adequately pay for their time, there will not be effective systemic change.[17]

Further, there will need to be effective public health initiatives to inform both individuals with developmental-behavioral disorders (and their families), as well as the clinicians who serve them, about the need for clinical planning and care coordination to provide a successful transition. The power of these programs cannot be underestimated in creating a true paradigm shift in the attitudes of the general public as well as the treating clinicians. Autism stands as a powerful example of a successful educational transformation. In a short period of time, the general public (and most clinicians) have shifted from having little knowledge about ASD to now having a significantly increased general awareness of the condition and methods of treatment (eg, there is now even a character on *Sesame Street* with ASD). These public health initiatives will need to help families and individuals come to understand that the world of possibilities is larger than ever before and to help them expand their expectations.

Finally, private and public funding programs will need to expand in the area of health care transitions. Past programs have been successful in targeting specific goals in regions of the country. To expand these successes, funding will need to be not only increased in amount but also distributed more generally across regions and across different models of care delivery. Health care systems that are already organized around population health and coordination of care are already in the lead, but their successes may not easily translate to other types of delivery systems. Also, research initiatives will need to be funded to explore the different models needed for different populations, including the differences due to race and ethnicity; underlying disability; rural, urban, and suburban locations; and differences in the subspecialty density (eg, there are clusters of developmental-behavioral subspecialists in the coastal areas but fewer in other parts of the country).

There have been many good programs created (see the following resource list), and the current situation is far better than in past eras. However, significant work remains to be done, especially in expanding the successes across the entire country and the subspecialties of clinicians who care for individuals with developmental-behavioral disorders.

Resources

"Life is one big transition."

Wilver Dornell "Willie" Stargell

Web Sites

Got Transition
www.gottransition.org
Starting a Transition Improvement Process Using the Six Core Elements of
Health Care Transition
http://www.gottransition.org/resourceGet.cfm?id=331

Integrating Young Adults with Intellectual and Developmental Disabilities into Your
Practice: Tips for Adult Health Care Providers
http://www.gottransition.org/resourceGet.cfm?id=367

American Academy of Pediatrics, Illinois Chapter
Transitioning Youth to Adult Health Care for Pediatric Providers Course
http://illinoisaap.org/projects/medical-home/transition/resources-for-physicians/

American Academy of Pediatrics
HealthyChildren.org Web site
https://www.healthychildren.org

Kids as Self Advocates (KASA)
http://www.fvkasa.org/index.php

Coding
American Academy of Pediatrics, *Standardized Screening/Testing Coding Fact
Sheet for Primary Care Pediatricians: Developmental/Behavioral/Emotional*
https://www.aap.org/en-us/Documents/coding_factsheet_
developmentalscreeningtestingandEmotionalBehvioraassessment.pdf

Department of Health and Human Services, Centers for Medicare & Medicaid Services,
Chronic Care Management Services Changes for 2017
https://www.cms.gov/Outreach-and-Education/
Medicare-Learning-Network-MLN/MLNProducts/Downloads/
ChronicCareManagementServicesChanges2017.pdf

American Academy of Pediatrics' Got Transition Web site, *2017 Coding and
Reimbursement Tip Sheet for Transition from Pediatric to Adult Health Care*
http://www.gottransition.org/resourceGet.cfm?id=352

References

1. McManus MA, Pollack LR, Cooley WC, et al. Current status of transition preparation among youth with special needs in the United States. *Pediatrics.* 2013;131(6):1090–1097

2. Cheak-Zamora NC, Yang X, Farmer JE, Clark M. Disparities in transition planning for youth with autism spectrum disorder. *Pediatrics.* 2013;131(3):447–454

3. Newacheck PW, Taylor WR. Childhood chronic illness: prevalence, severity, and impact. *Am J Public Health.* 1992;82(3):364–371

4. American Academy of Pediatrics, American Academy of Family Physicians, American College of Physicians, et al. Supporting the health care transition for adolescence to adulthood in the medical home. *Pediatrics.* 2011;128(1):182

5. Dinerstein RD, Herr SS, O'Sullivan JL. *A Guide to Consent.* Washington, DC: American Association on Mental Retardation; 1999

6. American Association on Intellectual and Developmental Disabilities (AAIDD). Autonomy, decision-making supports, and guardianship: Joint position statement of AAIDD and The Arc. http://aaidd.org/news-policy/policy/position-statements/autonomy-decision-making-supports-and-guardianship#.WiliU1WnGpo. Accessed January 10, 2018

7. Tassé MJ, Schalock R, Thompson JR, Wehmeyer M. *Guidelines for interviewing people with disabilities: Supports Intensity Scale.* Washington, DC: American Association on Intellectual and Developmental Disabilities; 2004–2009

8. Reiss JG, Gibson RW, Walker LR. Health care transition: youth, family, and provider perspectives. *Pediatrics.* 2005;115(1):112–1120

9. American Academy of Pediatrics, American Academy of Family Physicians, American College of Physicians-American Society of Internal Medicine. A consensus statement on health care transitions for young adults with special health care needs. *Pediatrics.* 2002;110(6 Pt 2):1304–1306

10. American Board of Pediatrics Inc. *2015–2016 Workforce Data.* Chapel Hill, NC: American Board of Pediatrics, Inc; 2016

11. American Board of Internal Medicine. *Internal Medicine: Certification Examination Blueprint.* http://www.abim.org/~/media/ABIM%20Public/Files/pdf/exam-blueprints/certification/internal-medicine.pdf. Accessed January 10, 2018

12. Accreditation Council for Graduate Medical Education (ACGME). *ACGME Program Requirements for Graduate Medical Education in Internal Medicine.* http://www.acgme.org/Portals/0/PFAssets/ProgramRequirements/140_internal_medicine_2017-07-01.pdf?ver=2017-06-30-083345-723. Accessed January 10, 2018

13. Peter NG, Forke CM, Ginsburg KR, Schwarz DF. Transition from pediatric to adult care: internists' perspectives. *Pediatrics.* 2009;123(2):417–423

14. Antonelli RC, Stile CJ, Antonelli DM. Care coordination for children and youth with special health care needs: a descriptive, multisite study of activities, personnel costs, and outcomes. *Pediatrics.* 2008;122(1):e209–e216

15. US Department of Health and Human Services. *Report to Congress: Young Adults and Transitioning Youth with Autism Spectrum Disorder: The Autism Collaboration, Accountability, Research, Education and Support Act (Autism CARES Act) of 2014. Report to the Congress.* Submitted by the National Autism Coordinator of the US Department of Health and Human Services, August 3, 2017. https://www.hhs.gov/sites/default/files/2017AutismReport.pdf. Accessed January 10, 2018

16. Antonelli RC, Antonelli DM. Providing a medical home: the cost of care coordination services in a community-based, general pediatric practice. *Pediatrics.* 2004;133(5):1522–1528

17. American Academy of Pediatrics Council on Children with Disabilities and Medical Home Implementation Project Advisory Committee. Patient- and family-centered care coordination: a framework for integrating care for children and youth across multiple systems. *Pediatrics.* 2014:133(5):e1451–1460

CHAPTER 27

Billing and Coding for Developmental and Behavioral Problems in Outpatient Primary Care

Lynn Mowbray Wegner, MD, FAAP

NOTE: All testing procedure codes discussed in this chapter will have different *Current Procedural Terminology* (*CPT*®) numbers at the time of this book's publication. The *CPT* numbers used are correct for *CPT 2017*.

Evolving and increasing interest by parents and professionals in areas of children's development and behavioral regulation has resulted in more medical care for children in these areas. Parents and professionals want early identification and ongoing supportive management to ensure optimal cognitive and behavioral development and social adaptation. Getting paid for this care can be problematic, as payers often view visits focusing on preventing problems and ongoing non–face-to-face services as difficult to manage from a cost-containment perspective. Published resources are available to inform medical providers and help them better understand the codes describing services and conditions.[1,2]

International Classification of Diseases

The *International Classification of Diseases, 10th Revision, Clinical Modification* (*ICD-10-CM*)[3] is used to classify diseases and operations and is universally used for claims submission. The World Health Organization published the 10th edition in 1993, but it was not adopted by the United States for general use until 2015. The *ICD-10* diagnostic codes are meant to completely and accurately describe the patient's clinical picture. These codes describe *why* the service was performed. Payers often use these codes as part of risk management (eg, to determine preexisting conditions and refuse payment for diagnoses). The reader is referred to online and printed published editions of *ICD-10-CM* for comprehensive review of these codes.[4–6]

Many of the diagnostic codes in *ICD-10-CM* Chapter 5, "Mental, Behavioral and Neurodevelopmental Disorders (**F01–F99**)," are also described in the *Diagnostic and Statistical Manual of Mental Disorders, Fifth Edition (DSM-5)*,[7] and the "mental health" codes are often referred to during discussions of parity. Just as payers may choose not to pay for some *CPT* services (such as non–face-to-face care services, eg, telephone calls, e-mail messages, and extended reports), payers also may exclude (in their contracts) care for certain *ICD-10* diagnostic codes, either individually or by groups, unless the medical provider is a designated "mental health provider."

Pediatric health care professionals providing a significant amount of developmental and behavioral care may overcome this obstacle by being paneled as a mental health provider by payers. However, some insurers continue to "carve out" mental health care panels, and there may be future changes in health care administration that might create new bureaucratic quagmires for mental health providers to handle.

Developmental and behavioral conditions often require several medical encounters before a diagnosis can be confirmed. *ICD-10-CM* has 2 chapters of "descriptive rather than diagnostic" codes; these are Chapter 18, "Symptoms, Signs and Abnormal Clinical and Laboratory Findings, Not Elsewhere Classified (**R00–R99**)," and Chapter 21, "Factors Influencing Health Status and Contact With Health Services (**Z00–Z99**)." The decision to pay for these codes is decided by each insurer, and while some may allow these codes to be used as the primary diagnosis, other payers will not allow them to be placed on the first line. Other payers may allow the R and Z codes to be the primary diagnosis but only for a specified number of visits. In any case, supportive documentation in the record must be provided.

Current Procedural Terminology (CPT®): Background

As another part of effective and efficient practice planning, it is important to understand how services for developmental/behavioral conditions are described in *CPT 2017*.[2] These procedure codes are Level I codes of the broader-based Healthcare Common Procedure Coding System (HCPCS).[8] Level II HCPCS codes, developed by the Centers for Medicare & Medicaid Services (CMS), are 5-digit alphanumeric codes with a letter as the first character and are used to report services and supplies not identified in *CPT*. *CPT* allows providers to concisely describe services provided at a patient encounter. If the provider understands the *CPT* system and stays current to additions and changes to *CPT*, it is possible to accurately "capture" most, if not all, of the work done. It must be remembered that payers are free to set their individual payment policies. Even when there are published relative value units (RVUs) for a procedure code, payers may refuse to pay for the services.

CMS has a process to assign values (RVUs) to medical service codes. The assumption is that service value is quantifiable, and each service has a relative value based on the resource costs needed to provide each service. Each code value comprises 3 elements: physician work, practice expense (direct and indirect costs), and medical liability expense. These 3 factors (each assigned an individual RVU or part thereof) are summed to get the total RVU. This total RVU is multiplied by a Medicare conversion factor ($ per RVU) and a geographic conversion factor (reflecting that expenses vary from community to community) to give the Medicare payment for that service. Medicare conversion factors are updated every 6 months (January 1 and July 1: 1/1–6/30; 7/1–12/31).

RVUs (either work RVUs or total RVUs) are increasingly being used by group practices and larger institutions to establish benchmarks for physician work and to determine individual salaries. RVUs are used in managed care contracts to determine the costs involved in providing the services. *CPT*® codes assigned to procedures often have higher RVUs per time unit than codes describing cognitive services.[9] This is a particularly relevant concern for pediatric health care professionals offering developmental-behavioral services, as most of this work does not involve procedures; such health care professionals may not be able to generate the same number of RVUs on a given day when compared with a provider who engages in more procedures. Developmental-behavioral specialists and generalists providing developmental and behavioral care can influence charges by advocating for more realistic RVU benchmarks by their administrators. Advocating stronger payment for cognitive services with payers during contract renewal discussions also can help level the playing field.

CPT for Developmental-Behavioral Services

Outpatient face-to-face codes pertinent to developmental-behavioral services describe new, established, consultation, and preventive evaluation and management (E/M) services. Appropriate inpatient hospital *CPT* codes are also used to describe inpatient services for developmental and behavioral conditions. Codes for developmental screening and objective developmental testing are also available. If a service was modified in some manner, modifiers may be appended to the basic service code to inform the payers that outpatient and/or inpatient services were modified, which may result in a change in charge or payment. Non–face-to-face services are also used when providing developmental and behavioral health care: Codes are available for those services as well as for telephone care, online medical evaluation, care plan oversight, extensive reports, and team conferences.

The current payment system may be used more effectively if providers understand "the system" and appropriately create clinical services in synchrony with the current reimbursement system. This does not mean abandoning *quality* care, but it does mean understanding *efficient* care. The following code descriptions are provided to improve code awareness and to link codes to efficient service delivery.

Outpatient Evaluation and Management (E/M) Codes

Outpatient developmental and behavioral care is provided using E/M services. These services include preventive health care (**99381–99384**; **99391–99394**), new (**99201–99205**) and established (**99211–99215**) patient office visits, and consultation (**99241–99245**) services on request of another appropriate professional. A patient is considered new if the provider or any other provider from the same specialty in the same medical group practice either has never provided care or has not seen the patient in the past 3 years in any clinical setting. All E/M services, with the exception of preventive visits, may be coded on the basis of either the complexity of the visit or on the amount of time required for counseling and case management on the date of service.

Nonpreventive E/M visit components are defined by 4 levels of service: problem focused, expanded problem focused, detailed problem focused, and comprehensive. Complexity entails consideration of 3 key components: history, physical examination, and the complexity of the medical decision-making required by the provider. Tables 27.1, 27.2, and 27.3 illustrate the 5 levels for consultation and for new and established patient visits.

Table 27.1. New Office Consultation[a]					
Component	99241	99242	99243	99244	99245
History	Problem focused	Expanded problem focused	Detailed	Comprehensive	Comprehensive
Examination	Problem focused	Expanded problem focused	Detailed	Comprehensive	Comprehensive
Medical Decision-making	Straightforward	Straightforward	Low complexity	Moderate complexity	High complexity
Time (min)	15	30	40	60	80

[a] Documentation of all components (history, examination, and medical decision-making) is required for all levels of care.

Table 27.2. New Patient Office Visit[a]					
Component	99201	99202	99203	99204	99205
History	Problem focused	Expanded problem focused	Detailed	Comprehensive	Comprehensive
Examination	Problem focused	Expanded problem focused	Detailed	Comprehensive	Comprehensive
Medical Decision-making	Straightforward	Straightforward	Low complexity	Moderate complexity	High complexity
Time (min)	10	20	30	45	60

[a] Documentation of all components (history, examination, and medical decision-making) is required for all levels of care.

Table 27.3. Established Patient Office Visit					
Component	99211	99212	99213	99214	99215
History	Not required	Problem focused	Expanded problem focused	Detailed	Comprehensive
Examination	Not required	Problem focused	Expanded problem focused	Detailed	Comprehensive
Medical Decision-making	Not required	Straightforward	Low complexity	Moderate complexity	High complexity
Time (min)	5	10	15	25	40

Note that the sole difference between the detailed problem-focused and comprehensive levels is the difficulty of medical decision-making. Determining the level of medical decision-making takes into consideration: (1) the number of possible diagnoses and/or potential treatments; (2) the amount and/or complexity of ancillary information (medical records, diagnostic tests, other information); and (3) the risk of complications, morbidity, and/or mortality associated with the patient's presenting problem.

The medical record documentation should always support both the *ICD-10* and *CPT*® codes selected. If the provider spends at least half of the visit in counseling or care coordination, then time may be used to determine the *CPT* code. A statement such as, "The visit took XXX minutes, and more than 50% of time was spent in counseling (and/or coordination of care)," should be included in the note. The clinician should code the diagnosis to the highest level of diagnostic *certainty* (the words in the descriptor) and *complexity* (the numbers in the *ICD-10* codes). The first diagnosis listed on the billing sheet should be the condition being actively managed on that date of service. A chronic condition, such as attention-deficit/hyperactivity disorder or depression, managed on an ongoing basis, may be coded and reported as many times as applicable to the patient's treatment.

There is no provision for "rule out" in *ICD-10,* but as noted earlier, there is a chapter of codes (Chapter 18, "Symptoms, Signs and Abnormal Clinical and Laboratory Findings, Not Elsewhere Classified [**R00–R99**]") which may be used if a more definite diagnosis is not possible. Similarly, in *ICD-10* Chapter 21, "Factors Influencing Health Status and Contact With Health Services (**Z00–Z99**)," the factors listed in the **Z03** and **Z04** ranges can be listed as a first-listed diagnosis only.

While these R and Z codes can be properly used, payers may not choose to pay if these codes (other than **Z03** and **Z04**) are listed first. Remember, payment is always dependent on each payer's decision.

Preventive Service E/M Codes and Developmental-Behavioral Care[10]
Health supervision (well-child checkups) and preventive medicine visits are properly described by the preventive medicine services codes (Table 27.4). These codes, like the other E/M codes, are subcategorized as new patient or established patient. Codes in these series are selected based on the age of the patient and not on the basis of time spent on the date of service.

If the pediatric health care professional wants to efficiently cover developmental and behavioral concerns in the typically busy primary care setting, developmental screening instruments and behavioral rating scales can be key procedures. These procedures may properly accompany the preventive service and be described to the payer by appending an appropriate modifier to either the preventive service code, the procedure code, or, in some circumstances, both.

Remember, too, there are preventive medicine visits when a separate medical service is provided, such as when a psychotropic medication refill is needed. These unique services may properly be coded separately provided the medical record shows the documentation of the required elements for the second E/M service.

Table 27.4. Preventive Services for New and Established Patients (99381–99384; 99391–99394)	
Code	**Description**
New Patient	
99381	Initial comprehensive preventive medicine evaluation and management; infant (<1 y of age)
99382	early childhood (age 1–4 y)
99383	late childhood (age 5–11 y)
99384	adolescent (age 12–17 y)
Established Patient	
99391	Periodic comprehensive preventive medicine evaluation and management; infant (<1 y of age)
99392	early childhood (age 1–4 y)
99393	late childhood (age 5–11 y)
99394	adolescent (age 12–17 y)

Modifiers

Modifiers are 2-digit suffixes appended to the end of a *CPT*® code to tell the payer that "this visit was different." The service may have been altered by a specific situation described by the modifier. Some modifiers may be used only with E/M codes, and others may only accompany procedures. Modifier use is extremely important, as modifiers enable the payer software to permit these special circumstances. When modifiers are used, however, the provider must take care to clearly document the circumstances supporting their use. Despite correct modifier use and supportive documentation in the medical record, not all payers recognize all modifiers. Listing modifiers on the billing sheet/electronic health record billing section will encourage their use!

The following modifiers may correctly be appended to E/M codes:

25—Significant, Separately Identifiable E/M Service by the Same Physician on the Same Day as the Procedure or Other Service: This modifier tells the payer the documentation requirements were met for a separate E/M service or procedure on that date. For example, at a preventive care visit, the discussion of current concerns, medication side effects, efficacy, etc, would contribute to the level of the separate E/M service selected. Modifier **25** would be properly appended to the E/M code to address the change in medication and not the preventive medical care visit. The medical record should have 2 separate sections documenting the 2 separate services.

Another example of correct modifier **25** use would be the situation when the parent completes a developmental screening instrument as part of a preventive medical care visit. In that situation, the procedure is described by code **96110** (developmental screening), modifier **25** would be properly appended to the selected **993XX** code, and **96110** also would be included as a separate service charge. Again, there must be separate sections in the medical record documenting the 2 provided services.

32—Mandated Services: This modifier is used when a third party requires the service being provided. For example, if a second opinion of a mental health or behavioral diagnosis is required before a child may receive treatment, modifier **32** would be appended to the E/M code describing the visit providing that evaluation service.

Modifiers used with procedures and not E/M codes include

52—Reduced Services: This is used when a procedure is started but then prematurely stopped at the physician's discretion. This might occur during developmental testing if the child became oppositional and refused to respond to the testing. In that case, **52** would be appended to **96111** (developmental testing, extended) to describe the premature termination of the testing session. The diagnosis code used at this visit should explain why the procedure was reduced. The physician is not required to reduce his or her charges for the reduced service, as the payer will make that decision.

53—Discontinued Service: This modifier might properly be appended to psychological and/or developmental testing codes if the child refused to participate in any of the testing. Why would one go to the trouble of documenting this for the payer? Using this modifier confirms the testing was needed, the test was selected, and time was taken to begin the testing. This may further support the selected level of complexity for medical decision-making. The medical records should, of course, provide documentation.

59—Distinct Procedural Service: This modifier is used when procedures not usually reported together do occur appropriately on the same date of service. It indicates the procedure was distinct from the other procedures performed on that same date of service. Coders refer to this modifier as the "modifier of last resort," and the physician should be satisfied that no other modifier would be more appropriate. Clear documentation is required to support payment of both procedures. An example of the use of modifier **59** would be a second office visit for developmental testing (**96111**) during which the parents also returned behavioral/emotional rating scales completed by the patient's child care provider for scoring and interpretation (**96127**). Modifier **59** would be appended to the second procedure marked on the billing sheet.

76—Multiple Procedures: Repeat procedures or services performed by the same physician on the same date of service. This code is used when the physician repeats a procedure on the same date. This modifier is appended to the second unit of the procedure to tell the payer more than one of that same procedure was performed. For instance, using **96110** (developmental screening) as an example, if a Pediatric Evaluation of Developmental Status (PEDS)[11] or an Ages and Stages Questionnaire[12] was completed, scored, and interpreted for a child's mother (custodial parent), father (has weekly visitation), and daily babysitter, then the 3 forms could be described as

96110 (modifier not put on the first unit)
96110 76
96110 76

Alternatively, as some payers do not want the modifier because they prefer units, the same example would be put on the billing sheet as

(3) **96110**

Always follow the payer guidelines!

Psychotherapy Services With E/M

Psychiatrists needed a set of procedure codes to describe medical encounters when both psychotherapy and medication management occurred during a single visit. Table 27.5 lists these services (**90833**, **90836**, and **90838**), published by CMS in 2013. These codes describe psychotherapy delivered with the medication E/M. While CMS understood that medication decisions occur while providing therapy, *CPT*® requires clear documentation of the therapy, the time devoted to therapy, and the key components of the selected E/M service. While any physician qualified to offer psychotherapy may use these codes, payers who "carve out" psychiatric services may require physicians coding psychotherapy to join their mental health panel.

Table 27.5. Psychotherapy Services Added on to Evaluation and Management[8]			
Code	**Descriptor**	**Official Time (min)**	**Actual Time Range**
90833	Individual psychotherapy; 30 minutes with patient and/or family member when performed with an evaluation and management service	30	16–37
90836	Individual psychotherapy; 45 minutes with patient and/or family member when performed with an evaluation and management service	45	38–52
90838	Individual psychotherapy; 60 minutes with patient and/or family member when performed with an evaluation and management service	60	At least 53

Behavioral Health Integration

The rising demand for improved access to medical care for mental and behavioral conditions is resulting in more models of collaboration between the patient's primary pediatric health care professional and mental health professionals. In 2017, CMS published codes for 4 services describing behavioral health integration, 3 of which describe services involving the primary qualified health care provider (MD/DO, physician assistant, nurse practitioner), a behavioral care manager, and the psychiatric consultant. Services include enhancing patient engagement, tracking response to interventions, and improved and documented communication with the patient, family members, and other professionals. In 2017, these are listed as G codes—payable by the government for Medicare services; however, it is anticipated these services, or other iterations of them, will eventually become Category I *CPT* codes.

Developmental and Behavioral Procedures: Screening and Objective Testing

Few procedure codes apply to physician provision of developmental-behavioral services, but those published and valued codes should not be ignored! These procedures include looking for possible areas of concern (screening) (see Chapter 9, Developmental and Behavioral Surveillance and Screening Within the Medical Home), as well as formally assessing performance in one or more areas of development (developmental testing, neurobehavioral status examination, and computerized neuropsychological testing; see Box 27.1).

Box 27.1. Standardized Test Examples for 96111, 96116, 96125[11,13–27]

CODE/TEST

96111: Developmental Testing; Extended

- Beery-Buktenica Test of Visual-Motor Integration (VMI)
- Peabody Developmental Motor Scales (PDMS)
- Bruininks-Oseretsky Test of Motor Proficiency (BOT)
- Clinical Evaluation of Language Fundamentals (CELF)
- Bayley Scales of Infant and Toddler Development
- Capute Scales (Cognitive Adaptive Test/Clinical Linguistic and Auditory Milestone Scale; CAT/CLAMS)
- Mullen Scales of Early Learning (MSEL)
- Parents' Evaluation[28,29] of Developmental Status: Developmental Milestones, assessment level (PEDS:DM, assessment level)
- Battelle Developmental Inventory (BDI)
- Brigance Inventory of Early Development
- Peabody Picture Vocabulary Test (PPVT)
- Kaufman Brief Intelligence Test (KBIT)
- Wide Range Achievement Test (WRAT)

96116: Neurobehavioral Status Examination

- Woodcock-Johnson Tests of Cognitive Abilities (WJ-TCA)
- Autism Diagnostic Observation Scale (ADOS)
- Psychoeducational Profile (PEP)

96125: Standardized Cognitive Performance Testing

- Comprehensive Test of Nonverbal Intelligence (C-TONI)
- Tests of Nonverbal Intelligence (TONI)
- Woodcock-Johnson Tests of Cognitive Abilities: Thinking Ability Index

Screening and Brief Standardized Assessment

Developmental surveillance and screening (see Chapter 9, Developmental and Behavioral Surveillance and Screening Within the Medical Home), as well as formal developmental evaluation (see Chapter 10, Developmental Evaluation), have been discussed elsewhere; therefore, comments about these 2 services will be restricted to coding for these services.

All screening and standardized brief assessment services pay only for the associated expenses to the practice and relevant medical liability expense. All physician work is captured in the associated E/M code. This work would include, but is not limited to, reviewing the results, explaining them to the patient (when appropriate) and/or caregiver, recording the results and how the results contribute to medical decision-making, and any actions performed after the service.

Developmental Screening

96110   Developmental screening (eg, developmental milestone survey, speech and language delay screen) with scoring and documentation, per standardized instrument

For examples, please refer to Chapter 9, Developmental and Behavioral Surveillance and Screening Within the Medical Home.

Behavioral/Emotional Brief Assessment

96127   Brief emotional/behavioral assessment (eg, depression inventory, attention-deficit/hyperactivity disorder [ADHD] scale), with scoring and documentation, per standardized instrument

For examples, please refer to Chapter 9, Box 9.5, and Chapter 12, Table 12.2.

Brief Health Risk Assessment

These codes were published by CMS on January 1, 2017. It is important to note that the assessment instruments for both services must meet the descriptor "standardized," and this would indicate statistically robust tools and not informally developed checklists. Additional requirements for reporting these codes include: the instrument is scorable and is documented in the medical record, and there is practice expense involved. This might be purchasing cost or staff time in explaining and collecting the tool.

Linking these to services to *ICD-10-CM* may be directly associated with previously identified conditions. These procedures also may be described through *ICD-10-CM* Z codes such as **Z13.89**, encounter for screening for other disorder; **Z81.3**, family history of psychoactive substance abuse, not elsewhere classifiable (NEC); **Z81.8**, family history of behavioral disorders, NEC; and **Z13.89**, encounter for screening for other disorder.

Public domain examples of **96160** and **96161** instruments are found in Table 27.6. The exact *CPT*® wording for **96160** and **96161** is as follows:

96160   Administration of patient-focused health risk assessment instrument (eg, health hazard appraisal) with scoring and documentation, per standardized instrument

Code **96160** replaced the previous code **99420** and is to be used to assess external factors potentially affecting the patient. Examples might include violence exposure or food insecurity.

96161 **Administration of a caregiver-focused health risk assessment instrument (eg, depression inventory) for the benefit of the patient, with scoring and documentation, per standardized instrument**

Code **96161** allows brief assessment of conditions in a person intimately involved in the patient's life. The service is billed under the patient and not the caregiver. Although there are alcohol-, substance-, and tobacco-use–specific *CPT*®, Medicare-specific, and Medicaid-specific codes, these codes are to be used when the patient is the informant. Code **96161** covers the use of assessment tools when administered to the caregiver for the benefit of the patient.

Table 27.6. Public-domain Health Risk Assessment Instruments		
Instrument	**96160**	**96161**
Alcohol Use Disorders Identification Test (AUDIT) https://www.drugabuse.gov/sites/default/files/files/AUDIT.pdf	X	X
Alcohol Screening and Brief Intervention for Youth (American Academy of Pediatrics/ National Institute on Alcohol Abuse and Alcoholism) https://pubs.niaaa.nih.gov/publications/Practitioner/YouthGuide/YouthGuide.pdf	X	
CRAFFT 2.0 Screening Interview and CRAFFT Self-administered Questionnaire 2.0 (Ages 12–18) http://www.childrenshospital.org/ceasar/crafft/crafft-publications		X
Drug Abuse Screening Test (DAST) (**96127** for patient) https://www.uspreventiveservicestaskforce.org/Home/GetFileByID/228		X
Edinburgh Postnatal Depression Scale (EPDS) (**96127** for patient) https://pesnc.org/wp-content/uploads/EPDS.pdf		X
Fagerström Test for Nicotine Dependence (FTND) (**96127** for patient) https://cde.drugabuse.gov/instrument/d7c0b0f5-b865-e4de-e040-bb89ad43202b https://www.emich.edu/uhs/documents/nicotine-dependence_adults.pdf		X
Fagerström Test for Nicotine Dependence-Smokeless Tobacco (FTND-ST) (**96127** for patient) https://www.emich.edu/uhs/documents/nicotine-dependence_smokeless.pdf		X
Patient Health Questionnaire (PHQ-9) http://www.cqaimh.org/pdf/tool_phq9.pdf		X
Patient Health Questionnaire-9 (PHQ-9) Modified for Teens (Use **96127**.) https://www.aacap.org/App_Themes/AACAP/docs/member_resources/toolbox_ for_clinical_practice_and_outcomes/symptoms/GLAD-PC_PHQ-9.pdf		X
Problem Oriented Screening Instrument for Parents (POSIP) http://adai.washington.edu/instruments/pdf/Problem_Oriented_Screening_ Instrument_for_Parents_409.pdf	X	
Problem Oriented Screening Instrument for Teenagers (POSIT) (Ages 12–19) http://adai.washington.edu/instruments/pdf/Problem_Oriented_Screening_ Instrument_for_Teenagers_188.pdf	X	
Safe Environment for Every Kid (SEEK) Parent Screening Questionnaire https://www.seekwellbeing.org/the-seek-parent-questionnaire-		X
Screening to Brief Intervention (S2BI) Tool http://massclearinghouse.ehs.state.ma.us/BSASSBIRTPROG/SA3542.html		

Developmental testing; limited (**96110**) may be properly coded in addition to the preventive service code to describe the services provided at the visit.[10]

When standardized developmental screening instruments are administered, scored, and interpreted as part of the preventive service visit, each screening instrument form is individually coded. For example, if an established 9-month-old patient is being cared for most of the time by the maternal grandmother while the child's mother is in school and working part-time, information from both the mother and grandmother may be needed for this child. Two units of **96110** would then be coded as follows:

2 x **96110**
(2) **96110**

It may be necessary to append modifier **25** (separate and identifiable service) to the preventive service code to alert the payer that the preventive service was a separate and identifiable service from the procedure (**96110**) also coded for at that visit. For the 9-month-old described, all services at that visit would thus be coded as

99391 25
(2) **96110**

Screening for autism spectrum disorder in children should include a formal measure, such as the Modified Checklist for Autism in Toddlers-R (M-CHAT-R).[30] Administration of such a formal autism screening instrument is recommended by the American Academy of Pediatrics at the 18- and 24-month visits. Administering, scoring, and interpreting this instrument also fulfills the description for the **96110** service and may be properly coded along with other standardized developmental screening instruments at a health visit. For example, if the child described previously was 18 months of age, and a PEDS and an M-CHAT-R both were given to the child's mother and grandmother to complete, these services would accurately be coded as

99391 25
(4) **96110**

Screening for development, autism, and behavioral regulation may occur during nonpreventive medical visits. If children miss their well-child checkups, office visits for other reasons can serve as opportunities for reviewing developmental, social, and communication status through caregiver reporting and completion of standardized screening instruments. If, for example, a child misses the 24-month anticipatory guidance visit and is not seen until a visit for otalgia and upper respiratory signs, the parent(s) may properly be asked to complete both a general developmental screening scale and an M-CHAT-R. The scored results would be reviewed by the medical provider and discussed with the family. If further action is needed, another visit could be scheduled, or if a referral for additional consultation by other professionals seems indicated, this could be made. Coding for this visit would include

992x4 (or 5) **25**
(2) **96110** (assuming one parent completed one developmental screening scale and one parent completed an M-CHAT-R)

It is important to note that the **96110** payment is based on the practice's expense of the screening instrument administration (cost of the protocol, clinic overhead, non-physician salary) and the malpractice expense. There is no physician work in this code. The payment is based on someone other than the physician administering and scoring the instrument. The physician's interpretation of the score, discussing the results with the family, acting on the results, and writing a brief summary of the results and action are included in the payment for the basic preventive or E/M service. If, however, the physician administers the screening instrument to the parent and scores and interprets the results, then this additional time and/or complexity of medical decision-making may be considered when selecting the proper code describing an E/M service. If more than 50% of the total visit time is devoted to counseling and/or care coordination, then the additional time needed to administer, score, and discuss the findings may add to the total time in this "counseling" service. Documentation of time counseling can be expressed as a fraction:

$$\frac{\text{time spent counseling}}{\text{total time of visit}}$$

If, however, the visit is being coded on the basis of complexity of the service, then the interpretation of the results of the rating scale and the integration of these findings into the medical decision-making may increase the medical decision-making complexity. Both examples show how developmental rating scales may contribute to a higher-level code (eg, **992x4→992x5**).

Rating scales are available to help identify those children and teens that need further evaluation for emotional conditions, such as anxiety. An anxiety scale in the public domain is the Screen for Child Anxiety Related Emotional Disorders (SCARED).[31] The physician often asks these questions directly during the visit and scores the results. In this instance, the separate code **(96127)** would not be appended to the visit, but the level of the service might be increased on either time or complexity of medical deci-sion-making (with appropriate documentation). If, however, a nurse (or other trained nonphysician) administers and scores the screening instrument and the physician inter-prets the results and reviews them with the family, then **96127** can be used, and the time and effort of the interpretation and discussion by the physician can be factored into the E/M code.

Objective Testing: 96111, 96116, 96125
Pediatric health care professionals who have been properly trained in the selection, administration, scoring, and interpretation of standardized tests assessing varying areas of developmental attainment may quite properly perform this service. The *CPT*® codes describing testing fall in the **96xxx** series. While all "psychological testing" codes (eg, **96101**, psychological testing; **96118**, neuropsychological testing) allow submission by physicians, the physician who uses these codes should be prepared to show very specific, specialty training in the administration and interpretation of these tests. Codes **96116** (neurobehavioral status examination) and **96125** (standardized cognitive perfor-mance testing) allow multiple-unit coding to cover test administration, scoring and interpretation, and report writing.

96111: Developmental Testing; Extended

This code was developed to include standardized testing for motor, language, social, adaptive, and/or cognitive functioning. It may be coded only once on each day of service and allows no additional units for test scoring, interpretation, or report writing. This code is applicable for testing sessions as brief as that needed for verbal fluency testing (eg, controlled oral word association test),[32] as well as testing lasting longer than an hour. It may also be properly used for administering objective developmental screening instruments such as the Brigance Early Childhood Screens.[29]

Some payers may not permit codes **96110** and **96111** to be charged together (developmental testing; limited and developmental testing; extended), as they interpret these services to be in conflict. They ask, "How can you bill for 'limited' developmental testing at the same time you are billing for 'extended' developmental testing? Isn't that 'unbundling'?" Addressing this will take additional clarification and advocacy with the individual payers.

96116: Neurobehavioral Status Examination

This code may be used for "clinical assessment" of thinking, reasoning, and judgment (ie, acquired knowledge, attention, language, memory, planning and problem-solving, and visual spatial abilities). Multiple units may be coded on the day of service to cover scoring and interpretation and report writing. While the descriptor does not specify use of standardized instruments, the physician who does not use a standardized test must be careful not to use this code to describe those tasks that would more customarily be included in the neurological or mental status examination (eg, serial 7s). When documenting activity, the actual time spent face-to-face with the patient and the time interpreting test results and preparing the report should be reported—it should exceed 31 minutes and be less than 60 minutes (for 1 unit of the code).

This service may properly be provided—and billed—in combination with **96110** and/or **96127**. For example, if rating scales are completed, scored, and interpreted at a visit during which the neurobehavioral status examination is performed, both codes may be documented on the billing sheet. For example, if a level 4 E/M visit occurs with rating scales administration and completion, this could be coded as

992X4 25
(x units) **96110**
(x units) **96116 59**

Alternatively, if a level 4 E/M visit occurs with rating scales and separate and identifiable developmental cognitive testing by a nonpsychologist, then appropriate coding for that visit could be

992X4 25
(x units) **96110**
(x units) **96125**

96125: Standardized Cognitive Performance Testing

This code was developed for other professionals who also do standardized testing but who were not included in the descriptors for **96101–96103** and **96118–96120**. As the descriptor says, "qualified health professional's time," this code could quite properly be used by physicians. This code permits multiple-unit coding on the day of service to allow payment for scoring, interpretation, and report writing.

Prolonged Services

Many times the visits for children with complex behavioral and developmental needs take longer than the time expected for the highest level of encounter. The average expected times are noted in Table 27.7, but the time may be more or less than noted, depending on the clinical circumstances.

Table 27.7. *Current Procedural Terminology*® Survey Time Guidelines for Highest-Level New and Established Outpatient Services		
Code	**Descriptor**	**Intraservice Time (min)**
99245	Consultation (new patient)	80
99205	New patient	60
99215	Established patient	45

If the time exceeds the time for the appropriate highest-level service by more than 29 minutes, prolonged service codes may be appended. This may describe both face-to-face and non–face-to-face prolonged time spent in care on the same day as the appointment occurred.

Table 27.8 shows time guidelines for prolonged outpatient services. To correctly account for prolonged time beyond that specified in the selected E/M code, the first 30 minutes exceeding the E/M time are still included in the initial E/M payment. Therefore, a prolonged service code may not be used until after the first 30 minutes of the prolonged services have been provided. The medical provider must spend 31 to 74 minutes with the patient and/or family in prolonged services before it is possible to correctly code for 31 minutes using code **99354**. What if the total prolonged services exceed 74 minutes? Code **99355** applies for each additional 30 minutes spent in face-to-face contact beyond the initial prolonged face-to-face 74 service minutes. To correctly use **99355**, however, the medical provider must spend at least 15 minutes beyond the initial 74 minutes of prolonged time.

Table 27.8. Guidelines for Prolonged Outpatient Services (99354, 99355 and 99358, 99359)	
Total Duration of Prolonged Services (min)	**Code(s)**
Face-to-face, <30	Not reported separately
Face-to-face, 31–74	**99354**
Face-to-face, 75–104	**99355**, each additional 30 minutes, past 74 minutes, use with **99354**
Face-to-face, 105–134	**99354** X 1 plus **99355** X 2
Before or after face-to-face, <30	Not reported separately
Before or after face-to-face, 31–74	**99358**
Before or after face-to-face, 75–104	**99359**, each additional 30 minutes, past 74 minutes, use with **99358**
Before or after face-to-face, 105–134	**99358** X 1 plus **99359** X 2

Providing medical care for developmental and behavioral health services often involves non–face-to-face work. Codes **99358** and **99359** can be used with any level of E/M service and may be reported on a date before or after the date of the associated service. Extended review of records, discussion with other professionals also providing care, and other services not described with existing codes all can have their time described by **99358** and **99359**.

It is essential to document the time and the services provided to substantiate the use of these prolonged service codes. Becoming familiar with these codes can help avoid the frequent (and disappointing!) situation of providing uncompensated care. Be aware, however, that even correct coding and documentation in the medical record may not result in payment. This is a payer issue. If request for payment is denied, ask for a written explanation of the denial from the insurer. If the patient is on a capitated plan, you may request authorization to bill the family directly for these noncovered services.

Non–Face-to-Face Services: Telephone Care (99441–99443) and Extended Reports (99080)

Providing a medical home for patients with complex medical and behavioral conditions necessitates many non–face-to-face services. Primary pediatric health care professionals often develop "virtual teams" of community-based specialists to create comprehensive care plans for their patients with complex developmental and behavioral conditions. Reviewing interim reports occurs regularly. Telephone and written communications between medical providers (both primary and specialty), professionals in other areas, and family members are a routine and expected aspect of ongoing care.

These services may be captured under the medical/behavioral care management *CPT*® codes if the patient meets their criteria.

99441–99443: Non–Face-to-Face Telephone Services

If care management codes are regularly submitted, it would not be appropriate to submit bills for individual telephone calls. Telephone care, however, is often a significant part of providing care for children with complex developmental and behavioral disorders. Communication between the primary medical clinician and therapists, teachers, school counselors, and family members can be important to optimal management. While telephone calls to nonfamily members might correctly be included in care management services, telephone care to the child's family can be billed very appropriately as a separate and justifiable service. There are 3 published telephone care codes for use when the physician is part of the call. RVUs for these 3 telephone care codes were published in 2008 (Table 27.9).

Table 27.9. Telephone Care (99441–99443)[a]	
Code	Time of Medical Discussion (min)
99441	5–10
99442	11–20
99443	21–30

[a] Telephone evaluation and management (E/M) service provided by a physician to an established patient, parent, or guardian not originating from a related E/M service provided within the previous 7 days nor leading to an E/M service or procedure within the next 24 hours or soonest available appointment.

Again, remember that even correct coding and documentation of the telephone call in the medical record may not result in payment. This is another payer issue. If request for payment is denied, the provider may ask for a written explanation of the denial by the insurer. If the patient is on a capitated plan, you may request authorization to bill the family directly for these noncovered services. Before you bill families for noncovered activities like telephone calls, it would be wise to let them know that your practice may be doing so, for example, by sending all families a letter explaining that payment will be expected from them for these services and providing a fee schedule.

99080: Special Reports Such as Insurance Forms, More Than the Information Conveyed in the Usual Medical Communications, or Standard Reporting Form

Finally, when parents purchase insurance coverage for their children with developmental or emotional/behavioral regulation conditions, insurers may require extensive documentation of need for this care on special forms. Self-contained schools and camps for children with significant developmental and behavioral conditions may require primary pediatric health care professionals to complete extensive forms for the child's admission. *CPT*® code **99080** is published and may be used for these services. There are no RVUs assigned to this code, and payers may not pay for this service. Clinicians should develop an office policy, similar to the decision for billing for telephone care, and advise families in advance if they will be expected to pay for this service.

Conclusion

Primary pediatric health care professionals have an important role in providing children's developmental and behavioral health care. Developmental and behavioral differences should be identified as early as possible, and the medical home can provide appropriate care and care coordination. Understanding the current codes to describe medical services and the documentation needed to support them, using efficient methods of care, and modifying practice habits to minimize services not currently supported by procedural codes will permit primary pediatric health care professionals to be paid in a more appropriate way for this medical care. Current medical procedure codes can legitimately be used to bill for care related to developmental and behavioral health needs, and consistent use of these codes will help address payment barriers.

Medical care guidelines and payer policies are constantly evolving. It cannot be over-emphasized how important it is for each medical provider to stay current with CMS policies and *CPT®* decisions.

This coding content was accurate as of August 21, 2017. CPT® copyright 2017 American Medical Association. All rights reserved.

Resources

Commercial Pediatric Coding Newsletters

American Academy of Pediatrics. *AAP Pediatric Coding Newsletter.* Itasca, IL: American Academy of Pediatrics

The Coding Institute. *Pediatric Coding Alert.* Durham, NC: Eli Research

Web Sites

Web site of the American Academy of Pediatrics Section on Developmental and Behavioral Pediatrics with coding information specific to developmental and behavioral health care for children
   www.dbpeds.org

Web site of the American Academy of Child and Adolescent Psychiatry with coding information specific to mental and behavioral health care for children
   www.aacap.org

Documentation guideline revisions by CMS and the American Medical Association
   www.cms.hhs.gov/MLNProducts

American Academy of Pediatrics updates on procedural and diagnostic coding
   www.coding.aap.org

Commercial site for coding information
   https://www.codinginstitute.com

References

1. American Academy of Pediatrics. *Coding for Pediatrics 2018.* Liechty EA, Hughes C, Dolan B, eds. 23rd ed. Elk Grove Village, IL: American Academy of Pediatrics; 2018

2. American Medical Association. *CPT 2018 Professional.* Chicago, IL: American Medical Association; 2017

3. Department of Health and Human Services. *ICD-10-CM Official Guidelines for Coding and Reporting: FY 2015.* https://www.cdc.gov/nchs/data/icd/icd10cm_guidelines_2015.pdf. Accessed February 12, 2018

4. Centers for Disease Control and Prevention. Classification of Diseases, Functioning, and Disability. https://www.cdc.gov/nchs/icd/index.htm. Accessed February 12, 2018

5. National Center for Health Statistics. *International Classification of Diseases, 10th Revision (ICD-10).* www.cdc.gov/nchs/data/dvs/icd10fct.pdf. Accessed February 12, 2018

6. ICD10Data.com. http://www.icd10data.com/ICD10CM/Codes. Accessed February 12, 2018

7. American Psychiatric Association. *Diagnostic and Statistical Manual of Mental Disorders.* 5th ed. Washington, DC: American Psychiatric Association; 2013

8. Center for Medicare & Medicaid Services. HCPCS—General Information. https://www.cms.gov/Medicare/Coding/MedHCPCSGenInfo/index.html. Accessed February 12, 2018

9. American Medical Association/Specialty Society. *Relative Value System Update Database: Reimbursement Update Committee Database 2017/Version 2.* Chicago, IL: American Medical Association; 2017

10. Bright Futures Steering Committee, Medical Home Initiatives for Children With Special Needs Project Advisory Committee. Identifying infants and young children with developmental disorders in the medical home: an algorithm for developmental surveillance and screening. *Pediatrics.* 2006;118(1):405–420

11. Glascoe FP. Parental Evaluation of Developmental Status. PEDStest.com Web site. http://www.pedstest.com/default.aspx. Accessed February 12, 2018

12. Squires J, Bricker D. *Ages & Stages Questionnaires (ASQ-3).* 3rd ed. Baltimore, MD: Brookes Publishing Company; 2009

13. Beery KE, Buktenica NA, Beery NA. *Beery-Buktenica Developmental Test of Visual-Motor Integration.* 6th ed. Minneapolis, MN: Pearson Assessments, Inc; 2010

14. Folio MR, Fewell RR. *Peabody Developmental Motor Scales.* 2nd ed. Austin, TX: PRO-ED Inc; 2000

15. Bruininks RH. *Bruininks-Oseretsky Test of Motor Proficiency (BOT-2).* Minneapolis, MN: Pearson Assessments, Inc; 2005

16. Semel EM, Wiig EH, Secord W. *CELF3: Clinical Evaluation of Language Fundamentals.* San Antonio, TX: Psychological Corporation, Harcourt Brace; 1995

17. Bayley N. *Bayley Scales of Infant and Toddler Development.* 3rd ed. Minneapolis, MN: Pearson Assessments, Inc; 2005

18. Capute A. *The Capute Scales: CAT/CLAMS.* Baltimore, MD: Kennedy Fellows Association; 1996

19. Mullen EM. *Mullen Scales of Early Learning.* Circle Pines, MN: Pearson Assessment, Inc; 1995

20. Dunn DM, Dunn LM. *Peabody Picture Vocabulary Test: Manual.* San Antonio, TX: Pearson; 2007

21. Kaufman AS, Kaufman NL. *Kaufman Brief Intelligence Test.* Wiley Online Library; 2004

22. Wilkinson GS, Robertson GJ. *Wide Range Achievement Test.* Psychological Assessment Resources; 2006

23. Schrank FA. Woodcock-Johnson III tests of cognitive abilities. In: Davis AS, ed. *Handbook of Pediatric Neuropsychology.* New York, NY: Springer; 2011:415–434

24. Lord C, Rutter M, DiLavore PC, Risi S, Gotham K, Bishop S. *Autism Diagnostic Observation Schedule: ADOS-2.* Los Angeles, CA: Western Psychological Services; 2012

25. Schopler E, Lansing MD, Reichler RJ, Marcus LM. *PEP-3: Psychoeducational Profile.* 3rd ed. Torrance, CA: Western Psychological Services; 2005

26. Hammill DD, Pearson NA, Wiederholt JL. *Comprehensive Test of Nonverbal Intelligence (CTONI-2).* 2nd ed. San Antonio, TX: Pearson; 2009

27. Brown L, Sherbenou RJ, Johnsen SK. *Test of Nonverbal Intelligence (TONI-4).* 4th ed. San Antonio, TX: Pearson; 2010

28. Newborg J, Stock JR, Wnek L, Guidubaldi J, Svinicki J. *Battelle Developmental Inventory.* Rolling Meadows, IL: Riverside; 2005

29. Brigance A. *Brigance Screens III, Technical Manual.* North Billerica, MA: Curriculum Associates, Inc; 2013

30. Robins DL, Fein D, Barton M. Modified Checklist for Autism in Toddlers, Revised with Follow-up (M-CHAT-R/F). MChat.org Web site. https://www.m-chat.org. Accessed February 12, 2018

31. Birmaher B, Brent DA, Chiappetta L, Bridge J, Monga S, Baugher M. Screen for Child Anxiety Related Emotional Disorders (SCARED). University of Pittsburgh Child and Adolescent Bipolar Spectrum Services Web site. http://pediatricbipolar.pitt.edu/resources/instruments. Accessed February 12, 2018

32. Lezak MD, Howieson DB, Bigler ED, Tanel D. *Neuropsychological Assessment.* 5th ed. Oxford, UK: Oxford University Press; 2012

INDEX

Page numbers followed by an *f*, a *t*, or a *b* denote a figure, a table, or a box, respectively.